HEMATOLOGICAL DISORDERS

Edited by:

Dr. Marie Hyacinth Chiong Tumara

ALLIED HEALTH PRESS

Hematological Disorders

Dr. Marie Hyacinth Chiong Tumara

Allied Health Press
4164 Lakeshore Road
Burlington ON L7L 1A4
Canada
www.alliedhealthpress.com
Email: orders@arclereducation.com

ISBN: 978-1-77956-804-5

ABOUT THE EDITOR

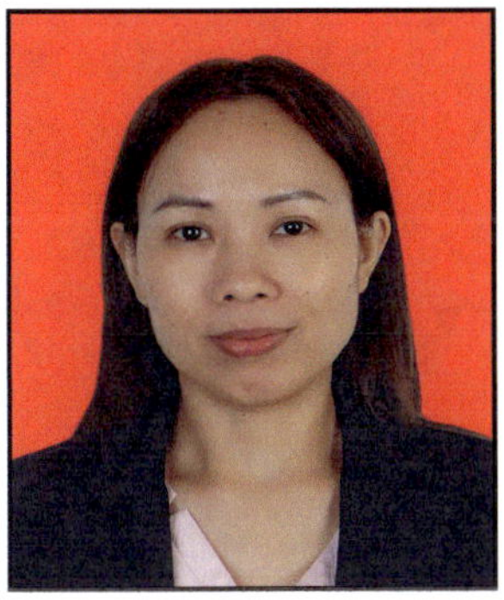

Dr. Marie Hyacinth Chiong Tumara, MD, FPCP, is an Internist with over 16 years of clinical practice and 11 years of government health service. She currently serves as Medical Director and OFW PEME Physician, with expertise in occupational and maritime medicine. A Fellow of the Philippine College of Physicians, she has authored research and medical reports and actively contributes to policy development in hospital and clinical settings. She is presently pursuing her Master's in Health and Hospital Management at Xavier University–Ateneo de Cagayan.

Brief Table of Contents

1. Introduction to Hematology and Hematopoiesis	1
2. Anemias: Pathophysiology and Classification	27
3. Iron Deficiency and Sideroblastic Anemia	55
4. Hemolytic Anemias	81
5. Hemoglobinopathies and Thalassemias	107
6. Megaloblastic and Aplastic Anemias	129
7. Disorders of Leukocytes	151
8. Platelet Disorders	179
9. Coagulation Disorders	207
10. Thrombotic Disorders	237
11. Acute Leukemias	267
12. Chronic Leukemias	295
13. Lymphomas	325
14. Plasma Cell Dyscrasias	353
15. Transfusion Medicine and Bone Marrow Transplantation	379
Index	405

Detailed Table of Contents

List of Figures *xvii*
Preface *xxxiii*

CHAPTER 1

Introduction to Hematology and Hematopoiesis 1

Introduction **1**
1.1. Blood Composition **2**
1.1.1. Components of Blood 2
1.1.2. Functions of Red Blood Cells (RBCs) 3
1.1.3. Role of White Blood Cells (WBCs) 3
1.1.4. Importance of Platelets 4
1.1.5. Plasma Composition and Functions 4
1.1.6. Blood Volume and Its Regulation 4
1.1.7. Hemoglobin and Oxygen Transport 5
1.1.8. Blood Types and Compatibility 5
1.1.9. Disorders Related to Blood Composition 6
1.2. Hematopoiesis **6**
1.2.1. Definition and Process of Hematopoiesis 7
1.2.2. Sites of Hematopoiesis in the Body 7
1.2.3. Stages of Hematopoietic Development 8
1.2.4. Role of Stem Cells in Hematopoiesis 8
1.2.5. Regulation of Hematopoiesis 9
1.2.6. Factors Influencing Hematopoiesis 9
1.2.7. Hematopoietic Growth Factors 10
1.2.8. Disorders of Hematopoiesis 11
1.2.9. Advances in Hematopoietic Research 11
1.3. Hematological Disorders **11**
1.3.1. Anemia: Types and Causes 12
1.3.2. Leukemia: Overview and Types 12
1.3.3. Lymphoma: Classification and Symptoms 13
1.3.4. Thrombocytopenia: Causes and Effects 13
1.3.5. Hemophilia: Genetic Basis and Treatment 14
1.3.6. Sickle Cell Disease: Pathophysiology 14
1.3.7. Myelodysplastic Syndromes (MDS) 15
1.3.8. Polycythemia Vera: Diagnosis and Management 15
1.3.9. Emerging Therapies for Hematological Disorders 16
1.4. Diagnostic Techniques in Hematology **16**
1.4.1. Complete Blood Count (CBC) 17
1.4.2. Bone Marrow Biopsy 17
1.4.3. Flow Cytometry 17
1.4.4. Hemoglobin Electrophoresis 18
1.4.5. Coagulation Studies 18
1.4.6. Blood Smear Analysis 19
1.4.7. Molecular Diagnostics in Hematology 19
1.4.8. Imaging Techniques in Hematology 20
1.4.9. Role of Laboratory Medicine in Hematology 20
Summary **22**
References **23**

CHAPTER 2

Anemias: Pathophysiology and Classification 27

Introduction 27

2.1. Pathophysiology of Anemia 28

2.1.1. Mechanisms of Red Blood Cell Production 28

2.1.2. Role of Hemoglobin in Oxygen Transport 29

2.1.3. Causes of Decreased Red Blood Cell Production 29

2.1.4. Causes of Increased Red Blood Cell Destruction 30

2.1.5. Impact of Nutritional Deficiencies 30

2.1.6. Genetic Factors Influencing Anemia 31

2.1.7. Role of Chronic Diseases in Anemia 31

2.1.8. Effects of Inflammation on Red Blood Cells 32

2.1.9. Compensatory Mechanisms in Anemia 33

2.2. Classification of Anemias 33

2.2.1. Microcytic Anemia 34

2.2.2. Macrocytic Anemia 34

2.2.3. Normocytic Anemia 35

2.2.4. Hemolytic Anemia 35

2.2.5. Aplastic Anemia 36

2.2.6. Anemia of Chronic Disease (ACD) 36

2.2.7. Iron Deficiency Anemia 37

2.2.8. Vitamin B12 Deficiency Anemia 37

2.2.9. Sickle Cell Anemia 38

2.3. Diagnosis of Anemia 38

2.3.1. Clinical Symptoms and Signs 39

2.3.2. Laboratory Tests for Anemia 39

2.3.3. Complete Blood Count (CBC) Analysis 39

2.3.4. Reticulocyte Count 40

2.3.5. Iron Studies and Ferritin Levels 40

2.3.6. Bone Marrow Biopsy 41

2.3.7. Genetic Testing for Hereditary Anemias 41

2.3.8. Differential Diagnosis Considerations 42

2.3.9. Importance of Accurate Diagnosis 42

2.4. Treatment and Management of Anemia 43

2.4.1. Dietary Modifications and Supplementation 43

2.4.2. Pharmacological Treatments 44

2.4.3. Blood Transfusions 44

2.4.4. Management of Underlying Conditions 45

2.4.5. Role of Erythropoietin-Stimulating Agents (ESAs) 45

2.4.6. Patient Education and Lifestyle Changes 45

2.4.7. Monitoring and Follow-up Care 46

2.4.8. Challenges in Treatment Adherence 46

2.4.9. Future Directions in Anemia Management 47

Summary 49

References 50

CHAPTER 3

Iron Deficiency and Sideroblastic Anemia 55

Introduction 55

3.1. Causes of Iron Deficiency 56

3.1.1. Dietary Insufficiency 56

3.1.2. Malabsorption Disorders 57

3.1.3. Chronic Blood Loss 57

3.1.4. Increased Iron Requirements 58

3.1.5. Pregnancy and Lactation 58

3.1.6. Gastrointestinal Conditions 59

3.1.7. Menstrual Cycle Impacts 59

3.1.8. Age-Related Factors 60

3.1.9. Genetic Predispositions 60

3.2. Pathophysiology of Sideroblastic Anemia 61

3.2.1. Mechanism of Sideroblasts Formation 61

3.2.2. Role of Mitochondria in Erythropoiesis 62

3.2.3. Iron Utilization in Hemoglobin Synthesis 62

3.2.4. Genetic Mutations Associated with Sideroblastic Anemia 62

3.2.5. Types of Sideroblastic Anemia 63

3.2.6. Impact of Lead Poisoning 63

3.2.7. Role of Vitamin B6 Deficiency 64

3.2.8. Interaction with Other Hematological Disorders 64

3.2.9. Consequences of Impaired Erythropoiesis 65

3.3. Symptoms and Diagnosis 66

3.3.1. Common Symptoms of Iron Deficiency 66

3.3.2. Symptoms Specific to Sideroblastic Anemia 67

3.3.3. Laboratory Tests for Diagnosis 67

3.3.4. Role of Complete Blood Count (CBC) 67

3.3.5. Iron Studies and Serum Ferritin Levels 68
3.3.6. Bone Marrow Biopsy Findings 68
3.3.7. Differential Diagnosis Considerations 69
3.3.8. Importance of Clinical History 69
3.3.9. Use of Genetic Testing 70
3.4. Treatment and Management 70
3.4.1. Dietary Modifications 70
3.4.2. Iron Supplementation 71
3.4.3. Treatment of Underlying Conditions 71
3.4.4. Use of Vitamin B6 in Sideroblastic Anemia 72
3.4.5. Blood Transfusions 72
3.4.6. Erythropoiesis-Stimulating Agents 73
3.4.7. Monitoring and Follow-Up Care 73
3.4.8. Patient Education and Support 73
Summary 76
References 77

CHAPTER 4

Hemolytic Anemias 81

Introduction 81
4.1. Causes of Hemolytic Anemias 82
4.1.1. Inherited Genetic Disorders 82
4.1.2. Acquired Conditions 83
4.1.3. Immune-Mediated Hemolysis 83
4.1.4. Infections Leading to Hemolysis 84
4.1.5. Drug-Induced Hemolytic Anemia 84
4.1.6. Mechanical Destruction of Red Blood Cells (RBCs) 84
4.1.7. Environmental Factors 85
4.1.8. Nutritional Deficiencies 86
4.1.9. Hemolytic Disease of the Newborn 86
4.2. Symptoms and Diagnosis 86
4.2.1. Common Symptoms of Hemolytic Anemias 87
4.2.2. Laboratory Tests for Diagnosis 87
4.2.3. Role of Blood Smears 88
4.2.4. Importance of Reticulocyte Count 88
4.2.5. Bilirubin Levels and Their Significance 89
4.2.6. Coombs Test and Its Implications 89
4.2.7. Bone Marrow Examination 90
4.2.8. Monitoring Disease Progression 90
4.3. Treatment and Management 91
4.3.1. General Treatment Strategies 91
4.3.2. Use of Corticosteroids 92
4.3.3. Blood Transfusions 92
4.3.4. Splenectomy and Its Indications 93
4.3.5. Management of Underlying Conditions 93
4.3.6. Role of Immunosuppressive Therapy 94
4.3.7. Nutritional Support and Supplementation 94
4.3.8. Patient Education and Support 95
4.4. Prognosis and Complications 95
4.4.1. Factors Influencing Prognosis 95
4.4.2. Potential Complications of Hemolytic Anemias 96
4.4.3. Long-Term Health Effects 96
4.4.4. Quality of Life Considerations 97
4.4.5. Psychological Impact on Patients 97
4.4.6. Importance of Regular Follow-Up 97
4.4.7. Risk of Secondary Conditions 98
4.4.8. Advances in Treatment and Their Impact 98
4.4.9. Case Studies Illustrating Outcomes 99
Summary 101
References 102

CHAPTER 5

Hemoglobinopathies and Thalassemias 107

Introduction 107
5.1. Types of Hemoglobinopathies 108
5.1.1. Sickle Cell Disease (SCD) 108
5.1.2. Hemoglobin C Disease 109
5.1.3. Hemoglobin E Disease 109
5.1.4. Hemoglobin D Disease 109
5.1.5. Hemoglobin H Disease 110
5.1.6. Thalassemia Major 110
5.1.7. Thalassemia Minor 110
5.1.8. Compound Hemoglobinopathies 111
5.1.9. Rare Hemoglobin Variants 111
5.2. Pathophysiology of Hemoglobin Disorders 112
5.2.1. Mechanism of Hemoglobin Synthesis 112

5.2.2. Genetic Mutations Involved 113
5.2.3. Impact on Red Blood Cell Morphology 113
5.2.4. Effects on Oxygen Transport 114
5.2.5. Consequences of Hemolysis 114
5.2.6. Complications of Chronic Anemia 115
5.2.7. Role of Iron Metabolism 115
5.2.8. Interaction with Other Diseases 116
5.2.9. Cellular and Molecular Consequences 116

5.3. Diagnosis and Screening 117

5.3.1. Clinical Presentation and Symptoms 117
5.3.2. Laboratory Tests for Diagnosis 118
5.3.3. Hemoglobin Electrophoresis 118
5.3.4. Genetic Testing Methods 118
5.3.5. Newborn Screening Programs 119
5.3.6. Importance of Family History 119
5.3.7. Role of Imaging Studies 120
5.3.8. Challenges in Diagnosis 120

5.4. Management and Treatment 120

5.4.1. Supportive Care Strategies 121
5.4.2. Blood Transfusion Therapy 121
5.4.3. Iron Chelation Therapy 122
5.4.4. Bone Marrow Transplantation (BMT) 122
5.4.5. Gene Therapy Advancements 122
5.4.6. Pharmacological Treatments 123
5.4.7. Nutritional Management 123
5.4.8. Psychological Support for Patients 124
5.4.9. Future Directions in Treatment 124

Summary 126

References 127

CHAPTER 6

Megaloblastic and Aplastic Anemias 129

Introduction 129

6.1. Megaloblastic Anemia 130

6.1.1. Definition and Characteristics 130
6.1.2. Causes of Megaloblastic Anemia 131
6.1.3. Role of Vitamin B12 Deficiency 131
6.1.4. Role of Folate Deficiency 132
6.1.5. Pathophysiology of Megaloblastic Anemia 132
6.1.6. Symptoms and Clinical Manifestations 133
6.1.7. Diagnostic Methods 133
6.1.8. Treatment Options 134
6.1.9. Complications Associated with Megaloblastic Anemia 134

6.2. Aplastic Anemia 134

6.2.1. Definition and Characteristics 135
6.2.2. Causes of Aplastic Anemia 135
6.2.3. Role of Bone Marrow Failure 135
6.2.4. Genetic Factors Contributing to Aplastic Anemia 136
6.2.5. Symptoms and Clinical Manifestations 136
6.2.6. Diagnostic Methods 137
6.2.7. Treatment Options 137
6.2.8. Prognosis and Long-Term Outcomes 138
6.2.9. Complications Associated with Aplastic Anemia 138

6.3. Current Research and Advances 139

6.3.1. Recent Studies on Megaloblastic Anemia 139
6.3.2. Recent Studies on Aplastic Anemia 140
6.3.3. Advances in Diagnostic Techniques 140
6.3.4. Innovations in Treatment Options 141
6.3.5. Genetic Research and Implications 141
6.3.6. Role of Nutrition in Prevention 142
6.3.7. Patient Education and Awareness 142
6.3.8. Future Directions in Research 143
6.3.9. Collaboration Between Healthcare Providers 143

Summary 145

References 146

CHAPTER 7

Disorders of Leukocytes 151

Introduction 151

7.1. Types of Leukocytes 152

7.1.1. Overview of Leukocyte Classification 152
7.1.2. Neutrophils: Function and Significance 153
7.1.3. Lymphocytes: Types and Roles 153
7.1.4. Monocytes: Characteristics and Functions 153

7.1.5. Eosinophils: Role in Allergic Reactions 154
7.1.6. Basophils: Functions in Inflammation 154
7.1.7. Natural Killer Cells: Importance in Immune Response 155
7.1.8. Dendritic Cells: Role in Antigen Presentation 155
7.2. Common Disorders of Leukocytes 156
7.2.1. Leukopenia: Definition and Causes 156
7.2.2. Leukocytosis: Definition and Causes 156
7.2.3. Lymphoma: Types and Implications 157
7.2.4. Leukemia: Types and Symptoms 157
7.2.5. Myelodysplastic Syndromes: Overview 158
7.2.6. Aplastic Anemia: Causes and Effects 158
7.2.7. Autoimmune Disorders Affecting Leukocytes 158
7.2.8. Infections Leading to Leukocyte Disorders 159
7.3. Diagnosis of Leukocyte Disorders 159
7.3.1. Importance of Blood Tests in Diagnosis 160
7.3.2. Complete Blood Count (CBC): Overview 160
7.3.3. Bone Marrow Biopsy: Procedure and Significance 161
7.3.4. Flow Cytometry: Role in Diagnosis 161
7.3.5. Genetic Testing: Applications in Leukocyte Disorders 162
7.3.6. Imaging Studies: When They Are Used 162
7.3.7. Clinical Symptoms and Their Relevance 162
7.3.8. Differential Diagnosis: Importance and Methods 163
7.4. Treatment and Management of Leukocyte Disorders 163
7.4.1. Overview of Treatment Options 164
7.4.2. Chemotherapy: Role in Treating Leukemias 164
7.4.3. Radiation Therapy: Applications and Effects 165
7.4.4. Immunotherapy: Types and Effectiveness 166
7.4.5. Stem Cell Transplantation: Procedure and Outcomes 166
7.4.6. Supportive Care: Importance in Management 167
7.4.7. Lifestyle Modifications: Role in Recovery 167
7.4.8. Emerging Therapies: Current Research Trends 168
Summary 170
References 171

CHAPTER 8

Platelet Disorders 179

Introduction 179
8.1. Types of Platelet Disorders 180
8.1.1. Thrombocytopenia: Definition and Causes 180
8.1.2. Thrombocytopathy: Definition and Mechanisms 181
8.1.3. Inherited Platelet Disorders 181
8.1.4. Acquired Platelet Disorders 182
8.1.5. Immune Thrombocytopenic Purpura (ITP) 182
8.1.6. Thrombotic Thrombocytopenic Purpura (TTP) 183
8.1.7. Bernard-Soulier Syndrome 183
8.1.8. Glanzmann Thrombasthenia 184
8.1.9. Essential Thrombocythemia 184
8.2. Pathophysiology of Platelet Disorders 184
8.2.1. Role of Bone Marrow in Platelet Production 185
8.2.2. Mechanisms of Platelet Activation 185
8.2.3. Genetic Mutations and Their Effects 186
8.2.4. Immune System Involvement 187
8.2.5. Environmental Factors Influencing Platelet Function 187
8.2.6. Interaction with Other Blood Components 188
8.2.7. Role of Cytokines in Platelet Disorders 188
8.2.8. Impact of Chronic Diseases on Platelet Function 189
8.2.9. Diagnostic Markers in Platelet Disorders 189
8.3. Diagnosis of Platelet Disorders 189
8.3.1. Clinical Symptoms and Signs 190
8.3.2. Laboratory Tests for Platelet Count 190
8.3.3. Platelet Function Tests 191
8.3.4. Bone Marrow Biopsy 191
8.3.5. Genetic Testing for Inherited Disorders 192
8.3.6. Imaging Studies in Diagnosis 192
8.3.7. Differential Diagnosis Considerations 193
8.3.8. Role of Hematologists in Diagnosis 193
8.3.9. Challenges in Accurate Diagnosis 193
8.4. Treatment and Management of Platelet Disorders 194
8.4.1. General Treatment Approaches 194

8.4.2. Medications for Thrombocytopenia 195
8.4.3. Platelet Transfusions: Indications and Risks 195
8.4.4. Immunosuppressive Therapy for ITP 195
8.4.5. Surgical Options for Severe Cases 196
8.4.6. Lifestyle Modifications and Patient Education 196
8.4.7. Role of Support Groups and Counseling 197
8.4.8. Long-Term Management Strategies 197
Summary **199**
References **200**

CHAPTER 9

Coagulation Disorders 207

Introduction **207**
9.1. Types of Coagulation Disorders **208**
9.1.1. Hemophilia A 209
9.1.2. Hemophilia B 209
9.1.3. Von Willebrand Disease (VWD) 209
9.1.4. Factor V Leiden Mutation 210
9.1.5. Antiphospholipid Syndrome (APS) 210
9.1.6. Disseminated Intravascular Coagulation (DIC) 211
9.1.7. Thrombocytopenia 211
9.1.8. Vitamin K Deficiency 211
9.1.9. Acquired Coagulation Disorders 212
9.2. Causes and Risk Factors **213**
9.2.1. Genetic Factors 213
9.2.2. Environmental Influences 213
9.2.3. Medications and Their Effects 214
9.2.4. Chronic Diseases and Conditions 214
9.2.5. Lifestyle Factors 215
9.2.6. Age-Related Changes 215
9.2.7. Gender Differences in Prevalence 216
9.2.8. Family History and Inheritance Patterns 216
9.2.9. Impact of Obesity on Coagulation 217
9.3. Symptoms and Diagnosis **217**
9.3.1. Common Symptoms of Coagulation Disorders 218
9.3.2. Diagnostic Tests for Coagulation Disorders 218
9.3.3. Role of Blood Tests in Diagnosis 219
9.3.4. Imaging Studies and Their Relevance 219
9.3.5. Clinical Evaluation and Patient History 219
9.3.6. Differential Diagnosis Considerations 220
9.3.7. Importance of Early Detection 220
9.3.8. Challenges in Diagnosing Coagulation Disorders 221
9.3.9. Advances in Diagnostic Technology 221
9.4. Treatment and Management **221**
9.4.1. Replacement Therapy for Hemophilia 221
9.4.2. Anticoagulant Medications 222
9.4.3. Lifestyle Modifications and Self-care 223
9.4.4. Role of Physical Therapy 223
9.4.5. Management of Bleeding Episodes 223
9.4.6. Education and Support for Patients 224
9.4.7. Emerging Therapies and Research 224
9.4.8. Psychological Support and Counseling 225
9.4.9. Importance of Regular Monitoring 225
Summary **228**
References **229**

CHAPTER 10

Thrombotic Disorders 237

Introduction **237**
10.1. Types of Thrombotic Disorders **238**
10.1.1. Deep Vein Thrombosis (DVT) 238
10.1.2. Pulmonary Embolism (PE) 239
10.1.3. Arterial Thrombosis 239
10.1.4. Thrombophilia 239
10.1.5. Antiphospholipid Syndrome (APS) 240
10.1.6. Cerebral Venous Sinus Thrombosis (CVST) 240
10.1.7. Myocardial Infarction 241
10.1.8. Stroke 241
10.1.9. Disseminated Intravascular Coagulation (DIC) 242
10.2. Pathophysiology of Thrombotic Disorders **242**
10.2.1. Coagulation Cascade Overview 243
10.2.2. Role of Platelets in Thrombosis 243
10.2.3. Endothelial Dysfunction 244
10.2.4. Genetic Factors Contributing to Thrombosis 245

10.2.5. Acquired Risk Factors 245
10.2.6. Inflammatory Processes in Thrombosis 245
10.2.7. Hemodynamic Changes Leading to Thrombus Formation 246
10.2.8. Interaction between Coagulation and Fibrinolysis 246
10.2.9. Impact of Lifestyle Factors on Thrombotic Risk 247
10.3. Diagnosis of Thrombotic Disorders 248
10.3.1. Clinical Assessment and History Taking 248
10.3.2. Imaging Techniques (e.g., Ultrasound, CT) 249
10.3.3. Laboratory Tests (e.g., D-dimer, Coagulation Profile) 249
10.3.4. Risk Assessment Models 250
10.3.5. Differential Diagnosis Considerations 250
10.3.6. Importance of Early Detection 250
10.3.7. Role of Biomarkers in Diagnosis 251
10.3.8. Challenges in Diagnosing Thrombotic Disorders 251
10.3.9. Guidelines for Diagnostic Protocols 252
10.4. Treatment and Management of Thrombotic Disorders 252
10.4.1. Anticoagulant Therapy 253
10.4.2. Thrombolytic Therapy 253
10.4.3. Surgical Interventions (e.g., Thrombectomy) 254
10.4.4. Long-Term Management Strategies 255
10.4.5. Patient Education and Lifestyle Modifications 255
10.4.6. Monitoring and Follow-Up Care 256
10.4.7. Management of Complications 256
10.4.8. Emerging Therapies and Research 257
10.4.9. Role of Multidisciplinary Teams in Management 257
Summary 259
References 260

CHAPTER 11

Acute Leukemias 267

Introduction 267
11.1. Types of Acute Leukemias 268
11.1.1. Acute Lymphoblastic Leukemia (ALL) 268
11.1.2. Acute Myeloid Leukemia (AML) 268
11.1.3. Differences between ALL and AML 269
11.1.4. Risk Factors Associated with Each Type 269
11.1.5. Age Demographics Affected by Each Type 270
11.1.6. Genetic Mutations Linked to Acute Leukemias 270
11.1.7. Subtypes of Acute Lymphoblastic Leukemia 271
11.1.8. Subtypes of Acute Myeloid Leukemia 271
11.1.9. Emerging classifications in Acute Leukemias 272
11.2. Symptoms and Diagnosis 272
11.2.1. Common Symptoms of Acute Leukemias 273
11.2.2. Diagnostic Tests Used for Identification 273
11.2.3. Role of Blood Tests in Diagnosis 274
11.2.4. Bone Marrow Biopsy Procedures 275
11.2.5. Imaging Studies and Their Significance 275
11.2.6. Differential Diagnosis Considerations 275
11.2.7. Importance of Early Symptom Recognition 276
11.2.8. Challenges in Diagnosing Acute Leukemias 276
11.3. Treatment Options 277
11.3.1. Overview of Treatment Modalities 277
11.3.2. Chemotherapy Regimens for Acute Leukemias 278
11.3.3. Role of Targeted Therapy 278
11.3.4. Stem Cell Transplantation Procedures 279
11.3.5. Radiation Therapy Applications 279
11.3.6. Clinical Trials and Experimental Treatments 280
11.3.7. Supportive Care and Symptom Management 280
11.3.8. Long-Term Management Strategies 281
11.3.9. Challenges in Treatment Adherence 281
11.4. Prognosis and Outcomes 281
11.4.1. Factors Influencing Prognosis 282
11.4.2. Survival Rates for Different Types 282
11.4.3. Impact of Age on Outcomes 283
11.4.4. Role of Genetic Factors in Prognosis 284
11.4.5. Quality of Life Considerations Post-Treatment 284
11.4.6. Recurrence Rates and Monitoring 285
11.4.7. Psychological Impact on Patients and Families 285

11.4.8. Advances in Research Affecting Outcomes 286
11.4.9. Future Directions in Improving Prognosis 286
Summary **288**
References **289**

CHAPTER 12

Chronic Leukemias 295

Introduction **295**
12.1. Types of Chronic Leukemias **296**
12.1.1. Chronic Lymphocytic Leukemia (CLL) 296
12.1.2. Chronic Myeloid Leukemia (CML) 297
12.1.3. Rare Types of Chronic Leukemias 297
12.1.4. Genetic Mutations Associated with Chronic Leukemias 297
12.1.5. Risk Factors for Developing Chronic Leukemias 298
12.1.6. Age and Gender Distribution 298
12.1.7. Geographic Variations in Incidence 299
12.1.8. Prognosis for Different Types 299
12.2. Pathophysiology of Chronic Leukemias **300**
12.2.1. Mechanisms of Leukemogenesis 300
12.2.2. Role of the Bone Marrow in Chronic Leukemias 300
12.2.3. Impact of the Immune System 301
12.2.4. Genetic and Epigenetic Changes 302
12.2.5. Microenvironmental Influences 302
12.2.6. Clonal Evolution in Chronic Leukemias 303
12.2.7. Interaction with Other Diseases 303
12.2.8. Biomarkers for Chronic Leukemias 303
12.2.9. Current Research on Pathophysiology 304
12.3. Diagnosis and Monitoring **305**
12.3.1. Initial Diagnostic Tests 305
12.3.2. Role of Blood Tests in Diagnosis 306
12.3.3. Bone Marrow Biopsy Procedures 306
12.3.4. Imaging Studies in Chronic Leukemias 306
12.3.5. Molecular Testing and Genetic Profiling 307
12.3.6. Staging of Chronic Leukemias 307
12.3.7. Monitoring Disease Progression 307
12.3.8. Challenges in Diagnosis 308
12.3.9. Importance of Early Detection 308
12.4. Treatment Options and Management **309**
12.4.1. Overview of Treatment Modalities 309
12.4.2. Chemotherapy Regimens 310
12.4.3. Targeted Therapies and Their Mechanisms 310
12.4.4. Role of Immunotherapy 311
12.4.5. Stem Cell Transplantation 311
12.4.6. Supportive Care and Symptom Management 312
12.4.7. Clinical Trials and Emerging Therapies 313
12.4.8. Long-Term Management Strategies 313
12.4.9. Patient Education and Involvement in Treatment 314
Summary **316**
References **317**

CHAPTER 13

Lymphomas 325

Introduction **325**
13.1. Types of Lymphomas **326**
13.1.1. Hodgkin Lymphoma (HL) 326
13.1.2. Non-Hodgkin Lymphoma (NHL) 327
13.1.3. Burkitt Lymphoma 327
13.1.4. Follicular Lymphoma 328
13.1.5. Diffuse Large B-Cell Lymphoma 328
13.1.6. Mantle Cell Lymphoma (MCL) 329
13.1.7. Peripheral T-Cell Lymphoma 329
13.1.8. Anaplastic Large Cell Lymphoma 330
13.1.9. Primary Mediastinal B-Cell Lymphoma (PMBCL) 330
13.2. Causes and Risk Factors **330**
13.2.1. Genetic Predisposition 331
13.2.2. Environmental Factors 331
13.2.3. Viral Infections (e.g., EBV, HIV) 332
13.2.4. Autoimmune Diseases 332
13.2.5. Age and Gender Considerations 333
13.2.6. Family History 333
13.2.7. Occupational Exposures 333
13.2.8. Lifestyle Factors (e.g., Smoking, Diet) 334
13.2.9. Previous Cancer Treatments 334
13.3. Diagnosis and Staging **335**
13.3.1. Initial Symptoms and Clinical Evaluation 335

13.3.2. Imaging Techniques (e.g., CT, PET Scans) 336
13.3.3. Biopsy Procedures 336
13.3.4. Blood Tests and Markers 336
13.3.5. Staging Systems (Ann Arbor, Lugano) 337
13.3.6. Prognostic Factors 337
13.3.7. Role of Pathologists 338
13.3.8. Importance of Accurate Diagnosis 338
13.3.9. Challenges in Diagnosis 338
13.4. Treatment Options 339
13.4.1. Chemotherapy Regimens 340
13.4.2. Radiation Therapy 340
13.4.3. Targeted Therapies 341
13.4.4. Immunotherapy 341
13.4.5. Stem Cell Transplantation 342
13.4.6. Clinical Trials and Research 343
13.4.7. Palliative Care Approaches 343
13.4.8. Side Effects and Management 344
13.4.9. Role of Multidisciplinary Teams 344
Summary 346
References 347

CHAPTER 14

Plasma Cell Dyscrasias 353

Introduction 353
14.1. Types of Plasma Cell Dyscrasias 354
14.1.1. Multiple Myeloma (MM) 354
14.1.2. Monoclonal Gammopathy of Undetermined Significance (MGUS) 355
14.1.3. Waldenström Macroglobulinemia 355
14.1.4. Primary Amyloidosis 356
14.1.5. Light Chain Deposition Disease 356
14.1.6. Plasma Cell Leukemia (PCL) 357
14.1.7. Solitary Plasmacytoma 357
14.1.8. Non-Secretory Multiple Myeloma (MM) 358
14.2. Pathophysiology of Plasma Cell Dyscrasias 358
14.2.1. Normal Plasma Cell Function 358
14.2.2. Genetic Mutations and Abnormalities 359
14.2.3. Role of the Bone Marrow Microenvironment 360
14.2.4. Mechanisms of Monoclonal Antibody Production 360
14.2.5. Immune Dysregulation 360
14.2.6. Cytokine Involvement 361
14.2.7. Tumor Microenvironment Interactions 361
14.2.8. Progression from Monoclonal Gammopathy of Undetermined Significance (MGUS) to Multiple Myeloma (MM) 362
14.2.9. Impact of Pathophysiology on Treatment Strategies 362
14.3. Diagnosis and Evaluation 363
14.3.1. Clinical Assessment and History Taking 363
14.3.2. Laboratory Tests and Biomarkers 364
14.3.3. Imaging Studies in Diagnosis 364
14.3.4. Bone Marrow Biopsy Techniques 365
14.3.5. Role of Flow Cytometry 365
14.3.6. Genetic Testing and Prognostic Factors 365
14.3.7. Differential Diagnosis Considerations 366
14.3.8. Staging Systems for Plasma Cell Dyscrasias 366
14.3.9. Importance of Multidisciplinary Approach 367
14.4. Treatment Options and Management 367
14.4.1. Chemotherapy Regimens 368
14.4.2. Targeted Therapies 368
14.4.3. Immunotherapy Approaches 369
14.4.4. Stem Cell Transplantation 369
14.4.5. Supportive Care and Symptom Management 370
14.4.6. Role of Clinical Trials 370
14.4.7. Long-term Management Strategies 371
14.4.8. Challenges in Treatment Adherence 371
14.4.9. Future Directions in Treatment Research 372
Summary 374
References 375

CHAPTER 15

Transfusion Medicine and Bone Marrow Transplantation 379

Introduction 379
15.1. Fundamentals of Transfusion Medicine 380
15.1.1. Types of Blood Components Used in Transfusions 380

15.1.2. Indications for Blood Transfusion 381
15.1.3. Blood Typing and Crossmatching Procedures 381
15.1.4. Risks and Complications Associated with Transfusions 382
15.1.5. Role of Blood Banks and Donation Centers 382
15.1.6. Advances in Blood Preservation Techniques 382
15.1.7. Ethical Considerations in Blood Donation 383
15.1.8. Regulations Governing Transfusion Practices 383
15.1.9. Future Directions in Transfusion Medicine 384
15.2. Bone Marrow: Structure and Function 384
15.2.1. Anatomy of Bone Marrow 384
15.2.2. Types of Cells Produced in Bone Marrow 385
15.2.3. Role of Bone Marrow in Hematopoiesis 385
15.2.4. Factors Affecting Bone Marrow Function 386
15.2.5. Diseases Affecting Bone Marrow Health 386
15.2.6. Diagnostic Techniques for Bone Marrow Disorders 387
15.2.7. Importance of Bone Marrow Microenvironment 387
15.2.8. Genetic Factors Influencing Bone Marrow Function 388
15.3. Bone Marrow Transplantation Procedures 388
15.3.1. Types of Bone Marrow Transplants (Autologous vs. Allogeneic) 389
15.3.2. Pre-Transplant Evaluation and Preparation 389
15.3.3. The Transplant Procedure: Step-by-Step 390
15.3.4. Post-Transplant Care and Monitoring 390
15.3.5. Complications and Management Strategies 390
15.3.6. Role of Graft-versus-Host Disease (GVHD) 391
15.3.7. Long-term Outcomes of Bone Marrow Transplantation (BMT) 391
15.3.8. Psychosocial Aspects of Bone Marrow Transplantation (BMT) 392
15.4. The Intersection of Transfusion Medicine and Bone Marrow Transplantation (BMT) 392
15.4.1. Role of Blood Products in Transplantation 393
15.4.2. Pre-Transplant Blood Management Strategies 393
15.4.3. Impact of Transfusion on Transplant Outcomes 394
15.4.4. Immunological Considerations in Transfusion and Transplantation 394
15.4.5. Case Studies of Transfusion in Bone Marrow Recipients 395
15.4.6. Research on Transfusion-Related Transplant Complications 395
15.4.7. Collaborative Approaches in Transfusion and Transplant Medicine 396
15.4.8. Education and Training for Healthcare Professionals 396
15.4.9. Future Research Directions at the Intersection 397
Summary 399
References 400

Index 405

LIST OF FIGURES

Figure 1.1. Blood is primarily composed of plasma, which accounts for about 55% of its volume, and formed elements, including red blood cells, white blood cells, and platelets

Figure 1.2. The primary function of red blood cells (RBCs), also known as erythrocytes, is to transport oxygen from the lungs to the tissues and return carbon dioxide from the tissues back to the lungs for exhalation

Figure 1.3. Platelets, or thrombocytes, are cellular fragments derived from megakaryocytes in the bone marrow and are primarily responsible for blood clotting, preventing excessive bleeding following vascular injury

Figure 1.4. Blood volume is intricately managed through various hormonal and renal mechanisms, primarily involving erythropoiesis, which is the process of red blood cell production

Figure 1.5. Blood types are classified primarily by the presence or absence of specific antigens on the surface of red blood cells, with the ABO and Rh systems being the most significant

Figure 1.6. Hematopoiesis

Figure 1.7. Initiating in the embryonic yolk sac, hematopoiesis transitions to the fetal liver and eventually to the bone marrow, delineating a clear timeline that reflects both spatial and temporal regulation

Figure 1.8. The regulation of hematopoiesis, the complex process of blood cell formation, relies on a sophisticated interplay of genetic and environmental factors

Figure 1.9. Hematopoietic growth factors play a pivotal role in regulating the proliferation, differentiation, and survival of hematopoietic stem cells (HSCs)

Figure 1.10. Development of allogeneic hematopoietic stem cell transplantation (HSCT)

Figure 1.11. Anemia represents a complex hematologic condition characterized by a deficiency in red blood cells or hemoglobin, leading to reduced oxygen transport within the body

Figure 1.12. Lymphoma, a pivotal focus within hematology, represents a diverse group of malignancies originating from lymphatic tissues, which are integral to the immune system

Figure 1.13. Hemophilia

Figure 1.14. Myelodysplastic syndromes (MDS)

Figure 1.15. The field of hematology is witnessing unprecedented advancements in therapeutic approaches, particularly concerning hematological disorders

Figure 1.16. The complete blood count (CBC) serves as an essential diagnostic tool in hematology, providing critical insights into an individual's hematopoietic health

Figure 1.17. Flow cytometry (FCM) is a pivotal technology in the realm of hematology, allowing for precise analysis of the cellular components within blood

Figure 1.18. Coagulation studies play a critical role in the field of hematology by providing insights into the hemostatic process, which is essential for maintaining vascular integrity and preventing excessive bleeding

Figure 1.19. The integration of molecular diagnostics into hematology has significantly enhanced the understanding and management of hematopoietic disorders

Figure 1.20. Laboratory medicine plays a pivotal role in the diagnosis, treatment, and monitoring of blood-related disorders, significantly enhancing the understanding of hematopoiesis

Figure 2.1. Anemia

Figure 2.2. The production of red blood cells (RBCs), a process known as erythropoiesis, involves intricate mechanisms that are closely regulated to maintain adequate oxygen transport in the body

Figure 2.3. Decreased red blood cell (RBC) production can arise from a variety of pathophysiological mechanisms, leading to different forms of anemia

Figure 2.4. The impact of nutritional deficiencies on anemia is profound, particularly in populations with limited access to diverse food sources

Figure 2.5. Chronic diseases significantly contribute to the prevalence and complexity of anemia, illustrating a compelling intersection between various pathological processes

Figure 2.6. The body employs several compensatory mechanisms in response to anemia, which serves as a critical adaptive strategy to maintain oxygen delivery despite reduced hemoglobin levels

Figure 2.7. Microcytic anemia represents a classification of anemia characterized by smaller-than-normal red blood cells, primarily linked to reduced hemoglobin synthesis

Figure 2.8. Normocytic anemia, characterized by red blood cells that are of normal size and appearance but deficient in number, presents a unique diagnostic challenge within the broader framework of anemia classification

Figure 2.9. Aplastic anemia is a critical condition characterized by the failure of the bone marrow to produce adequate blood cells, leading to profound consequences across hematological health

Figure 2.10. Iron deficiency anemia, one of the most prevalent forms of anemia worldwide, significantly impacts individual's health and functionality

Figure 2.11. Sickle cell anemia, classified under inherited anemias, presents significant challenges due to its complex pathophysiology and multi-organ effects

Figure 2.12. The clinical symptoms and signs of anemia present a complex tapestry of manifestations that can vary widely depending on the underlying cause and severity

Figure 2.13. The complete blood count (CBC) analysis is a fundamental diagnostic tool in hematology, particularly in the assessment of anemias

Figure 2.14. Low serum iron and ferritin levels are hallmark indicators of iron deficiency anemia, which is particularly prevalent among specific populations, such as menstruating women and children suffering from nutritional challenges

Figure 2.15. Genetic testing has emerged as a pivotal tool in the diagnosis and management of hereditary anemias (HAs), a diverse group of disorders characterized by their genetic underpinnings

Figure 2.16. Accurate diagnosis is crucial in the management of anemias, as misclassification can lead to inappropriate treatment strategies with potentially detrimental results

Figure 2.17. Dietary modifications and supplementation play a crucial role in the management of various types of anemia, particularly iron-deficiency anemia

Figure 2.18. Blood transfusions play a critical role in managing various types of anemia, particularly in situations where rapid restoration of red blood cell (RBC) levels is necessary

Figure 2.19. Erythropoietin-stimulating agents (ESAs) play a crucial role in the management of various types of anemia

Figure 2.20. Regular assessments of hematological parameters, including hemoglobin levels and red cell indices, are crucial for evaluating treatment efficacy and identifying potential complications

Figure 3.1. Inadequate dietary intake of iron, particularly in populations with limited access to iron-rich foods, remains a prevalent factor contributing to this deficiency

Figure 3.2. Dietary insufficiency plays a significant role in the prevalence of iron deficiency and sideroblastic anemia, particularly affecting vulnerable populations such as pregnant women and young children

Figure 3.3. The process of heme biosynthesis is critically dependent on iron, as it is incorporated into hemoglobin within erythrocytes, facilitating oxygen transport

Figure 3.4. During pregnancy, the increased demands for iron are driven by fetal growth, placental development, and the expansion of maternal blood volume, which can lead to a notable depletion of iron stores

Figure 3.5. Regular menstrual bleeding can lead to substantial iron loss, which, if not adequately compensated through dietary intake, may precipitate or exacerbate anemia

Figure 3.6. Genetic factors contribute significantly to an individual's susceptibility to both iron deficiency and anemia, where inherited conditions can disrupt normal erythropoiesis

Figure 3.7. Mechanism of sideroblast formation

Figure 3.8. Iron plays a crucial role in the synthesis of hemoglobin, the protein responsible for oxygen transport in erythrocytes

Figure 3.9. Sideroblastic anemia is a heterogeneous group of disorders characterized by the impaired utilization of iron in heme synthesis, leading to the accumulation of ring sideroblasts in the bone marrow

Figure 3.10. Vitamin B6, as a cofactor for enzymes that facilitate the production of heme, is crucial for the effective incorporation of iron into hemoglobin

Figure 3.11. Effects of inflammation on iron recycling

Figure 3.12. The common symptoms of iron deficiency often present a complex and multi-faceted challenge that can significantly impact daily functioning and overall health

Figure 3.13. The diagnosis of iron deficiency and sideroblastic anemia relies heavily on a range of laboratory tests that provide critical insights into the underlying mechanisms of these disorders

Figure 3.14. Iron studies, aimed at evaluating the body's iron levels, are critical in understanding conditions such as iron deficiency and sideroblastic anemia

Figure 3.15. Bone marrow biopsy findings are critical in diagnosing iron deficiency and sideroblastic anemia, as they provide insight into erythropoiesis and hematopoietic function

Figure 3.16. In patients presenting with symptoms of anemia, such as fatigue or pallor, a detailed account of dietary habits, family history, and prior medical conditions is invaluable

Figure 3.17. Individuals suffering from iron deficiency anemia often benefit from an increased intake of iron-rich foods, such as red meats, poultry, and legumes, which provide heme and non-heme iron, respectively

Figure 3.18. Understanding the underlying pathologies of anemia can guide clinicians in selecting appropriate interventions, thereby reducing morbidity associated with these conditions

Figure 3.19. Blood transfusions play a crucial role in the management of various anemias, including those associated with iron deficiency and sideroblastic anemia

Figure 3.20. Regular assessment of hematological parameters, including hemoglobin levels, mean corpuscular volume (MCV), and reticulocyte counts, is critical to gauge the efficacy of iron supplementation and to detect potential complications

Figure 4.1. Hemolytic anemias are characterized by the premature destruction of red blood cells, resulting from a variety of underlying causes

Figure 4.2. Acquired conditions play a significant role in the pathophysiology of hemolytic anemias, where external factors contribute to the destruction of red blood cells (RBCs)

Figure 4.3. Infections represent a substantial etiology of hemolytic anemias, often causing direct damage to red blood cells (RBCs) or indirectly triggering immune responses that compromise RBC integrity

Figure 4.4. Mechanical destruction of red blood cells (RBCs) is a significant contributor to hemolytic anemias, wherein the integrity of the erythrocyte membrane is compromised, resulting in premature cell lysis

Figure 4.5. Nutritional deficiencies are a significant contributor to the onset and development of hemolytic anemias, as they impair the body's ability to produce healthy red blood cells

Figure 4.6. Hemolytic anemias present a variety of symptoms that directly result from the premature destruction of red blood cells

Figure 4.7. Traditional blood smears provide direct visual insights into red blood cell morphology, which can reveal characteristic changes associated with specific disorders

Figure 4.8. The measurement of bilirubin levels serves as a vital diagnostic tool in understanding hemolytic anemias, as elevated bilirubin indicates increased breakdown of red blood cells

Figure 4.9. The Coombs test, or direct antiglobulin test, is a critical diagnostic tool for identifying autoimmune hemolytic anemia (AIHA), a condition characterized by the premature destruction of red blood cells

Figure 4.10. Non-invasive diagnostic approaches, such as smartphone applications utilizing colorimetric analysis, are emerging as practical tools to evaluate hemoglobin concentrations and monitor changes over time

Figure 4.11. Supportive care is a cornerstone of treatment, encompassing measures such as blood transfusions to alleviate severe anemia and intravenous immunoglobulin (IVIG) for autoimmune cases

Figure 4.12. Corticosteroids are employed explicitly in cases of warm AIHA, where autoantibodies target red blood cells, facilitating their destruction

Figure 4.13. The surgical procedure known as splenectomy, defined as the removal of the spleen, holds significant therapeutic potential in the management of various hemolytic anemias

Figure 4.14. The role of immunosuppressive therapy in managing hemolytic anemias is pivotal, particularly in cases where autoimmune mechanisms drive red blood cell destruction

Figure 4.15. Patient education and support are crucial components in the management of hemolytic anemias, as they empower individuals to understand their condition and play an active role in treatment decisions

Figure 4.16. Key determinants include the underlying etiology of the anemia, the patient's age, and their overall health status before diagnosis

Figure 4.17. Chronic hemolytic anemias, such as β thalassemia, pose significant long-term health effects that extend beyond the immediate symptoms of anemia

Figure 4.18. The management of hemolytic anemias necessitates the critical practice of regular follow-up appointments, which play an essential role in monitoring patient progress and adjusting treatment plans as needed

Figure 4.19. Reblozyl

Figure 5.1. Sickle cell disease (SCD)

Figure 5.2. Hemoglobin E disease

Figure 5.3. Hemoglobin H disease (Hb H disease)

Figure 5.4. Thalassemia minor

Figure 5.5. The vast spectrum of hemoglobinopathies includes not only prominent disorders such as alpha and beta thalassemia but also rare hemoglobin variants that can complicate diagnosis and management

Figure 5.6. Hemoglobin is primarily composed of four polypeptide chains—two alpha and two beta chains—encoded by genes located on different chromosomes

Figure 5.7. The impact of hemoglobinopathies and thalassemias on red blood cell morphology is profound and multifaceted, leading to various structural abnormalities in erythrocytes

Figure 5.8. Hemolysis results in the premature destruction of red blood cells, which in turn precipitates anemia, often characterized by fatigue, pallor, and increased heart rate

Figure 5.9. Iron metabolism plays a crucial role in the pathophysiology of hemoglobinopathies and thalassemias, as iron is an essential component of hemoglobin, which is responsible for oxygen transport in the bloodstream

Figure 5.10. The cellular and molecular consequences of hemoglobinopathies and thalassemias are profound, affecting oxygen transport and leading to a spectrum of clinical manifestations

Figure 5.11. The clinical presentation of hemoglobinopathies, including thalassemias and sickle cell disease (SCD), is characterized by a spectrum of symptoms that vary in severity and manifestation

Figure 5.12. Hemoglobin electrophoresis serves as a pivotal diagnostic tool in the investigation of hemoglobinopathies, particularly in differentiating various types of thalassemia's

Figure 5.13. Newborn screening programs play a critical role in the early detection of hemoglobinopathies and thalassemias, allowing for timely intervention that can significantly improve health outcomes for affected infants

Figure 5.14. Techniques such as magnetic resonance imaging (MRI) and ultrasound are instrumental in evaluating organ damage caused by iron overload, a common consequence of frequent blood transfusions in patients with conditions like beta thalassemia

Figure 5.15. Patient education is crucial for fostering adherence to treatment protocols and empowering patients to manage their health effectively

Figure 5.16. The management of hemoglobinopathies, particularly beta-thalassemia, often necessitates iron chelation therapy due to the risks associated with excessive iron accumulation from repeated blood transfusions

Figure 5.17. Gene editing techniques, such as CRISPR-Cas9, which enable precise alterations to the faulty globin genes responsible for these conditions

Figure 5.18. Iron and folic acid supplements form the bedrock of anemia prevention during pregnancy, a significant concern given that pregnant women are particularly susceptible to anemia due to increased nutritional demands

Figure 5.19. In the management of hemoglobinopathies, particularly thalassemias, the provision of psychological support is an essential component that greatly influences patient outcomes

Figure 6.1. Megaloblastic anemia, commonly attributed to deficiencies in vitamin B12 or folate, disrupts DNA synthesis, leading to ineffective erythropoiesis and the production of abnormally large red blood cells

Figure 6.2. Hypersegmented neutrophils

Figure 6.3. Vitamin B12 deficiency plays a critical role in the pathophysiology of megaloblastic anemia, a condition characterized by large, abnormal red blood cells resulting from impaired DNA synthesis

Figure 6.4. Production of megaloblasts

Figure 6.5. Bone marrow aspiration (BMA) and trephine biopsy are complementary techniques that provide critical cytological and histological insights into hematological disorders

Figure 6.6: Health Pancytopenia

Figure 6.7. Aplastic anemia is marked by the bone marrow's failure to produce adequate blood cells due to autoimmune destruction, exposure to toxins, or genetic predispositions

Figure 6.8. Bone marrow failure (BMF) plays a crucial role in the pathology of both megaloblastic and aplastic anemias, highlighting the intricate relationship between hematopoietic cell production and hematological health

Figure 6.9. Patients suffering from megaloblastic anemia typically present with symptoms such as fatigue, pallor, and shortness of breath, which stem from the ineffective production of erythrocytes

Figure 6.10. Treatment for aplastic anemia, characterized by bone marrow failure, may involve immunosuppressive therapy or hematopoietic stem cell transplantation, depending on the severity of the patient's condition

Figure 6.11. Patients may experience severe anemia, leading to fatigue, pallor, and even heart complications as the body struggles to deliver sufficient oxygen to tissues

Figure 6.12. Ocular manifestations that often accompany blood dyscrasias

Figure 6.13. Diamond-blackfan anemia

Figure 6.14. Advancements in genetic profiling have revealed how mutations and deficiencies in specific genes, such as those involved in DNA metabolism, are linked to the pathogenesis of megaloblastic anemia

Figure 6.15. Effective patient education and awareness are crucial components in managing megaloblastic and aplastic anemias, as these conditions often arise from nutritional deficiencies and a lack of appropriate healthcare practices

Figure 6.16. Fostering a collaborative environment enables healthcare professionals to engage in shared problem-solving, drawing on each other's expertise to navigate the intricacies of these anemias

Figure 7.1. Agranulocytes

Figure 7.2. Neutrophils serve as essential components of the immune system, primarily tasked with identifying and eliminating pathogens

Figure 7.3. Monocytes, a critical component of the leukocyte family, exhibit unique characteristics and multifaceted functions that influence various disorders, including inflammatory and autoimmune diseases

Figure 7.4. Basophils

Figure 7.5. Dendritic cells

Figure 7.6. Leukopenia

Figure 7.7. Lymphoma

Figure 7.8. Myelodysplastic syndromes (MDS)

Figure 7.9. Autoimmune diseases often involve the aberrant activation of leukocytes, leading to tissue damage and chronic inflammation

Figure 7.10. The role of blood tests in diagnosing disorders of leukocytes cannot be overstated, as these diagnostic tools provide critical insights into the functionality and health of the immune system

Figure 7.11. The bone marrow biopsy is a critical diagnostic procedure that provides essential insights into various disorders of leukocytes, particularly those related to hematological malignancies and other bone marrow pathologies

Figure 7.12. Genetic testing plays a crucial role in the diagnosis and management of leukocyte disorders, significantly enhancing our understanding of various hematological conditions

Figure 7.13. Symptoms often manifest as a result of dysregulation in leukocyte function, leading to various clinical presentations, including recurrent infections, chronic inflammation, or hematological malignancies

Figure 7.14. Understanding the biological mechanisms at play allows clinicians to optimize treatment plans, integrating pharmacological and supportive interventions to improve patient outcomes and quality of life effectively

Figure 7.15. Radiation therapy has emerged as a pivotal component in the treatment of various leukocyte disorders, particularly in cancers such as chronic lymphocytic leukemia (CLL), where it addresses the abnormal proliferation of leukocytes

Figure 7.16. In treating disorders of leukocytes, stem cell transplantation has emerged as a pivotal procedure, particularly in addressing hematologic malignancies and genetic disorders

Figure 7.17. Adopting nutritional strategies, engaging in regular physical activity, and minimizing stress through mindfulness practices can promote overall immune function, directly impacting leukocyte behavior and health

Figure 8.1. Anomalies in platelet production, activation, or survival can lead to a spectrum of conditions, from thrombocytopenia to thrombocytopathy, highlighting the importance of accurate diagnosis and treatment modalities

Figure 8.2. Thrombocytopenia

Figure 8.3. Inherited platelet disorders (IPDs)

Figure 8.4. Immune thrombocytopenic purpura (ITP) represents a complex platelet disorder characterized by a markedly low platelet count, resulting from both accelerated destruction and inadequate production of platelets

Figure 8.5. Bernard-Soulier syndrome (BSS)

Figure 8.6. Essential thrombocythemia (ET)

Figure 8.7. The bone marrow plays a crucial role in the production of platelets, acting as the primary site for thrombopoiesis—the process through which platelets are generated from megakaryocytes

Figure 8.8. Von Willebrand disease (VWD) arises from mutations affecting the von Willebrand factor (VWF), which is crucial for platelet adhesion

Figure 8.9. The interplay between environmental factors and platelet function is crucial in understanding platelet disorders

Figure 8.10. Cytokines, as signaling molecules in the immune system, significantly influence platelet production and activation

Figure 8.11. Diagnostic markers in platelet disorders

Figure 8.12. Patients experiencing abnormal bleeding patterns, such as easy bruising or prolonged bleeding from minor cuts, often present with symptoms indicative of underlying platelet dysfunction

Figure 8.13. Platelet function tests

Figure 8.14. Conditions like immune thrombocytopenic purpura (ITP) can sometimes present with thrombocytopenia linked to malignancies, making a biopsy essential for ruling out neoplastic processes and ensuring appropriate management

Figure 8.15. Techniques such as ultrasonography and magnetic resonance imaging (MRI) are often employed to visualize vascular abnormalities or complications arising from these disorders

Figure 8.16. The role of hematologists in the diagnosis of platelet disorders is crucial, especially given their expertise in evaluating blood components and identifying hematological abnormalities

Figure 8.17. Hematopoietic stem cell therapy

Figure 8.18. Platelet transfusions

Figure 8.19. Surgical interventions may involve splenectomy, particularly for conditions like immune thrombocytopenic purpura (ITP), where the spleen's role in platelet destruction necessitates removal to increase platelet counts

Figure 8.20. Counseling can address the psychological impacts of living with a platelet disorder, helping patients manage issues related to pain and emotional well-being

Figure 9.1. Coagulation disorders

Figure 9.2. Types of hemophilia

Figure 9.3. Hemophilia B

Figure 9.4. Factor V Leiden mutation

Figure 9.5. Disseminated intravascular coagulation (DIC)

Figure 9.6. Vitamin K deficiency is a critical factor in the development of coagulation disorders, primarily because it impairs the synthesis of vitamin K-dependent proteins essential for effective blood clotting

Figure 9.7. Numerous genetic mutations can lead to deficiencies or dysfunctions in key coagulation factors, resulting in either excessive bleeding or thrombosis

Figure 9.8. The use of clotting factor replacements is crucial for individuals with conditions such as hemophilia, where the body lacks specific factors necessary for proper coagulation

Figure 9.9. A diet high in omega-3 fatty acids and low in saturated fats has been shown to promote healthier blood coagulation profiles

Figure 9.10. The influence of gender on the prevalence of coagulation disorders reveals significant disparities that warrant closer examination

Figure 9.11. Obesity significantly influences the coagulation system, contributing to an increased risk of thrombosis

Figure 9.12. Hemarthrosis, or bleeding into joints, is another alarming symptom, leading to severe pain and swelling, which can impede mobility

Figure 9.13. Blood tests play a critical role in the diagnosis of coagulation disorders, providing essential information that guides clinical management

Figure 9.14. Ecchymoses

Figure 9.15. Early detection of coagulation disorders is paramount for improving patient outcomes and minimizing complications

Figure 9.16. Replacement therapy for hemophilia represents a cornerstone in the management of this coagulation disorder, primarily involving the infusion of clotting factors VIII or IX to mitigate the risk of bleeding episodes

Figure 9.17. Lifestyle modifications and self-care play a pivotal role in managing coagulation disorders, as these conditions often require patients to implement daily practices that enhance their overall health and well-being

Figure 9.18. Management of bleeding episodes

Figure 9.19. The introduction of gene therapy has shown promise in addressing genetic factors underlying conditions like Hemophilia A, which is characterized by factor VIII deficiency and can lead to severe complications such as hemophilic arthropathy and thrombosis

Figure 9.20. Coagulation self-monitoring

Figure 10.1. Thrombotic disorders

Figure 10.2. Deep vein thrombosis (DVT)

Figure 10.3: Arterial thrombosis

Figure 10.4. Antiphospholipid syndrome (APS)

Figure 10.5. Myocardial infarction

Figure 10.6. Disseminated intravascular coagulation (DIC)

Figure 10.7. The coagulation cascade is a fundamental aspect of hemostasis, orchestrating the complex process of blood clot formation in response to vascular injury

Figure 10.8. Endothelial dysfunction is a crucial factor contributing to thrombotic disorders, as it disrupts the delicate balance between prothrombotic and anticoagulant mechanisms within the vascular system

Figure 10.9. Antiphospholipid syndrome (APS)

Figure 10.10. Formation of DVT is a complex process that is affected by three factors: endothelial damage/vascular injury, blood flow turbulence, and hypercoagulability of blood

Figure 10.11. A high body mass index (BMI) is associated with increased levels of inflammatory markers and endothelial dysfunction, which are known precursors to thrombosis

Figure 10.12. Tools like the CHA2DS2-VASc and HAS-BLED scores can be utilized during this assessment to systematically classify the thrombotic and bleeding risks associated with individual patients

Figure 10.13. D-dimer test

Figure 10.14. Atypical hemolytic uremic syndrome (aHUS)

Figure 10.15. C-reactive protein (CRP)

Figure 10.16. Diagnostic tests should not be standardized across the board; rather, they must be tailored to individual patient circumstances

Figure 10.17. Anticoagulant therapy plays a crucial role in managing thrombotic disorders, particularly in patient populations who are at heightened risk of thromboembolic events

Figure 10.18. Surgical interventions, particularly thrombectomy, play a crucial role in the management of thrombotic disorders, especially in cases involving acute ischemic stroke

Figure 10.19. Engaging patients in understanding their condition enhances adherence to prescribed health regimens and fosters proactive behavior, such as managing weight and increasing physical activity

Figure 10.20. Complications like renal vein thrombosis (RVT) in MN patients require prompt recognition and management, often involving anticoagulation and immunosuppressive therapy to mitigate acute kidney injury

Figure 11.1. Acute Lymphoblastic Leukemia (ALL) represents a heterogeneous group of hematological malignancies characterized by the rapid proliferation of immature lymphoid cells

Figure 11.2. Acute myeloid leukemia (AML)

Figure 11.3. Understanding the risk factors associated with different types of acute leukemias is essential for effective management and treatment strategies

Figure 11.4. The thymic TME promotes survival and proliferation of T-ALL cells by providing pro-leukemic signals such as IL-7, NOTCH ligands, and IGF1

Figure 11.5. Advancements in genetic profiling provide a promising avenue for better management of these subtypes, facilitating more personalized therapeutic approaches and improving patient outcomes

Figure 11.6. Patients may experience fatigue, fever, and recurrent infections due to the compromised bone marrow function that hampers blood cell production

Figure 11.7. Initially, a complete blood count (CBC) can reveal essential variations, including increased white blood cell counts, reduced red blood cells, and abnormal platelets, indicating hematological disturbance

Figure 11.8. Techniques such as magnetic resonance imaging (MRI) and computed tomography (CT) scans provide critical insights into the central nervous system

Figure 11.9. Delayed diagnosis can lead to disease progression and exacerbate treatment challenges, emphasizing the crucial role of heightened awareness among both healthcare providers and patients

Figure 11.10. Therapy-related myeloid neoplasms (t-MN)

Figure 11.11. By focusing on specific molecular abnormalities within cancer cells, targeted therapies aim to inhibit the growth of malignant cells more effectively while sparing healthy tissues

Figure 11.12. Radiation is primarily utilized as a part of the preparative regimen for hematopoietic stem cell transplantation, effectively eradicating malignant cells and enabling the engraftment of healthy hematopoietic stem cells

Figure 11.13. As new therapies emerge, particularly in acute lymphoblastic leukemia (ALL) and acute myeloid leukemia (AML), the spectrum of toxic effects becomes increasingly complex, necessitating a robust framework for addressing these challenges

Figure 11.14. The necessity for multifaceted support strategies—encompassing education, symptom management, and addressing barriers to care—is crucial for fostering adherence

Figure 11.15. Specific genetic mutations, such as those identified in acute myeloid leukemia (AML), play a pivotal role in determining treatment responsiveness and overall outcomes

Figure 11.16. Age significantly influences the outcomes of acute leukemias, particularly in the context of treatment effectiveness and overall survival rates

Figure 11.17. Survivors often contend with long-term side effects, including oral health complications like mucositis, xerostomia, and gingival bleeding, which significantly impact their overall well-being and life satisfaction

Figure 11.18. The psychological impact of acute leukemias on patients and their families can be profound and multifaceted, shaping their daily lives and emotional well-being

Figure 12.1. Chronic lymphocytic leukemia (CLL)

Figure 12.2. Chronic lymphocytic leukemia (CLL) is increasingly recognized for its diverse prognostic groups, largely determined by various genetic and molecular factors

Figure 12.3. Chronic myelomonocytic leukemia (CMML)

Figure 12.4. Environmental exposures, particularly to hazardous chemicals like benzene, have been strongly linked to an increased risk of such hematologic malignancies

Figure 12.5. Chronic lymphocytic leukemia (CLL), for instance, often presents with an indolent course and a relatively favorable overall survival rate, especially in early-stage cases

Figure 12.6. Chronic myeloid leukemia (CML)

Figure 12.7. Aberrant signaling pathways, such as NOTCH1, are frequently activated in leukemias, thereby disrupting normal immune functions and promoting malignant cell survival

Figure 12.8. The microenvironment plays a crucial role in the progression and treatment response of chronic leukemias, significantly influencing patient outcomes

Figure 12.9. The interaction of chronic leukemias with other diseases plays a significant role in shaping the clinical management and outcomes for affected patients

Figure 12.10. Current research delves into the molecular and cellular mechanisms driving the disease, revealing how genetic mutations and epigenetic alterations contribute to the leukemic transformation of hematopoietic cells

Figure 12.11. Initial diagnostic tests are crucial in the assessment of chronic leukemias, particularly in distinguishing between various subtypes such as chronic myeloid leukemia (CML)

Figure 12.12. Bone marrow biopsy procedures are critical in the diagnosis and evaluation of chronic leukemias, providing necessary insights into the hematological landscape of affected patients

Figure 12.13. Molecular testing and genetic profiling have revolutionized the landscape of chronic leukemias, particularly in their diagnosis, treatment, and monitoring

Figure 12.14. Effective monitoring of disease progression in chronic leukemias is crucial for optimizing patient outcomes and tailoring therapeutic interventions

Figure 12.15. The early detection of chronic leukemias plays a crucial role in patient prognosis and treatment efficacy

Figure 12.16. The cornerstone of CML treatment involves the use of tyrosine kinase inhibitors (TKIs), such as imatinib, which directly inhibit the activity of the BCR-ABL fusion protein that drives the disease pathology

Figure 12.17. The development of targeted therapies has revolutionized the treatment landscape for chronic leukemias, particularly chronic myeloid leukemia (CML) and chronic lymphocytic leukemia (CLL)

Figure 12.18. As a pivotal therapeutic intervention for chronic leukemias, stem cell transplantation offers a potential cure by replenishing the hematopoietic system and enabling the eradication of malignancies

Figure 12.19. Clinical trials and emerging therapies for chronic leukemias

Figure 12.20. Effective patient education and involvement are critical components in managing chronic leukemias, as they empower patients to participate in their care actively

Figure 13.1. Lymphomas primarily originate in the lymphatic system, a vital component of the immune system responsible for combating infections

Figure 13.2. Hodgkin lymphoma classification

Figure 13.3. Burkitt lymphoma

Figure 13.4. Diffuse large B-cell lymphoma (DLBCL)

Figure 13.5. Peripheral T-cell lymphoma (PTCL) represents a diverse category of non-Hodgkin lymphomas that arise from mature T-cells, often exhibiting aggressive clinical behavior and a poor prognosis

Figure 13.6. Primary mediastinal B-cell lymphoma (PMBCL)

Figure 13.7. B-cell lymphoma

Figure 13.8. Epstein-Barr virus (EBV)

Figure 13.9. Age and gender are critical factors in understanding the epidemiology and prognosis of lymphomas

Figure 13.10. Occupational exposures play a significant role in the etiology of lymphomas, as specific industries and work environments present increased risk factors for these malignancies

Figure 13.11. Mechanism of action of mosunetuzumab

Figure 13.12. In cases where lymphomas are suspected, diagnostic techniques such as flow cytometry can provide crucial insights, mainly when atypical cells are observed in blood or effusions

Figure 13.13. Fine-needle aspiration (FNA) biopsy has emerged as a critical method, particularly for evaluating lymphadenopathy, enabling pathologists to obtain cellular material with minimal invasiveness

Figure 13.14. The staging systems

Figure 13.15. Pathologists play an indispensable role in the diagnosis and management of lymphomas

Figure 13.16. The diagnosis of lymphomas presents numerous challenges that significantly impact patient outcomes and treatment approaches

Figure 13.17. Chemotherapy regimens are critical in the management of lymphomas, serving as the cornerstone of treatment for both Hodgkin and non-Hodgkin lymphoma

Figure 13.18. Recent advancements have revealed specific targets, such as the CCR4 receptor, which is crucial in cutaneous T-cell lymphoma (CTCL) due to its role in tumor immune evasion

Figure 13.19. Stem cell transplantation has emerged as a pivotal strategy in the management of lymphomas, particularly for patients facing relapsed or refractory disease

Figure 13.20. Palliative care approaches play a critical role in improving the quality of life for patients, particularly when curative treatments have been exhausted or deemed inappropriate

Figure 13.21. The management of lymphomas necessitates a comprehensive approach, which is where multidisciplinary teams (MDTs) play a vital role

Figure 14.1. Plasma cell dyscrasias

Figure 14.2. Multiple myeloma (MM)

Figure 14.3. Waldenström Macroglobulinemia (WM)

Figure 14.4. Light Chain Deposition Disease (LCDD) represents a significant manifestation of plasma cell dyscrasias, characterized by the abnormal accumulation of light chains produced by malignant plasma cells, primarily impacting renal function

Figure 14.5. Solitary plasmacytoma

Figure 14.6. Plasma cells, derived from B lymphocytes, play a pivotal role in the adaptive immune response by producing high-affinity antibodies specific to antigens

Figure 14.7. The characterization of non-coding RNAs within this ecosystem has unveiled new mechanisms of gene expression regulation that significantly contribute to the aberrant behavior of plasma cells, thus highlighting potential therapeutic targets

Figure 14.8. The phenomenon of immune dysregulation plays a crucial role in the pathogenesis of plasma cell dyscrasias, particularly as it relates to multiple myeloma (MM)

Figure 14.9. The tumor microenvironment (TME) plays a crucial role in the progression and treatment resistance of plasma cell dyscrasias, particularly multiple myeloma (MM)

Figure 14.10. Understanding the pathophysiology of plasma cell dyscrasias, particularly multiple myeloma, is crucial for developing effective treatment strategies

Figure 14.11. Laboratory tests, such as serum protein electrophoresis and immunofixation, are essential in identifying the presence of monoclonal proteins indicative of plasma cell disorders

Figure 14.12. Serum-free light chains (FLC)

Figure 14.13. Trephine biopsy

Figure 14.14. Venetoclax

Figure 14.15: The International Staging System (ISS) remains a cornerstone, stratifying multiple myeloma patients based on serum albumin and beta-2 microglobulin levels, thus providing crucial insights into overall survival outcomes

Figure 14.16. The treatment landscape for plasma cell dyscrasias has evolved significantly, particularly concerning chemotherapy regimens

Figure 14.17. Daratumumab

Figure 14.18. Effective supportive care and symptom management are crucial components in the treatment of plasma cell dyscrasias, particularly as patients often experience complex symptomatology

Figure 14.19. Long-term management strategies for plasma cell dyscrasias are critical in optimizing patient outcomes and enhancing quality of life

Figure 15.1. Transfusion medicine serves as a critical cornerstone within the healthcare system, particularly in the context of BMT

Figure 15.2. Indications for blood transfusion typically encompass severe anemia, significant blood loss from trauma or surgery, and specific hematological disorders, most notably thalassemia and sickle cell disease

Figure 15.3. Transfusions, while often life-saving, are not without inherent risks and complications that can arise during or after the procedure

Figure 15.4. The evolution of blood preservation techniques has significantly impacted the efficiency and safety of transfusion medicine and bone marrow transplantation

Figure 15.5. The regulations governing transfusion practices are pivotal for ensuring patient safety, particularly in the context of bone marrow transplantation, where immunocompromised patients face heightened risks

Figure 15.6. The anatomy of bone marrow plays a crucial role in understanding its function within the framework of transfusion medicine and bone marrow transplantation

Figure 15.7. Within the complex hierarchy of blood cell production, bone marrow plays an indispensable role in hematopoiesis, the process through which all blood components, including RBCs, white blood cells, and platelets, are generated

Figure 15.8. The health of bone marrow is critically significant, as it is the site of hematopoiesis—the process of blood cell formation

Figure 15.9. The bone marrow microenvironment plays a critical role in hematopoiesis, influencing the development and function of various blood cell lineages essential for maintaining systemic homeostasis

Figure 15.10. Bone marrow transplants, a critical therapeutic intervention in transfusion medicine, are classified into two primary types: autologous and allogeneic

Figure 15.11. The transplant procedure represents a critical aspect of modern medical practice, particularly in the context of transfusion medicine and bone marrow transplantation

Figure 15.12. Common complications such as infections, graft-versus-host disease (GVHD), and transplant rejection pose significant risks that require vigilant monitoring and timely interventions

Figure 15.13. One of the significant concerns post-transplantation is the management of thrombocytopenia, particularly in patients with hematological malignancies

Figure 15.14. Blood components, including red blood cells, platelets, and plasma, are critical during perioperative management to address issues such as anemia, coagulopathy, and thrombocytopenia, which patients may experience due to underlying conditions or surgical interventions

Figure 15.15. Repeated blood transfusions, while often necessary for managing severe anemia, can lead to complications that adversely affect transplant survival rates

Figure 15.16. Techniques like adoptive T cell transfer (ACT) have been introduced in transfusion medicine, expanding possibilities for treatment in oncology and autoimmune conditions

Figure 15.17. Ivosidenib

Figure 15.18. The education and training of healthcare professionals are critical components in ensuring optimal outcomes in transfusion medicine and bone marrow transplantation

PREFACE

Hematologic disease refers to various illnesses that can alter the cells and plasma in blood, and these changes can affect nearly all the body's organs. The failure of the body's complex process for blood cell formation, function, or removal results in diseases that can range from mild fatigue to severe emergencies. It is necessary to understand blood formation and circulation to appreciate how various abnormalities in this process result in a wide range of clinical symptoms. From the development of bone marrow stem cells to the relationship between coagulation factors and leukocytes, the emergence of blood disorders reveals the beauty and weaknesses of the circulatory system.

Blood not only provides oxygen, nutrients, and removes waste from the body but also acts as a strong defender against harmful infections and injuries. When red blood cells cannot deliver enough oxygen, patients may feel weak and pale. With weakened white blood cells, the body's defenses are no longer effective. If platelets or clotting proteins are not functioning correctly, patients may experience bleeding or clotting problems. Every disease class, such as anemia, leukocyte abnormality, platelet disorder, or coagulation imbalance, requires different diagnostic and treatment approaches. With the aid of molecular diagnostics, immunophenotyping, and targeted therapies, we can now diagnose and treat various diseases in ways that were previously impossible.

The textbook *"Hematological Disorders"* provides a clear outline of the causes, types, diagnosis, and management of blood diseases. The purpose is to support practitioners and help students of hematology, internal medicine, and similar disciplines learn. By using scientific evidence and practical tips, this book aims to bridge the gap between science and patient care.

Chapter 1 describes hematology and hematopoiesis, illustrating how stem cells are differentiated and the factors that guide them to become various types of blood cells. Chapter 2 discusses anemias, categorizing them by main categories, providing a summary of common symptoms, and outlining the laboratory tests used to identify them. Chapter 3 describes iron deficiency and sideroblastic anemia, examining how iron is absorbed, utilized, and how pathological ring sideroblasts develop in the latter disorder.

In Chapter 4, the author explains hemolytic anemias, highlighting the differences between immune and non-immune causes, and describes how membrane defects, enzyme deficiencies, and mechanical trauma can lead to red cell destruction. The fifth chapter deals with hemoglobinopathies and thalassemias, explaining the genetic reasons for abnormal hemoglobin and chain synthesis, and discussing both current treatment and genetic counseling.

Chapter 6 explains megaloblastic and aplastic anemias, pointing out that errors or problems in DNA synthesis or bone marrow can halt the production of red blood cells. It also discusses the clinical role of vitamin B_{12}, folate, and marrow cellularity.

Chapter 7 covers problems related to leukocytes, starting with a lack of white blood cells in neutropenia and ending with an excess in leukocytosis. It emphasizes infectious, autoimmune, and neoplastic causes. Chapter 8 discusses platelet disorders, low blood platelet counts, and issues with their function, and explains the use of platelet aggregation studies for diagnosis.

Chapter 9 deals with coagulation disorders and describes the clotting cascade, standard tests for coagulation, and how to manage hemophilia and von Willebrand disease. Chapter 10 addresses thrombotic disorders, outlining the causes of these conditions and detailing treatment and prevention strategies.

Chapter 11 explains acute leukemias and explains how immunophenotyping, cytogenetics, and molecular markers are used to distinguish between acute myeloid leukemia and acute lymphoblastic leukemia. Chapter 12 explains that chronic lymphocytic leukemia grows slowly and is less aggressive than chronic myeloid leukemia, which has a varied outcome.

Chapter 13 describes lymphomas, including both Hodgkin and non-Hodgkin types, their staging, and the use of immunotherapy as a new treatment approach. Chapter 14 addresses plasma cell dyscrasias, ranging from monoclonal gammopathy of undetermined significance to multiple myeloma, and explains the primary methods for diagnosing, stratifying risk, and utilizing new drugs that target survival pathways in plasma cells.

The last chapter, Chapter 15, focuses on bone marrow and transfusion medicine, covering donor selection, various types of therapy, potential transfusion reactions, graft-versus-host disease, and post-transplant issues for patients.

In the book, real-life case examples and informative graphics help explain important concepts and illustrate where decisions should be made in everyday situations. Important details about diagnoses, various conditions, and treatments are presented in tables, and each chapter concludes with a summary for quick reference and to aid in learning.

This text will be helpful for hematology fellows, internal medicine residents, medical students, nurse practitioners, and physician assistants who wish to learn about blood disorders in a structured and organized manner. Practicing hematologists, oncologists, laboratory directors, and transfusion medicine specialists will find a single resource to learn about the latest best practices.

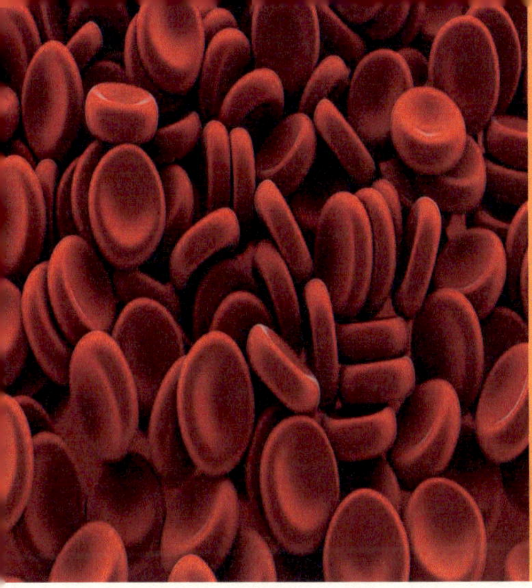

Chapter 1

INTRODUCTION TO HEMATOLOGY AND HEMATOPOIESIS

Contents

Introduction........1

1.1. Blood Composition........2

1.2. Hematopoiesis........6

1.3. Hematological Disorders........11

1.4. Diagnostic Techniques in Hematology........16

Summary........22

References........23

Introduction

Hematology encompasses the study of blood, blood-producing organs, and hematological diseases as a key field of study in medical science. Hematology not only addresses the structure and function of blood but also the intricate processes of hematopoiesis, which is the formation of blood cells. It is essential to know about hematopoiesis since it involves hematopoietic stem cells (HSCs) responsible for the life-long production of blood cells and maintaining normal physiological conditions. Abnormalities in this process will lead to various disorders, like leukemia, that critically affect patient health, particularly in populations that are aging, since the risk of hematological malignancies increases immensely (Winik et al., 2020). Additionally, the niche in which HSCs operate, referred to as the bone marrow niche, plays a crucial role in regulating these cells and their interactions, thereby playing a pivotal role in both healthy and leukemic hematopoiesis (Dolinska et al., 2019).

1.1. Blood Composition

Understanding the composition of blood lies at the heart of hematology and hematopoiesis, as the cellular and biochemical constituents of the blood have crucial functions in maintaining physiological homeostasis. Blood is comprised predominantly of plasma, which constitutes approximately 55% of its volume, and formed elements, including red cells, white cells, and platelets. Red blood cells, or erythrocytes, carry oxygen, while leukocytes play a role in immunity. Additionally, the significance of adequate blood composition is reflected in studies on the effect of nutritional deficiency on hematologic parameters. For instance, maternal subnutrition during pregnancy has been reported to negatively impact the hematologic health of the offspring, suggesting a link between nutrition and hematopoiesis (Almaguer et al., 2019). Furthermore, genetic factors can also affect the blood composition, for instance, in congenital sideroblastic anemias (CSAs) caused by mutations related to the metabolism of iron and hemoglobinization (Crispin et al., 2017) (Figure 1.1).

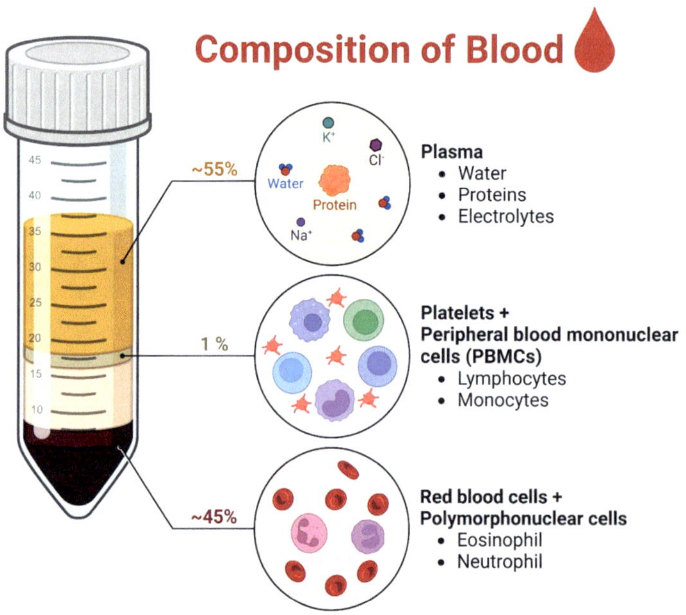

Figure 1.1. Blood is primarily composed of plasma, which accounts for about 55% of its volume, and formed elements, including red blood cells, white blood cells, and platelets.

Source: https://microbenotes.com/wp-content/uploads/2023/04/Composition-of-Blood.jpg.

1.1.1. Components of Blood

Blood is an evolved fluid composed of numerous essential elements that collectively perform crucial physiological functions. The major components include red blood cells (erythrocytes), which deliver oxygen; white blood cells (leukocytes), an integral part of the immune system; and platelets (thrombocytes), required for blood coagulation. Additionally, plasma, the liquid extracellular environment, is comprised of water, electrolytes, nutrients, and proteins essential in maintaining osmotic balance and cell-to-cell communication. The hematopoietic process of generating these components by pluripotent cells in the bone marrow is behind the continuous replacement of these components. The failure of any of these cellular components, as seen in CSAs, serves as a reminder of the integrated nature of the relationship between blood components and overall health. Research indicates that mutations affecting hematopoiesis may result in pathologies characterized by the atrophy of hematopoietic tissue and the production of abnormal blood, underscoring the importance of research on blood components in medical science (Frisch et al., 1987; Crispin et al., 2017) (Figure 1.2).

1.1.2. Functions of Red Blood Cells (RBCs)

The primary role of red blood cells (RBCs), also known as erythrocytes, is to transport oxygen from the lungs to the tissues and return carbon dioxide from the tissues to the lungs for exhalation.

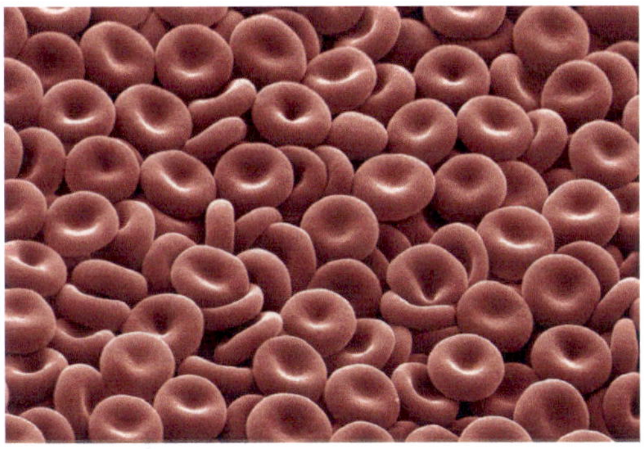

Figure 1.2. The primary function of red blood cells (RBCs), also known as erythrocytes, is to transport oxygen from the lungs to the tissues and return carbon dioxide from the tissues back to the lungs for exhalation.

Source: https://www.thoughtco.com/thmb/RIWieAd8xKjbo9yOHkrrovfKkhQ=/1500x0/filters:no_upscale():max_bytes(150000):strip_icc()/red_blood_cells_1-57b20c583df78cd39c2f8e15.jpg.

This is made possible through hemoglobin, a protein complex that efficiently incorporates oxygen molecules. Besides oxygen transport, RBCs also contribute to maintaining the acid-base balance in blood, thereby playing a role in homeostasis. Stress, aging, and environmental factors can significantly impact RBC mass. For instance, research has revealed that decreases in RBC mass were observed following sustained microgravity exposure, with astronauts losing 10 to 15% of their red cell mass during space missions lasting weeks, which take weeks to recover from upon completion of the flight. It is essential to know these functions and limitations if hematological understanding and therapies are to be developed for numerous medical illnesses (Li et al., 2018).

1.1.3. Role of White Blood Cells (WBCs)

The role of white blood cells (WBCs), also known as leukocytes, is indispensable in the body's immune defense mechanism and response to infection, underscoring their importance in hematology and hematopoiesis. These multifunctional cell types, including lymphocytes, neutrophils, monocytes, eosinophils, and basophils, work together as a high-level defense mechanism against infection and foreign matter. Lymphocytes, particularly T and B cells, are key players in adaptive immunity, affecting pathogen-specific targeting, while neutrophils are innate immunity's first line of defense that rapidly phagocytose and kill entering microbes. Recent studies continue to elucidate the intricate regulatory networks governing WBC development and function, highlighting their importance in immune competence and disease pathogenesis. Notably, genetic research into the pathophysiology of such diseases as leukemias and neutropenia brings to the forefront the significant contributions WBCs make towards disease and health, a testament to their central place in hematologic studies (Erik et al., 2019; Naldini et al., 2022).

1.1.4. Importance of Platelets

In hematology, platelets are recognized as more than simply playing their widely valued role in hemostasis; they are key players in a variety of physiological and pathological processes. Platelets, or thrombocytes, are cytoplasmic fragments of megakaryocytes in the bone marrow and are essentially responsible for blood clotting, which prevents excessive blood loss when there is a vascular injury. However, their function is not limited to coagulation but is also involved in inflammation, wound healing, and tumor metastasis. The European Hematology Association Roadmap prioritizes platelet disorders as a critical area of research, emphasizing the need for targeted therapies in managing these disorders (Allard et al., 2016). It is essential to understand the multifunctionality of platelets in disease and health, as advancements in this area can lead to more effective diagnostic and therapeutic strategies tailored to specific diseases, such as thrombocytopathies and related blood disorders (Allard et al., 2016).

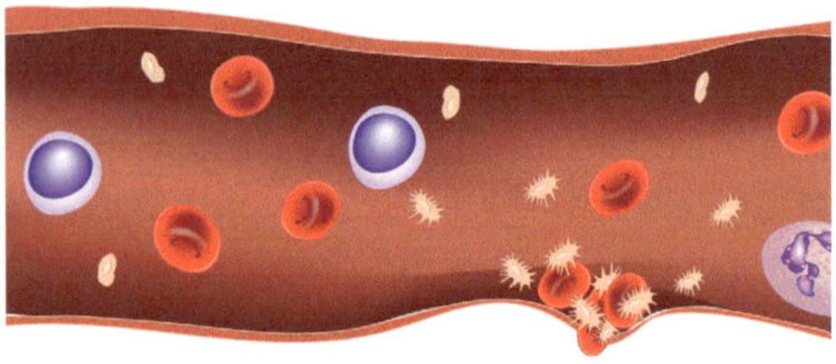

Figure 1.3. Platelets, or thrombocytes, are cellular fragments derived from megakaryocytes in the bone marrow and are primarily responsible for blood clotting, preventing excessive bleeding following vascular injury.

Source: https://myhematology.com/wp-content/uploads/2023/12/Primary-hemostasis.jpg.

1.1.5. Plasma Composition and Functions

The plasma, which accounts for approximately 55% of blood volume, plays a vital role in the body's homeostasis. It is not just a solvent; it is also a medium for transporting proteins, hormones, and waste materials. Plasma contains mostly water, electrolytes, proteins, and other solutes, the most common of which is albumin, responsible for maintaining osmotic pressure and transporting various molecules. Plasma also contains fibrinogen, a component essential for blood coagulation, and immunoglobulins, which play a crucial role in immune defense. Dynamic plasma content can control hematopoiesis, particularly the balance of bone marrow mesenchymal stem cells (BMSCs), maintaining the hematopoietic niche and regulating differentiation of HSCs (Li et al., 2018). Understanding these complexities is crucial, particularly when considering the context of plasma composition in relation to bone marrow transplantation (BMT) recovery (Chaviano et al., 2017).

1.1.6. Blood Volume and Its Regulation

Among the most significant roles of hematology is regulating blood volume, which is necessary to maintain homeostasis and optimize physiological function. Erythropoiesis, i.e., the generation of RBCs, primarily regulates blood volume through various hormonal and renal mechanisms. HSCs play an essential role in this process, as they become erythrocytes responsible for transporting oxygen throughout the body and therefore influencing blood volume and viscosity. Variations in blood volume can lead to severe medical conditions, such as anemia or polycythemia. Current research suggests that signaling pathways, such as those regulated by the cAMP-responsive element binding protein (CREB), are essential for the regulation of myelopoiesis and cell proliferation of the HSC, indicating sophisticated interactions among cellular events and control of systemic blood volume (Akashi et al., 2008). Additionally, iron metabolism disorders, such as those seen in CSAs, highlight the importance of effective blood control for optimal hematopoiesis (Crispin et al., 2017) (Figure 1.4).

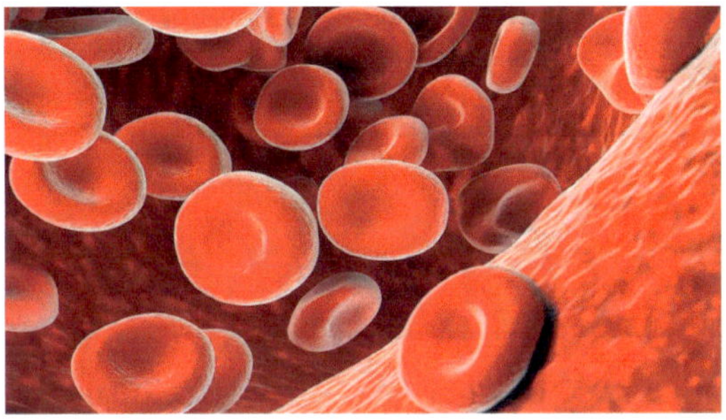

Figure 1.4. Blood volume is intricately managed through various hormonal and renal mechanisms, primarily involving erythropoiesis, which is the process of red blood cell production.

Source: https://myhematology.com/wp-content/uploads/2023/11/RBC-flowing-in-a-vein.jpg.

1.1.7. Hemoglobin and Oxygen Transport

The intricate role of hemoglobin in carrying oxygen underscores its importance in the field of hematology. Hemoglobin is a tetrameric protein consisting of four subunits that capture oxygen in the lungs and release it to tissues to facilitate cellular respiration. Not only essential to sustain cellular metabolism, but this oxygen-carrying process is responsive to various physiological conditions, including those of spaceflight. Research has indicated that astronauts experience a significant reduction in the mass of RBCs, averaging 10 to 15%, which can complicate oxygen delivery when they return to Earth's gravitational field. Furthermore, genetic mutations in hemoglobin synthesis, including those in CSA, cause impaired iron homeostasis and defective production of RBCs, resulting in clinical symptoms of anemia (Crispin et al., 2017). Therefore, knowledge of hemoglobin's function guides both physiological responses and pathophysiological states that influence oxygen transport.

1.1.8. Blood Types and Compatibility

In hematology, it is crucial to have knowledge of blood types and their compatibility, particularly when performing transfusions and organ transplants. Blood types are classified primarily based on the presence or absence of specific antigens on the surface of RBCs, with the ABO and Rh systems being the most significant. Incompatible blood transfusion can lead to severe immune reactions, hemolytic reactions being one of them that could be lethal. With ongoing research, new techniques such as direct cell reprogramming to induced pluripotent stem cells (iPSCs) are proving to be increasingly hopeful in tailored medicine and hematological therapies (Cascino et al., 2017). Further, diseases like Acute Myeloid Leukemia (AML) necessitate careful evaluation of compatibility between blood types since such has a direct role in the determination of treatment progress and recovery of patients; therefore, awareness of these forces is imperative for ensuring optimal care for affected populations (Blanco et al., 2009) (Figure 1.5).

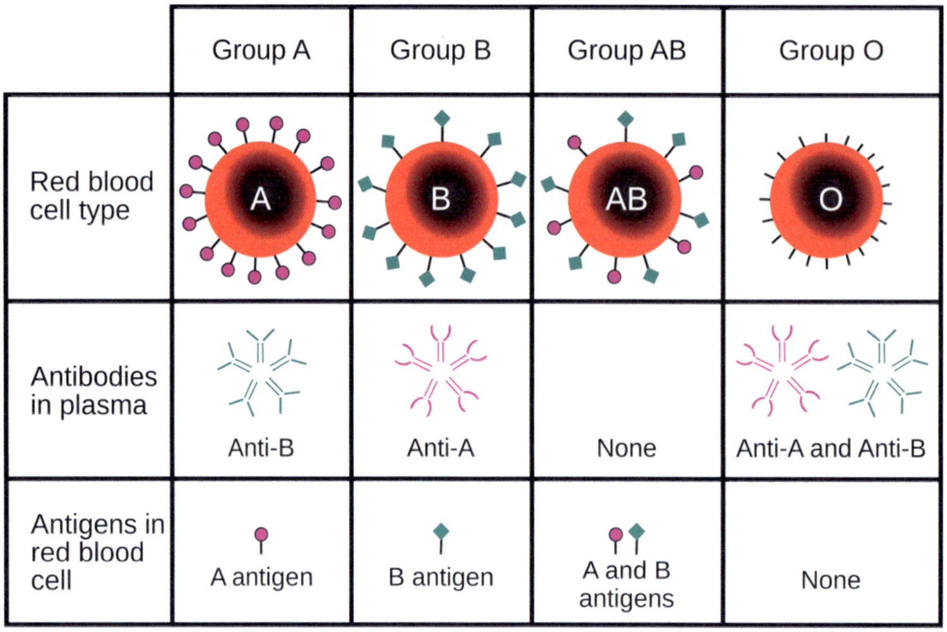

Figure 1.5. Blood types are classified primarily by the presence or absence of specific antigens on the surface of red blood cells, with the ABO and Rh systems being the most significant.

Source: https://upload.wikimedia.org/wikipedia/commons/thumb/3/32/ABO_blood_type.svg/1200px-ABO_blood_type.svg.png.

1.1.9. Disorders Related to Blood Composition

Disorders of blood composition pose a significant challenge in hematology, affecting both immune function and oxygen transport. Some of the disorders like CSA are due to defects in heme biosynthesis and iron-sulfur cluster assembly and result in pathologic iron accumulation within bone marrow erythroblasts. Recent studies have uncovered mutations in genes like HSCB as being central to the identification of such diseases; in particular, HSCB mutations lead to diminished protein expression and profound hematopoietic defects in model organisms, mirroring clinical observations noted in CSA patients (Crispin et al., 2017). Aside from anemia, other hematological disorders derived from blood cells, including rare tumors related to the composition of blood, illustrate the intricacy of blood-cell-derived cancers. These rare cancers are not appropriately addressed in clinical practice but account for a high percentage of cancer diagnoses and require concerted treatment standards as well as collaborative studies to improve patient outcomes (Chaviano et al., 2017).

1.2. Hematopoiesis

Hematopoiesis, the process of blood cell development, occurs predominantly in the bone marrow and is controlled by a complex interplay of intrinsic and extrinsic regulators. BMSCs, in addition to HSCs, which give rise to various lineages of blood cells, also play a pivotal role in creating the supportive microenvironments necessary for hematopoiesis. BMSC differentiation into stromal cells is responsible for the majority of hematopoietic niches that maintain HSCs and, hence, control their proliferation and fate decisions (Li et al., 2018). Current studies indicate that genetic alterations, such as those in CSAs, can disrupt this balance, leading to impaired hematopoiesis. For instance, protein mutations necessary for heme synthesis can result in defects in hematologic function, such as the HSCB variants that have a marked influence on erythropoiesis (Crispin et al., 2017). Thus, awareness of such dynamics informs about the complex regulation of blood cell development.

1.2.1. Definition and Process of Hematopoiesis

Hematopoiesis, the process responsible for generating all blood cells, is a crucial part of human physiology that ensures the continuous production of erythrocytes, leukocytes, and thrombocytes to maintain homeostasis. Hematopoiesis occurs predominantly in the bone marrow, where pluripotent HSCs differentiate into various progenitor cells, which ultimately lead to mature blood cells. The regulation of hematopoiesis is complex signaling networks and transcription factors that are sensitive to physiological demand, e.g., erythrocyte-stimulated production following extensive loss of blood or hypoxia. Significantly, derangements of hematopoiesis can lead to diseases such as myelodysplastic syndromes (MDS), which are defined by dyscrasias of hematopoiesis and associated cytopenias that typically require transfusion to manage anemia (Rydén et al., 2021). Furthermore, hematopoietic function can be influenced by outside factors, as evidenced by the temporary reduction of RBC mass in astronauts following space travel (Figure 1.6).

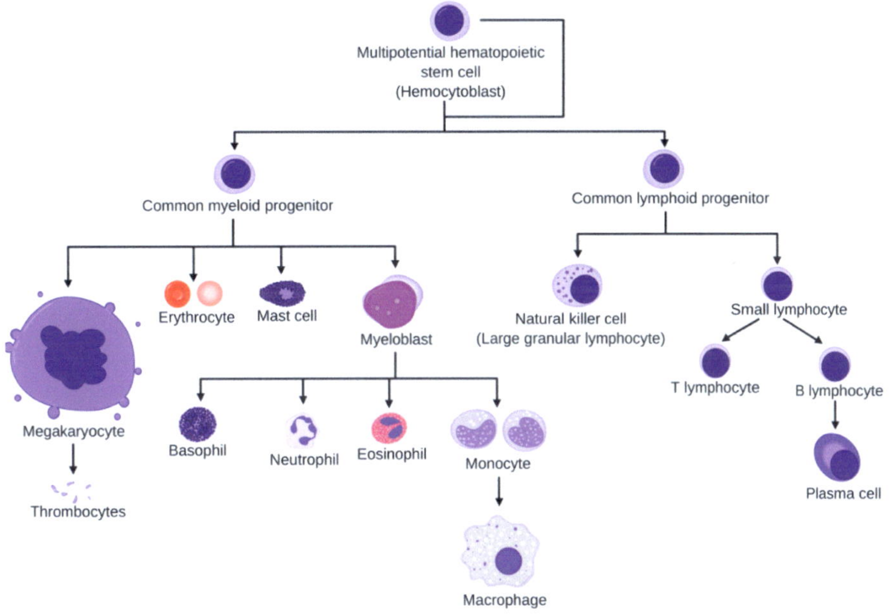

Figure 1.6. Hematopoiesis.

Source: https://upload.wikimedia.org/wikipedia/commons/thumb/f/f0/Hematopoiesis_simple.svg/1200px-Hematopoiesis_simple.svg.png.

1.2.2. Sites of Hematopoiesis in the Body

Hematopoiesis, or the formation of blood cells, is a process that occurs in distinct areas of the body, varying from infancy through adulthood. In early life, hematopoiesis is largely fetal and occurs in the yolk sac, eventually being succeeded by the liver and spleen, which are essential organs for blood cell production until birth. Postnatally, the bone marrow is the primary site of hematopoiesis, a process that remains active in adulthood. Interestingly, while the bone marrow cannot do without, organs like the spleen assist in hematological processes, like sequestration of faulty erythrocytes, as suggested by evidence pointing toward a participative role of the reactive state of the reticuloendothelial system (RES) of liver and spleen in the pathogenesis of hematological disorders (Hasegawa et al., 1969). Additionally, presence of reticulonodular patterns in the spleen indicates involvement and may be interpreted to signify normal variations because of age and lymphoid development (Capps et al., 2024). Descriptions of these locations provide us with further knowledge on hematological disease and health.

1.2.3. Stages of Hematopoietic Development

The hematopoietic complexity arises through a series of well-defined steps required for blood cell production. From the embryonic yolk sac, hematopoiesis develops into the fetal liver and then into the bone marrow, establishing a clear chronology that corresponds to spatial and temporal regulation. This progression is tightly controlled by various transcription factors and gene signaling pathways, including the highly important microRNAs controlling B cell maturation and function. Experiments have determined that some of the miRNAs play crucial roles in normal bone marrow B cell development and are significantly involved in their activation and terminal differentiation in the periphery (Fernando et al., 2012). Additionally, genetic disorders during these developmental stages may lead to diseases such as CSA, which constitute disruptions in hematopoiesis and iron metabolism, highlighting the significance of precise molecular interactions in hematopoietic development (Crispin et al., 2017) (Figure 1.7).

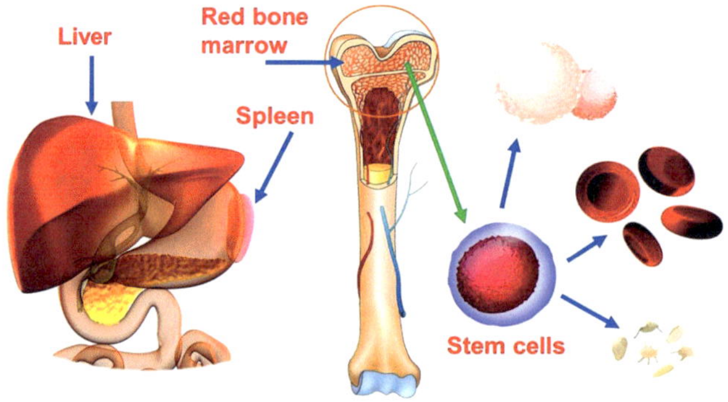

Figure 1.7. Initiating in the embryonic yolk sac, hematopoiesis transitions to the fetal liver and eventually to the bone marrow, delineating a clear timeline that reflects both spatial and temporal regulation.

Source: https://interactivebiology.com/wp-content/uploads/2022/01/sites-of-blood-formation.jpg.

1.2.4. Role of Stem Cells in Hematopoiesis

The role of stem cells in hematopoiesis is also significant as they are the precursors from which all blood cells develop. HSCs are characterized by their ability to self-renew and differentiate into various blood cell lineages, including erythrocytes, leukocytes, and platelets. Recent studies highlight the function of transcription factors, such as CREB, in regulating HSC function. Increased expression of CREB has been implicated in myeloid leukemia, wherein it sustains cell proliferation in both stem cells and leukemia cells, establishing evidence that controlling this may offer therapeutic potential for preventing malignant transformations (Akashi et al., 2008). Genetic mutations that affect processes in hematopoietic cells can also lead to diseases such as CSAs, exhibiting the complex interaction between hematological diseases and stem cell biology. Research also highlights the irreversibility of determinants such as HSCB in maintaining normal hematopoiesis, underscoring the central role of stem cells in maintaining blood homeostasis (Crispin et al., 2017).

1.2.5. Regulation of Hematopoiesis

Regulation of hematopoiesis, the complex process of blood cell generation, is based on a complex interaction of genetic and environmental signals. The transcription factor CREB is integral to the proliferation and differentiation of HSCs. Higher levels of CREB have been linked to myeloid leukemias and have demonstrated its critical role in normal and tumor hematopoiesis; studies have determined that CREB knockdown in HSCs leads to decreased proliferation and cell-cycle pathology, as evidenced by diminished committed progenitor populations in mouse models (Akashi et al., 2008). Secondly, gene mutations in genes such as HSCB also disrupt fundamental pathways of iron homeostasis and erythropoiesis, which contribute to CSAs and highlight the intricacy of hematopoiesis control (Crispin et al., 2017). Overall, all these discoveries, put together, emphasize the importance of transcriptional regulation and genetic integrity in maintaining hematopoietic balance and preventing hematologic disorders (Figure 1.8).

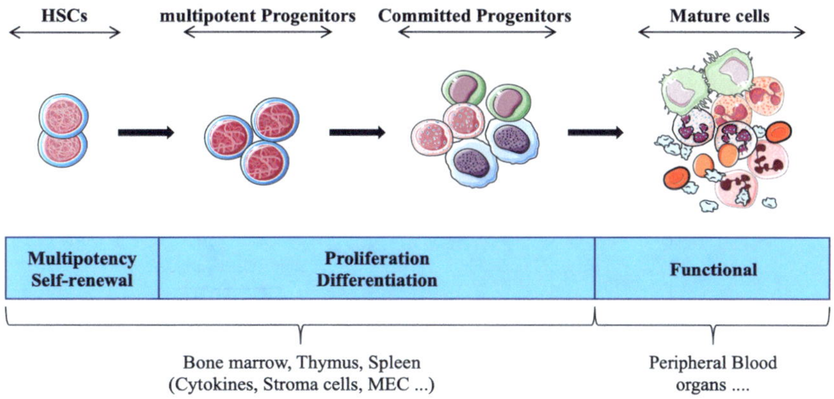

Figure 1.8. The regulation of hematopoiesis, the complex process of blood cell formation, relies on a sophisticated interplay of genetic and environmental factors.

Source: https://images-provider.frontiersin.org/api/ipx/w=1200&f=png/https://www.frontiersin.org/files/Articles/1151343/fonc-13-1151343-HTML/image_m/fonc-13-1151343-g001.jpg.

1.2.6. Factors Influencing Hematopoiesis

The intricate hematopoiesis process is orchestrated by a complex network of factors that regulate HSC development and differentiation. The role of BMSCs is among the most important factors contributing to the formation of essential hematopoietic niches that nurture HSCs. The differentiation of BMSCs is important; alterations in their lineage of differentiation can have a dramatic impact on hematopoiesis, particularly under situations such as aging or chemotherapy, which can bias their differentiation and hinder recovery after BMT (Li et al., 2018). The epigenetic profile also plays a vital role in impacting hematopoietic outcomes. Above all, iPSCs possess an epigenetic memory derived from their tissue of origin, which affects their differentiation capability. These characteristics demonstrate the need for a balanced microenvironment and suggest that knowledge of this is imperative to proceed with therapeutic strategies in hematology (Aryee et al., 2010).

1.2.7. Hematopoietic Growth Factors

In the complex processes of hematopoiesis, the hematopoietic growth factors are a pivotal element in regulating the growth, differentiation, and survival of HSCs. These factors, like erythropoietin, thrombopoietin, and the colony-stimulating factors, ensure the efficacy of the microenvironment of the bone marrow, thereby ensuring the production of blood cell lineages. Interestingly, alterations of the signaling pathways regulated by these growth factors may lead to hematological disorders, including leukemias, in which CREB plays a crucial role. CREB is found to be extensively expressed in lineage-negative HSCs, and its inhibition causes decreased proliferation and cell-cycle aberrations in HSCs and myeloid leukemia cells (Akashi et al., 2008). Furthermore, the equilibrium of BMSCs differentiation is crucial for optimal hematopoiesis and significantly impacts recovery after bone marrow transplant (Li et al., 2018). Hence, understanding of such growth factors comes into play when designing therapeutic mechanisms for hematological therapies (Figure 1.9).

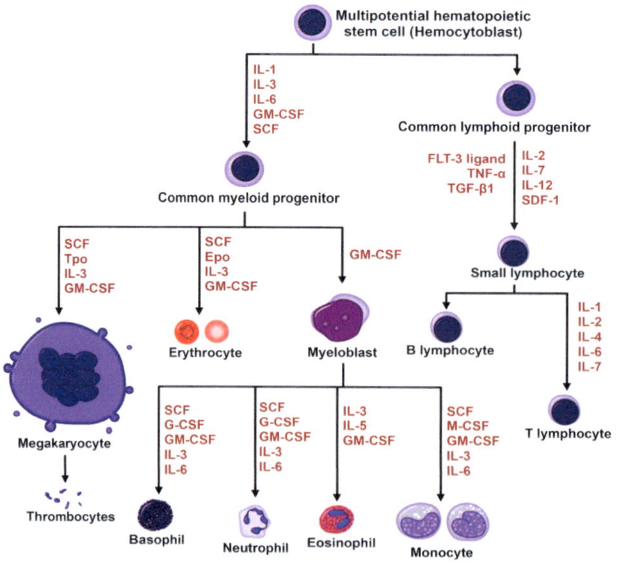

Figure 1.9. Hematopoietic growth factors play a pivotal role in regulating the proliferation, differentiation, and survival of hematopoietic stem cells (HSCs).

Source: https://upload.wikimedia.org/wikipedia/commons/thumb/a/a1/Hematopoietic_growth_factors.png/1200px-Hematopoietic_growth_factors.png.

1.2.8. Disorders of Hematopoiesis

Hematopoietic disorders comprise a range of diseases impacting the development and function of blood cells with a severe clinical presentation. Gaucher disease (GD) is one condition where the accumulation of glucocerebrosidase in macrophages leads to cytopenias and hepatosplenomegaly, which can initially mimic primary myelofibrosis (PMF) due to overlapping clinical presentations (Cardarelli et al., 2018). Similarly, CSA are caused by mutations in the genes controlling heme biosynthesis and mitochondrial function to lead to aberrant iron deposits and impaired erythropoiesis (Crispin et al., 2017). The severity of such disorders effectively highlights the intricacy involved in hematopoietic regulation, as well as the need for careful diagnostic methodology. Misdiagnosis could result in inefficient treatment programs, further accentuating the importance of understanding these disorders within the context of hematological research. Lastly, advancements in hematopoiesis are critical in improving patient outcomes with targeted interventions and therapies.

1.2.9. Advances in Hematopoietic Research

Key advances in hematopoietic research have revolutionized the treatment models of hematological diseases, primarily by way of introducing allogeneic hematopoietic stem cell transplantation (HSCT). A curative treatment regimen, wherein stem cells are transfused from various sources—mobilized peripheral blood, bone marrow, and umbilical cord blood—has emerged as the standard for patients without an HLA-identical sibling donor. Interestingly enough, the development of fully comprehensive cord blood banks and donor registries has greatly enhanced donor availability and consequently patient outcomes for diverse patient populations. However, as much promise as HSCT holds, it poses challenges, particularly on the clinical and ethical fronts in terms of donor safety and informed consent (Russa et al., 2017). Additionally, it has been demonstrated that the patients with a history of invasive fungal infections prior to pre-transplantation have lower progression-free survival as well as overall survival significantly, indicating the intricacy of pre-transplant status (Aljurf et al., 2017) (Figure 1.10).

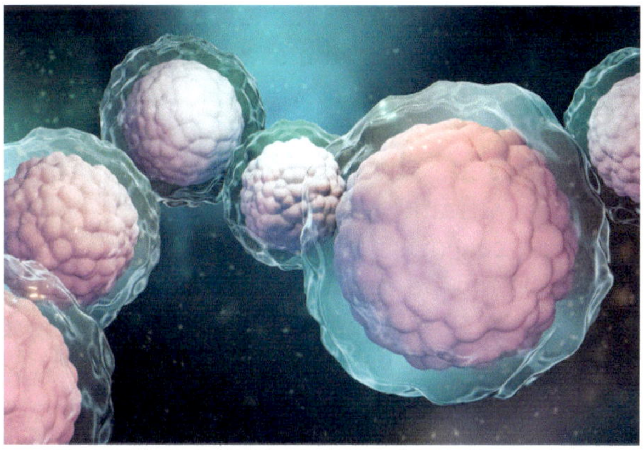

Figure 1.10. Development of allogeneic hematopoietic stem cell transplantation (HSCT).

Source: https://vertassets.blob.core.windows.net/image/e5f842ff/e5f842ff-8258-416d-aaa5-7e3ffb4b442b/istock_1218436078.jpg.

1.3. Hematological Disorders

Pathophysiology of hematological disorders is a multistep interplay between environmental and genetic factors impinging on the normal process of blood cell production and function. CSA is an example where the underlying genetic etiology of such disorders can be demonstrated, as gene mutations for heme biosynthesis result in abnormal iron deposition in erythroblasts, which ultimately leads to disturbed erythropoiesis and anemia. Studies on such patients have identified certain mutations, such as those present in HSCB, which are crucial for maintaining hematopoiesis and erythropoiesis (Crispin et al., 2017). In contrast, chronic myeloid leukemia (CML) highlights the role of tumor suppressor genes, such as PTPRG, in hematopoietic cancers, where their suppression contributes to disease development and treatment resistance (Sayab et al., 2017). These results not only enhance our understanding of hematological disorders but also create possibilities for future therapeutic interventions aimed at the actual molecular processes.

1.3.1. Anemia: Types and Causes

Anemia is a complex hematologic disorder characterized by a deficiency in RBCs or hemoglobin and reduced oxygen transportation within the body. Anemia may be broadly categorized into various types based on its etiology, including iron deficiency anemia, which occurs as a result of inadequate iron; megaloblastic anemia, which is caused by the deficiency of vitamin B12 or folate; and hemolytic anemia, which is due to the premature destruction of RBCs. Additionally, bone marrow disorders, such as aplastic anemia, can severely impair hematopoiesis, or the production of blood. It is critical to recognize the varied etiologies of anemia, especially because RBC mass can be significantly impaired under certain conditions, such as manned space flight, where there is no red cell mass loss mean of 10 to 15%. Additionally, BMSCs' contribution to hematopoietic health cannot be ruled out, as their differentiation dictates hematopoietic recovery after stress (Li et al., 2018) (Figure 1.11).

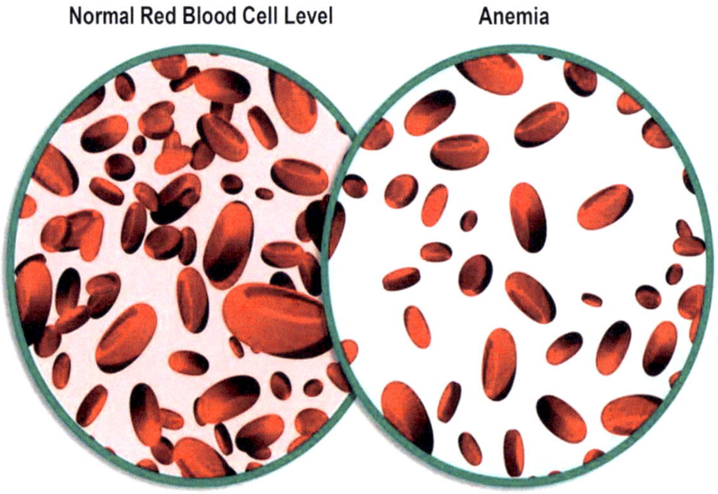

Figure 1.11. Anemia represents a complex hematologic condition characterized by a deficiency in red blood cells or hemoglobin, leading to reduced oxygen transport within the body.

Source: https://img.lb.wbmdstatic.com/vim/live/webmd/consumer_assets/site_images/articles/health_tools/guide_to_blood_disorders_slideshow/1800ss_getty_rf_normal_blood_vs_anemia.jpg?resize=750px:*&output-quality=75.

1.3.2. Leukemia: Overview and Types

Leukemia is a heterogeneous and multiform set of malignancies caused by genetic alterations of the HSCs that lead to uncontrolled growth of the cells and impaired cell differentiation. The common forms of leukemia are divided into acute and chronic, and the acute forms present with the rapid progression and expansion of immature blood cells, while the chronic ones consist of more mature cells and typically develop over an extended period. Of special interest to mention is T cell acute lymphoblastic leukemia (T-ALL), which symbolizes the complexity of leukemias' oncogenic events and those resulting from probing the functions of noncoding RNAs and the transformation process and normal T cell development (Durinck et al., 2017). Moreover, therapeutic techniques such as allogenic hematopoietic progenitor cell transplantation (allo-HSCT) have evolved to allow for exposure to varied stem cell sources and the weighing of ethical issues encompassing donor selection and recipient care (Russa et al., 2017). Consequently, identification of the nature of leukemia plays a key role in the advancement of hematology therapeutic techniques.

1.3.3. Lymphoma: Classification and Symptoms

Lymphoma, a primary concern in hematology, is a heterogeneous group of lymphoid tissue malignancies that are a vital component of the immune system. The World Health Organization classifies lymphomas primarily into two categories: Hodgkin lymphoma (HL) and non-Hodgkin lymphoma (NHL). Both share typical histological characteristics, clinical presentations, and prognosis. The symptoms are typically nonspecific and consist of lymphadenopathy, fever, night sweats, and unexplained weight loss. These presentations may vary significantly based on the type of lymphoma. For instance, while HL usually is more localized in its dissemination, NHL is more aggressive in behavior and systemic in presentation as observed in patterns of transfusion and prognosis of patients in hematological malignancies (Rydén et al., 2021). Besides, as the nature of such disorders is not straightforward, their classification not only facilitates diagnosis but also guides therapeutic interventions, justifying the effort to conduct ongoing research in hematopoiesis (Landtblom et al., 2023) (Figure 1.12).

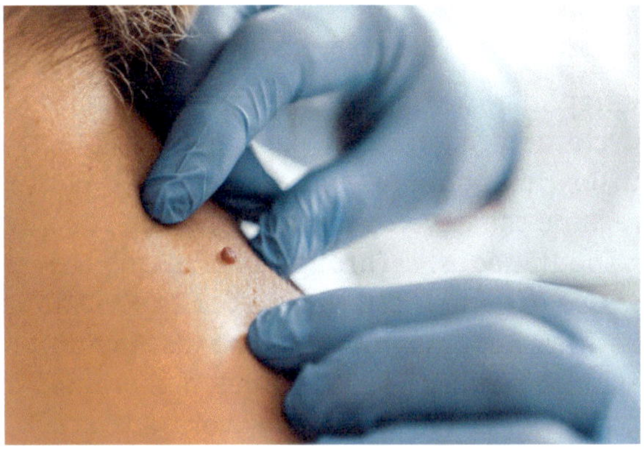

Figure 1.12. Lymphoma, a pivotal focus within hematology, represents a diverse group of malignancies originating from lymphatic tissues, which are integral to the immune system.

Source: https://www.jeffersonhealth.org/content/dam/health2021/images/photos/stock/people/clinical/dermatologist-checking-mole.jpg.

1.3.4. Thrombocytopenia: Causes and Effects

Thrombocytopenia, or a decreased platelet count, can result from several underlying conditions, each of which poses significant health threats. Among the frequent causes are bone marrow disorders, including aplastic anemia, which leads to an inefficient production of platelets due to a deficiency in adequate megakaryocyte formation. Some autoimmune disorders, including immune thrombocytopenic purpura (ITP), also lead to platelet destruction, further aggravating this condition. The physiological effects of thrombocytopenia are severe, and decreased platelets can cause increased tendencies of bleeding, for example, petechiae and more serious hemorrhagic events. As such, awareness of such causes is vital in hematology because prompt detection and treatment are essential to prevent life-threatening complications. Thrombocytopenia complexity is significant in underscoring the importance of ongoing research and development in treatment modalities, which have significantly improved patient outcomes in malignancies and hematological disease, as emphasized in Hematology – Science and Practice discussions (Hebbelinck et al., 2016).

1.3.5. Hemophilia: Genetic Basis and Treatment

Hemophilia is a genetic bleeding disorder caused most frequently by mutations in genes that code for clotting factors that participate in blood clotting. A deficiency of factor VIII, most commonly causes Hemophilia A and hemophilia B is caused by the deficiency of factor IX. These gene defects preclude the development of blood clots so that bleeding occurs uncontrollably from trivial trauma or spontaneously. Through continuous research, treatment interventions have evolved to include the use of gene therapy, with the expectation of bringing a cure to the genetic etiology of diseases. The EHA Roadmap outlines the justification for research in hematology, emphasizing the need for genomic profiling-based targeted therapies and innovation in gene therapy (Allard et al., 2016). Such specific research endeavors are crucial in enhancing the quality of life for patients with hemophilia and ultimately revolutionizing treatment models (Figure 1.13).

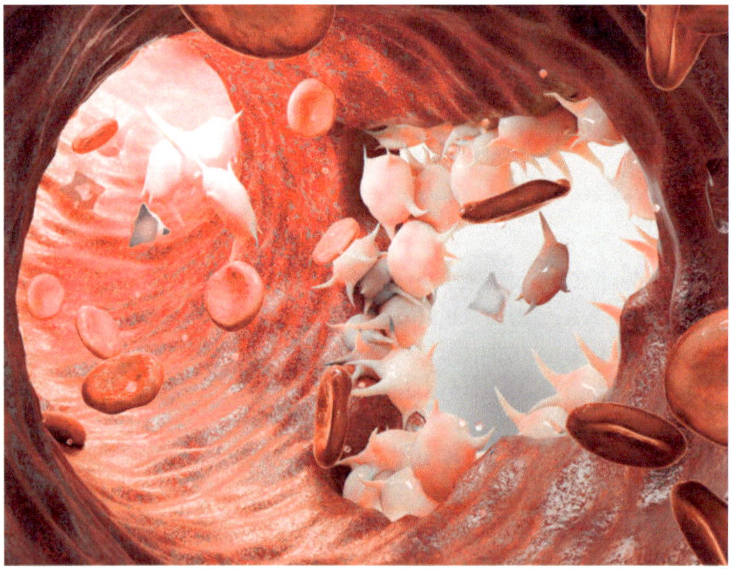

Figure 1.13. Hemophilia.

Source: https://www.bioworld.com/ext/resources/Stock-images/Therapeutic-topics/Hematologic/Hematologic-hemostasis-hemophilia-injury-wound-vessel.jpg?height=488&t=1743196293&width=650.

1.3.6. Sickle Cell Disease: Pathophysiology

The pathophysiology of Sickle Cell Disease (SCD) is directly associated with the abnormal polymerization of hemoglobin S in conditions of reduced oxygen. This abnormal hemoglobin sickles the RBCs, leading to obstruction of the blood vessels and ultimately to ischemia in organs. Clinical manifestations of SCD are multifarious and vary from acute pain crises to long-term hemolytic anemia and increased susceptibility to infections. Patients over time may develop organ damage as a result of recurrent vaso-occlusive crises. importantly, whereas SCD uniquely attacks the erythropoietic process, the disease's complications extend to other systems, and its management requires a multidisciplinary approach. More recent research has identified potential therapeutic agents, such as gene therapy and agents that induce fetal hemoglobin, as ways to mitigate the disease's effects and improve patient outcomes. Additionally, it is worthwhile to study analogous conditions, such as thalassemia, which may offer analogous pathophysiological insights, as noted in Cappellini et al. (2009). Additionally, the metabolic pathways regulated by V-ATPase would provide further insights on the treatment side, akin to findings in cancer, as discussed in McConnell et al. (2016).

1.3.7. Myelodysplastic Syndromes (MDS)

Myelodysplastic syndromes (MDS) are a group of heterogeneous hematological disorders that interfere with normal hematopoiesis, causing dysplasia in the lineages of blood cells. MDS largely affects the patient population of advanced age, with the median age at diagnosis being approximately 75 years, thereby validating the emergent need for effective interventions in this population. Severe anemia is most commonly encountered in patients requiring repeated RBC transfusions associated with deleterious effects on overall survival and quality of life, as discussed in transfusion patterns studies in MDS patients (Rydén et al., 2021). Furthermore, the risk of further development to acute myeloid leukemia (AML) is a severe threat, particularly in those with germline mutations or being subjected to cytotoxic therapy, making MDS a preleukemic status (Koeffler et al., 2017). Consequently, our understanding of MDS has to be enhanced to provide an improved prognosis in patients and the design of targeted therapies (Figure 1.14).

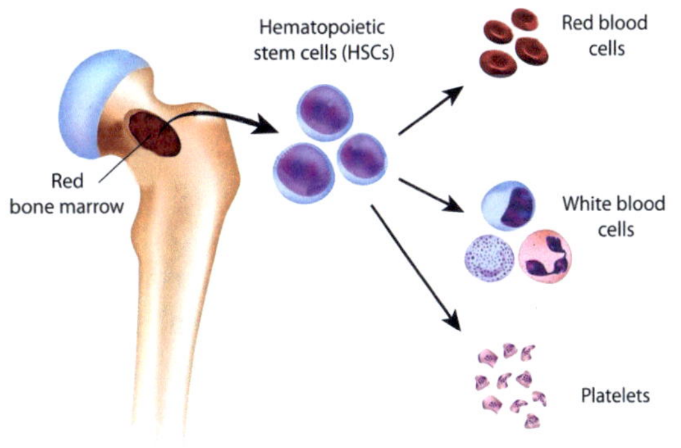

Figure 1.14. Myelodysplastic syndromes (MDS).

Source: https://www.parkwaycancercentre.com/images/default-source/cancer-type/shutterstock_126428768690707b7-2939-45a2-8da0-2569c22808b0.webp?sfvrsn=812ad513_1.

1.3.8. Polycythemia Vera: Diagnosis and Management

Polycythemia Vera (PV) is a field of greatest investigation in hematology where there is overproduction of RBCs due to a mutation of the JAK2 gene. Diagnosis is based on clinical evaluation, laboratory results, and genetic analysis, as PV can appear without any symptoms at all or with very few, such as fatigue, dizziness, and an increased risk of thro mbotic complications. Management strategies typically entail decreasing hematocrit levels through phlebotomy and administering cytoreductive therapies to avert complications in the form of cardiovascular incidents and second malignancies (Landtblom et al., 2023). Apart from this, patients with myeloproliferative neoplasm (MPN), such as PV, also carry a higher risk of infection and second malignancies, which are reasons for regular monitoring and supportive therapy (Landtblom et al., 2023). Effective management, therefore, aims not only to control the hematologic features of PV but also to address broader general health effects and safeguard patients' quality of life and overall prognosis in the long run.

1.3.9. Emerging Therapies for Hematological Disorders

The field of hematology is witnessing unprecedented advances in therapeutic approaches, particularly in the context of hematological disorders. Emerging therapies like gene editing and precision immunotherapies are being accorded the highest priority to address the complexity of the disease. For instance, CAR-T cell therapies have received considerable attention, as they have proven remarkably effective against malignant neoplasms of the lymphoid line, as highlighted in the updated EHA Research Roadmap, which underscores the urgent clinical needs for hematology research (Anagnou et al., 2021). Additionally, it has recently been discovered that non-receptor tyrosine kinases, including the JAK family, have emerged as central regulators of essential cellular functions that contribute to the pathogenesis of MPNs (Azevedo et al., 2019). The new therapies not only promise to help patients but also redefine the practice of hematological medicine, highlighting the importance of continued research efforts and funding in this vital discipline. Therefore, the blend of these new therapies marks a watershed in the management of hematological diseases (Figure 1.15).

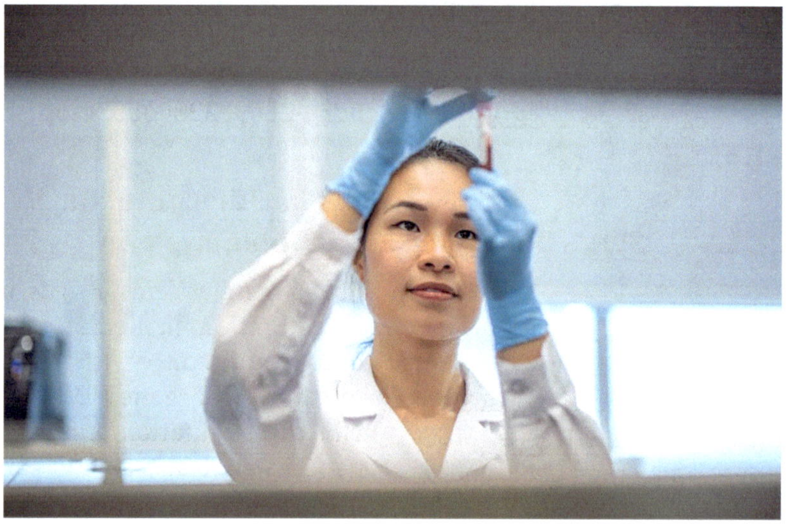

Figure 1.15. The field of hematology is witnessing unprecedented advancements in therapeutic approaches, particularly concerning hematological disorders.

Source: https://www.hemoncnc.com/wp-content/uploads/2023/11/medical-professional-with-new-cancer-treatement.jpg.

1.4. Diagnostic Techniques in Hematology

Hematology practice encompasses a series of diagnostic technologies that are very crucial in determining and managing blood disorders effectively. These include conventional practices such as complete blood counts and blood smears, as well as advanced technologies like flow cytometry and molecular diagnostics. For instance, the EHA Roadmap emphasizes the importance of germline and somatic genetic profiling, enabling the design of targeted treatments and the optimization of personalized treatment modalities in hematologic malignancies (Allard et al., 2016). The ability to detect minimal residual disease (MRD) using sensitive assays is also essential for monitoring treatment outcomes and guiding therapeutic decision-making (Allard et al., 2016). The integration of these diagnostic techniques not only improves patient management but also directs future research initiatives towards addressing the current unmet clinical and scientific needs in hematology, as reflected in the EHA Roadmap results.

1.4.1. Complete Blood Count (CBC)

Complete Blood Count (CBC) is a hematology diagnostic test that provides crucial information regarding an individual's hematopoietic status. By assessing various parameters like RBC count, hemoglobin level, hematocrit level, WBC count, and platelet count, the CBC provides a comprehensive view of cellular blood components.

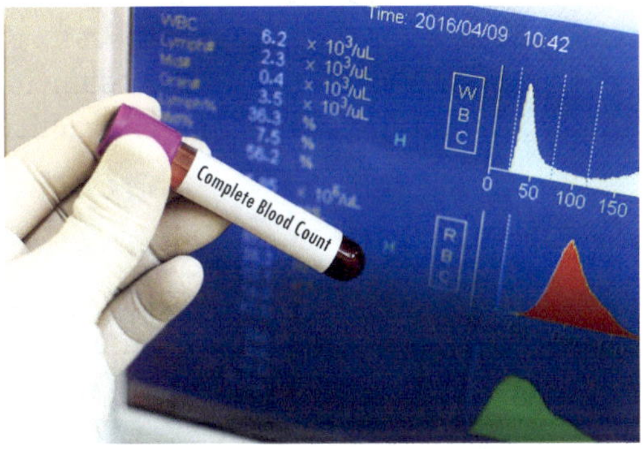

Figure 1.16. The complete blood count (CBC) serves as an essential diagnostic tool in hematology, providing critical insights into an individual's hematopoietic health.

Source: https://www.lalpathlabs.com/blog/wp-content/uploads/2016/12/complete-blood-count.jpg.

Abnormalities in these measurements may be indicative of various hematologic disorders, ranging from anemia and leukopenia to thrombocytopenia. For instance, the significance of somatic mutations, as seen in primary myelofibrosis, can be appreciated by putting CBC results into context. Patients who present with cytopenias may also be evaluated for conditions like Diamond-Blackfan anemia, in which there are genetic mutations that make clinical presentation more complex. Thus, the CBC not only aids in diagnosis but also serves as a vital point of reference for monitoring both the response to treatment and disease course in hematologic disorders (Anton et al., 2023; Fathpour et al., 2024) (Figure 1.16).

1.4.2. Bone Marrow Biopsy

Bone marrow biopsy is a significant clinical tool in hematology, providing detailed information on hematopoiesis and hematologic malignancies. With the procurement of a bone marrow specimen, physicians can analyze its cellular composition and morphology and use this to make a diagnosis of MDS and other anemias. For instance, a case study highlighted the emergence of acquired elliptocytosis in a patient with MDS, which was diagnosed following a bone marrow biopsy, emphasizing the role of the biopsy in explaining complex hematologic abnormalities (Dwyre et al., 2017). Moreover, bone marrow evaluation is essential in the diagnosis of pancytopenia cases, where accurate diagnosis leads to personalized treatment regimens. In an etiology research of pancytopenia, such breakdown in detail as bone marrow morphology was critical in setting up megaloblastic anemia as a common etiology, with the biopsies taking center stage in clinical tests (Mansuri et al., 2017). A bone marrow biopsy is thus key to advancing our understanding and care of hematological disorders.

1.4.3. Flow Cytometry

Flow cytometry (FCM) is a key technology in hematology, enabling the precise analysis of cellular constituents in blood. By employing fluorescent-labeled antibodies to mark the desired cell surface antigens, FCM allows researchers and clinicians to quantify and delineate several blood cell populations, including HSCs. These cells are crucial in hematopoiesis, as they are self-renewing and can differentiate into other lineages through a process regulated by microRNAs, such as miR-15b, which are responsible for HSC growth and maintenance (Rahnama et al., 2015). Additionally, flow cytometry is also used in determining measurable residual disease (MRD) in conditions like AML, which serves as an accurate predictor (Bachas et al., 2021). In this way, flow cytometry not only increases our understanding of hematopoiesis but also significantly improves clinical diagnosis and treatment strategies (Figure 1.17).

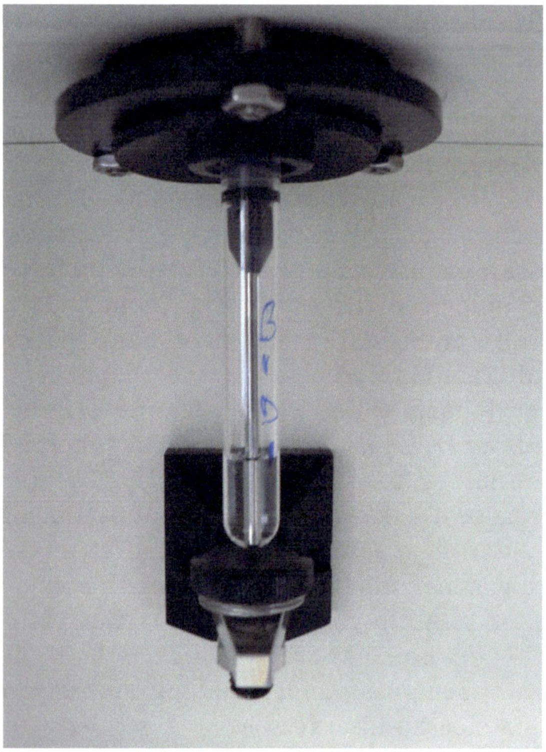

Figure 1.17. Flow cytometry (FCM) is a pivotal technology in the realm of hematology, allowing for precise analysis of the cellular components within blood.

Source: https://upload.wikimedia.org/wikipedia/commons/d/d1/FACS-buisje.JPG.

1.4.4. Hemoglobin Electrophoresis

In hematology, electrophoresis of hemoglobin is a crucial diagnostic tool that enables clinicians to differentiate and detect various hemoglobin variants and pathologies. The technique is based on the fractionation of hemoglobin molecules in terms of size and charge and thus provides valuable information about diseases such as SCD and thalassemia. Identification of such hemoglobinopathies is critical since beta thalassemia disorders affect millions of people around the globe, and thousands of infants are born with the disorder each year, creating a significant public health problem. In addition, advancements in hemoglobin electrophoresis have followed developments in other areas of hematology, ensuring enhanced understanding of blood diseases. These innovations underscore the importance of evidence-based practice in hematology to achieve effective diagnosis and management of hemoglobinopathies. The role of hemoglobin electrophoresis, therefore, is at the center of the ongoing advancement of hematological research and clinical practice.

1.4.5. Coagulation Studies

The coagulation tests are a vital part of hematology because they illuminate the pathway of hemostasis that is required to maintain vascular integrity and prevent excessive blood loss. Coagulation tests comprise a range of assessments that examine the components of the coagulation cascade, including platelets, clotting factors, and the intrinsic and extrinsic pathways. As outlined in the EHA Roadmap, the significance of the study of blood coagulation and hemostatic disorders is emphasized by its identification as one of the nine obligatory parts of hematology research. This all-encompassing strategy not only adds to the diagnosis of such diseases as hemophilia and thrombosis but also to the therapeutic approach, in the guise of creating target therapies and treatments that optimize patient outcomes. Through the clarification of our understanding of coagulation mechanisms, hematology studies seek to decrease the economic burden of estimated blood disorders with a cost of Euro 23 billion yearly, ultimately improving health care (Allard et al., 2016) (Figure 1.18).

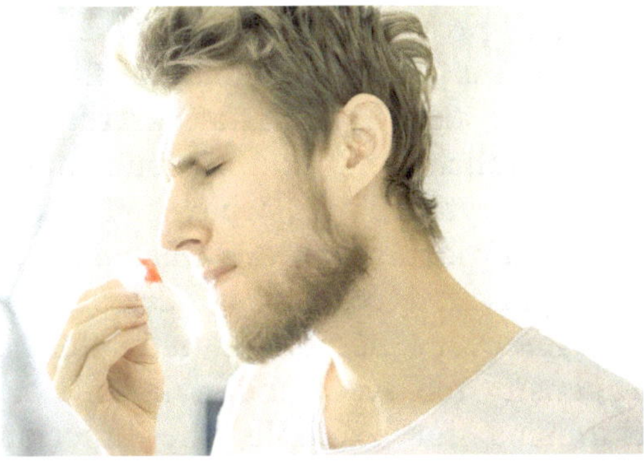

Figure 1.18. Coagulation studies play a critical role in the field of hematology by providing insights into the hemostatic process, which is essential for maintaining vascular integrity and preventing excessive bleeding.

Source: https://cdn-prod.medicalnewstoday.com/content/images/articles/323/323671/nosebleed-from-hemophiia.jpg.

1.4.6. Blood Smear Analysis

Blood smear analysis is a crucial hematology diagnostic test that enables one to view blood cell morphology and identify various hematological abnormalities. The test provides significant information on the pathology and characteristics of blood cells, which could be indicative of related pathologies such as MDS or leukemia. For example, acquired elliptocytosis, while infrequent, has been described in MDS, illustrating its potential association with severe hematologic diseases (Dwyre et al., 2017). Furthermore, analysis of the blood smear may aid in differentiating between neoplastic and reactive processes, such as chronic neutrophilic leukemia, where accurate differential diagnosis is also crucial (Dietze et al., 2008). By examining cellular morphology and proportions, physicians can make significant correlations between clinical symptomatology and specific blood diseases, ultimately refining diagnosis and treatment methodologies within the discipline of hematology and hematopoiesis. Blood smear examination is thus a cornerstone in the general assessment of blood disease.

1.4.7. Molecular Diagnostics in Hematology

The integration of molecular diagnostics in hematology has significantly enhanced the understanding and management of hematopoietic conditions. These advancements have enabled more precise detection of genetic mutations, which are at the core of the pathogenesis of most hematological cancers. For instance, the identification of the JAK2 p.V617F mutation has emerged as a crucial biomarker in the diagnosis and monitoring of MPN (Siebolts et al., 2011).

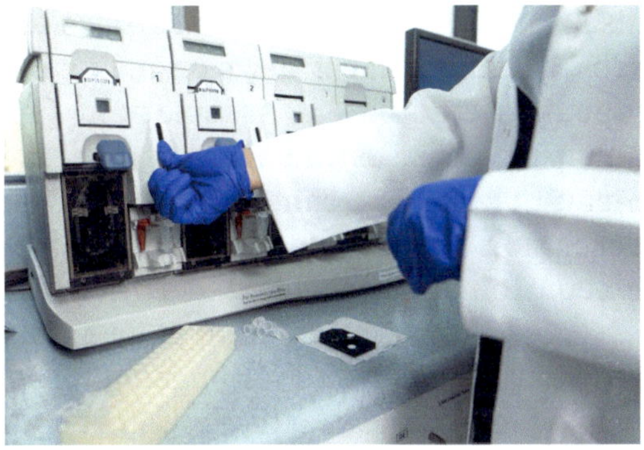

Figure 1.19. The integration of molecular diagnostics into hematology has significantly enhanced the understanding and management of hematopoietic disorders.

Source: https://advancementsinhematology.com/wp-content/uploads/2024/06/Flow_Cytometry_dreamstime_m_306796305.jpg.

In addition, new culture systems have been designed to support and expand hematopoietic stem/progenitor cells (HSPCs), promoting research on their regulation and potential therapeutic applications (Huang et al., 2016). These approaches not only direct treatment regimes but also facilitate the detection of MRD, crucial for assessing the efficacy of treatment and potential relapse. Therefore, molecular diagnostics is a precious tool in continuing to advance hematology as a science, enabling individualized patient care and clinical improvement (Figure 1.19).

1.4.8. Imaging Techniques in Hematology

Imaging techniques are a cornerstone of the treatment and evaluation of hematological disorders, significantly enhancing prognosis and diagnosis. Current modalities, such as magnetic resonance imaging (MRI), computed tomography (CT), and positron emission tomography (PET), have revolutionized hematologists' capabilities to visualize hematologic diseases, particularly malignancies like lymphoma and leukemia. These imaging modalities permit the assessment of disease severity and response to therapy, thereby guiding clinical decision-making. The European Hematology Association (EHA) Roadmap emphasizes the value of integrating high-end diagnostic technology in hematology research for the development of improved patient outcomes and targeted therapies (Allard et al., 2016). With the evolution of hematology, there is always a demand for ongoing research in imaging modalities to address unmet clinical needs and optimize therapeutic interventions (Allard et al., 2016). In general, the application of advanced imaging technology is an important advancement in hematology and hematopoiesis.

1.4.9. Role of Laboratory Medicine in Hematology

In hematology, laboratory medicine is a key component in the diagnosis, treatment, and monitoring of hematopoietic diseases, significantly enhancing the understanding of hematopoiesis. Laboratory tests, which analyze cellular components and identify genetic mutations, provide important information about diseases such as anemia and leukemia. For example, CSA have mutations that affect iron metabolism and exhibit abnormal iron storage in erythroblasts, which indicates the role played by laboratory tests when diagnosing these aggravated conditions (Crispin et al., 2017). Moreover, laboratory investigations have a propensity to reveal underlying molecular mechanisms, for example, the function of transcription factors like CREB, which are key to typical myelopoiesis and potentially mark leukemic transformations if aberrantly expressed (Akashi et al., 2008). Thus, in this manner, by allowing precise diagnosis and guiding therapies, laboratory medicine is at the forefront of advancing the field of hematology and improving patient care (Figure 1.20).

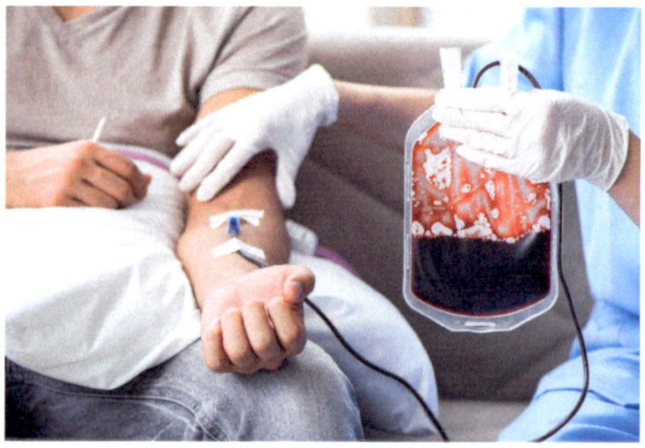

Figure 1.20. Laboratory medicine plays a pivotal role in diagnosis, treatment, and monitoring of blood-related disorders, significantly enhancing the understanding of hematopoiesis.

Source: https://d2jx2rerrg6sh3.cloudfront.net/images/Article_Images/ImageForArticle_745_16624283204238538.jpg.

A CLOSER LOOK

RED BLOOD CELLS

RBCs or erythrocytes are the most prevalent cells present in human blood. They are the cells that transport oxygen from the lungs to the tissues and carbon dioxide from the tissues to the lungs, allowing it to be expelled. RBCs have a distinctive biconcave disc shape that maximizes their surface area to promote proper gas transfer. They have hemoglobin, a protein that picks up oxygen and is responsible for the red color of blood. Mature RBCs do not have a nucleus, which provides more room for hemoglobin and increases their capacity to carry oxygen.

SUMMARY

In short, hematology and hematopoiesis emphasize the intricacy of blood cell formation and function and underscore the relevance of the HSC to health and disease. The monoclonal antibody approach has been essential in investigations, most prominently in the characterization of hematopoietic progenitor cells. However, the limitations encountered with species-specific antibodies, as with those against CD34 in sheep, indicate that there is still room for improvement in this area (Antuofermo et al., 2010). Moreover, the physiological acclimatization to external environments, as evident in the reorganization of red cell mass following flight, is also a reflection of the adaptive challenges faced by the hematology system. Taken together, these findings validate the merit of ongoing hematology research, not only to expand our understanding of the dynamics of blood, but also to establish therapeutic interventions capable of effectively overcoming hematology afflictions.

Good understanding of hematology and hematopoiesis is of great importance in the explanation of blood diseases and their etiologic cause. A fundamental facet in this field is how genetic mutations affect erythropoiesis, as evident from CSA. New data have implicated HSCB mutations in the central role of heme biosynthesis, leading to pathologic iron accumulation and hematopoietic disorders in patient populations (Crispin et al., 2017). Furthermore, physiological adjustments of RBC mass in unorthodox environments, such as space, exemplify the dynamic flexibility of hematopoiesis. Experiments have demonstrated that upon return from space flights, astronauts may experience a significant loss of red blood cells, which can take weeks to regain. Individually, these experiments demonstrate the intricacies of hematological studies and their importance for both genetic diseases and environmental stressors affecting blood production.

REFERENCES

1. Cheng, J. C., Kinjo, K., Judelson, D. R., Chang, J., Wu, W. S., Schmid, I., Shankar, D. B., Kasahara, N., Stripecke, R., Bhatia, R., Landaw, E. M., & Sakamoto, K. M. (2007). CREB is a critical regulator of normal hematopoiesis and leukemogenesis. *Blood, 111*(3), 1182–1192. https://doi.org/10.1182/blood-2007-04-083600Akhavan Rahnama, M., Anbarlou, A., Atashi, A., Movassaghpour, A., et al. (2015). *microRNA-15b Target Sall4 and Diminish in vitro UCB-Derived HSCs Expansion.* https://core.ac.uk/download/46917140.pdf (accessed on 12th June 2025).
2. Al Sayab, A., Al-Dewik, N., Fiorini, S., Zeno, I., Holyoake, T., et al. (2017). *A New Monoclonal Antibody Detects Downregulation of Protein Tyrosine Phosphatase Receptor Type Γ In Chronic Myeloid Leukemia Patients.* https://core.ac.uk/download/84148497.pdf (accessed on 12th June 2025).
3. Aljurf, M., Auletta, J. J., Battiwalla, M., Boeckh, M., et al. (2017). *Pre-Existing Invasive Fungal Infection Is Not a Contraindication for Allogeneic HSCT for Patients with Hematologic Malignancies: A CIBMTR Study.* https://core.ac.uk/download/323072284.pdf (accessed on 12th June 2025).
4. Allard, S., Anagnou, N., Andolfo, I., Andrau, J. C., et al. (2016). *The European Hematology Association Roadmap for European Hematology Research: A Consensus Document.* https://core.ac.uk/download/79516495.pdf (accessed on 12th June 2025).
5. Almaguer, C., Civelek, T., Fay, R. A., García-Belenguer, S., Krimer, P. M., Lozano, M., Schafer, S., et al. (2019). *Effects of Maternal Sub Nutrition During Early Pregnancy on Cow Hematological Profiles and Offspring Physiology and Vitality in Two Beef Breeds.* https://core.ac.uk/download/322890174.pdf (accessed on 12th June 2025).
6. Anagnou, N. P., Andolfo, I., Barcellini, W., Camaschella, C., et al. (2021). *The EHA Research Roadmap: Anemias.* https://core.ac.uk/download/478721871.pdf (accessed on 12th June 2025).
7. Anton, G., Ataman, M., Bleotu, C., Botezatu, A., et al. (2023). *Leukemic Conversion Involving RAS Mutations of Type 1 CALR-Mutated Primary Myelofibrosis in A Patient Treated for HCV Cirrhosis: A Case Report.* https://core.ac.uk/download/591440959.pdf (accessed on 12th June 2025).
8. Antuofermo, E., Bonelli, P., Dattena, M., Manetti, M., et al. (2010). *Monoclonal Antibodies Against Human CD34 Antigens Do Not Cross-React with Ovine Umbilical Cord Blood Cells.* https://core.ac.uk/download/11691727.pdf (accessed on 12th June 2025).
9. Aryee, M. J., Cahan, P., Cunniff, K. C., Daley, G. Q., et al. (2010). *Epigenetic Memory in Induced Pluripotent Stem Cells.* https://core.ac.uk/download/323071670.pdf (accessed on 12th June 2025).
10. Azevedo, A., Rueff, J., & Silva, S. (2019). *Non-Receptor Tyrosine Kinases Role and Significance in Hematological Malignancies.* https://core.ac.uk/download/322441613.pdf (accessed on 12th June 2025).
11. Bachas, C., Bene, M. C., Buccisano, F., Buecklein, V., et al. (2021). *Technical Aspects of Flow Cytometry-Based Measurable Residual Disease Quantification in Acute Myeloid Leukemia: Experience of the European LeukemiaNet MRD Working Party.* https://core.ac.uk/download/541504941.pdf (accessed on 12th June 2025).

12. Bao, E. L., Cheng, A., & Sankaran, V. G. (2019). The genetics of human hematopoiesis and its disruption in disease. *EMBO Molecular Medicine, 11*. https://doi.org/10.15252/emmm.201910316 (accessed on 12th June 2025).

13. Cappellini, M. D., Musallam, K. M., & Taher, A. T. (2009). *Thalassemia Intermedia: An Update.* https://core.ac.uk/download/pdf/8522728.pdf (accessed on 12th June 2025).

14. Capps, C. M. (2024). *Ultrasonographic Appearance of The Spleen of Growing Kittens Using a High Frequency Linear Transducer.* https://core.ac.uk/download/618318727.pdf (accessed on 12th June 2025).

15. Cardarelli, L., Foà, R., Giona, F., Mariani, S., et al. (2018). *Gaucher Disease and Myelofibrosis: A Combined Disease or A Misdiagnosis?* https://core.ac.uk/download/188825657.pdf (accessed on 12th June 2025).

16. Cascino, P., Di Ruscio, A., Li, M., Ummarino, S., et al. (2017). *Application of Induced Pluripotent Stem Cell Technology to The Study of Hematological Diseases.* https://core.ac.uk/download/287153741.pdf (accessed on 12th June 2025).

17. Chaviano, F., Orazi, A., Pizzi, M., Rugge, M., et al. (2017). *A Lucky Mistake: The Splenic Glands of Marcello Malpighi.* https://core.ac.uk/download/154325705.pdf (accessed on 12th June 2025).

18. Crispin, A. (2017). *HSCB, a Co-Chaperone in Mitochondrial Iron-Sulfur Cluster Biogenesis, Is A Novel Candidate Gene for Congenital Sideroblastic Anemia.* https://open.bu.edu/bitstream/2144/26669/5/Crispin_bu_0017N_13280.pdf (accessed on 12th June 2025).

19. Dietze, O., Faber, V., Greil, R., Kemmerling, R., et al. (2008). *Differential Diagnostic Challenge of Chronic Neutrophilic Leukemia in A Patient with Prolonged Leukocytosis.* https://core.ac.uk/download/pdf/8307668.pdf (accessed on 12th June 2025).

20. Dolinska, M. (2019). *Understanding the Role of Bone Marrow Niche in Myeloid Malignancies.* https://core.ac.uk/download/185614393.pdf (accessed on 12th June 2025).

21. Durinck, K., Speleman, F., Taghon, T., Van Vlierberghe, P., et al. (2017). *T-ALL and Thymocytes: A Message of Noncoding RNAs.* https://core.ac.uk/download/84047020.pdf (accessed on 12th June 2025).

22. Dwyre, D. M., Jonas, B. A., & Kjelland, J. D. (2017). *Acquired Elliptocytosis as A Manifestation of Myelodysplastic Syndrome with Ring Side Oblasts and Multilineage Dysplasia.* https://core.ac.uk/download/323069593.pdf (accessed on 12th June 2025).

23. Fathpour, G., Gharehdaghi, Z., Obeidi, N., & Rostamipoor, et al. (2024). Undiagnosed anemia after 9 years: Diamond-Blackfan (homozygous variant c.140G>T; p.Gly47Val in *ADA2* gene). https://core.ac.uk/download/618356597.pdf (accessed on 12th June 2025).

24. Fernando, T. R., Rao, D. S., & Rodriguez-Malave, N. I. (2012). MicroRNAs in B cell development and malignancy. https://core.ac.uk/download/4894914.pdf (accessed on 12th June 2025).

25. Fisher, K. D., & Talbot, J. M. (2025). Research opportunities in loss of red blood cell mass in space flight. https://core.ac.uk/download/pdf/42845286.pdf (accessed on 12th June 2025).

26. Foa, R., Giona, F., Larocca, L. M., & Teofili, L. (2008). Childhood polycythemia vera and essential thrombocythemia: Does their pathogenesis overlap with that of adult patients? https://core.ac.uk/download/54259489.pdf (accessed on 12th June 2025).

27. Frisch, B., Mallmann, B., Breslow, R., Burkhardt, H., Burkhardt, R., Burkhardt, M., Burkhardt,

H., et al. (1987). *Changes in Trabecular Bone, Hematopoiesis and Bone Marrow Vessels in Aplastic Anemia, Primary Osteoporosis, And Old Age.* https://core.ac.uk/download/12167710.pdf (accessed on 12th June 2025).

28. Hasegawa, M. (1969). Studies on the relationship between the function of reticuloendothelial system and the hematopoiesis. I. Experimental studies on the RES functions using 51Cr-labelled heat-damaged iso-erythrocytes in the induced hematological disorders of mice. https://core.ac.uk/download/12546986.pdf (accessed on 12th June 2025).
29. Hebbelinck, L., Kitshoff, A., Paepe, D., et al. (2016). Feminization and severe pancytopenia caused by testicular neoplasia in a cryptorchid dog. https://core.ac.uk/download/84041954.pdf (accessed on 12th June 2025).
30. Huang, X., Wang, C., Wang, X., et al. (2016). Three-dimensional co-culture of mesenchymal stromal cells and differentiated osteoblasts on human bio-derived bone scaffolds supports active multi-lineage hematopoiesis *in vitro*: Functional implication of the biomimetic HSC niche. https://core.ac.uk/download/323075326.pdf (accessed on 12th June 2025).
31. Koeffler, H. P., & Leong, G. (2017). Preleukemia: One name, many meanings. https://core.ac.uk/download/323076596.pdf (accessed on 12th June 2025).
32. La Russa, R., Liso, A., Pascale, N., et al. (2017). Donor selection for allogenic hemopoietic stem cell transplantation: Clinical and ethical considerations. https://core.ac.uk/download/141694739.pdf (accessed on 12th June 2025).
33. Li, S. C., Li, Z., Ran, Q., et al. (2018). The differentiation balance of bone marrow mesenchymal stem cells is crucial to hematopoiesis. https://core.ac.uk/download/323062656.pdf (accessed on 12th June 2025).
34. Mansuri, B., & Thekdi, K. P. (2017). A prospective study among cases of the pancytopenia on the basis of clinic-hematological analysis and bone marrow aspiration. https://core.ac.uk/download/539910417.pdf (accessed on 12th June 2025).
35. McConnell, M. J. (2016). *Atp6v1c1* enhances breast cancer growth by activating V-ATPase mediated mTORC1 signaling and metastasis by increasing V-ATPase activity in cancer cells. https://core.ac.uk/download/640976129.pdf (accessed on 12th June 2025).
36. Mortera Blanco, T. (2009). *Development of an Ex Vivo Three-Dimensional (3-D) Model of Acute Myeloid Leukemia (AML).* https://core.ac.uk/download/323076596.pdf (accessed on 12th June 2025).
37. Naldini, L., Cicalese, M. P., Bernardo, M. E., Gentner, B., Gabaldo, M., Ferrari, G., & Aiuti, A. (2022). The EHA research roadmap: Hematopoietic stem cell gene therapy. *HemaSphere, 6*, e671–e671. https://doi.org/10.1097/hs9.0000000000000671 (accessed on 12th June 2025).
38. Ravn Landtblom, A. (2023). *Morbidity and Childbirth in Myeloproliferative Neoplasms.* https://core.ac.uk/download/560711311.pdf (accessed on 12th June 2025).
39. Rydén, J. (2021). *Chronic Bone Marrow Failure and Transfusion Patterns: Epidemiological Studies of Blood Transfusions and Outcomes in Patients with Myelodysplastic Syndromes.* https://core.ac.uk/download/365939211.pdf (accessed on 12th June 2025).
40. Siebolts, U. (2011). *New Aspects into Pathophysiology and Molecular Diagnostics of Myeloproliferative Neoplasms.* https://core.ac.uk/download/12011132.pdf (accessed on 12th June 2025).

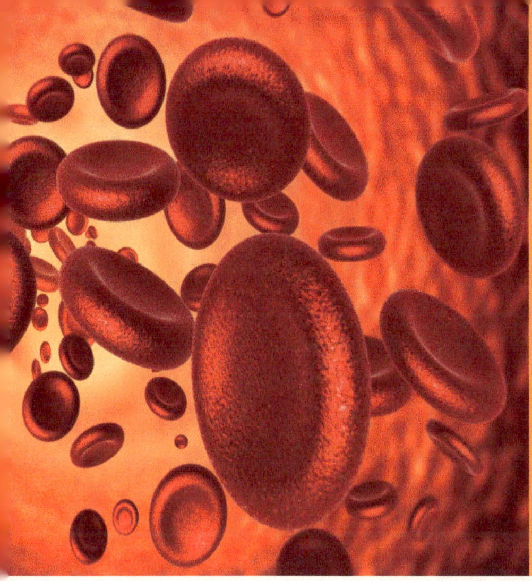

Chapter 2

ANEMIAS: PATHOPHYSIOLOGY AND CLASSIFICATION

Contents

Introduction........27
2.1. Pathophysiology of Anemia........28
2.2. Classification of Anemias........33
2.3. Diagnosis of Anemia........38
2.4. Treatment and Management of Anemia........43
Summary........49
References........50

Introduction

Anemia is a heterogeneous and multifactorial category of disease characterized by a decrease in the number or quality of red blood cells (RBCs), which can present with a spectrum of clinical findings. Understanding the classification and pathophysiology of anemias is necessary for optimal diagnosis and therapy. The conditions can result from a wide range of etiologies, including nutrient deficiencies, chronic diseases, genetic disorders, and immune system abnormalities. In particular, beta-thalassemia and sickle cell disease highlight the dominant role of hemolysis and ineffective erythropoiesis in disease progression, particularly in instances where complement system activation has emerged as a pivotal factor in their pathophysiology (Maciel et al., 2024). In addition, the discrimination between the various anemias not only facilitates their identification of causes, but also promotes therapeutic interventions in use, developing clinical practice on the basis of a solid evidence base of scientific knowledge (Garci et al., 2024) (Figure 2.1).

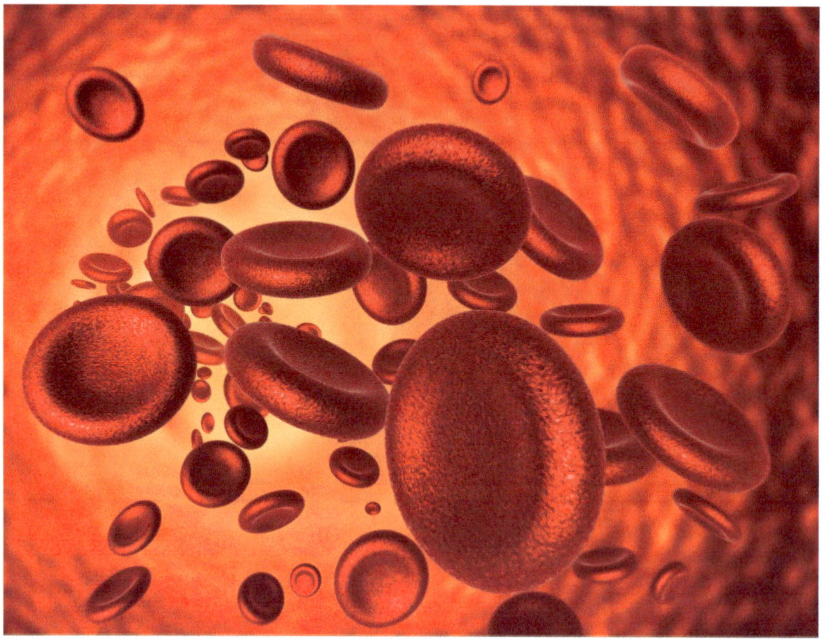

Figure 2.1. Anemia.

Source: https://www.viplab.in/uploads/blog/1446214083_anemia.jpg.

2.1. Pathophysiology of Anemia

Pathophysiology of anemia is a complex interplay of mechanisms that can lead to reduced red blood cell (RBC) mass or ineffective hemoglobin. Insufficient production of RBCs is the leading cause of anemia, and it can be due to failure of the bone marrow, deficiency in nutrients, or chronic inflammation. For instance, aplastic anemia disrupts hematopoietic potential, while deficiency of iron, vitamin B12, or folate prevents maximum erythropoiesis. Conversely, increased RBC destruction, as seen in autoimmune hemolytic anemias (AIHAs), exhibits a unique pathophysiological mechanism where the immune system mistakenly targets its RBCs for destruction. Through the mechanism of action of autoantibodies, AIHA causes the phagocytosis of dysfunctional cells, creating a state of chronic hemolysis that exacerbates anemia (Loriamini et al., 2024). Such different mechanisms support the significance of broad classification in appreciating the complex nature of anemias (Garci et al., 2024).

2.1.1. Mechanisms of Red Blood Cell Production

The process of RBC formation in the body, called erythropoiesis, is a sophisticated and tightly regulated process to facilitate the appropriate delivery of oxygen in the body. This occurs predominantly in the bone marrow and requires the highly coordinated interaction of growth factors, nutrients, and hormones. Most prominent among them is erythropoietin, which triggers the proliferation and differentiation of erythroid progenitor cells. In addition, iron metabolism is also involved in the production of hemoglobin, where an equilibrium between iron and erythropoietic demand is necessary. The hormone hepcidin plays a central role in this regulation, as it controls iron homeostasis by acting on ferroportin, thereby influencing iron uptake and mobilization from stores (Ganz et al., 2023). In inherited diseases such as congenital sideroblastic anemia (CSA), abnormalities in the use of iron disrupt RBC generation with resulting ineffective erythropoiesis (Crispin et al., 2017). Thus, these mechanisms also explain the pathophysiology of anemias (Figure 2.2).

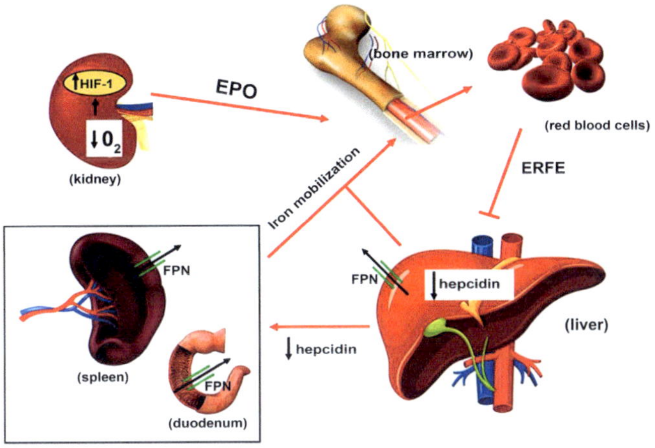

Figure 2.2. The production of red blood cells (RBCs), a process known as erythropoiesis, involves intricate mechanisms that are closely regulated to maintain adequate oxygen transport in the body.

Source: https://pub.mdpi-res.com/ijms/ijms-23-05341/article_deploy/html/images/ijms-23-05341-g001.png?1652257335.

2.1.2. Role of Hemoglobin in Oxygen Transport

Hemoglobin serves a crucial role in oxygen delivery across the body, being the primary oxygen-transport molecule in RBCs. Its quaternary structure enables it to pick up oxygen when the partial pressure is elevated in the lungs and deliver oxygen to tissues with low oxygen pressure. This is crucial for cellular respiration and the maintenance of metabolic processes. However, hemoglobin disorders may produce other anemias, such as CSAs, which result from defects that disrupt heme biosynthesis and ultimately influence hemoglobin synthesis (Crispin et al., 2017). Moreover, extracellular hemoglobin pathophysiology becomes relevant for hemolytic anemias, where circulating free hemoglobin can produce oxidative stress and reduce the efficiency of oxygen transport (Allhorn et al., 2012). A perception of these mechanisms highlights the importance of hemoglobin as not only a transport molecule for oxygen but as a regulator of a range of disease processes.

2.1.3. Causes of Decreased Red Blood Cell Production

Many pathophysiologic mechanisms and results in many forms of anemia cause decreased RBC production. Perhaps the most distinctive cause is ineffective erythropoiesis, which is most frequently linked with disorders such as CSA, where genetic mutations are responsible for the failure of heme synthesis and result in aberrant iron accumulation in bone marrow erythroblasts. Mutations in the HSCB gene, which plays a crucial role in erythropoiesis, have been found to result in decreased RBC production by way of impaired iron metabolism and aberrant hemoglobinization in patients

(Crispin et al., 2017). Also significant is the role of hepcidin, an iron-regulatory hormone; increasing hepcidin can lead to iron-limiting anemias by limiting the availability of iron for erythropoiesis during inflammation or iron overload states (Ganz et al., 2023). Treatment of such causes is central to effective anemia management (Figure 2.3).

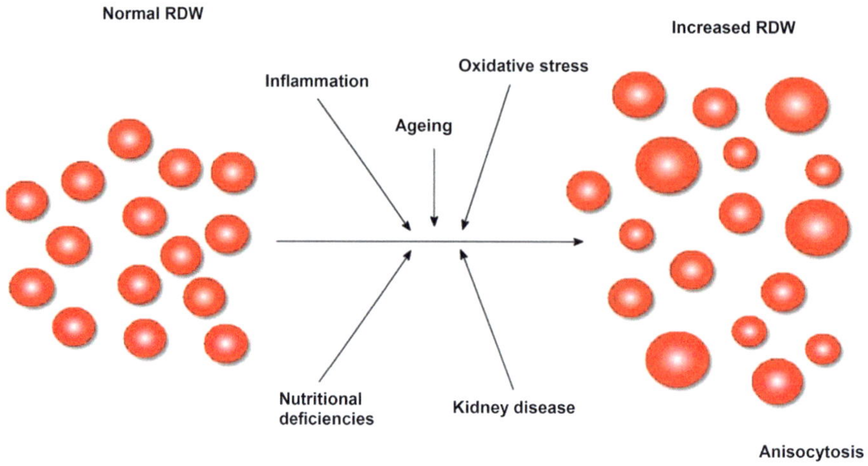

Figure 2.3. Decreased red blood cell (RBC) production can arise from a variety of pathophysiological mechanisms, leading to different forms of anemia.

Source: https://www.researchgate.net/publication/323388271/figure/fig2/AS:597863662882819@1519553213687/Pathophysiological-mechanisms-causing-anisocytosis-RDW-Red-blood-cell-distribution.png.

2.1.4. Causes of Increased Red Blood Cell Destruction

Accelerated RBC breakdown, a significant etiology of numerous anemias, may be due to a myriad of factors, either intrinsic or extrinsic. Intrinsic disorders, such as sickle cell anemia and hereditary spherocytosis, weaken the structural competence and viability of erythrocytes, leading to their premature removal from the circulation. Extrinsic causes typically involve immune-mediated diseases, such as AIHA, in which the body's immune system mistakenly targets its RBCs for destruction. Furthermore, infection, particularly in immunocompromised patients, can promote hemolysis, as in cases of HIV, where anemia due to increased RBC destruction presents problems in control (Groer et al., 2002). It becomes necessary to learn more about such mechanisms, as they significantly influence the clinical presentation and therapy of these hematological conditions, thereby precluding late diagnosis and intervention to avert the complications of these hematological disorders (Suhasini et al., 2017).

2.1.5. Impact of Nutritional Deficiencies

The impact of nutritional deficits on anemia is crucial, particularly in populations with limited access to diverse food supplies. Deficiencies of the essential nutrients, such as iron, vitamin B12, and folate, may induce alterations in various types of anemia with varied pathophysiological mechanisms. As a case in point, iron-deficiency anemia disrupts erythropoiesis due to a deficiency in hemoglobin synthesis, resulting in impaired oxygen delivery to tissues. Also, based on recent findings, 60% of rural pregnant Indian women suffer from anemia caused by nutritional deficiencies, added to socio-economic barriers that block access to quality nutrition and healthcare (Premnivas, 2025). Moreover, the pathogenic effect of malnutrition, as observed in heart failure patients with anemia resulting from congestive processes, underscores the correlation between nutrition and overall health (Mocan et al., 2025). Therefore, the management of nutritional deficiency becomes a priority not only to treat anemia but also to prevent its occurrence through public health interventions that promote better dietary practices (Figure 2.4).

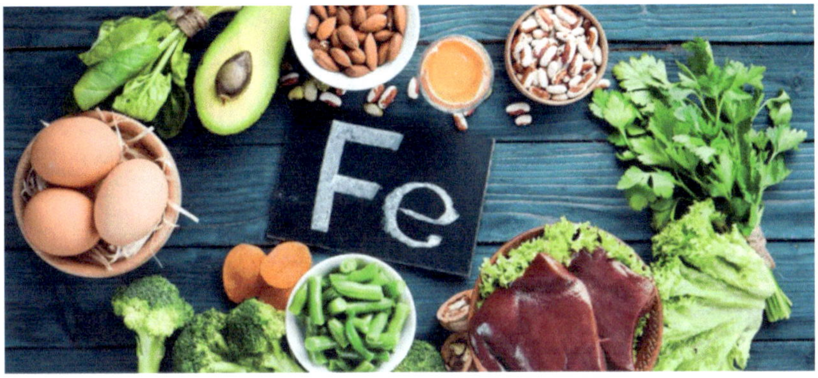

Figure 2.4. The impact of nutritional deficiencies on anemia is profound, particularly in populations with limited access to diverse food sources.

Source: https://abmedia.co.in/wp-content/uploads/2024/03/Ways-You-Can-Prevent-Iron-Deficiency-Anemia-11707899200.webp.

2.1.6. Genetic Factors Influencing Anemia

The etiologic foundation of anemia is a multifactorial interaction of several hematologic diseases, of which sickle cell anemia and thalassemia are the most notable. These genetic diseases, characterized by anomalous hemoglobin synthesis or structure, cause defective erythropoiesis and increased erythrocyte destruction, resulting in varying degrees of anemia severity. The recent advances in hematological research bring to the fore the role of genomic profiling in the identification of the target therapies for these genetic anemias, which are being viewed increasingly as global health concerns swamping populations disproportionately (Allard et al., 2016). Additionally, the World Health Organization requires robust definitions and frameworks to diagnose anemia, particularly among genetically heterogeneous populations, to improve public health interventions. The fight against these genetic etiologies not only propels research in the pathophysiology of anemia but also facilitates the creation of individualized treatment strategies and ultimately results in better health outcomes among affected populations.

2.1.7. Role of Chronic Diseases in Anemia

Chronic diseases contribute significantly to the prevalence and multifactorial etiology of anemia, illustrating a striking intersection between various pathological processes. For instance, in CKD, erythropoietin deficiency, coupled with iron dysregulation and systemic inflammation, induces anemia, worsening the health status and quality of life in patients (Badura et al., 2024). Similarly, ankylosing spondylitis patients tend to develop anemia of chronic disease (ACD) and iron deficiency anemia (IDA), presenting diagnostic challenges that need careful consideration of hepcidin's contribution towards these conditions (Zviahina et al., 2023). Such complexity necessitates the need for healthcare practitioners to implement specific diagnostic and therapeutic measures to effectively address anemia in patients with chronic conditions. Through the analysis of the underlying pathophysiology and discrimination between the different anemias, more appropriate management protocols can be developed, eventually improving patient care and outcomes for those suffering from these multifaceted diseases (Figure 2.5).

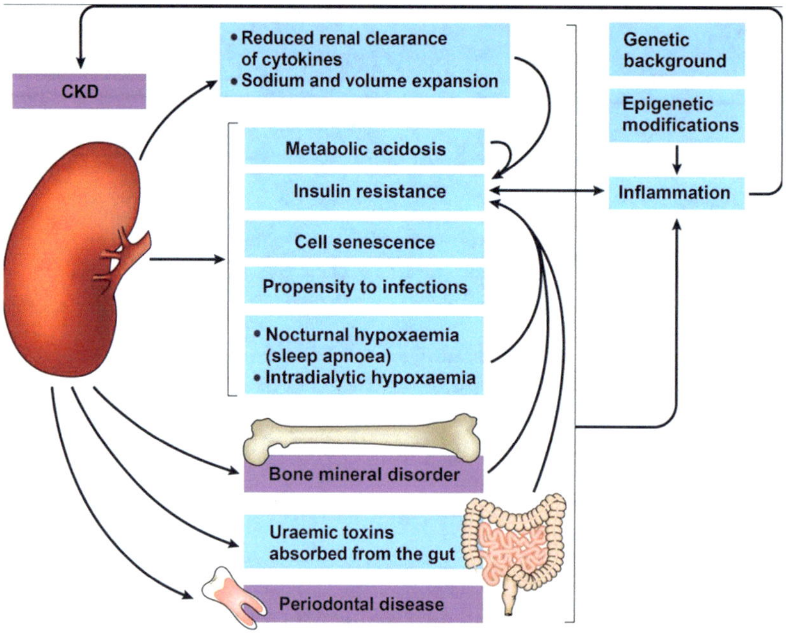

Figure 2.5. Chronic diseases significantly contribute to the prevalence and complexity of anemia, illustrating a compelling intersection between various pathological processes.

Source: https://media.springernature.com/lw1200/springer-static/image/art%3A10.1038%2Fnrneph.2017.52/MediaObjects/41581_2017_Article_BFnrneph201752_Fig2_HTML.jpg.

2.1.8. Effects of Inflammation on Red Blood Cells

Inflammation plays a crucial role in anemia pathophysiology, particularly through its effects on RBCs and iron metabolism. The liver increases the synthesis of the regulatory hormone hepcidin in response to inflammation, a hormone that maintains body iron homeostasis. Higher hepcidin inhibits ferroportin, a protein required for iron export by macrophages and enterocytes, resulting in less available iron for erythropoiesis and consequently anemia of inflammation (Ganz et al., 2023). Additionally, inflammation can lead to oxidative stress, which in turn impairs hemoglobin stability and function. The presence of extracellular hemoglobin due to hemolysis or overload with iron may also enhance oxidative damage to promote cellular dysfunction and the resultant pathological condition leading to anemia (Allhorn et al., 2012). The knowledge of such inflammatory processes is hence crucial in establishing effective therapeutic choices for controlling anemia following chronic inflammatory conditions.

2.1.9. Compensatory Mechanisms in Anemia

The body utilizes several compensatory mechanisms to counteract anemia, an effective adaptive mechanism to maintain oxygen delivery in the face of reduced hemoglobin. Primarily, the heart increases blood flow through enhanced contractility and heart rate to provide adequate tissue perfusion. Additionally, there is a physiological response in the bone marrow to elevate erythropoiesis, caused by erythropoietin due to the decreased oxygen-carrying capacity of the blood. There are other adaptations that involve shifting the oxygen dissociation curve, allowing for the effective release of oxygen to tissues in cases of hypoxia. Along with these responses, RBC distribution width (RDW) variations can indicate variances in RBC production and lifespan. They may be associated with more global pathophysiological significance in other anemic states (Mutlaq et al., 2024). All in all, all of these compensatory mechanisms demonstrate the body's superb ability to respond to the stress of anemia (Andrew et al., 2022) (Figure 2.6).

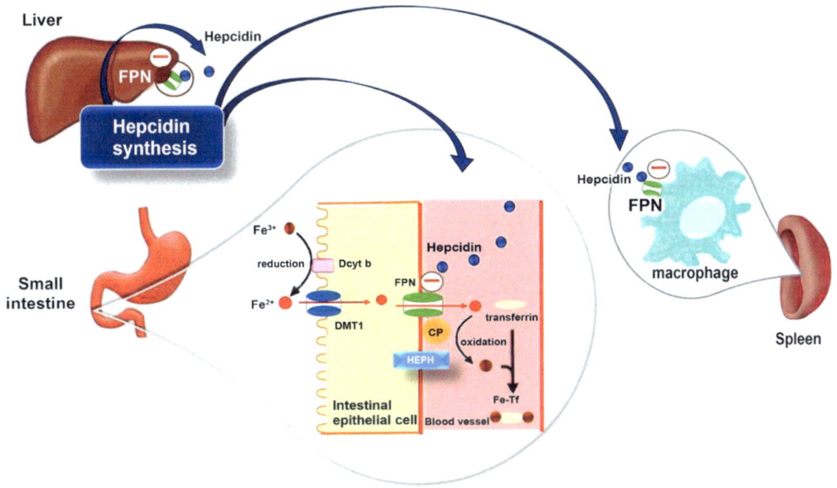

Figure 2.6. The body employs several compensatory mechanisms in response to anemia, which serves as a critical adaptive strategy to maintain oxygen delivery despite reduced hemoglobin levels.

Source: https://www.mdpi.com/immuno/immuno-04-00017/article_deploy/html/images/immuno-04-00017-g001.png.

2.2. Classification of Anemias

Anemia can be classified into several categories based on its etiological basis and pathophysiology, which is of paramount importance for determining the appropriate treatment modalities. The most frequent categories are microcytic, normocytic, and macrocytic anemias, referring to the size of the erythrocytes and being typically related to various etiologies. Microcytic anemia is frequently secondary to iron deficiency or thalassemia, whereas normocytic anemia can be caused by chronic disease or acute blood loss. Macrocytic anemia with large red cells usually suggests a deficiency of vitamin B12 or folate and highlights the predominant role of nutrition in erythropoiesis. Recent findings also link anemia with other pathologic disorders of the heart, further complicating patient care and outcomes (Kraevsky-Phillips et al., 2024). Additionally, the rare presentations of anemia, such as atypical hemolytic uremic syndrome, draw attention to genetic insights into disease mechanisms, as seen in recent studies employing next-generation sequencing (Dervla et al., 2023).

2.2.1. Microcytic Anemia

Microcytic anemia refers to a form of anemia in which the RBCs are smaller than they should be, most commonly associated with reduced hemoglobin production. It is commonly associated with a deficiency of iron, which interferes with the development of hemoglobin, the critical protein responsible for oxygen carriage. While its apparently simple etiology, it can have a multifactorial underlying cause, from nutritional factors such as inadequate dietary iron, vitamin B12, or folic acid to more advanced disorders like CSA. The latter is a consequence of heme biosynthesis defects and has been attributed to mutations in genes that participate in iron metabolism, as indicated by recent research establishing that decreased protein levels of HSCB impair erythropoiesis and hematopoiesis (Crispin et al., 2017). It highlights the importance of early detection and complete treatment in pediatric populations, where untreated anemia has severe consequences for general health and development (Muthuraman et al., 2010) (Figure 2.7).

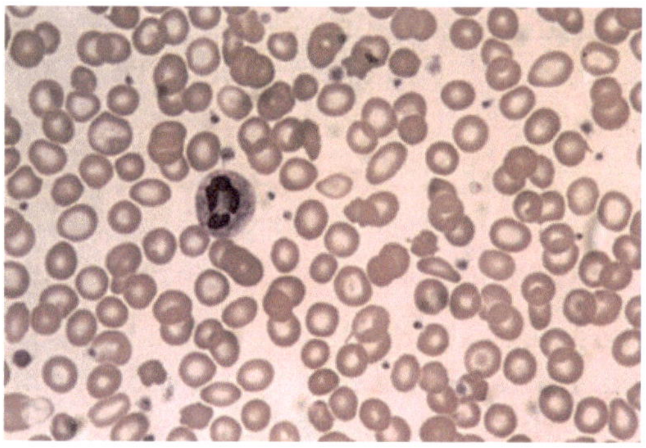

Figure 2.7. Microcytic anemia represents a classification of anemia characterized by smaller than normal red blood cells, primarily linked to reduced hemoglobin synthesis.

Source: https://cached.imagescaler.hbpl.co.uk/resize/scaleWidth/815/cached.offlinehbpl.hbpl.co.uk/news/PGH/AC32E678-ED5B-4229-D4232596E83DD0DC.gif.

2.2.2. Macrocytic Anemia

Macrocytic anemia is a specific form of anemia that is characterized by the presence of unusually large erythrocytes, commonly the result of either a vitamin B12 or folate deficiency. Macrocytic anemia disrupts normal RBC maturation, leading to ineffective erythropoiesis and consequently a reduction of proper oxygen delivery throughout the body. During a clinical trial, case evaluations identified macrocytic hyperchromic anemias as a significant category within the spectrum, with individual occurrences noted among patients who exhibited mismatches in their hematological parameters (Mardari et al., 2017). Causes of macrocytic anemia are also diverse and can range from nutritional deficiencies to more severe conditions, such as bone marrow failure or hematologic malignancies (Muthuraman et al., 2010). The etiologic heterogeneity emphasizes the need for accurate diagnosis and classification, in which macrocytic anemia is not only considered an independent disorder but also a significant clinical marker of more widespread systemic pathologies.

2.2.3. Normocytic Anemia

Normocytic anemia, where RBCs usually are shaped and sized but fewer in number, presents a particular diagnostic challenge in the broader scheme of anemia classification. Unlike microcytic or macrocytic types, normocytic anemia generally reflects underlying conditions, such as concurrent chronic disease, acute blood loss, or renal insufficiency, that compromise erythropoiesis but do not alter the morphology of RBCs. The pathophysiologic mechanisms usually follow a combination of reduced RBC production and increased destruction, making the clinical picture more complex. Recent advances in diagnostic technology, however, indicate a promising avenue of using machine learning models to further subclassify anemia subtypes, including normocytic ones, into more specific and detailed etiologies (Gómez et al., 2025). It is essential to understand the multifactorial pathogenesis of normocytic anemia, as it affects a substantial portion of the global population and requires tailored therapeutic strategies to enhance patient care (Mutlaq et al., 2024) (Figure 2.8).

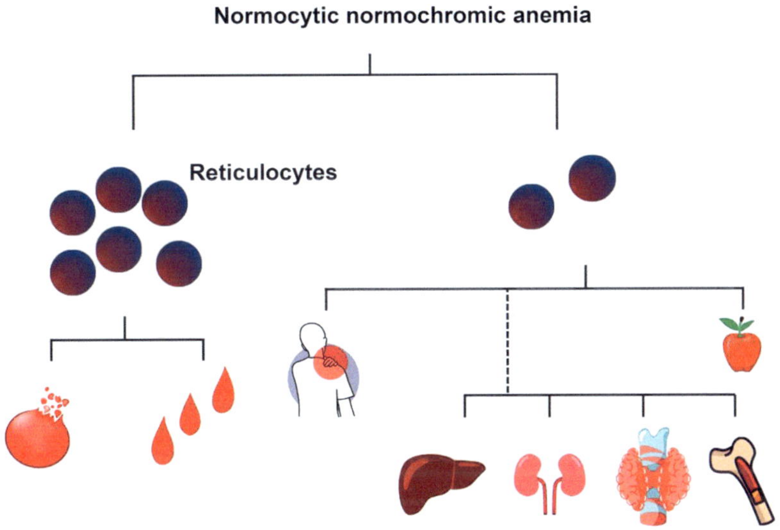

Figure 2.8. Normocytic anemia, characterized by red blood cells that are of normal size and appearance but deficient in number, presents a unique diagnostic challenge within the broader framework of anemia classification.

Source: https://www.thebloodproject.com/wp-content/uploads/2022/07/Normocytic-anemia_2.svg.

2.2.4. Hemolytic Anemia

Hemolytic anemia is a severe type of anemia in which RBCs are destroyed prematurely, leading to decreased hemoglobin content and overall oxygen-carrying capacity. Hemolytic anemia can be caused by various etiologies, including autoimmune mechanisms, in which the immune system produces antibodies against the RBCs of the same patient, such as AIHAs (Loriamini et al., 2024). Of these, warm-antibody and cold-antibody AIHAs are unique in their pathophysiologic features, as expected for the heterogeneity of this category. More recent studies have also established a potential association between viral infections, such as COVID-19, and the development of hemolytic anemia, highlighting the significance of preventing and controlling this complication in the affected population (Julia et al., 2023). Understanding of the pathophysiology and proper classification of hemolytic anemia is required to start specific treatment regimens, thereby maximizing patient outcomes and quality of care.

2.2.5. Aplastic Anemia

Aplastic anemia is a dangerous condition in which the bone marrow cannot produce adequate blood cells, with far-reaching implications for hematological well-being. In comparison to other anemias, which can be attributed to nutritional deficiency or chronic disease response, aplastic anemia is a severe, potentially life-threatening illness that may suggest the presence of more serious underlying pathology, such as infiltrative bone marrow processes or autoimmune disease (Muthuraman et al., 2010). Clinical presentations often include signs and symptoms of reduced numbers of RBCs, WBCs, and platelets, with some examples including fatigue, susceptibility to infections, and bleeding diatheses. There are also ocular manifestations, as seen in research, where a high rate of patients with blood dyscrasias, such as aplastic anemia, exhibit retinal hemorrhage and cotton-wool spots (Suhasini et al., 2017). Hence, while aplastic anemia may appear as a solitary hematologic issue, it actually indicates a complex interaction involving the overall health of the system, which requires sophisticated diagnostic evaluation and management (Figure 2.9).

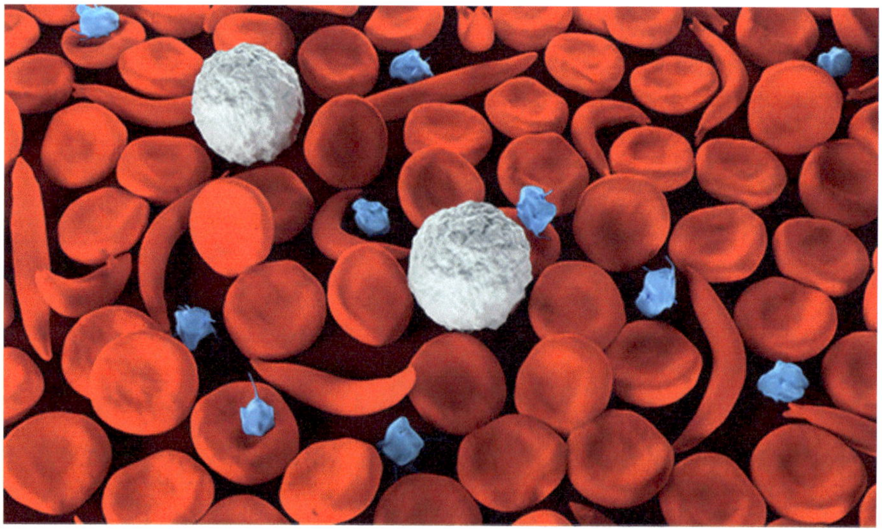

Figure 2.9. Aplastic anemia is a critical condition characterized by the failure of the bone marrow to produce adequate blood cells, leading to profound consequences across hematological health.

Source: https://www.hopkinsmedicine.org/-/media/images/health/1_-conditions/heart-and-vascular/aplastic-anemia-teaser-image.jpg.

2.2.6. Anemia of Chronic Disease (ACD)

Anemia of chronic disease (ACD) is a multifaceted disorder commonly found in patients with chronic inflammatory disorders, such as autoimmune diseases, infections, or malignancies. A combination of disordered iron metabolism and cytokine-mediated inflammation brings about the anemia in ACD. Cytokines like interleukin-6 and tumor necrosis factor-alpha bring about interference with erythropoiesis and sequestration of iron in macrophages, and hence render it unavailable for the synthesis of hemoglobin. This contrasts with iron deficiency anemia, in which iron is depleted. Although treatment involves controlling the underlying disease, an understanding of ACD pathophysiology is essential for implementing effective interventions. Of note is that ACD is chronic and tends to worsen underlying conditions since patients can present with reduced quality of life from resulting fatigue and weakness. This highlights the importance not only of treating the anemia itself, but also of addressing the underlying chronic conditions that contribute to its persistence (Abdolrahim et al., 2017; Ballas et al., 2018).

2.2.7. Iron Deficiency Anemia

Iron deficiency anemia, the most prevalent form of anemia worldwide, significantly impacts an individual's overall health and functioning. Iron deficiency anemia occurs due to a lack of sufficient iron to synthesize hemoglobin, resulting in decreased oxygen transport in the blood. The involved groups characteristically exhibit weakness, pallor, and impaired mental function, which are particularly disabling in pregnant women and growing children. As the complex interaction of all factors in iron homeostasis, hepcidin is a critical regulatory hormone that controls systemic iron availability by regulating the mobilization of iron from stores and iron absorption from the diet (Ganz et al., 2023). In certain clinical conditions, such as rare hereditary anemias, the pathophysiology can be complex, and treatment outcomes may need to be adjusted, along with the necessity for individualized therapeutic interventions (Iolascon et al., 2020). With growing recognition of the holism of iron deficiency anemia, sound management measures may become more sophisticated to address this widespread health condition holistically (Figure 2.10).

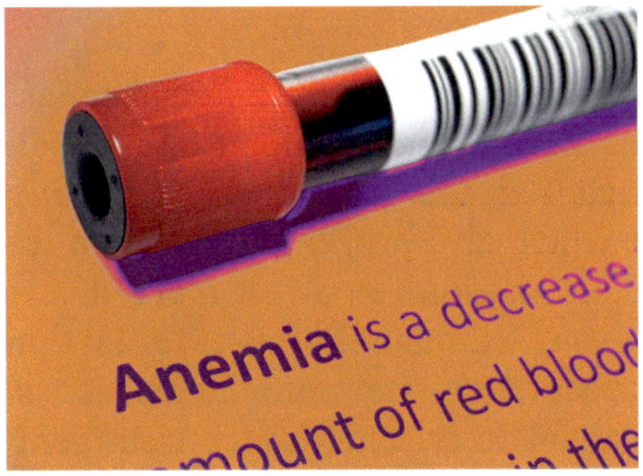

Figure 2.10. Iron deficiency anemia, one of the most prevalent forms of anemia worldwide, significantly impacts individuals health and functionality.

Source: https://nivarana.org/images/1711002829.png.

2.2.8. Vitamin B12 Deficiency Anemia

Vitamin B12 deficiency anemia constitutes a large subcategory of megaloblastic anemia due to cobalamin insufficiency, a critical vitamin in RBC and neurological metabolism. While formerly associated with pernicious anemia secondary to intrinsic factor deficiency, it is nowadays often secondary to food-bound malabsorption phenomena, emphasizing the need for increased diagnostic acuity. Symptoms can be nonspecific and include fatigue, pallor, and neurological impairment, particularly if untreated, placing the patient at risk of irreversible damage, such as degeneration of the spinal cord. The clinical response to vitamin B12 injection, whether administered intramuscularly or through oral supplementation, highlights the importance of early intervention in preventing severe complications (Sakshi et al., 2024). Additionally, there is growing worry about the interaction between high doses of folic acid and B12 deficiency, as the folate supplementation may mask anemia but exacerbate neurological complications, and hence, careful monitoring in at-risk groups is necessary (Joshua et al., 2024).

2.2.9. Sickle Cell Anemia

Sickle cell anemia, as an inherited anemia, is a problematic disease due to its complex pathophysiology and multi-organ involvement. Sickle cell anemia, resulting from a mutation of the hemoglobin gene, leads to the production of defective hemoglobin, and it makes RBCs assume a rigid sickle shape, which also prevents them from traversing narrow blood vessels. The issues that arise from this malformation can affect more than one organ system, resulting in both acute and long-term conditions. Although its relatively low prevalence in America, approximately 100,000 cases, does not attract much attention, the disease is typically under-studied, and different clinical definitions and diagnostic criteria hinder treatment approaches (Adams et al., 2009). Moreover, as ongoing initiatives by professionals in the field, comprehensive guidelines have been established to enhance the management and therapeutic interventions for patients with sickle cell disease (SCD) and other rare inherited anemias (Iolascon et al., 2020) (Figure 2.11).

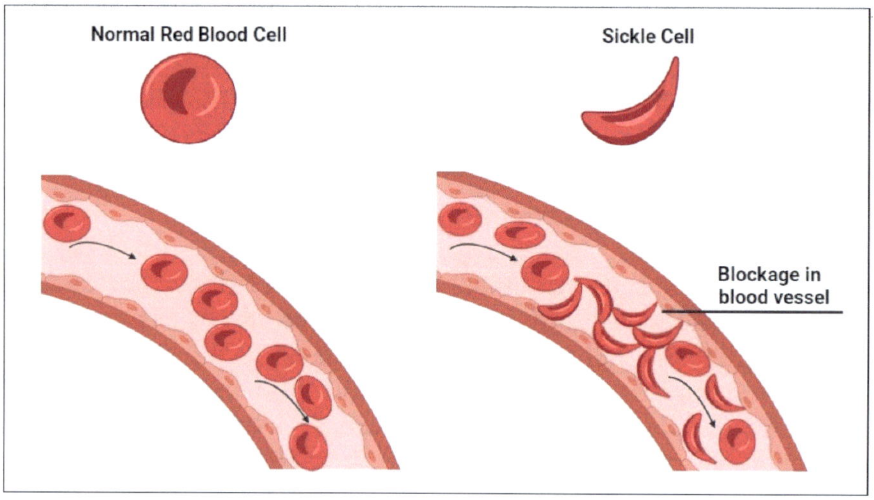

Figure 2.11. Sickle cell anemia, classified under inherited anemias, presents significant challenges due to its complex pathophysiology and multi-organ effects.

Source: https://www.mdpi.com/cimb/cimb-46-00349/article_deploy/html/images/cimb-46-00349-g001.png.

2.3. Diagnosis of Anemia

Diagnosis of anemia requires a comprehensive approach taking into consideration both physical and laboratory parameters to determine the cause. The cornerstone of this is the complete blood count (CBC), which quantifies hemoglobin, hematocrit, and RBC indices. These are employed to classify anemia as microcytic, macrocytic, or normocytic, leading to differential diagnosis by etiology. For example, iron deficiency anemia is typically microcytic in type, while vitamin B12 deficiency is characterized by microcytic RBCs, and vitamin B12 deficiency is characterized by macrocytic RBCs. Reticulocyte counts also provide insight into the bone marrow's response to anemia, further narrowing down the diagnostic process. Biochemical markers, such as serum ferritin, total iron-binding capacity, and vitamin B12 levels, also play a significant role in identifying specific deficiencies responsible for anemia. Thus, diagnosis relies on both clinical assessment and specific laboratory procedures, attesting to the complexity of managing this prevalent condition (Konorev et al., 2008; Abdolrahim et al., 2017).

2.3.1. Clinical Symptoms and Signs

The manifestations and clinical presentation of anemia are a complex interlaced tapestry of symptoms, highly variable depending on the cause and degree.

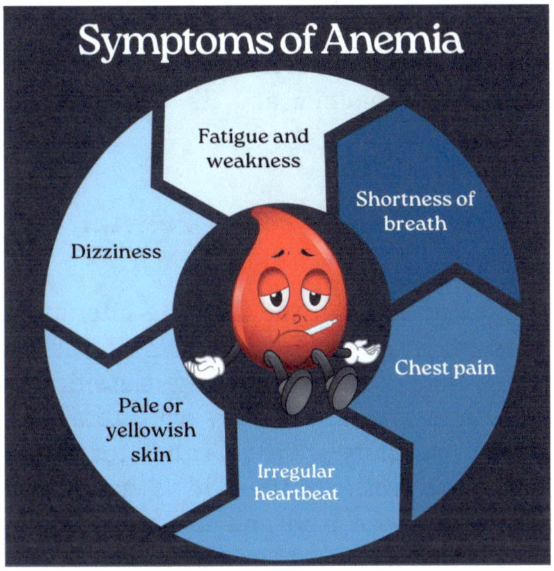

Figure 2.12. The clinical symptoms and signs of anemia present a complex tapestry of manifestations that can vary widely depending on its underlying cause and severity.

Source: https://continentalhospitals.com/uploads/mceu_98999565211701163526573.jpg.

Although pallor, weakness, and dyspnea are common signs, these occur as the body struggles to compensate for diminished tissue oxygenation. In AIHA, the patient's clinical presentation is jaundice and tea-colored urine resulting from increased bilirubin levels due to hemolysis, requiring clinical presentation for diagnosis and prompt treatment (Furmiga, 2024). Furthermore, Loeffler's cardiac syndrome, a more deleterious expression of eosinophilia, can lead to cardiac impairment in the symptoms of weakness and chest pain, emphasizing the systemic effects of hematological disorders (Silva et al., 2024). Recognition of these signs is important as they guide the clinician towards effective management, which is the core of managing the pathophysiology of anemia and enhancing patient outcome (Figure 2.12).

2.3.2. Laboratory Tests for Anemia

The diagnosis of anemia relies heavily on a variety of laboratory exams, which provide essential information regarding the pathophysiology behind the condition. Several are the CBC, serum ferritin, and reticulocyte count, all of which aid in categorizing the type of anemia and establishing its etiology. The CBC offers invaluable information about hemoglobin status and RBC indices. At the same time, the determination of serum ferritin levels is employed to evaluate the body's iron stores to distinguish ACD from iron deficiency anemia. Recent advances, such as machine learning algorithms, have also enabled the prediction of serum ferritin levels with higher precision by taking into account additional clinical parameters, thereby enhancing diagnostic accuracy (Varekha et al., 2025). Additionally, novel supervised learning methods have achieved very high precision in subclassifying anemia types, which provides an enormous advancement over traditional binary classifications (Gómez et al., 2025). These developments underscore the evolving situation of laboratory diagnostics in anemia treatment.

2.3.3. Complete Blood Count (CBC) Analysis

The CBC test is a fundamental diagnostic test in hematology, particularly for the diagnosis of anemias. Through the measurement of various blood components, including RBCs, hemoglobin, and hematocrit levels, the CBC provides valuable information about a person's hematologic status. This broad analysis proves its worth in identifying not just the occurrence of anemia, but also its likely causes, ranging from dietary insufficiencies to genetic conditions such as CSA with genetic mutations in heme synthesis pathways and iron metabolism routes (Crispin et al., 2017). Additionally, technological advances in CBC have transformed the analytical process from manual to sophisticated automated systems capable of gathering large amounts of multiparameter data (d'Onofrio et al., 2021). Consequently, CBC analysis not only aids in anemia categorization but also improves understanding of their pathophysiology, ultimately culminating in appropriate therapeutic interventions (Figure 2.13).

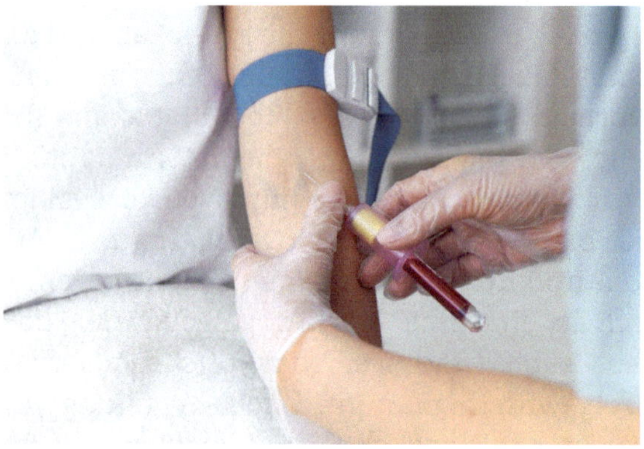

Figure 2.13. The complete blood count (CBC) analysis is a fundamental diagnostic tool in hematology, particularly in the assessment of anemias.

Source: https://www.makatimed.net.ph/wp-content/uploads/2024/06/viber_image_2024-06-20_09-42-21-814.jpg.

2.3.4. Reticulocyte Count

Reticulocyte count is a critical laboratory result in the workup of anemias, and it is a measure of the bone marrow's response to erythropoietic stimuli. The reticulocyte count generally increases when there is increased RBC production, such as in compensatory states, such as hemolytic anemia or acute blood loss. A low reticulocyte count may sometimes reflect ineffective erythropoiesis, secondary to chronic disease or nutritional insufficiency. In HIV disease, anemia is usually a complication, and reticulocyte count is enlightening regarding the pathophysiology, particularly for differentiating among conditions of anemia, for example, ACD (Groer et al., 2002). Furthermore, reticulocyte counts can be influenced by sample handling and the measurement method employed, emphasizing the importance of optimized measurement processes in accurately estimating reticulocyte counts (Bauer et al., 2016). This multi-dimensioned assessment of reticulocyte counts makes anemia and its subtypes more clinically relevant.

2.3.5. Iron Studies and Ferritin Levels

An understanding of the intricate interactions of iron studies and ferritin levels is crucial to anemia diagnosis as well as its classification. Iron studies include serum iron, total iron-binding capacity (TIBC), and ferritin, a protein that reflects the body's iron stores. Decreased serum iron and ferritin levels are characteristic findings in iron deficiency anemia, particularly in specific groups of individuals, such as menstruating women and children with nutritional problems. Recent research highlights the importance of serum tests, revealing strong statistical correlations between reduced ferritin concentrations and various diseases, including early childhood caries and anemia (Atri et al., 2023; Farrokhnia et al., 2024). The ability to use these iron indicators within clinics enables the early detection and treatment of anemia, underscoring the importance of regular screenings in high-risk groups. As research advances, the pooling of data from multiple studies will increasingly clarify the role of iron metabolism in anemia classifications (Figure 2.14).

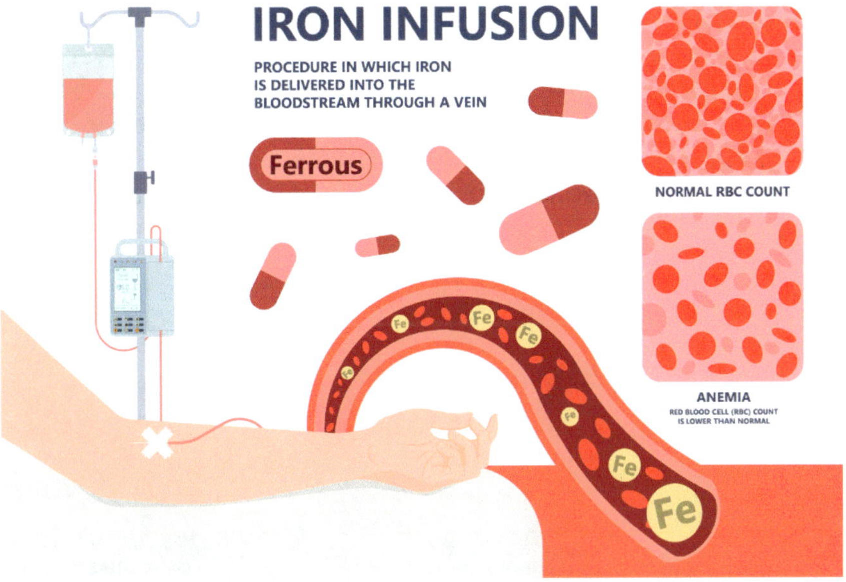

Figure 2.14. Low serum iron and ferritin levels are hallmark indicators of iron deficiency anemia, which is particularly prevalent among specific populations, such as menstruating women and children suffering from nutritional challenges.

Source: https://www.parsemus.org/wp-content/uploads/2022/08/shutterstock_1928198045.png.

2.3.6. Bone Marrow Biopsy

Bone marrow biopsy is an essential diagnostic procedure in the assessment of anemia, particularly when the pathogenic mechanisms are not obviously visible or are multifactorial. Bone marrow sampling involves the collection of bone marrow samples, allowing clinicians to assess hematopoietic cell populations, cell morphology, and the marrow microenvironmental architecture. Such precise analysis is necessary to distinguish between various forms of anemia—aplastic anemia to those secondary to malignancies, such as leukemias. It is also required for identifying secondary causes, such as myelodysplastic syndromes or chemotherapy-induced effects on blood cell production. Understanding the pathophysiology of these changes is essential, especially in consideration of the correlation between immune responses at a systemic level and hematology disorders, as exemplified by studies concerning the immune-mediated etiology of conditions like graft-versus-host disease, which underscore the complexity of anemic presentations (Baloglu et al., 2014). Bone marrow biopsy thus remains a mainstay in the precise classification and management of anemia (Konorev et al., 2008).

2.3.7. Genetic Testing for Hereditary Anemias

Genetic evaluation has become a pivotal tool in the diagnosis and management of hereditary anemias (HAs), a clinically heterogeneous group of diseases that share a unifying genetic etiology. These disorders, such as congenital dyserythropoietic anemias (CDAs) and SCD, generally present with complex clinical findings that are challenging for traditional diagnostic methods. The application of next-generation sequencing (NGS) has significantly enhanced diagnostic accuracy, revealing that a substantial number of patients initially presumed to have CDAs may, in fact, have other types of HAs, such as pyruvate kinase deficiency (Marra et al., 2021). Moreover, genetic testing not only enables the identification of specific mutations, thereby providing the basis for personalized therapeutic interventions, but also elucidates the pathophysiologic processes of these disorders (Iolascon et al., 2020). Therefore, the integration of genetic testing into clinical practice is crucial for effective management and treatment of hereditary anemias, leading to improved patient outcomes (Figure 2.15).

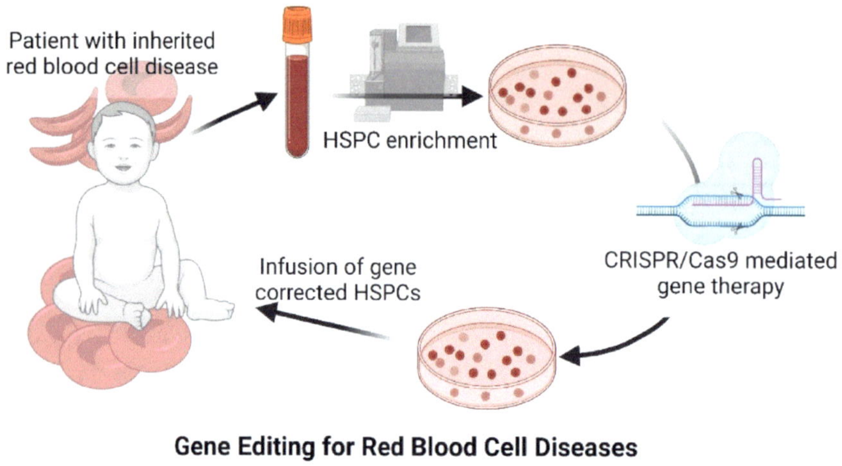

Figure 2.15. Genetic testing has emerged as a pivotal tool in the diagnosis and management of hereditary anemias (HAs), a diverse group of disorders characterized by their genetic underpinnings.

Source: https://www.frontiersin.org/files/Articles/848261/fphys-13-848261-HTML/image_m/fphys-13-848261-g001.jpg.

2.3.8. Differential Diagnosis Considerations

Careful differential diagnosis is crucial in the identification of the cause of anemia in a patient, as various causes have different management strategies. Anemia may be produced by various mechanisms, including nutritional deficits, chronic diseases, or genetic disorders. For instance, iron deficiency anemia, characterized by low serum ferritin and high total iron-binding capacity, must be distinguished from ACD, where iron stores are typically normal but bioavailability is impaired due to inflammatory mechanisms. Furthermore, congenital disorders like the CSA highlight the complexity of diagnosis; disruptions in heme biosynthesis can lead to distinctive findings of a peripheral blood smear and bone marrow biopsy, e.g., aberrant iron deposition in erythroid precursors (Crispin et al., 2017). As put by the World Health Organization, explicit case definitions are essential in documenting epidemiology and guiding appropriate clinical interventions.

2.3.9. Importance of Accurate Diagnosis

Accurate diagnosis is critical in the management of anemia since misclassification can lead to inappropriate treatment interventions with damaging consequences. Anemias can result from many different underlying mechanisms, including nutritional deficiencies, chronic illness, and genetic disorders. They must thus be known correctly in terms of their causes for proper management. For instance, misclassifying iron deficiency anemia as ACD can lead to excessive delays in administering appropriate iron supplementation, with adverse outcomes for the patient. Additionally, diagnostic tests for other conditions, such as diabetes mellitus, highlight the function of advanced diagnostic agents. Glycosylated proteins, such as Hemoglobin A1c, provide data on long-term conditions, and it is argued that they could also enable anemia classification and management (Abdolrahim et al., 2017). In complex cases where there are unorthodox presentations, complete diagnostic tests can prevent missing underlying disorders, thereby improving patient care and outcomes overall (Bateni et al., 2018) (Figure 2.16).

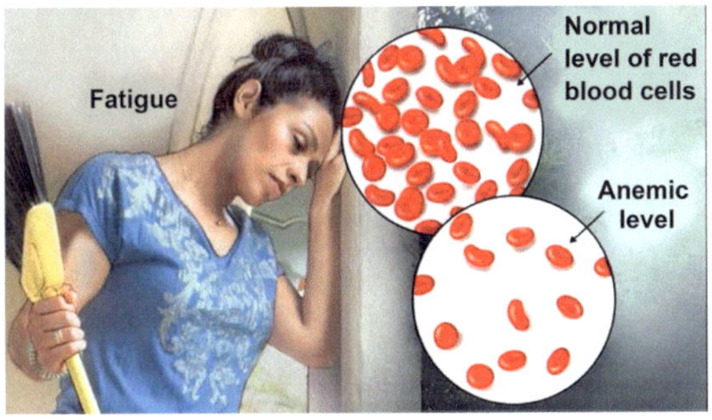

Figure 2.16. Accurate diagnosis is crucial in the management of anemias, as misclassification can lead to inappropriate treatment strategies with potentially detrimental results.

Source: https://healthjade.net/wp-content/uploads/2018/01/anemia.jpg.

2.4. Treatment and Management of Anemia

Its management and therapy demand a proper understanding of its underlying pathophysiology and etiologies. For anemia associated with chronic kidney disease (CKD), for instance, anemia is due primarily to erythropoietin deficiency and dysregulation of iron (Badura et al., 2024). Therapy typically consists of erythropoiesis-stimulating agents (ESAs) plus iron supplementation to correct deficiencies and improve hemoglobin levels. Furthermore, new developments point towards the promise of the utilization of hypoxia-inducible factor-prolyl hydroxylase inhibitors (HIF-PHI) as novel therapeutic approaches that induce erythropoiesis through the body's response to hypoxia. More generally, awareness of the patient's individual anemia etiology—whether due to nutritional deficits, chronic inflammation, or other causes—is also helpful in directing therapy. Conducting a thorough assessment enables a patient-tailored treatment plan, resulting in enhanced patient outcomes and quality of life (Siopi et al., 2024).

2.4.1. Dietary Modifications and Supplementation

Dietary modifications and supplements play a crucial role in managing the majority of cases of anemia, particularly iron-deficiency anemia. Clinical practice guidelines recommend a first-line approach that involves enhancing dietary iron intake through the consumption of red meat, green leafy vegetables, and fortified cereals to sustainably increase hemoglobin levels. Nutritional education is required; awareness of factors impacting iron absorption, such as the synergistic effect of vitamin C when co-ingested with iron, can enhance therapeutic outcomes. Ferrous sulfate or other iron salts supplementation is also typically prescribed for individuals who cannot obtain sufficient iron from their diet. Recent studies have also demonstrated that molecular docking techniques can be utilized to identify specific nutrients in the diet that are likely to interact with the biochemical pathways of anemia (Agu et al., 2023), potentially leading to personalized nutritional treatments. Lastly, incorporating dietary intervention with appropriate supplementation is a comprehensive method for combating anemia and achieving overall health benefits (José et al., 2023) (Figure 2.17).

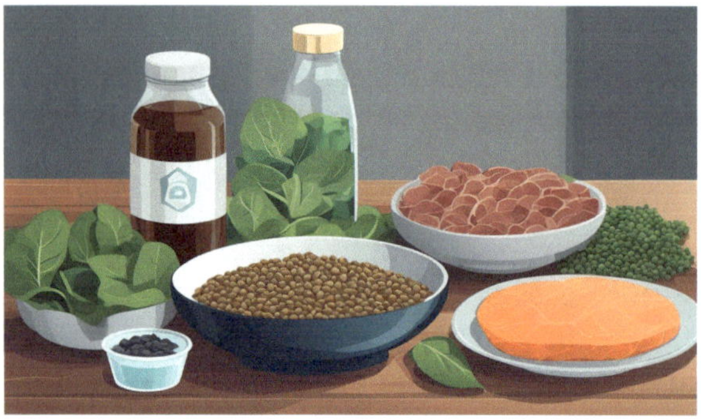

Figure 2.17. Dietary modifications and supplementation play a crucial role in the management of various types of anemia, particularly iron-deficiency anemia.

Source: https://images.squarespace-cdn.com/content/v1/62e7a92f066fa3730dcd4604/aab30672-6c13-4d95-9c3b-9c0c70348e91/4.jpg.

2.4.2. Pharmacological Treatments

Pharmacologic treatments of anemias target the pathophysiologic mechanisms responsible for restoring erythropoiesis and improving patient outcomes. In diseases like myelodysplastic syndromes (MDS), studies have demonstrated the utility of iron modulation; more specifically, treatment with vamifeport has been found to be effective in alleviating anemia and enhancing RBC maturation by mitigating oxidative stress and apoptosis in erythroid progenitors (Antypiuk et al., 2024). This therapy approach not only alleviated iron overload, a common issue in the majority of anemias, but also underscored the importance of individualized treatment protocols. In addition, in anemia related to heart failure, surveillance and therapy using erythropoiesis-stimulating agents can significantly enhance both hemoglobin levels and quality of life (Siopi et al., 2024). Thus, the application of pharmacologic therapy to treat anemia not only improves hematologic parameters but also considers the complex interplay between various disease processes, highlighting their multifactorial nature.

2.4.3. Blood Transfusions

Blood transfusions are highly crucial in the management of many forms of anemia, particularly in situations where it is critically needed to augment RBC counts. It is a medical therapy that rapidly improves tissue oxygenation, thereby eliminating symptoms of anemia such as weakness and breathlessness. Blood transfusions are essential in the treatment of acute anemia, in which patients receive profound physiological deficits that must be treated quickly in order not to develop complications.

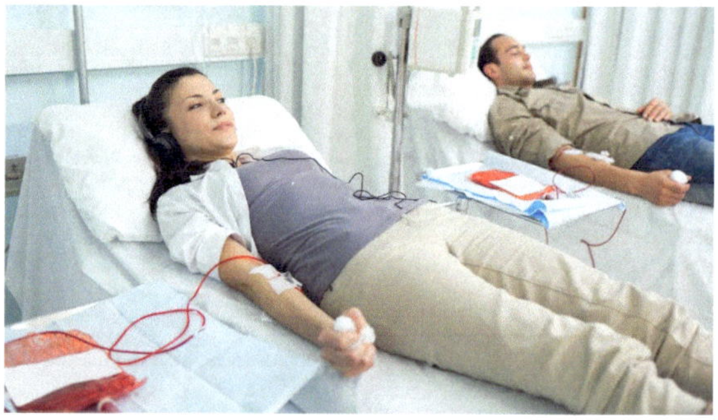

Figure 2.18. Blood transfusions play a critical role in managing various types of anemia, particularly in situations where rapid restoration of red blood cell (RBC) levels is necessary.

Source: https://i0.wp.com/post.medicalnewstoday.com/wp-content/uploads/sites/3/2020/06/GettyImages-151340032_header-1024x575.jpg?w=1155&h=1528.

Furthermore, the progress made in the field of transfusion medicine, as outlined in the EHA Roadmap, points to the importance of individualized strategies according to the specific hematological features of the patient and the type of treated anemia, including orphan genetic anemias and acquired anemias (Iolascon et al., 2020). These target therapies, combined with conventional transfusions, represent a systemic approach to anemia therapy that highlights the need for ongoing research to further improve these practices (Allard et al., 2016) (Figure 2.18).

2.4.4. Management of Underlying Conditions

Management of underlying diseases is most important in the case of anemias, since these diseases are usually caused by or exacerbated by chronic conditions. For example, patients with chronic cardiovascular disease or chronic renal disease often present with multiple forms of anemia, and treatment should address both the anemia and the underlying causes (Schwartz et al., 2005). In the case of SCD, where anemia is a consequence of a genetic disorder, an understanding of the complexity of the disease's pathophysiology becomes central to effective management (Adams et al., 2009). Tailoring interventions to incorporate consideration of comorbidities not only improves patient outcomes but enhances the overall understanding of anemia's multifactorial nature. Therefore, a multimodal strategy that addresses, first and foremost, the management of these underlying illnesses is necessary to prevent the exacerbation of anemia and enhance quality of life in affected individuals.

2.4.5. Role of Erythropoietin-Stimulating Agents (ESAs)

Erythropoietin-stimulating agents (ESAs) play a critical role in the management of most types of anemia, particularly those caused by the absence of normal erythropoiesis, such as ACD and certain MDSs. ESAs are mimics of the action of the hormone erythropoietin, which is secreted nearly exclusively by the kidneys, and that acts to stimulate erythropoiesis in the bone marrow. By stimulating erythropoiesis, ESAs can improve symptoms related to anemia, including fatigue and reduced exercise capacity. Their use is not, however, free of complications, as ESA administration has been associated with adverse effects related to iron metabolism. Higher hepcidin levels, for instance, can be caused by inflammation or iron overload, leading to a restriction of iron availability for hemoglobin synthesis and compromised erythropoietin-stimulated action (Ganz et al., 2023). Also, blood-transfusion subjects who are frequently subjected to it will acquire toxic iron with additional effects and reduced survival (Bagguley et al., 2017). Thus, while ESAs are an essential part of the treatment of anemia, careful regulation of iron status and monitoring of the patient are crucial to optimize outcomes (Figure 2.19).

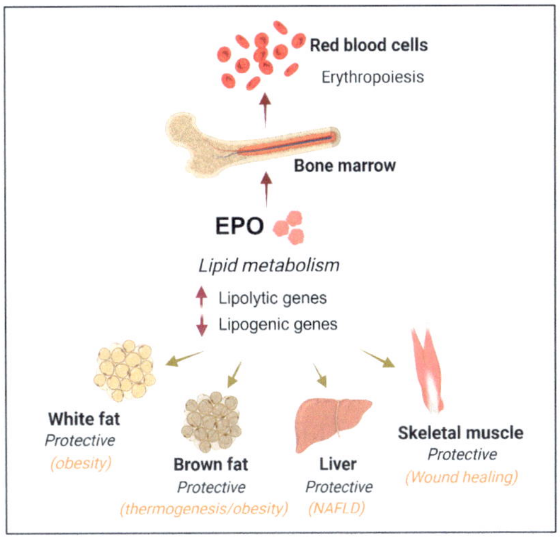

Figure 2.19. Erythropoietin-stimulating agents (ESAs) play a crucial role in the management of various types of anemia.

Source: https://www.mdpi.com/cells/cells-14-00280/article_deploy/html/images/cells-14-00280-g001.png.

2.4.6. Patient Education and Lifestyle Changes

Effective patient education is an integral aspect of managing anemia since it enables patients to make well-informed decisions about their well-being and enact significant lifestyle adjustments. Education regarding the nature of the type of anemia, whether iron deficiency or vitamin B12 deficiency, can significantly impact dietary intake and adherence to recommended interventions. Dietary counseling should focus on consuming iron-rich foods, such as red meat, legumes, and iron-enriched cereals, which can help alleviate the symptoms of low hemoglobin. Healthy lifestyle modifications, such as a daily exercise regimen and avoiding known iron-blocking substances, including excessive caffeine consumption and certain medications, are also critical. Alongside dietary adjustments, understanding the role of follow-up care and monitoring can convert patients into active participants in their therapy and thus improve clinical outcomes. Coordination of these educational components forms a comprehensive strategy for treating anemia and enhances patient quality of life (Araujo et al., 2006; Konorev et al., 2008).

2.4.7. Monitoring and Follow-up Care

Careful monitoring and follow-up after treatment are active components in the management of anemia, as they directly impact patient outcomes and allow for individualized therapeutic approaches. Regular checking of hematological parameters, including hemoglobin concentration and red blood cell indices, is valuable in monitoring both cure and complications. Particularly, conditions such as Rh isoimmunization highlight the need for close monitoring since secondary issues result in severe perinatal and neonatal care problems that detract from both maternal and fetal health. Preventive strategies, such as the administration of Rho (D) immune globulin (RIG), reflect the need for follow-up interventions to mitigate the risks of hemolytic disease of the newborn. Hence, the inclusion of overall surveillance strategies in the plan for anemia management not only ensures safety but also encourages better clinical outcomes, substantiating the merit of continuous patient evaluation (Hanson et al., 2003; Konorev et al., 2008) (Figure 2.20).

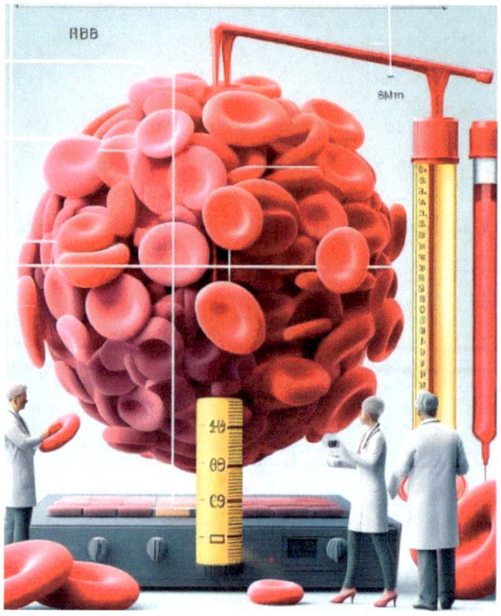

Figure 2.20. Regular assessments of hematological parameters, including hemoglobin levels and red cell indices, are crucial for evaluating treatment efficacy and identifying potential complications.

Source: https://www.mdpi.com/medicina/medicina-59-02124/article_deploy/html/images/medicina-59-02124-g001.png.

2.4.8. Challenges in Treatment Adherence

Adherence to treatment in the situation of various anemias, particularly illnesses like beta-thalassemia, is a cause of grave concern with adverse effects on patient outcomes. These are more likely to result from long-term treatment, which may require multiple blood transfusions and iron chelation to prevent iron overload. For instance, while diagnostic and therapeutic advances have improved the prognosis of transfusion-dependent thalassemia, disparities in treatment access remain, especially in resource-limited regions (Farmakis et al., 2022).

Moreover, psychological burden and frequent follow-up needs may lead to non-adherence, which makes clinical management more difficult and reduces the effectiveness of treatment. In addition, the American Diabetes Association guidelines emphasize patient-centered care, aiming to address not only the medical but also the psychosocial determinants of adherence. Thus, multifaceted care models are to be developed in an effort to enhance treatment adherence and improve patient health outcomes for anemias.

2.4.9. Future Directions in Anemia Management

The direction of anemia treatment in the future is poised for revolution with the help of advancements in research and innovation. An increased understanding of anemia's multifactorial etiology will enable clinicians to tailor treatment even more effectively for different patient groups. More recent therapeutic approaches will utilize genomic profiling to select patient-specific therapy, thereby increasing efficacy and minimizing adverse effects. Furthermore, initiatives such as the European Hematology Association (EHA) Roadmap emphasize the importance of targeted research in addressing unmet clinical needs in treating anemia. This research may include the development of new therapies and the personalization of therapy regimens based on individual genetic backgrounds (Allard et al., 2016). In addition, the establishment of standard definitions and diagnostic criteria will make possible more precise comparisons of treatment results, crucial for better anemia care methods (Adams et al., 2009). Together, these developments underscore the need for ongoing advancements in anemia management paradigms as scientific knowledge evolves.

A CLOSER LOOK

ERYTHROPOIESIS

Erythropoiesis is the production of red blood cells (erythrocytes) within the body. It occurs primarily in the bone marrow and is regulated by the hormone erythropoietin, which is mainly produced by the kidneys in response to low blood oxygen levels. The procedure begins from HSCs, which become erythroid progenitor cells and then mature into fully functional RBCs. These cells are released into the bloodstream and live for about 120 days. Erythropoiesis plays a crucial role in supplying adequate oxygenation to tissues and responding to situations like anemia or blood loss.

SUMMARY

An understanding of the pathophysiology and classification of anemias is key to the effective diagnosis and management of this multifaceted group of conditions. Anemias can be caused by diverse etiologic factors, including nutritional factors, chronic conditions, and genetic causes, each contributing a variable degree of hematological impairment. Classification based on the etiology not only helps in directed treatment methods but also enhances the clinician's capability to predict complications and the outcome of the patient. Furthermore, emerging research is increasingly clarifying the intricate mechanisms involved, as demonstrated by recent studies defining vascular involvement in similar pathologies, including bulbar urethral necrosis (Joshi et al., 2025) and neurophysiological changes in patients with migraines (Sebastianelli et al., 2025). As our understanding of anemia evolves, so too should the approaches to treating it, so that they are attuned to underlying biology and to the individual patient's needs.

The data on the pathophysiology and classification of anemias indicate a complex interaction between the determinants of clinical presentation and etiology of this blood disorder. Most relevant are the arguments that indicate anemias occur due to either the lack of RBC production or loss in excess, and that there exist certain classifications, such as microcytic, macrocytic, and normocytic anemias, that can guide diagnosis and treatment. Recent literature emphasizes the importance of identifying pathogen-specific processes in anemia etiology, suggesting that secondary causes, such as chronic infection, can lead to a complex presentation (Ramesh et al., 2025). Additionally, in certain congenital conditions, such as congenital portosystemic shunts (CPSS), anemia often accompanies other systemic derangements, including liver dysfunction (Konstantinidis et al., 2023). These findings underscore the necessity for a multidisciplinary approach in diagnosing and treating anemias, so that both primary and secondary causes are adequately addressed to optimally treat the patient.

REFERENCES

1. Yazdanpanah, S., Rabiee, M., Tahriri, M., Abdolrahim, M., Rajab, A., Jazayeri, H. E., & Tayebi, L. (2017). Evaluation of glycated albumin (GA) and GA/HbA1c ratio for diagnosis of diabetes and glycemic control: A comprehensive review. Critical Reviews in Clinical Laboratory Sciences, 54(4), 219–232. https://doi.org/10.1080/10408363.2017.1299684
2. Agu, P. C., Afiukwa, C. A., Orji, O. U., Ezeh, E. M., Ofoke, I. H., Ogbu, C. O., Ugwuja, E. I., et al. (2023). Molecular docking as a tool for the discovery of molecular targets of nutraceuticals in diseases management. Scientific Reports, 13. https://doi.org/10.1038/s41598-023-40160-2 (accessed on 12th June 2025).
3. Allhorn, M., Bülow, L., Gram, M., et al. (2012). Pathological conditions involving extracellular hemoglobin: Molecular mechanisms, clinical significance, and novel therapeutic opportunities for alpha(1)-microglobulin. https://core.ac.uk/download/83748016.pdf (accessed on 12th June 2025).
4. Antypiuk, A., Vance, S., Sharma, R., Passos, S. T., Asperti, M., Navaneethabalakrishnan, S., Durrenberger, F., et al. (2024). Genetic iron overload aggravates and pharmacological iron restriction improves MDS pathophysiology in a preclinical study. Blood. https://www.semanticscholar.org/paper/057592c91e192012ac25a2f6af6268acdf6bd709 (accessed on 12th June 2025).
5. Araujo, L. F., de Matos Soeiro, A., Fernandes, J. L., et al. (2006). Coronary artery disease in women: A review on prevention, pathophysiology, diagnosis, and treatment. https://core.ac.uk/download/pdf/7711531.pdf (accessed on 12th June 2025).
6. Atri, Y., Garg, N., Pathivada, L., Kaur, H., & Yeluri, R. (2023). Association between serum iron, serum ferritin levels, and severe early childhood caries: A case–control study. International Journal of Clinical Pediatric Dentistry, 16, 288–292. https://www.semanticscholar.org/paper/d81bfeac9c27731d1148fd6dee18cdbc26b8a607 (accessed on 12th June 2025).
7. Badura, K., Janc, J., Wąsik, J., Gnitecki, S., Skwira, S., Młynarska, E., Rysz, J., et al. (2024). Anemia of chronic kidney disease—A narrative review of its pathophysiology, diagnosis, and management. Biomedicines, 12. https://www.semanticscholar.org/paper/47c222851a11c0973dca7c2d04170d1ffc5b7833 (accessed on 12th June 2025).
8. Bagguley, T., Blijlevens, N., Bowen, D., et al. (2017). Labile plasma iron levels predict survival in patients with lower-risk myelodysplastic syndromes. https://core.ac.uk/download/132212833.pdf (accessed on 12th June 2025).
9. Ballas, S. K. (2018). Comorbidities in aging patients with sickle cell disease. https://core.ac.uk/download/213438652.pdf (accessed on 12th June 2025).
10. Ballas, S. K., Lieff, S., Benjamin, L. J., Dampier, C. D., Heeney, M. M., Hoppe, C., Johnson, C. S., Rogers, Z. R., Smith-Whitley, K., Wang, W. C., Telen, M. J., & Investigators, Comprehensive Sickle Cell Centers. (2010). Definitions of the phenotypic manifestations of sickle cell disease. American Journal of Hematology, 85(1), 6–13. https://doi.org/10.1002/ajh.21550 (accessed on 12th June 2025).
11. Baloglu, O., McArthur, J., & Rowan, C. (2014). Non-infectious pulmonary complications of hematopoietic stem cell transplantation. https://core.ac.uk/download/228066089.pdf (accessed on 12th June 2025).

12. Bateni, C. P., Canter, R. J., Darrow, M. A., et al. (2018). Retroperitoneal extramedullary hematopoietic pseudotumor in ataxia-telangiectasia. https://core.ac.uk/download/323070540.pdf (accessed on 12th June 2025).

13. Bauer, N., Ginder, M., Johannes, S., et al. (2016). Optimized gating and reference ranges of reticulated platelets in dogs for the Sysmex XT-2000iV. https://core.ac.uk/download/84118343.pdf (accessed on 12th June 2025).

14. Coello García, B. E., Cantos Pesántez, M. P., Yascaribay González, J. P., Cobos Calle, J. I., Ortiz Álvarez, S. B., Berrezueta Rodríguez, D. M., Cabrera Castillo, B. X., et al. (2024). Updated analysis and review of hallux valgus, clinical case description, etiology, epidemiology, pathophysiology, clinical evaluation, concomitant disorders, radiographic approach, imaging classification systems, treatment, prognosis and complications. EPRA International Journal of Multidisciplinary Research (IJMR). https://www.semanticscholar.org/paper/d5a17125a12a73bfef7a608e3d1faaad85146be0 (accessed on 12th June 2025).

15. Connaughton, D. M., Bhai, P., Isenring, P., Mahdi, M., Sadikovic, B., & Schenkel, L. (2023). Genotypic analysis of a large cohort of patients with suspected atypical hemolytic uremic syndrome. Journal of Molecular Medicine (Berlin, Germany), 101, 1029–1040. https://www.semanticscholar.org/paper/ed20cc93e0fef2c06297ddfcafa2ec4541b0ef02 (accessed on 12th June 2025).

16. Crispin, A. (2017). HSCB, a co-chaperone in mitochondrial iron-sulfur cluster biogenesis, is a novel candidate gene for congenital sideroblastic anemia. https://open.bu.edu/bitstream/2144/26669/5/Crispin_bu_0017N_13280.pdf (accessed on 12th June 2025).

17. d'Onofrio, G. (2021). Full-field hemocytometry. Forty years of progress seen through Clinical and Laboratory Hematology and the International Journal of Laboratory Hematology. https://core.ac.uk/download/604623263.pdf (accessed on 12th June 2025).

18. Engert, A., Balduini, C., Brand, A., Coiffier, B., Cordonnier, C., Döhner, H., Duyvené de Wit, T., Eichinger, S., Fibbe, W., Green, T., de Haas, F., Iolascon, A., Jaffredo, T., Rodeghiero, F., Salles, G., Schuringa, J. J., & EHA Roadmap for European Hematology Research. (2016). The European Hematology Association roadmap for European hematology research: A consensus document. Haematologica, 101(2), 115–208. https://doi.org/10.3324/haematol.2015.136739 (accessed on 12th June 2025).

19. Farmakis, D., Porter, J. B., Taher, A., Cappellini, M. D., Angastiniotis, M., & Eleftheriou, A. (2022). 2021 Thalassemia International Federation guidelines for the management of transfusion-dependent thalassemia. Hemisphere, 6, e732–e732. https://doi.org/10.1097/hs9.0000000000000732 (accessed on 12th June 2025).

20. Farrokhnia, T., Shoorgashti, R., Sadeghian, M., Hasanzade, S., Lesan, S., & Hedayati, M. (2024). Comparative analysis of serum and saliva iron, ferritin, and TIBC in women with iron deficiency anemia: Highlighting saliva's screening potential. Middle East Journal of Rehabilitation and Health Studies. https://www.semanticscholar.org/paper/761377847ad3387f5080e687b0acd3d68e2b059e (accessed on 12th June 2025).

21. Furmiga, I. S. L. (2024). Diagnostic laboratorial das anemias hemolytic autoimmune. Absolute Review. https://www.semanticscholar.org/paper/650d9fbd233b20ccab47d3b595a9c1138c5a82dc (accessed on 12th June 2025).

22. Ganz, T., & Nemeth, E. (2023). Hepcidin and iron in health and disease. https://core.ac.uk/download/573387980.pdf (accessed on 12th June 2025).

23. Gómez, J., Parra Urueta, C., Salas-Álvarez, D., Hernández Riaño, V., & Ramírez-González, G. A. (2025). Anemia classification system using machine learning. Informatics, 12, 19. https://www.semanticscholar.org/paper/135f4f046e648306d69794def187091bcde76482 (accessed on 12th June 2025).

24. Hanson, L., Harrod, K. S., Heywood, P., et al. (2003). Rh negative status and isoimmunization update: A case-based approach to care. https://core.ac.uk/download/213075292.pdf (accessed on 12th June 2025).

25. Iolascon, A., Taher, A. T., Gulbis, B., Matar, C. F., Bencaiova, G. A., Forni, G., Tamary, H., et al. (2020). Recommendations for pregnancy in rare inherited anemias. https://core.ac.uk/download/373375214.pdf (accessed on 12th June 2025).

26. Jajoo, S. S., Zamwar, U. M., & Nagrale, P. H. (2024). Etiology, clinical manifestations, diagnosis, and treatment of cobalamin (vitamin B12) deficiency. Cureus, 16. https://www.semanticscholar.org/paper/2e77987419d7e283622343383f16122439676b13 (accessed on 12th June 2025).

27. Joglar, J. A., Chung, M. K., Armbruster, A. L., Benjamin, E. J., Chyou, J. Y., Cronin, E. M., Deswal, A., et al. (2023). 2023 ACC/AHA/ACCP/HRS guideline for the diagnosis and management of atrial fibrillation: A report of the American College of Cardiology/American Heart Association Joint Committee on Clinical Practice Guidelines. Circulation, 149. https://doi.org/10.1161/cir.0000000000001193 (accessed on 12th June 2025).

28. Joshi, P., Navarro, J., Ocampo, M. A., De Win, G., Filip, T., Wood, D., Bhadranavar, S., et al. (2025). Bulbar urethral necrosis: Current concept and novel comprehensive classification. BJU International. https://www.semanticscholar.org/paper/6ef420ff4f3bda38ec9a96bd069677dd08b00d29 (accessed on 12th June 2025).

29. Kononowicz, J. E., Ali, M. F., Palko, W., Pyper, S., & Agasthya, N. (2023). Rapidly progressing autoimmune hemolytic anemia in a pediatric patient with COVID-19. Cureus, 15. https://www.semanticscholar.org/paper/78c01c4d73b4089ccfa195afa98713e3cecb75ac (accessed on 12th June 2025).

30. Konorev, M. R. (2008). Lecture Notes by Internal Diseases. https://core.ac.uk/download/80150474.pdf (accessed on 12th June 2025).

31. Konstantinidis, A., Patsikas, M., Papazoglou, L., & Adamama-Moraitou, K. (2023). Congenital portosystemic shunts in dogs and cats: Classification, pathophysiology, clinical presentation and diagnosis. Veterinary Sciences, 10. https://www.semanticscholar.org/paper/dea163e17634fc2e03834f9701ec52d7b96f99a9 (accessed on 12th June 2025).

32. Kraevsky-Phillips, K., Ji, R. Q., Thangavel, S., & Al-Zaiti, S. (2024). Abstract 4139307: Machine learning identifies predictors of poor outcomes in patients with heart failure presenting to the emergency department for chest pain. Circulation. https://www.semanticscholar.org/paper/d65837f96687917d6815ff4f73adcbc9281b44cf (accessed on 12th June 2025).

33. Loriamini, M., Cserti-Gazdewich, C., & Branch, D. R. (2024). Autoimmune hemolytic anemias: Classifications, pathophysiology, diagnoses and management. International Journal of Molecular Sciences, 25. https://www.semanticscholar.org/paper/c078553c98f1f6ffca39999103ec7c95b9657ec8 (accessed on 12th June 2025).

34. Maciel, T. T., Sbeih, N., Rignault-Bricard, R., Chevalme, I., Allali, S., Brochier, C., Kiialainen, A., et al. (2024). Complement activation and its implication in the pathophysiology of hemolytic anemia and aging in mouse models of sickle cell disease and beta-thalassemia. Blood. https://www.semanticscholar.org/paper/ad026d73aa6982d6946ea368841cf75b3cee51cf (accessed on 12th June 2025).

35. Mardari, I. I., Mălăncuș, R., & Pavel, G. (2017). Hematological diagnosis of anemia in dogs and cats. https://core.ac.uk/download/428341947.pdf (accessed on 12th June 2025).

36. Marra, R. (2021). Dissecting the Molecular Genetics and Pathogenesis of Hereditary Dyserythropoietic Anemias. https://core.ac.uk/download/574199335.pdf (accessed on 12th June 2025).

37. Miller, J. W., Smith, A., Troen, A., Mason, J. B., Jacques, P. F., & Selhub, J. (2024). Excess folic acid and vitamin B12 deficiency: Clinical implications? Food and Nutrition Bulletin, 45, S67–S72. https://www.semanticscholar.org/paper/39fd33b1102e0ccc01dfd5c5c82db5381bc10a97 (accessed on 12th June 2025).

38. Mocan, D., Jipa, R., Jipa, D. A., Lala, R., Rasinar, F. C., Groza, I. M., Sabau, R., et al. (2025). Unveiling the systemic impact of congestion in heart failure: A narrative review of multisystem pathophysiology and clinical implications. Journal of Cardiovascular Development and Disease, 12. https://www.semanticscholar.org/paper/aaba71583513782a192175f71351f4d2a0df1a69 (accessed on 12th June 2025).

39. Muthuraman, M. (2010). Evaluation of morphological patterns of anemia in children. https://core.ac.uk/download/235652851.pdf (accessed on 12th June 2025).

40. Premnivas, G. C. (2025). Understanding the impact of nutritional deficiencies on maternal health in India. JTH: Journal of Technology and Health. https://www.semanticscholar.org/paper/ca2a0c4e9129da22daf1656d6cb1718dddd7083b (accessed on 12th June 2025).

41. Ramesh, R., & Ranganathan, L. N. (2025). Headache in infections. Current Opinion in Neurology, 38, 281–287. https://www.semanticscholar.org/paper/e3bba95445a682693aff6422c785f65c7f354b01 (accessed on 12th June 2025).

42. Schwartz, J. D. (2005). The Prevalence of Comorbid Chronic Disease in Virginia's Adult Patient Population During the Years 2001 and 2004. https://core.ac.uk/download/51292489.pdf (accessed on 12th June 2025).

43. Sebastianelli, G., Secci, D., Casillo, F., Abagnale, C., Di Lorenzo, C., Serrao, M., Wang, S. J., et al. (2025). Artificial neural networks applied to somatosensory evoked potentials for migraine classification. The Journal of Headache and Pain, 26. https://www.semanticscholar.org/paper/10794c7da4915afd2357dd28833a679dc94c1748 (accessed on 12th June 2025).

44. Shukhayr Mutlaq, H., Alotaibi, K. A. T., Husaykan, I. M., Alotaibi, S. S. F., Alotaibi, F. H. H., Alotibi, F. A. A., Alotaibi, E. S. E., et al. (2024). Anemia: An updated review for healthcare professionals. Journal of Eco Humanism. https://www.semanticscholar.org/paper/6c44d2ea3daad8c7976360d006e13e11138ba621 (accessed on 12th June 2025).

45. Silva López, D. E., & Contreras Montes, A. E. (2024). Loeffler's cardiac syndrome: An in-depth review of pathophysiology, clinical manifestations, diagnostic strategies, and management approaches. International Journal of Medical Science and Clinical Research Studies. https://www.semanticscholar.org/paper/ad64df923fe61aa06fb7106ec767a3d6c9d78d10 (accessed on 12th June 2025).

46. Siopi, S. A., Antonitsis, P., Karapanagiotidis, G., Tagarakis, G., Voucharas, C., & Anastasiadis, K. (2024). Cardiac failure and cardiogenic shock: Insights into pathophysiology, classification, and hemodynamic assessment. Cureus, 16. https://www.semanticscholar.org/paper/d7186d00765939a8dee82f4beb66daed105661e5 (accessed on 12th June 2025).

47. Suhasini, S. (2017). Ocular Manifestations of Blood Dyscrasias. https://core.ac.uk/download/288215952.pdf (accessed on 12th June 2025).

48. Varekha, N. V., Stuklov, N., Gordienko, K. V., Gimadiev, R., Shchegolev, O. B., Kislaya, S. N., Gubina, E. V., et al. (2025). Development of a method for differential diagnosis of iron deficiency anemia and anemia of chronic disease based on demographic data and routine laboratory tests using machine learning technologies. Onomatology. https://www.semanticscholar.org/paper/930c05038b73760229db40ada827a2c95efa0f34 (accessed on 12th June 2025).

49. Xanthopoulos, A. V., Giamouzis, G., Dimos, A., Skoularigki, E., Starling, R., Skoularigis, J., & Triposkiadis, F. (2022). Red blood cell distribution width in heart failure: Pathophysiology, prognostic role, controversies and dilemmas. Journal of Clinical Medicine, 11. https://www.semanticscholar.org/paper/30881371fc22fb05d254a1653e7cf0131f3d1706 (accessed on 12th June 2025).

50. Zviahina, O., Shevchuk, S., & Pavliuk, O. (2023). AB1068: The role of hepcidin in the formation of anemia syndrome in patients with ankylosing spondylitis and its significance in the differentiation of anemia of chronic disease, iron deficiency anemia and their combination. Annals of the Rheumatic Diseases. https://www.semanticscholar.org/paper/49a5c49f77bf8b3ffa8e9293d956607de5791c48 (accessed on 12th June 2025).

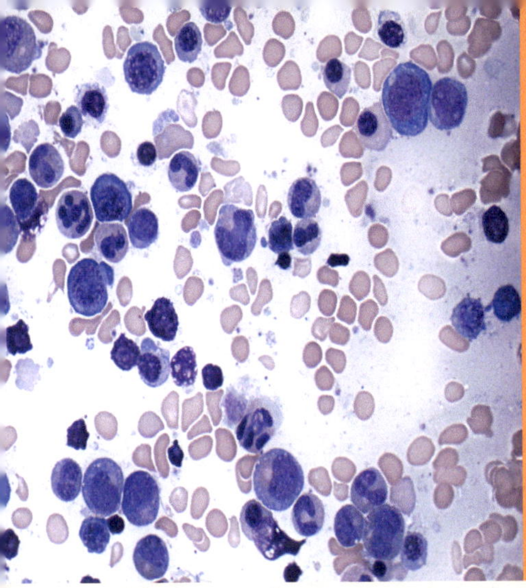

Chapter 3

IRON DEFICIENCY AND SIDEROBLASTIC ANEMIA

Contents

Introduction....55
3.1. Causes of Iron Deficiency....56
3.2. Pathophysiology of Sideroblastic Anemia....61
3.3. Symptoms and Diagnosis....66
3.4. Treatment and Management....70
Summary....76
References....77

Introduction

Iron deficiency and sideroblastic anemia are significant hematological disorders that indicate the complexity of iron metabolism and its influence on human health. Iron deficiency, resulting from nutritional deficiency, chronic blood loss, or malabsorption, leads to defective hemoglobin synthesis, which can lead to fatigue, pallor, and reduced exercise tolerance. Conversely, sideroblastic anemia is also characterized by impaired erythropoiesis, wherein iron accumulates in mitochondria due to genetic changes or environmental factors, thereby causing unregulated hemoglobin production. The intricacy between these conditions is the reason one needs to know everything about iron homeostasis, particularly in cases such as COVID-19, where iron metabolism can be greatly deranged, resulting in secondary conditions such as sideroblastic-like anemia and systemic hypoxia (Cavezzi et al., 2020). Thus, learning about both of the disorders using what is already known indicates not just their clinical significance but also their mechanisms of pathophysiology (Fern Eández-Vizarra et al., 2020).

3.1. Causes of Iron Deficiency

The etiology of iron deficiency is multifactorial, encompassing dietary deficiencies, increased physiological requirements, and underlying medical conditions. Inadequate dietary intake of iron, particularly in populations without access to foods rich in iron, remains a common cause of deficiency. Increased physiological requirements during growth periods, pregnancy, and lactation may be in excess of the dietary iron absorption, leading to severe deficits. In sideroblastic anemia, genetic mutations in the pathways of iron metabolism, including those in the NDUFB11 gene, can also cause the inappropriate use and storage of iron. The gene is related to complex I deficiency and possesses characteristic clinical features, including the early development of sideroblastic anemia, which reflects the significance of genetic factors in iron homeostasis (Bertini et al., 2017). In addition, iron-sulfur cluster biogenesis defects have been linked to several disorders, further complicating the etiology of iron deficiency (Cardenas-Rodriguez et al., 2018). It is clear, therefore, that iron deficiency etiology extends beyond the presence of nutrients (Figure 3.1).

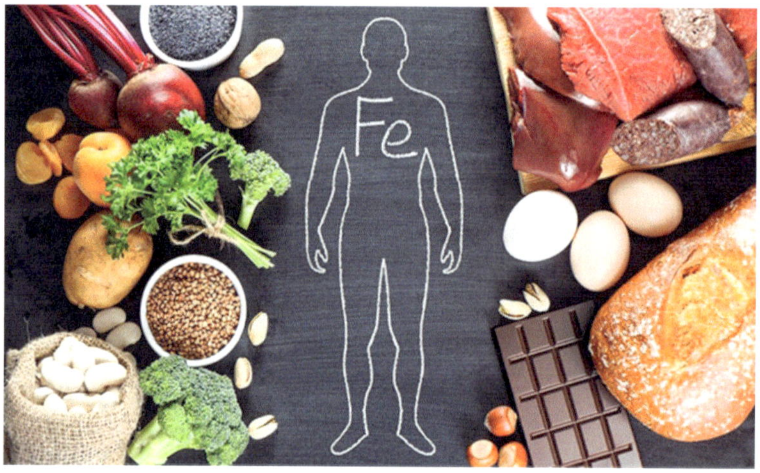

Figure 3.1. Inadequate dietary intake of iron, particularly in populations with limited access to iron-rich foods, remains a prevalent factor contributing to this deficiency.

Source: https://www.asknestle.in/sites/default/files/2024-01/640x380_7_Iron%20deficiency%20and%20its%20impact%20on%20immunity.jpg.

3.1.1. Dietary Insufficiency

Nutritional deficiency is a crucial determinant for the occurrence of sideroblastic anemia and iron deficiency, particularly in vulnerable populations such as pregnant women and infants. Inadequate dietary iron and lower ability to absorb iron effectively can lead to depletion of the stores of iron that contribute to anemia risk. (Li et al., 2017) Iron deficiency anemia remains the most common nutritional disorder globally, with the worst prevalence occurring in pregnant women, where there is a high priority on balanced consumption of iron for both maternal and fetal well-being. Inadequate dietary iron, coupled with increased physiological requirements during pregnancy, can cause not only anemia but also other issues in neonatal development. Besides, studies indicate that effective public health interventions that are based on dietary modification and iron supplementation are critical to the prevention of this disease in areas of high burden, emphasizing the need for multiple-level nutritional interventions (Abdulraheem et al., 2023) (Figure 3.2).

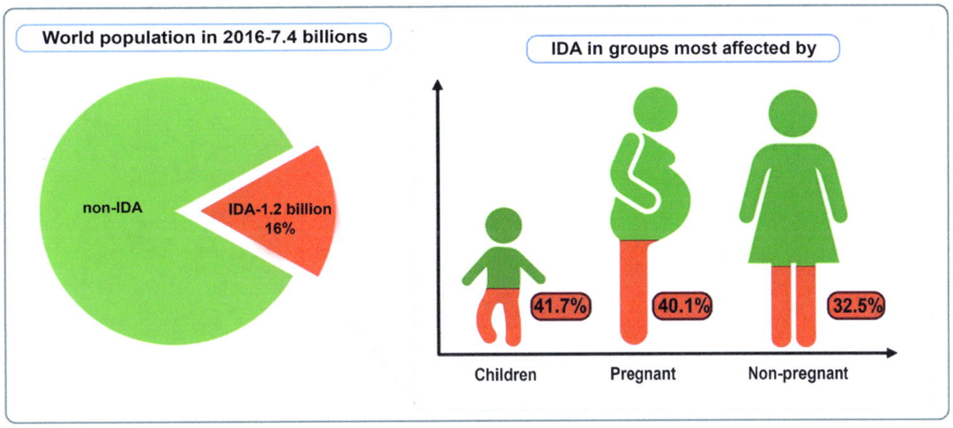

Figure 3.2. Dietary insufficiency plays a significant role in the prevalence of iron deficiency and sideroblastic anemia, particularly affecting vulnerable populations such as pregnant women and young children.

Source: https://www.researchgate.net/publication/362912021/figure/fig1/AS:11431281080886274@1661430156295/Occurrence-of-iron-deficiency-anemia-IDA-iron-deficiency-anemia-Non-IDA-anemia-without.png.

3.1.2. Malabsorption Disorders

Malabsorption illnesses can significantly impair the nutritional status of patients, particularly their ability to absorb essential minerals such as iron, which is crucial for hemoglobin production. Illnesses like celiac disease, Crohn's disease, and post-operative anatomical change, like alterations following Roux-en-Y gastric bypass surgery (RYGB), tend to lead to decreased intestinal absorption of nutrients. According to studies, RYGB subjects often suffer from iron deficiency, as well as deficiencies in other essential nutrients such as zinc and copper, which play a crucial role in the effective metabolism of iron and overall health (Wright et al., 2014). An interaction of these deficiencies results in a greater risk of developing sideroblastic anemia, where iron is present but not utilized effectively due to disrupted hematopoiesis. Therefore, identification and treatment of malabsorption disorders become essential in the management of iron deficiency as well as its consequent complications (Kelly et al., 2017).

3.1.3. Chronic Blood Loss

Malabsorption disorders can severely impair a patient's nutritional condition, particularly their ability to absorb essential minerals such as iron, which is necessary for hemoglobin formation. Conditions such as celiac disease, Crohn's disease, and postoperative anatomical changes, e.g., following RYGB, are likely to lead to less than normal absorption of nutrients in the intestine. Research has shown that RYGB patients often suffer from iron deficiency, as well as other deficiencies such as zinc and copper, which are essential for the normal metabolism of iron and overall health (Wright et al.,

2014). Their cumulative interaction results in a greater risk of sideroblastic anemia, wherein the presence of iron is seen but is not utilized effectively because of defective hematopoiesis. Therefore, identification of malabsorption disorder and treatment become crucial in the management of iron deficiency as well as its resultant complications (Kelly et al., 2017) (Figure 3.3).

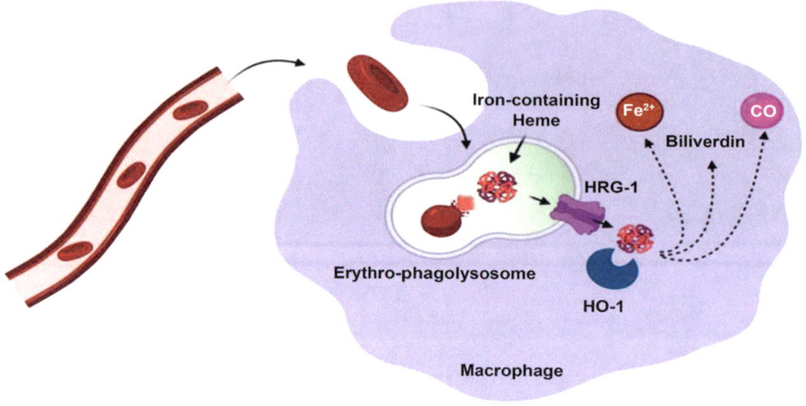

Figure 3.3. The process of heme biosynthesis is critically dependent on iron, as it is incorporated into hemoglobin within erythrocytes, facilitating oxygen transport.

Source: https://www.mdpi.com/ijms/ijms-22-04591/article_deploy/html/images/ijms-22-04591-g005.png.

3.1.4. Increased Iron Requirements

The translation of increased iron requirements is critical in the context of iron deficiency and sideroblastic anemia. Situations such as growth spurts, pregnancy, and blood loss significantly augment the body's iron requirement, perhaps exacerbating underlying deficits if unmet. With accelerated growth or augmented erythropoiesis, the body's iron demands increase, necessitating greater dietary absorption or supplementation to maintain acceptable hemoglobin levels. Additionally, conditions like congenital sideroblastic anemia (CSA), which have pathologies in heme biosynthesis and disturbed iron metabolism, illustrate the need for adequate iron supply. As Crispin et al. (2017) state, there exist genetic determinants that can severely affect the utilization of iron, thereby leading to high requirements that, if not met, trigger extraordinary health risks. Furthermore, the one-third population prevalence of anemia worldwide underscores the need to address these increased iron needs on a systematic scale through the use of nutritional care and medical management (Tuli et al., 2017).

3.1.5. Pregnancy and Lactation

The physiological changes during pregnancy and lactation significantly increase the risk for iron deficiency and related conditions, e.g., sideroblastic anemia. Pregnancy is accompanied by a heightened demand for iron to accommodate fetal growth, placental enlargement, and the increase in maternal blood volume, leading to significant iron storage loss. Postpartum anemia affects up to 27% of women, mostly because of iron deficiency along with other conditions such as poor supplementation and blood loss during delivery. Moreover, lactating women continue to require large amounts of iron for milk production, thereby complicating their nutritional status if dietary requirements are not properly met (et al., 2019). This precarious balance makes timely close observation and intervention important to ensure maternal and fetal welfare during these critical periods (Figure 3.4).

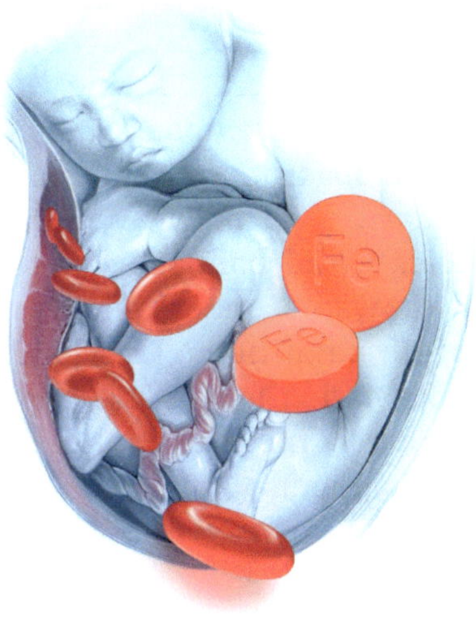

Figure 3.4. During pregnancy, the increased demands for iron are driven by fetal growth, placental development, and the expansion of maternal blood volume, which can lead to a notable depletion of iron stores.

Source: https://cdn.mdedge.com/files/s3fs-public/Image/November-2017/obgm291208_fig.jpg.

3.1.6. Gastrointestinal Conditions

Gastrointestinal disorders significantly impact iron deficiency and sideroblastic anemia, particularly in patients who are candidates for bariatric surgery such as RYGB. Following RYGB, patients are at a higher risk of developing iron deficiency due to abnormal nutrient absorption, which can result in various hematological complications, including anemia. Research has indicated that a high proportion of RYGB patients report various micronutrient deficiency disorders, including iron deficiency, zinc deficiency, copper deficiency, and deficiencies in vitamins B6 and B12, all of which are critical to normal erythropoiesis and iron metabolism (Wright et al., 2014).

Other instances of CSA indicate the importance of mitochondrial function and iron homeostasis in the pathogenesis of anemia. Iron-sulfur cluster mutations that interfere with cluster assembly compromise erythropoiesis and underlie disease iron deposits, illustrating the complex interplay between gastrointestinal disease and iron dysregulation (Crispin et al., 2017).

3.1.7. Menstrual Cycle Impacts

Menstrual bleeding is a significant physiological process that can have very significant impacts on women's iron status, particularly concerning sideroblastic anemia and total iron deficiency. Menstrual bleeding leads to a significant loss of iron, which, if not adequately replenished by dietary iron intake, can cause or aggravate anemia. Specifically, as iron is crucial in erythropoiesis and central in heme biosynthesis, iron loss during menstruation can jeopardize hemoglobin production, which may lead to the characteristic ring sideroblasts of sideroblastic anemia (Ricci et al., 2022).

Moreover, diet is also key to determining iron status, highlighting the importance of personalized nutrition counseling to avoid iron-deficiency risks (Abrams et al., 2011). Hence, information regarding the interaction between menstrual cycle effects and iron metabolism is crucial in the development of effective interventions for women at risk of these hematological disorders (Figure 3.5).

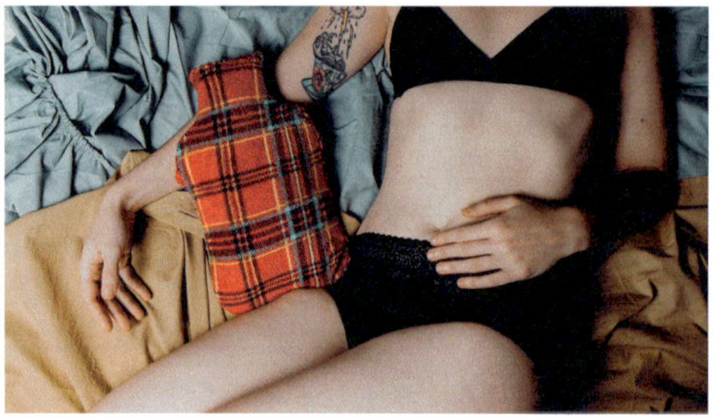

Figure 3.5. Regular menstrual bleeding can lead to substantial iron loss, which, if not adequately compensated through dietary intake, may precipitate or exacerbate anemia.

Source: https://post.healthline.com/wp-content/uploads/2020/11/menstration-period-cramps-heating-pad-1296x728-header.jpg.

3.1.8. Age-Related Factors

The interaction of iron metabolism with hematologic health becomes more complex as people age, particularly in cases of diseases such as sideroblastic anemia. Aging affects the utilization and absorption of iron, which will exacerbate deficiencies and lead to anemia. Mitochondrial aging-related dysfunction, as suggested in cases of mitochondrial translation disorders, highlights how imperfections can lead to defective heme biosynthesis and clinically manifest as sideroblastic anemia, myopathy, lactic acidosis, and iron overload (Cleary et al., 2013). In addition, heme synthesis control is also strictly regulated to the supply of iron, and disruption in this balance has the potential to lead to the formation of ring sideroblasts within the bone marrow, which is the characteristic feature in sideroblastic anemia (Ricci et al., 2022). Unraveling these mechanisms associated with aging is crucial for developing effective interventions that can improve the treatment and prognosis in older adults suffering from these diseases.

3.1.9. Genetic Predispositions

The relationship between genetic predispositions and iron deficiency, particularly in sideroblastic anemia, highlights the complexity of hematological disease. Genetic factors play a significant role in a person's predisposition to both iron deficiency and anemia, with hereditary diseases commonly disrupting normal erythropoiesis. Specifically, inherited bone marrow failure syndromes such as Diamond Blackfan anemia are not only linked to gene mutations but also with deficiencies that impact essential cellular functions in iron metabolism and erythropoiesis. Such genetic defects can lead to failure in hemoglobin production, thereby exacerbating iron-related diseases (Henson et al., 2013). Furthermore, food intake and how it impacts iron absorption, as identified in the Scientific Advisory Committee on Nutrition's report, indicate the contribution of genetic background towards understanding anemia's multifactorial condition. This background provides information for disease management and treatment, including diseases like sideroblastic anemia (Abrams et al., 2011) (Figure 3.6).

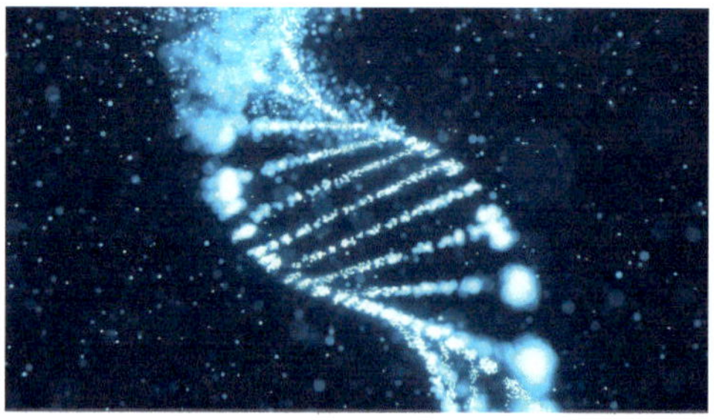

Figure 3.6. Genetic factors contribute significantly to an individual's susceptibility to both iron deficiency and anemia, where inherited conditions can disrupt normal erythropoiesis.

Source: https://i0.wp.com/post.medicalnewstoday.com/wp-content/uploads/sites/3/2021/11/iron_deficiency_GettyImages1193685570_Header-1024x575.jpg?w=1155&h=1528.

3.2. Pathophysiology of Sideroblastic Anemia

Sideroblastic anemia is predominantly characterized by ineffective erythropoiesis, where ringed sideroblasts are produced in the bone marrow due to disrupted iron metabolism and failure of iron uptake in hemoglobin. Sideroblastic anemia occurs due to various genetic mutations that affect heme biosynthesis or mitochondrial activity, leading to the inappropriate deposition of iron in erythrocytes. Surprisingly, mutations in genes such as NDUFB11, which are essential for mitochondrial complex I assembly, have been linked to sideroblastic anemia and may present with other phenotypes, including complex I deficiency, illustrating the close relationship between mitochondrial failure and anemic diseases (Bertini et al., 2017). Similarly, CSAs illustrate how alterations in the heme biosynthetic pathway and mitochondrial iron-sulfur cluster assembly can lead to ineffective erythropoiesis, underscoring the significance of proteins such as HSCB in maintaining iron homeostasis and promoting proper red blood cell (RBC) development (Crispin et al., 2017). Therefore, these molecular processes are essential in the development of targeted therapeutic strategies.

3.2.1. Mechanism of Sideroblasts Formation

Sideroblast generation is a crucial process in the pathogenesis of sideroblastic anemia, characterized by a morphologic abnormality of iron accumulation in erythroblast mitochondria. Incorporation of iron into heme molecules during normal erythropoiesis is intimately linked with mitochondrial function as well as iron metabolism.

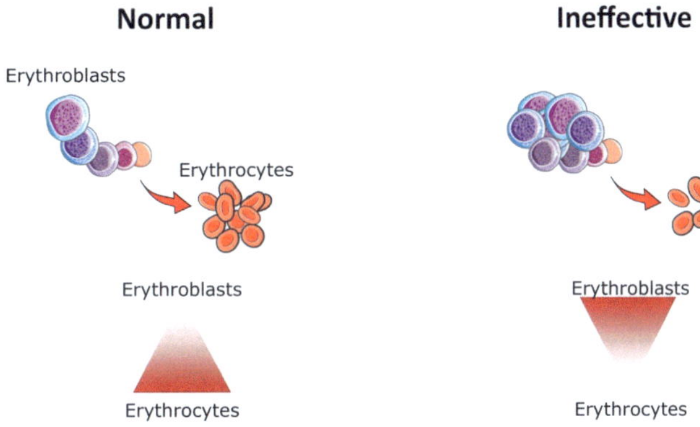

Figure 3.7. Mechanism of sideroblast formation.

Source: https://iiif.elifesciences.org/lax:90189%2Felife-90189-fig6-v2.tif/full/1500,/0/default.jpg.

The disturbances observed in CSAs are often attributed to defects in heme biosynthesis or mitochondrial iron-sulfur cluster assembly, as suggested by recent studies linking mutations in genes such as HSPA9 and HSCB to sideroblast development (Crispin et al., 2017). In addition, hormonal regulation by hepcidin is the core of this process; underproduction of hepcidin may lead to iron overload and, consequently, inefficient erythropoiesis (Nai et al., 2020). In general, understanding these mechanisms clarifies the pathophysiology of sideroblastic anemia and offers prospects for selective therapeutic interventions in the treatment of iron disorders (Figure 3.7).

3.2.2. Role of Mitochondria in Erythropoiesis

Mitochondria play a pivotal role in erythropoiesis, particularly in the context of iron metabolism and the pathophysiology of sideroblastic anemia. These organelles are integral to heme biosynthesis, where iron is chelated and incorporated into protoporphyrin IX, ultimately forming heme, a crucial component of hemoglobin in mature erythrocytes. In cases of CSA, mitochondrial dysfunction disrupts iron utilization by erythroid precursors, leading to iron overload within the mitochondria and the characteristic accumulation of ring sideroblasts in the bone marrow (Crispin et al., 2017). Furthermore, iron's dual nature as both an essential nutrient and a potentially toxic element necessitates careful regulation; it is well established that impairments in heme biosynthesis can result in various hematologic disorders (Ricci et al., 2022). Thus, understanding mitochondrial dynamics and their influence on erythropoiesis is essential for elucidating the mechanistic underpinnings of iron-related anemias.

3.2.3. Iron Utilization in Hemoglobin Synthesis

Iron plays a crucial role in the synthesis of hemoglobin, the protein responsible for oxygen transport in erythrocytes. Inadequate iron availability can impede hemoglobin production, leading to various types of anemia, including sideroblastic anemia. Sideroblastic anemia is characterized by the ineffective incorporation of iron into hemoglobin, resulting in the accumulation of iron-laden mitochondria within precursor RBCs, a condition known as ringed sideroblasts. Genetic defects affecting heme biosynthesis or mitochondrial iron-sulfur cluster assembly can cause this disorder, with mutations in genes such as HSPA9 identified as culprits that disrupt iron metabolism and erythropoiesis (Crispin et al., 2017). Moreover, recent findings regarding the NDUFB11 gene highlight the complexity of iron utilization in hemoglobin synthesis; mutations can lead to complex I deficiency and concomitant sideroblastic anemia (Bertini et al., 2017). Understanding these mechanisms is essential for developing targeted strategies to address anemia related to iron deficiency (Figure 3.8).

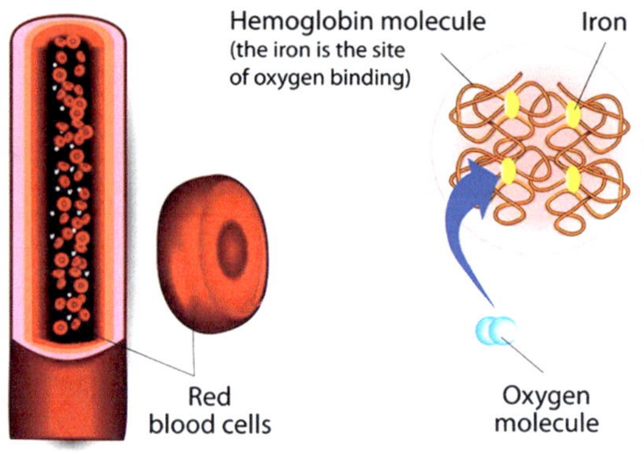

Figure 3.8. Iron plays a crucial role in the synthesis of hemoglobin, the protein responsible for oxygen transport in erythrocytes.

Source: https://d18x2uyjeekruj.cloudfront.net/wp-content/uploads/2023/11/haemoglobin.jpg.

3.2.4. Genetic Mutations Associated with Sideroblastic Anemia

Sideroblastic anemia is intricately linked to genetic mutations that disrupt heme biosynthesis and iron metabolism. Notably, mutations in the NDUFB11 gene, which encodes a component of mitochondrial complex I, have been associated with early-onset sideroblastic anemia as a distinct clinical feature. This mutation exemplifies how complex mitochondrial defects can manifest primarily as blood disorders, thereby expanding the understanding of the molecular underpinnings of sideroblastic anemia (Bertini et al., 2017). Additionally, defects in the HSPA9 gene and its binding partner HSCB have been reported as significant contributors to CSAs.

Studies have shown that mutations in these genes lead to impaired iron-sulfur cluster assembly and mitochondrial dysfunction, ultimately resulting in pathological iron deposition in erythroblasts (Crispin et al., 2017). Such genetic insights underscore the diverse mechanisms through which sideroblastic anemia can arise, offering pathways for potential therapeutic interventions.

3.2.5. Types of Sideroblastic Anemia

Sideroblastic anemia is a heterogeneous group of disorders characterized by impaired utilization of iron in heme synthesis, resulting in the accumulation of ring sideroblasts in the bone marrow. This condition can be classified into several types, including hereditary and acquired forms. Hereditary sideroblastic anemia is often associated with genetic mutations that affect the enzymes involved in heme biosynthesis, whereas acquired forms may result from various factors, including exposure to toxins, infections, or other diseases. Notably, the role of iron in these disorders is complex; not only does it contribute to the production of hemoglobin, but it also poses cellular risks due to oxidative stress when iron homeostasis is disrupted (Ricci et al., 2022). The interplay between iron and heme metabolism ultimately dictates the clinical outcomes of sideroblastic anemia and underscores the significance of understanding these underlying mechanisms (Cardenas-Rodriguez et al., 2018) (Figure 3.9).

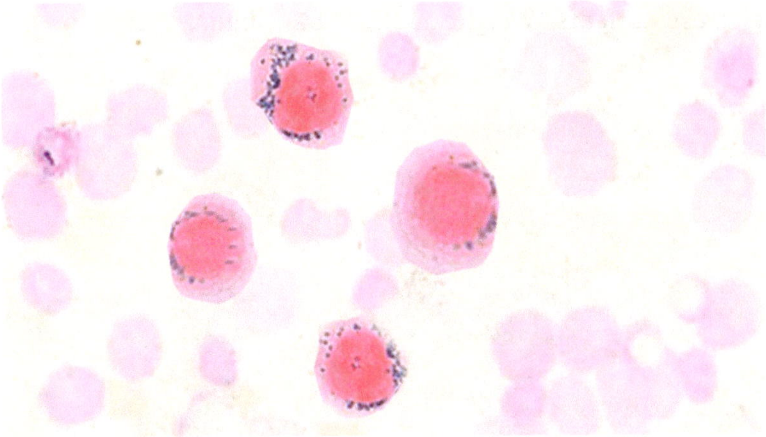

Figure 3.9. Sideroblastic anemia is a heterogeneous group of disorders characterized by the impaired utilization of iron in heme synthesis, leading to the accumulation of ring sideroblasts in the bone marrow.

Source: https://d1irpg7po1rqdm.cloudfront.net/page/J72Sd9e2zQbHlyvkjRG1miblZNOHdGHSS0AxlXbE.webp.

3.2.6. Impact of Lead Poisoning

Lead poisoning is a powerful argument in the context of iron deficiency and sideroblastic anemia because it represents the multifactorial interaction between environmental toxins and hematological disorders. The lead's hematotoxic effect on hematopoiesis disrupts the normal production of RBCs, leading to peripheral cytopenias of blood and ultimately increased risk for myelodysplastic syndromes (MDS) (Pyatt et al., 2013). By inhibiting enzymes involved in heme synthesis, lead exposure results in defective hemoglobin synthesis, producing typical symptoms of sideroblastic anemia, in which iron accumulation occurs in precursors to RBCs due to the misutilization of iron (Berman et al., 2016). The consequences of lead poisoning are not limited to acute health complications since chronic exposure can trigger persistent genetic defects and enhance the risk of progressing towards acute myeloid leukemia (AML), which underscores the urgent need for prevention measures and effective interventions to mitigate the incidence of lead on public health.

3.2.7. Role of Vitamin B6 Deficiency

The role of Vitamin B6 deficiency in iron deficiency and sideroblastic anemia cannot be overemphasized, as it plays a central role in various biochemical reactions with regard to hemoglobin formation and iron metabolism. Vitamin B6, as an enzyme cofactor that renders heme production feasible, is critical for the effective incorporation of iron into hemoglobin. In its deficiency state, the body is unable to produce functional hemoglobin, leading to ineffective erythropoiesis, characteristic of sideroblastic anemia. One of the most notable examples of this is in patients with complex I deficiency due to mutations within the NDUFB11 gene, in which early-onset sideroblastic anemia is a prevalent clinical feature (Bertini et al., 2017). Additionally, Vitamin B6 deficiencies are one of the collections of nutritional issues that may worsen iron deficiency anemia in gastric bypass surgery patients. A study indicates a high prevalence of not only iron deficiency but also Vitamin B6 deficiency among these patients (Wright et al., 2014) (Figure 3.10).

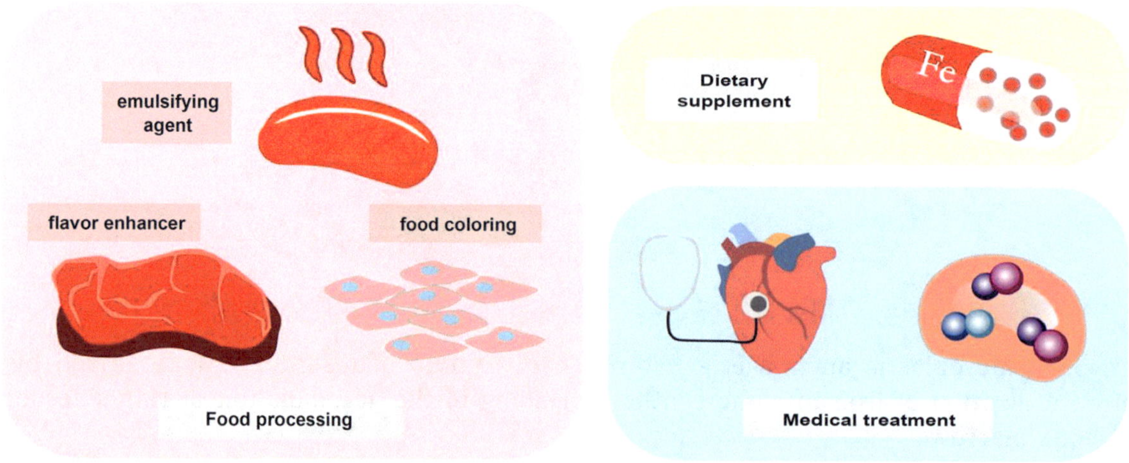

Figure 3.10. Vitamin B6, as a cofactor for enzymes that facilitate the production of heme, is crucial for the effective incorporation of iron into hemoglobin.

Source: https://www.mdpi.com/ijms/ijms-24-08384/article_deploy/html/images/ijms-24-08384-g001.png.

3.2.8. Interaction with Other Hematological Disorders

The interrelationship between iron deficiency and other hematologic disorders, such as CSA and DBA, creates a fine context crucial to the investigation of erythropoiesis. In CSA, mitochondrial impairment in iron utilization is associated with iron overload and the characteristic finding of ring sideroblasts, directly linking iron metabolism with hematologic disease (Ricci et al., 2022). In contrast, DBA, more associated with RPL11 mutations, highlights other interactions, as disturbed hematopoiesis also involves the dysregulation of iron metabolism genes, underscoring the complexity of the function performed by iron during hemoglobin biosynthesis (Jia et al., 2013). Both conditions demonstrate that iron regulation is not only imperative for the production of erythrocytes in optimal conditions but that dysregulation will result in an overlapping syndrome manifesting as a shared vulnerability in hematopoietic processes. It is essential to unravel these interactions to create targeted therapeutic approaches.

3.2.9. Consequences of Impaired Erythropoiesis

Impaired erythropoiesis, as seen in sideroblastic anemia, presents with severe physiologic consequences due to deranged heme biosynthesis and altered iron metabolism. As iron is a critical element in hemoglobin synthesis, any disruption in its metabolism can lead to ineffective erythropoiesis, which is characterized by the observation of ring sideroblasts in the bone marrow and subsequent anemia. Its failure to efficiently incorporate iron into heme creates a cycle of oxidative stress in erythrocytes that may hasten cellular damage and result in hemolytic anemia, as demonstrated through experimentation with irradiated mice lacking significant mitochondrial enzymes (May et al., 2011). Additionally, the abnormal regulation of iron metabolism not only impacts hematopoiesis but also triggers ancillary metabolic disorders, ultimately disrupting systemic oxygen supply and leading to multifocal organ dysfunction (Ricci et al., 2022). The relationship between iron and heme biosynthesis, therefore, identifies a critical element of sideroblastic anemia's pathophysiology and its broader health implications (Figure 3.11).

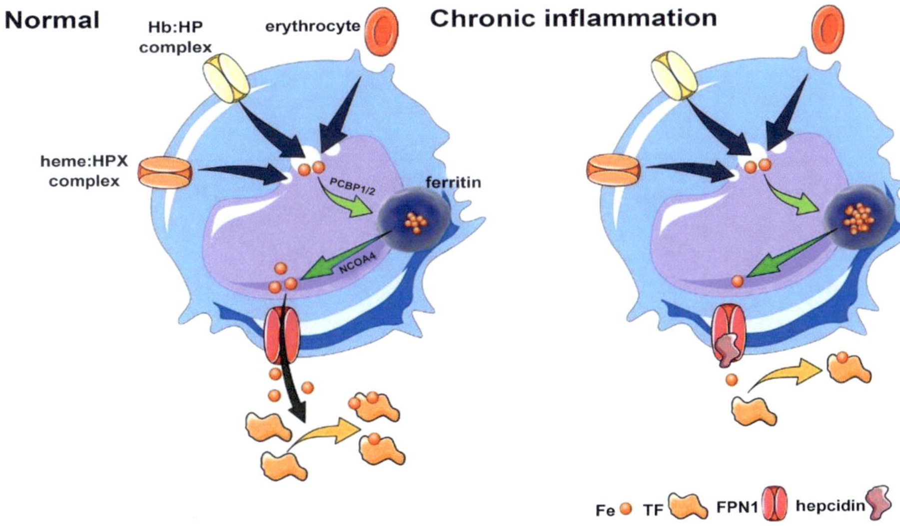

Figure 3.11. Effects of inflammation on iron recycling.

Source: https://iiif.elifesciences.org/lax:90189%2Felife-90189-fig5-v2.tif/full/1500,/0/default.jpg.

3.3. Symptoms and Diagnosis

Iron deficiency and sideroblastic anemia are typically diagnosed based on a careful evaluation of the clinical presentation and laboratory findings. The most frequent presentation is characterized by typical anemia features, including fatigue, pallor, and dyspnea, as well as other symptoms resulting from dysregulation of iron metabolism. For instance, in sideroblastic anemia, ring sideroblasts in the bone marrow are a distinctive diagnostic feature, distinguishing this from other anemias. Additionally, elevated serum ferritin levels can indicate iron overload, rather than iron deficiency, which is typically characterized by low ferritin levels. Their heterogeneity is highlighted through the variances in the underlying mechanisms: while sideroblastic anemia involves mitochondrial iron overload and impaired erythropoiesis, iron deficiency primarily results from inadequate iron supply for hemoglobin production (Bertini et al., 2017; Ricci et al., 2022). Proper diagnosis is of utmost importance in guiding effective treatment interventions for patients.

3.3.1. Common Symptoms of Iron Deficiency

The typical signs of iron deficiency often represent a complex, multifaceted problem that has the potential to significantly impact everyday functioning and overall well-being. Some of the most frequent signs include fatigue and weakness, both of which are consequences of the body's impaired ability to generate hemoglobin, a key constituent for transporting oxygen in the blood. In addition, pallor, brittle nails, and alopecia may occur in patients, indicating deficiencies in the delivery of necessary nutrients and cellular processes. In severe cases, more extreme diseases, such as sideroblastic anemia, may occur. This disease suggests alterations in iron metabolism and erythropoiesis, as seen through mutations of factors like NDUFB11, leading to complex I deficiencies (Bertini et al., 2017). Moreover, iron-sulfur cluster biosynthesis defects also demonstrate how disturbances in iron utilization can present clinically, emphasizing the importance of proper diagnosis and treatment of iron deficiency (Coster et al., 2018) (Figure 3.12).

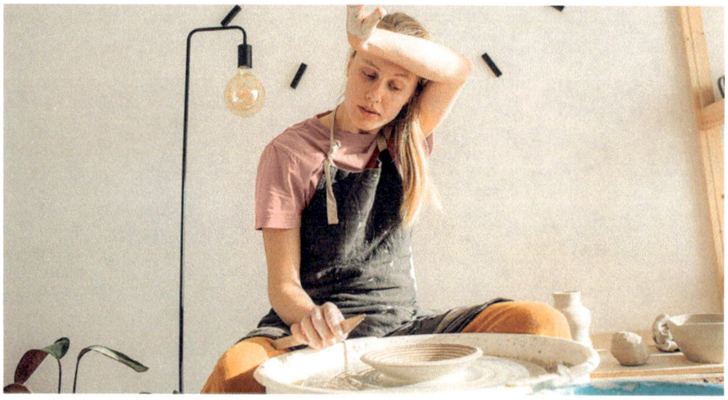

Figure 3.12. The common symptoms of iron deficiency often present a complex and multi-faceted challenge that can significantly impact daily functioning and overall health.

Source: https://media.post.rvohealth.io/wp-content/uploads/2021/11/female-tired-at-pottery-wheel-1200-628-facebook-1200x628.jpg.

3.3.2. Symptoms Specific to Sideroblastic Anemia

Sideroblastic anemia is characterized by a spectrum of typical symptoms due to impaired hemoglobin synthesis as a consequence of faulty erythroid precursors in the bone marrow. Anemia-related symptoms, like weakness, fatigue, and pallor, may present in patients with various forms of anemia. However, a characteristic feature of sideroblastic anemia is the presence of ring sideroblasts in the bone marrow, indicating pathologic iron accumulation in erythroid cells. Pathologic accumulation leads to organ damage and complications. On rare occasions, inherited mutations related to iron-sulfur cluster biosynthesis, as documented in recent literature, have been linked to the form of early-onset sideroblastic anemia, demonstrating the genetic basis of the condition (Bertini et al., 2017). Furthermore, mutations in subunits essential for the assembly of mitochondrial complex I have also been described, which reinforces its multi-dimensional pathogenesis (Coster et al., 2018). Therefore, identifying the characteristic symptoms of sideroblastic anemia is crucial for early diagnosis and management.

3.3.3. Laboratory Tests for Diagnosis

The diagnosis of sideroblastic anemia and iron deficiency relies heavily on a range of laboratory tests that are critical for uncovering the mechanisms of these conditions. Complete blood counts (CBC) are often the initial step of a comprehensive blood work, which can identify anemia with reduced RBC count and pathologic morphology of cells. Subsequently, iron and serum ferritin tests quantify iron transport and storage, which establishes the specific nature of anemia. Importantly, hemoglobin electrophoresis and bone marrow biopsy can be used to differentiate between sideroblastic anemia and iron deficiency anemia, as the former typically demonstrates characteristic ringed sideroblasts in the marrow. The delicate balance of these tests serves as a critical diagnostic compass by which doctors can steer the multifaceted nature of anemia and embark on corresponding treatment strategies (Bertini et al., 2017; Tuli et al., 2017) (Figure 3.13).

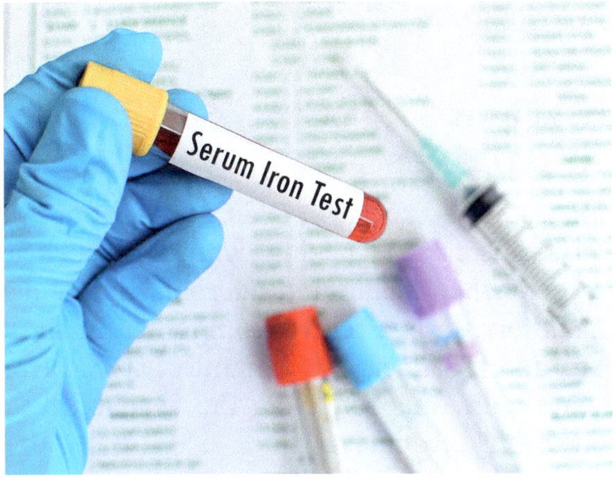

Figure 3.13. The diagnosis of iron deficiency and sideroblastic anemia relies heavily on a range of laboratory tests that provide critical insights into the underlying mechanisms of these disorders.

Source: https://labs.selfdecode.com/app/uploads/2019/12/bigstock-142428056-min.jpg.

3.3.4. Role of Complete Blood Count (CBC)

CBC has a critical role in the diagnosis and management of various hematological diseases, including iron deficiency anemia and sideroblastic anemia. A single blood test provides valuable information regarding RBC parameters such as hemoglobin, hematocrit, and mean corpuscular volume (MCV), which play a pivotal role in assessing erythropoiesis and identifying deficiencies. In anemia due to iron deficiency, a CBC would typically reveal microcytic anemia with a reduced MCV, whereas sideroblastic anemia has a heightened severity of normocytic or microcytic RBCs, as well as an abnormal reticulocyte count. Furthermore, CBC also distinguishes between different types of anemia to enable appropriate interventions. The combination of CBC findings with other tests, such as bone marrow examination and iron levels, is crucial for gaining a holistic understanding of the underlying pathophysiology of these conditions (Pawsat et al., 2021; Blau et al., 2023).

3.3.5. Iron Studies and Serum Ferritin Levels

Iron tests are crucial in evaluating the body's iron stores for diagnosing conditions such as iron deficiency anemia and sideroblastic anemia. Serum ferritin is a central component of these tests, and it reflects the amount of stored iron in the body, thus reflecting the availability of iron for erythropoiesis.

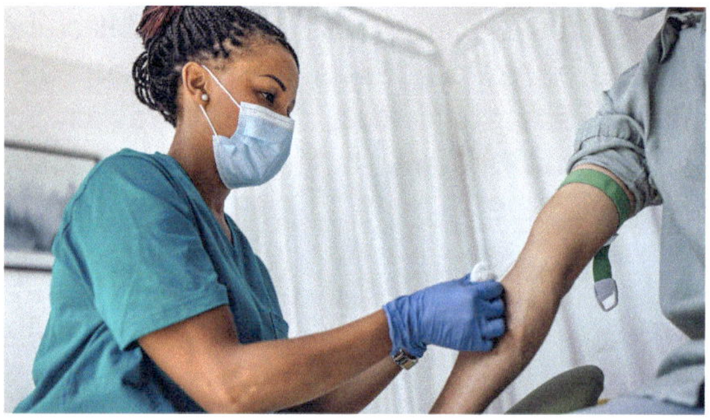

Figure 3.14. Iron studies, aimed at evaluating the body's iron levels, are critical in understanding conditions such as iron deficiency and sideroblastic anemia.

Source: https://post.healthline.com/wp-content/uploads/2023/02/nurse-taking-blood-from-patient-1296x728-header-1296x729.jpg.

In sideroblastic anemia, there is impaired use of mitochondrial iron that results in ineffective erythropoiesis, resulting in accumulation of ring sideroblasts and, characteristically, elevated ferritin levels despite overall body iron deficiency (Ricci et al., 2022). Hence, serum ferritin may be misleading in presenting the true iron status, and thus, diagnosis and management become challenging. Furthermore, the dysregulation of iron homeostasis in diseases such as Friedreich ataxia and sideroblastic anemia, resulting from glutaredoxin 5 deficiency, illustrates the intricacy of the interaction between mitochondrial function and iron metabolism, underscoring the need for combined studies on iron to develop effective therapeutic interventions (Abboud et al., 2010). Such understanding supports the establishment of treatment modalities for the affected patients (Figure 3.14).

3.3.6. Bone Marrow Biopsy Findings

Bone marrow biopsy findings are crucial for diagnosing iron deficiency anemia and sideroblastic anemia, as they provide insight into erythropoiesis and hematopoietic function. In anemia of iron deficiency, the bone marrow in most cases will contain depleted or vacant iron stores that confirm inadequate available iron for hemoglobin production. Conversely, sideroblastic anemia is linked with ringed sideroblasts developed due to the accumulation of surplus iron in mitochondria in the setting of aberrant erythroid precursors. There has been recent research into genetic aberrations, such as the NDUFB11 gene mutation, which has been implicated with deficiency of complex I and early-onset sideroblastic anemia as the characteristic finding (Bertini et al., 2017). Also noteworthy is the fact that inherited metabolic disorders are typically characterized by hematological complications, such as anemia, hence the necessity of a thorough evaluation of bone marrow findings in light of these diseases (Blau et al., 2023). Extensive evaluations must be carried out in such hematologic conditions for effective management plans (Figure 3.15).

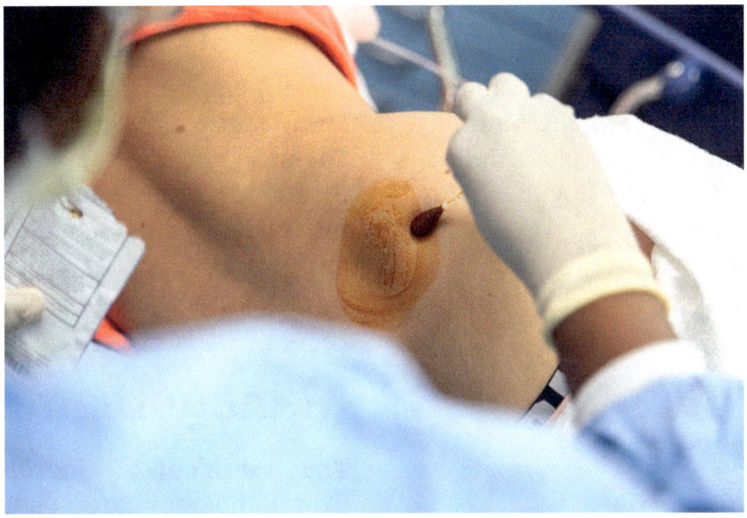

Figure 3.15. Bone marrow biopsy findings are critical in diagnosing iron deficiency and sideroblastic anemia, as they provide insight into erythropoiesis and hematopoietic function.

Source: https://stjude.scene7.com/is/image/stjude/patient-anna-00207239-068?fit=crop,1&wid=1200.

3.3.7. Differential Diagnosis Considerations

In patient anemia clinical assessment, the meticulous process of differential diagnosis is crucial to achieve appropriate management. Iron deficiency anemia is the most prevalent hematologic disease; therefore, differentiating the condition from other microcytic anemias, such as thalassemia, chronic disease anemia, and sideroblastic anemia, among others, is important (Figueiredo et al., 2010). Interestingly, congenital or acquired sideroblastic anemia is distinguished by pathologic iron accumulation in erythrocyte precursors, often secondary to disorders in heme biosynthesis or mitochondrial dysfunction (Crispin et al., 2017). Identifying these distinctions enables practitioners to initiate targeted interventions, as different etiologies may require differential interventions. By considering these differential diagnoses, clinicians can prevent misdiagnosis and ensure that underlying conditions are effectively treated, ultimately improving patient outcomes in both iron deficiency and sideroblastic anemia contexts.

3.3.8. Importance of Clinical History

A thorough clinical history is of utmost value in treating and diagnosing iron deficiency and sideroblastic anemia, as it provides the clinician with important information regarding the etiology of these two hematologic disorders. A thorough history of diet intake, previous medical illnesses, and family history is invaluable in patients presenting with symptoms of anemia, such as pallor or fatigue. For instance, sideroblastic anemia patients can be initially misattributed to iron deficiency, which is why their separation through clinical history and further diagnosis is required. Identification of inherited metabolic disorders (IMDs) that complicate hematological status may also guide appropriate treatment. For example, studies affirm that the majority of IMDs are capable of manifesting as anemia; therefore, comprehensive investigation beyond standard tests must be ensured to obtain the optimal result (Blau et al., 2023). Moreover, awareness of clinical history can accelerate genetic testing for specific conditions, which is invaluable for early interventions and treatment planning, particularly as seen in the example of MLASA syndrome (Cleary et al., 2013) (Figure 3.16).

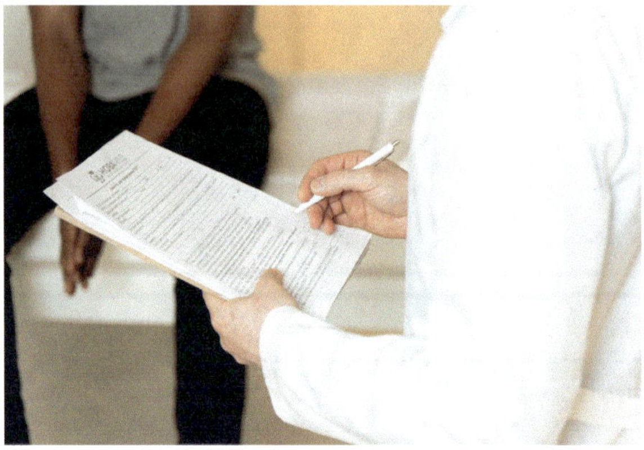

Figure 3.16. In patients presenting with symptoms of anemia, such as fatigue or pallor, a detailed account of dietary habits, family history, and prior medical conditions is invaluable.

Source: https://classicalhematology.com/wp-content/uploads/2024/04/pexels-photo-7088834.jpeg.

3.3.9. Use of Genetic Testing

In sideroblastic anemia and iron deficiency, the use of genetic testing has emerged as an essential tool for enhancing diagnostic sensitivity and determining correct treatment. Through genetic testing, doctors can identify specific mutations associated with sideroblastic anemia in cases where the clinical presentation is rare or the diagnosis is challenging. For example, patients with specific congenital mutations often present with ringed sideroblasts on their bone marrow examination, a classic finding that triggers further investigation for potential genetic etiologies of their disease (Campagna et al., 2016). By gaining a greater understanding of the genetic etiology of sideroblastic anemia, clinicians can more precisely tailor interventions, thereby improving patient outcomes. Furthermore, the identification of the genetic cause of such disorders will aid in screening families, thereby emphasizing the contribution of genetic knowledge to the diagnosis and treatment of anemia (Fisher et al., 2007). Thus, genetic testing is at the center of understanding the intricacies of such hematologic disorders.

3.4. Treatment and Management

The treatment of sideroblastic anemia and iron deficiency focuses on addressing the underlying etiology, in addition to correcting the dysregulation of iron metabolism. Supplementation with oral iron is generally the first-line therapy for patients with iron deficiency, aiming to replenish iron stores and stimulate hemoglobin synthesis. Sideroblastic anemia is more challenging to treat because it is accompanied by mitochondrial iron accumulation and impaired heme synthesis. Treatment in these cases can involve the use of pyridoxine (vitamin B6), which is effective in certain inherited conditions by stimulating heme production in spite of the underlying enzymatic alterations. In addition, long-term transfusion therapy may be necessary to correct severe anemia in patients and avoid iron overload through chelation therapy, especially in light of the pivotal role played by iron in cellular homeostasis as highlighted in recent literature (Crispin et al., 2017; Ricci et al., 2022). Ongoing monitoring of iron load and clinical symptoms is crucial for planning individualized treatment plans.

3.4.1. Dietary Modifications

Dietary intervention is of primary concern in the prevention and management of iron deficiency and sideroblastic anemia. Iron deficiency anemia patients commonly receive an increased diet consisting of food rich in iron, such as red meats, chicken, and legumes, which supply heme and non-heme iron, respectively. Moreover, the availability of iron may affect its bioavailability through the consumption of vitamin C-rich foods with iron-rich foods since vitamin C enhances absorption. Given the complexity of heme biosynthesis, as exemplified by the interaction of iron and cellular functions, dietary modification may impact not only the quantity of iron but also erythropoiesis in general (Ricci et al., 2022). It is essential that healthcare providers educate patients about the importance of maintaining long-term healthy eating habits and avoiding nutritional deficiencies. Pediatric populations require adequate dietary iron to prevent developmental issues and anemia, with particular emphasis on ongoing monitoring and supplementation where appropriate (Galati et al., 2018) (Figure 3.17).

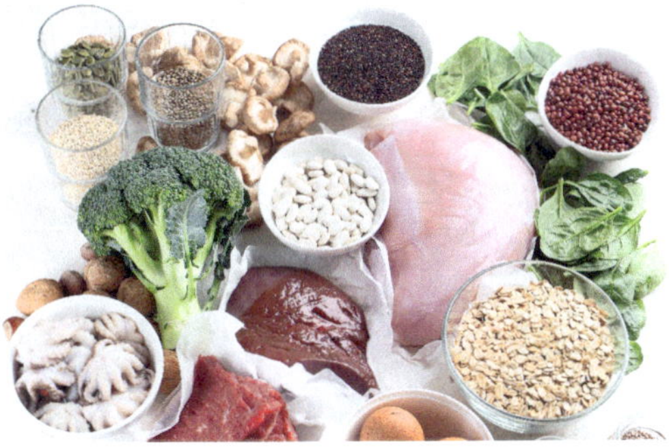

Figure 3.17. Individuals suffering from iron deficiency anemia often benefit from an increased intake of iron-rich foods, such as red meats, poultry, and legumes, which provide heme and non-heme iron, respectively.

Source: https://nutritionsource.hsph.harvard.edu/wp-content/uploads/2019/09/shutterstock_1187637787-copy.jpg.

3.4.2. Iron Supplementation

Iron supplementation then becomes a critical intervention for iron deficiency and accompanying disorders, such as sideroblastic anemia. The disorder is caused by an inappropriateness in the utilization of mitochondrial iron in erythroid precursors, resulting in the accumulation of ring sideroblasts within the bone marrow, a direct consequence of disrupted heme biosynthesis pathways (Ricci et al., 2022). In iron administration, it is not only essential to consider dosage and duration but also the individual patient's needs as well as underlying conditions. Effective iron supplementation may enhance erythropoiesis and thereby increase hemoglobin levels, as well as overall health. Furthermore, the complexities of anemia demand that clinicians have knowledge of potential side effects and drug interactions with other treatments, emphasizing the need for continuous clinician education on anemia's pathophysiology and management approaches in children (Fisher et al., 2007). Consequently, iron supplementation is crucial in alleviating deficiencies and preventing complications associated with sideroblastic anemia.

3.4.3. Treatment of Underlying Conditions

Effective management of primary conditions is crucial in the treatment of both iron deficiency anemia and sideroblastic anemia, as these anemias often indicate more serious underlying health conditions. Iron deficiency anemia is typically caused by chronic blood loss, insufficient dietary intake, or problems with malabsorption; as such, correcting normal erythropoiesis demands treating these underlying situations. In a study, decreased activity of δ-aminolevulinic acid (ALA) synthetase was noted in iron deficiency anemia, as opposed to its effect on erythropoiesis. Sideroblastic anemia, which involves ineffective hematopoiesis, is, however, responsive to therapeutic approaches towards correcting certain deficiencies, such as pyridoxal phosphate, and it can be observed to stimulate ALA synthetase activity when depressed. Ultimately, understanding the pathologies underlying anemia can help clinicians select the most effective interventions and potentially mitigate associated morbidity (Figure 3.18).

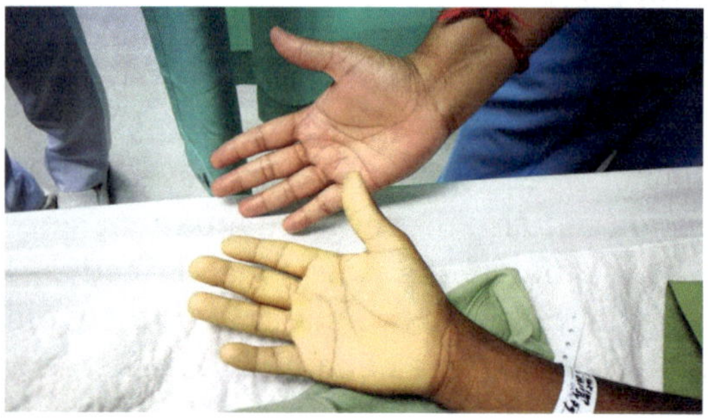

Figure 3.18. Understanding the underlying pathologies of anemia can guide clinicians in selecting appropriate interventions, thereby reducing morbidity associated with these conditions.

Source: https://pharmaceutical-journal.com/wp-content/uploads/2022/02/Learning_CPD_iron-deficiency-anaemia-Lead-Art-scaled-e1644856219520.jpg.

3.4.4. Use of Vitamin B6 in Sideroblastic Anemia

Sideroblastic anemia (SA) is a complex cross-talk between iron metabolism and other nutrient deficiency syndromes, with the pivotal role of vitamin B6 (pyridoxine). In SA, due to cases of acquired conditions, vitamin B6 is essential for the proper functioning of enzymes involved in heme synthesis—a critical activity because defective heme synthesis leads to the accumulation of iron in the mitochondria of erythroid precursors, resulting in the formation of ring sideroblasts characteristic of the disorder. Additionally, vitamin B6 deficiency exacerbates the clinical manifestations of anemia by disrupting hemoglobin synthesis and promoting iron accumulation, thereby complicating therapy. Clinical observations in patients with sideroblastic anemia reveal, in addition to iron deficiency, a high prevalence of vitamin B6 deficiency, necessitating careful nutritional assessment. Because the individuals with deficiency tend to have more than one micronutrient deficiency, like copper and folate, physicians need to initially evaluate and supplement these nutrients to improve global hematologic status, particularly in those with known deficiencies relative to iron nutriture (Wright et al., 2014; Amer et al., 2022).

3.4.5. Blood Transfusions

Blood transfusion is crucial for the management of most anemias, including iron deficiency and sideroblastic anemia. In particular, blood transfusion provides immediate relief from acute anemia symptoms by replenishing hemoglobin stores and enhancing oxygen delivery to the entire body. However, the therapeutic intervention carries intrinsic risks, particularly about iron metabolism. Routinely transfused patients are subject to iron overload, and this is particularly problematic in patients with RHA because their homeostasis for iron is compromised.

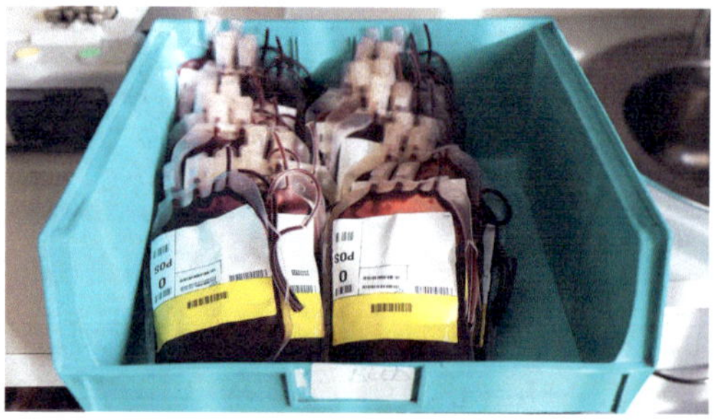

Figure 3.19. Blood transfusions play a crucial role in the management of various anemias, including those associated with iron deficiency and sideroblastic anemia.

Source: https://i0.wp.com/post.healthline.com/wp-content/uploads/2023/02/blood-bags-1296-728-header.jpg?w=1155&h=1528.

There needs to be vigilance regarding the reality that while transfusions may be lifesaving, they must be carefully managed to avoid exacerbating existing iron overload problems. The therapeutic target should not only address correcting hematological levels but also achieve a proper balance in iron levels to prevent secondary deleterious effects of iron loading, as observed by Galati et al. (2018) and Bartels et al. (2021) (Figure 3.19).

3.4.6. Erythropoiesis-Stimulating Agents

Erythropoiesis-stimulating agents (ESAs) play a central role in the treatment of anemia, particularly in conditions characterized by ineffective erythropoiesis, such as sideroblastic anemia. ESAs induce RBC production, which addresses one of the main issues of this condition, i.e., the insufficiency of erythroid proper output despite access to ample iron stores. For Erythropoiesis-Stimulating Agents, this becomes a matter of concern when the mechanisms involved are understood, as evidence shows complex interactions between iron regulation and erythropoietic processes. For instance, MDS patients with ring sideroblasts often have reduced expression of significant genes, such as ABCB7, leading to aberrant iron deposition that compromises productive RBC production (Conte et al., 2016). Furthermore, the findings of toxic iron species—presenting as labile plasma iron—in transfusion-dependent patients underscore the need for careful monitoring of iron status during ESA treatment to achieve optimal patient benefits and prevent complications (Bagguley et al., 2017).

3.4.7. Monitoring and Follow-Up Care

Close monitoring and follow-up are essential for managing iron deficiency, as well as sideroblastic anemia, both of which require constant evaluation to achieve optimal treatment outcomes. Hematological indices, such as hemoglobin concentration, mean corpuscular volume (MCV), and reticulocyte count, must be constantly evaluated to assess the efficacy of iron supplementation and detect potential complications. As the literature emphasizes, an integrated management strategy can significantly contribute to enhancing the outcomes of patients with inherited metabolic disorders, many of which are characterized by hematologic presentations (Blau et al., 2023). Moreover, following the normalization of hemoglobin, iron therapy should be extended for an additional three months to regain iron stores and prevent recurrences of anemia (Galati et al., 2018). This systematic follow-up enables health care providers to make timely treatment plan modifications so patients receive the best possible care based on their individual needs (Figure 3.20).

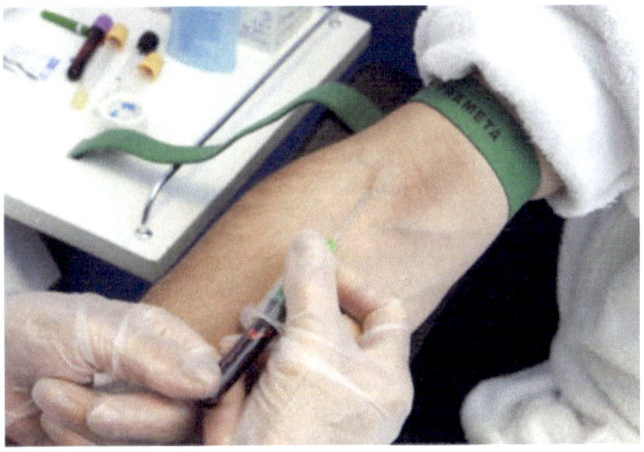

Figure 3.20. Regular assessment of hematological parameters, including hemoglobin levels, mean corpuscular volume (MCV), and reticulocyte counts, is critical to gauge the efficacy of iron supplementation and to detect potential complications.

Source: https://cached.imagescaler.hbpl.co.uk/resize/scaleWidth/815/cached.offlinehbpl.hbpl.co.uk/news/PGH/55353170-FF0D-DCF5-44DADA5B57EDE11B.jpg.

3.4.8. Patient Education and Support

Effective patient education and support are crucial components in managing iron deficiency and sideroblastic anemia. Patients often experience confusion regarding their conditions, necessitating an educational framework that demystifies the complexities of hematologic disorders. Through tailored educational programs, healthcare providers can equip patients with knowledge about the pathophysiology of their illness, especially as highlighted by research on CSAs, which show a clear genetic basis affecting iron metabolism and erythropoiesis (Crispin et al., 2017). This knowledge empowers patients to actively participate in their treatment regimens actively, thus enhancing adherence to therapies such as iron supplementation and vitamin B6 administration. Moreover, support groups can provide vital emotional and psychological assistance, fostering a community environment where patients share experiences and coping strategies. Integrating both education and supportive measures not only improves patient outcomes but also cultivates a proactive attitude towards managing chronic conditions such as iron deficiency and sideroblastic anemia.

A CLOSER LOOK

YARS2 GENE

The YARS2 gene (Tyrosyl-tRNA synthetase 2, mitochondrial) codes for an enzyme involved in protein synthesis within the mitochondria—the components within cells used to generate energy. Specifically, the enzyme enables the addition of the amino acid tyrosine to its corresponding transfer RNA (tRNA), a crucial step in mitochondrial protein synthesis.

YARS2 gene mutations can lead to impaired mitochondrial function and are associated with a condition called MLASA (Myopathy, Lactic Acidosis, and Sideroblastic Anemia), an uncommon genetic syndrome. The clinical presentation of this condition typically involves muscle weakness, lethargy, exercise intolerance, and disturbances in RBC production. Being crucial for energy metabolism, YARS2 mutations have the potential to affect energy-demanding tissues, such as muscles and bone marrow.

YARS2 diseases usually arise in an autosomal recessive manner; thus, the person would have to inherit two dysfunctional copies of the gene (one from each of their parents) in order to develop the disease.

SUMMARY

The intricate relationship between sideroblastic anemia and iron deficiency reflects the complexity of the processes involved in heme biosynthesis and iron metabolism. Both conditions indicate critical pathways of erythropoiesis, that is, how iron serves as a fundamental cofactor for enzymatic reactions playing critical roles in redox reactions and oxygen transport. The malfunctioning utilization of iron in sideroblastic anemia results in mitochondrial iron overload, which affects predominantly erythroid precursors and leads to characteristic ring sideroblastic accumulation in the bone marrow. The process is well illustrated by the function of the iron-sulfur clusters, which are required by many mitochondrial enzymes and are directly related to the pathology of such diseases (Coster et al., 2018). In addition, the dysregulation of heme synthesis underscores the complex role iron plays in cellular processes and highlights the need for an integrated strategy to understand and treat these interrelated disorders (Ricci et al., 2022).

An appreciation of the intricacies of iron deficiency and sideroblastic anemia necessitates an understanding of the molecular mechanisms underlying these conditions. Iron deficiency anemia typically occurs as a result of inadequate iron intake or absorption, leading to reduced hemoglobin production. On the contrary, sideroblastic anemia is characterized by the body's inability to use iron for hemoglobin synthesis, which leads to iron accumulation in erythroid precursors. Current research has also indicated essential factors involved in the biosynthesis of heme, including more than one mitochondrial transporter and regulatory proteins, which are important for iron insertion into protoporphyrin IX, a precursor to heme iron (Baughman et al., 2009). Additionally, genetic factors, such as pathogenic variants of the YARS2 gene, have been found to be implicated in sideroblastic anemia cases, indicating the involvement of mitochondrial function in the disease (Carreño-Gago et al., 2021). Together, these observations give a critical insight into the pathophysiologic interaction between anemia and iron metabolism and provide avenues for the creation of targeted therapeutic strategies.

REFERENCES

1. Ye, H., & Rouault, T. A. (2010). Human Iron–Sulfur cluster assembly, cellular iron homeostasis, and disease. Biochemistry, 49(24), 4945–4956. https://doi.org/10.1021/bi1004798Abdulraheem, A. L., Faraj, R. K., Hama Amin, G. S., et al. (2023). Prevalence of anemia, iron deficiency anemia and its socio-demographic factors among pregnant women in Garmian Province, Kurdistan region of Iraq. https://core.ac.uk/download/568376974.pdf (accessed on 12th June 2025).
2. Amer, A., Soliman, D. S., Ibrahim, F., El-Omri, H., Ganwo, I., Chandra, P., Kohla, S., et al. (2022). Acquired sideroblastic anemia: An exploratory comparative statistical analysis between clonal and non-clonal cases. https://core.ac.uk/download/552045528.pdf (accessed on 12th June 2025).
3. Bagguley, T., Blijlevens, N., Bowen, D., et al. (2017). Labile plasma iron levels predict survival in patients with lower-risk myelodysplastic syndromes. https://core.ac.uk/download/132212833.pdf (accessed on 12th June 2025).
4. Bangal, B., Baheti, V., Deshpande, T., Podey, S., et al. (2019). Efficacy, tolerability and safety of intravenous iron sucrose in postpartum anemia. https://core.ac.uk/download/327998962.pdf (accessed on 12th June 2025).
5. Bartels, M., de Wilde, J., Grootendorst, S., et al. (2021). The interplay between drivers of erythropoiesis and iron homeostasis in rare hereditary anemias: Tipping the balance. https://core.ac.uk/download/613938469.pdf (accessed on 12th June 2025).
6. Baughman, J. M., Culotta, V. C., Kaplan, J., et al. (2009). Discovery of genes essential for heme biosynthesis through large-scale gene expression analysis. https://core.ac.uk/download/pdf/81196499.pdf (accessed on 12th June 2025).
7. Berman, J., Coombs, A., Dufay, J. N., et al. (2016). Glycine and folate ameliorate models of congenital sideroblastic anemia. https://core.ac.uk/download/76420276.pdf (accessed on 12th June 2025).
8. Bertini, E., Bianchi, M., Carrozzo, R., et al. (2017). A novel mutation in NDUFB11 unveils a new clinical phenotype associated with lactic acidosis and sideroblastic anemia. https://core.ac.uk/download/54531084.pdf (accessed on 12th June 2025).
9. Bertino, F., Chiabrando, D., & Tolosano, E. (2020). Hereditary ataxia: A focus on heme metabolism and Fe-S cluster biogenesis. https://core.ac.uk/download/385864070.pdf (accessed on 12th June 2025).
10. Blau, N., Cotter, M., Crushell, E., et al. (2023). Clinical and biochemical footprints of inherited metabolic disease. XVI. Hematological abnormalities. https://core.ac.uk/download/636779735.pdf (accessed on 12th June 2025).
11. Campagna, D. R., Caruso Brown, A. E., Cattivelli, K., et al. (2016). Ringed sideroblasts in β-thalassemia. https://deepblue.lib.umich.edu/bitstream/handle/2027.42/136352/pbc26324.pdf?sequence=1&isAllowed=y (accessed on 12th June 2025).
12. Cardenas-Rodriguez, M., Chatzi, A., & Tokatlidis, K. (2018). Iron–sulfur clusters: From metals through mitochondria biogenesis to disease. https://core.ac.uk/download/153444555.pdf (accessed on 12th June 2025).

13. Carreño-Gago, L., Garcia-Arumí, E., Garrabou Tornos, G., et al. (2021). Two novel variants in YARS2 gene are responsible for an extended MLASA phenotype with pancreatic insufficiency. https://core.ac.uk/download/479276381.pdf (accessed on 12th June 2025).
14. Cavezzi, A., Troiani, E., & Corrao, S. (2020). COVID-19: Hemoglobin, iron, and hypoxia beyond inflammation. A narrative review. Clinics and Practice, 10, 1271–1271. https://doi.org/10.4081/cp.2020.1271 (accessed on 12th June 2025).
15. Cleary, M. A., Lindley, K. J., Rahman, S., et al. (2013). A distinct mitochondrial myopathy, lactic acidosis and sideroblastic anemia (MLASA) phenotype associates with YARS2 mutations. https://core.ac.uk/download/16264866.pdf (accessed on 12th June 2025).
16. Conte, S. (2016). Genotype-phenotype relations in SF3B1 mutated myelodysplastic syndromes with ring sideroblasts. https://core.ac.uk/download/70344139.pdf (accessed on 12th June 2025).
17. Crispin, A. (2017). HSCB, a co-chaperone in mitochondrial iron-sulfur cluster biogenesis, is a novel candidate gene for congenital sideroblastic anemia. https://open.bu.edu/bitstream/2144/26669/5/Crispin_bu_0017N_13280.pdf (accessed on 12th June 2025).
18. Fernández-Vizarra, E., & Zeviani, M. (2020). Mitochondrial disorders of the OXPHOS system. FEBS Letters, 595, 1062–1106. https://doi.org/10.1002/1873-3468.13995 (accessed on 12th June 2025).
19. Figueiredo, M. S., & Vicari, P. (2010). Differential diagnosis of iron deficiency. https://core.ac.uk/download/37709174.pdf (accessed on 12th June 2025).
20. Fisher, M. (2007). Anemia in PEDs. https://core.ac.uk/download/62771891.pdf (accessed on 12th June 2025).
21. Galati, M. C., Giancotti, L., Miniero, R., et al. (2018). Iron deficiency and iron deficiency anemia in children. https://core.ac.uk/download/322438447.pdf (accessed on 12th June 2025).
22. Geissler, C., & Singh, M. (2011). Iron, meat and health. Nutrients, 3(3), 283–316. https://doi.org/10.3390/nu3030283 (accessed on 12th June 2025).
23. Henson, A. L. (2013). Molecular Bases of Inherited Bone Marrow Failures: Schwachman-Diamond Syndrome and Diamond Black Fan Anemia. https://core.ac.uk/download/143834116.pdf (accessed on 12th June 2025).
24. Jia, H., Zhang, Q., Jia, Q., Cheng, T., Zhang, W., Yuan, W., Fang, X., et al. (2013). Assessment of hematopoietic failure due to Rpl11 deficiency in a zebrafish model of Diamond-Black fan anemia by deep sequencing. https://core.ac.uk/download/19838210.pdf (accessed on 12th June 2025).
25. Kelly, A. U., McSorley, S. T., Patel, P., et al. (2017). Interpreting iron studies. https://core.ac.uk/download/83960582.pdf (accessed on 12th June 2025).
26. Li, C., Pei, L., Yan, H., Zeng, et al. (2017). Iron deficiency anemia. https://core.ac.uk/download/322431331.pdf (accessed on 12th June 2025).
27. May, A., Yunis, A. A., Bergmann, A. K., Spiegelman, B. M., Camaschella, C., Wallace, D. C., Wallace, D. C., et al. (2011). SOD2 deficient erythroid cells up-regulate transferrin receptor and down-regulate mitochondrial biogenesis and metabolism. https://core.ac.uk/download/pdf/8523211.pdf (accessed on 12th June 2025).

28. Nai, A., Camaschella, C., & Silvestri, L. (2020). Iron metabolism and iron disorders revisited in the hepcidin era. https://core.ac.uk/download/616505330.pdf (accessed on 12th June 2025).

29. Pawsat, G. A. (2021). Investigation of Semiquantitative Marrow Iron Scoring and Reticulocyte Hemoglobin Content (CHr) in Healthy and Ill Canines with And Without Clinical Evidence of Blood Loss. https://core.ac.uk/download/524887883.pdf (accessed on 12th June 2025).

30. Pyatt, D., & Natelson, E. A. (2013). Acquired myelodysplasia or myelodysplastic syndrome: Clearing the fog. https://core.ac.uk/download/206710539.pdf (accessed on 12th June 2025).

31. Ricci, A., Buzzetti, E., Corradini, E., Bergamini, E., Di Betto, G., & Ventura, P. (2022). Iron metabolism in the disorders of heme biosynthesis. https://core.ac.uk/download/543263252.pdf (accessed on 12th June 2025).

32. Tuli, A., & Yenilmez, E. D. (2017). Laboratory approach to anemia. https://core.ac.uk/download/322432622.pdf (accessed on 12th June 2025).

33. Van Coster, R., & Vanlander, A. (2018). Clinical and genetic aspects of defects in the mitochondrial iron-sulfur cluster synthesis pathway. https://core.ac.uk/download/210534359.pdf (accessed on 12th June 2025).

34. Wright, B. N. (2014). Iron Nutriture Following Roux-En-Y Gastric Bypass Surgery. https://core.ac.uk/download/77955417.pdf (accessed on 12th June 2025).

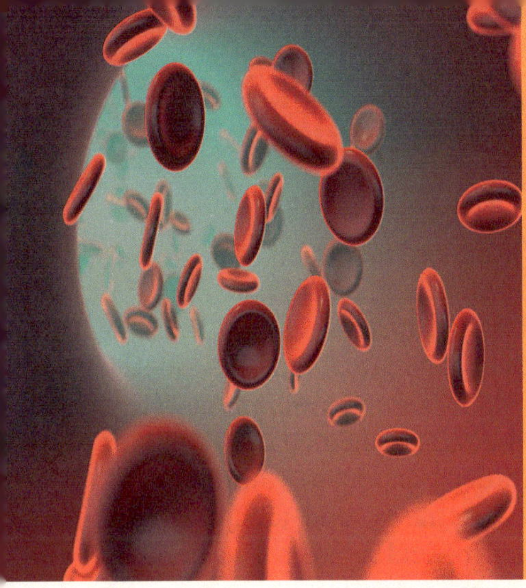

Chapter 4

HEMOLYTIC ANEMIAS

Contents

Introduction.....81
4.1. Causes of Hemolytic Anemias.....82
4.2. Symptoms and Diagnosis.....86
4.3. Treatment and Management.....91
4.4. Prognosis and Complications.....95
Summary.....101
References.....102

Introduction

Among the hematological diseases, hemolytic anemias constitute a significant group, characterized by premature red blood cell (RBC) lysis, which results in compromised oxygen-carrying capacity and secondary clinical manifestations. Understanding this condition involves considering its etiology, which can be broadly classified into intrinsic and extrinsic causes. The inherent causes could be genetic mutations that affect RBC integrity, such as β-thalassemia syndromes, where defects in genes substantially impact the production of hemoglobin and lead to the requirement for chronic transfusions (Lal et al., 2021). On the other hand, extrinsic causes could be autoimmune mechanisms or drug hypersensitivities to certain drugs, which can cause hemolysis. Resolution of hemolytic anemias on an overall scale requires a multidisciplinary approach that incorporates expert opinion and evidence-based practices for effective treatment of the condition (Bryan et al., 2021). Awareness of the linked mechanisms and clinical presentations of hemolytic anemias is thus needed for improving patient outcomes.

4.1. Causes of Hemolytic Anemias

Hemolytic anemias are characterized by the earlier destruction of RBCs, caused by a large variety of etiologies. They are generally categorized into immune and non-immune mechanisms. Immune-mediated hemolytic anemias are those that occur when antibodies inappropriately target RBCs for destruction, perhaps in the context of diseases such as systemic lupus erythematosus, as described in the antiphospholipid antibody syndrome (Alarcón-Segovia et al., 2020). However, non-immune causes involve genetic factors such as membrane dysfunction, enzymatic deficits, or hemoglobinopathies, as well as acquired conditions like infection, systemic disease, and drug exposure (Phillips et al., 2018). The clinical presentation may be characterized by jaundice, lethargy, and tachycardia, in addition to laboratory findings consistent with hemolysis, including reticulocytosis and elevated lactate dehydrogenase levels. Identification of these different etiological determinants is crucial in the diagnosis as well as treatment of hemolytic anemias (Figure 4.1).

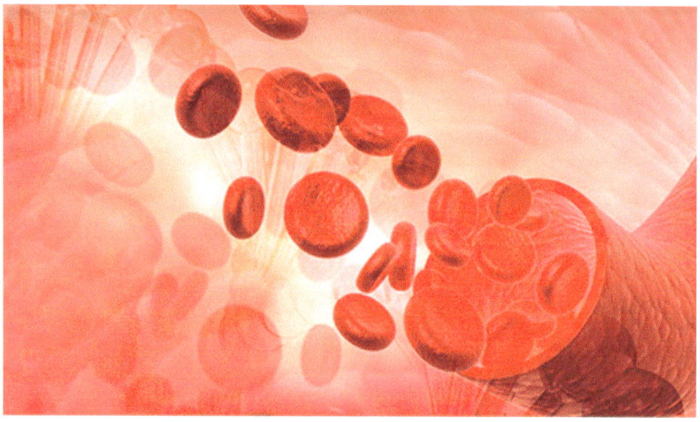

Figure 4.1. Hemolytic anemias are characterized by the premature destruction of red blood cells, resulting from a variety of underlying causes.

Source: https://www.hopkinsmedicine.org/-/media/images/health/1_-conditions/heart-and-vascular/hemolytic-anemia-teaser-image.jpg.

4.1.1. Inherited Genetic Disorders

Inherited genetic disorders are the leading cause of hemolytic anemias, highlighting the complex interaction between genetic variations and the production of blood cells. For instance, β-thalassemia is a paradigm of an autosomal recessive disease characterized by the reduced production of the beta-globin chains of hemoglobin, resulting in ineffective erythropoiesis and chronic hemolytic anemia. This disease focuses on the consequences of specific genetic mutations, for example, when alterations in the HBB gene lead to disturbances in the production of alpha and beta globin chains, ultimately causing RBC deterioration. Furthermore, an understanding of the molecular mechanisms that underlie these disorders, including the regulation of iron homeostasis related to hepcidin and ferroportin, is necessary to improve therapeutic treatments for patients suffering from these conditions. Results from gene research have the potential to open up promising routes for gene-targeted therapy, thereby enhancing the treatment of inherited hemolytic anemias (Erik et al., 2019; Camaschella et al., 2020).

4.1.2. Acquired Conditions

Acquired disorders are key factors in the pathophysiology of hemolytic anemias, where the external environment plays a role in the destruction of RBCs. Unlike inherited anemias, acquired hemolytic anemias have many etiologies and encompass disorders caused by autoimmune diseases, infections, and exposure to certain medications or toxins. In autoimmune hemolytic anemia (AIHA), the body's immune system mistakenly attacks RBCs, leading to their premature destruction. This condition may vary in severity, making it essential to employ integrated assessment methods to identify causative factors, given that it is merely a symptom and not a disease in itself (Tuli et al., 2017). Moreover, recent developments in hematology research have clarified the necessity for more robust diagnostic and treatment procedures in this field (Anagnou et al., 2021). Understanding these acquired conditions is crucial for managing and treating hemolytic anemias effectively (Figure 4.2).

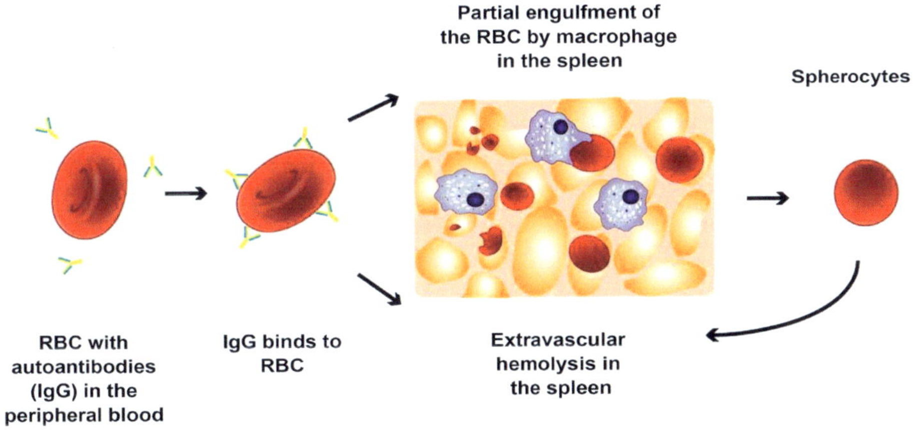

Figure 4.2. Acquired conditions play a significant role in the pathophysiology of hemolytic anemias, where external factors contribute to the destruction of red blood cells (RBCs).

Source: https://myhematology.com/wp-content/uploads/2024/03/warm-AIHA.jpg.

4.1.3. Immune-Mediated Hemolysis

Immune-mediated hemolysis is one of the primary forms of hemolytic anemias, characterized by the body's immune system mistakenly attacking and destroying RBCs. It tends to do so via autoantibody formation, which can trigger direct hemolysis or complement system activation, leading to RBC destruction. One of the typical subtypes is cold agglutinin disease, in which cold agglutinins can cause hemolysis, especially in cold weather, and present with symptoms such as acrocyanosis and severe anemia (Tvedt et al., 2021).

Besides, immune-mediated hemolysis management is complex and requires a thorough understanding of immunotherapy, particularly in identifying the risks associated with immune checkpoint inhibitors. These can cause dangerous immune responses (Bryan et al., 2021). Hence, an understanding of the mechanisms and management strategies for immune-mediated hemolysis is paramount for effective clinical treatment of hemolytic anemias.

4.1.4. Infections Leading to Hemolysis

Infections are a significant etiology of hemolytic anemias and often cause direct damage to RBCs or activate immune processes that compromise RBC integrity. Intravascular hemolysis is caused by pathogens such as the malaria parasite and certain bacterial toxins, resulting in sudden hemoglobin loss. The presentation may be sudden and include jaundice and anemia, necessitating urgent diagnostic tests. Laboratory testing will reflect increased reticulocytes as the marrow attempts to replace the lost cells, as well as elevated lactate dehydrogenase (LDH) and decreased haptoglobin levels, consistent with hemolytic activity (Fattizzo et al., 2015). Because infections could potentially be complicated by other conditions such as thrombocytopenia and organ dysfunction as well, adequate clinical and laboratory assessment must be done for optimal management. Lastly, understanding the mechanisms by which infections cause hemolysis is essential for designing effective interventions and enhancing patient outcomes (To et al., 2018) (Figure 4.3).

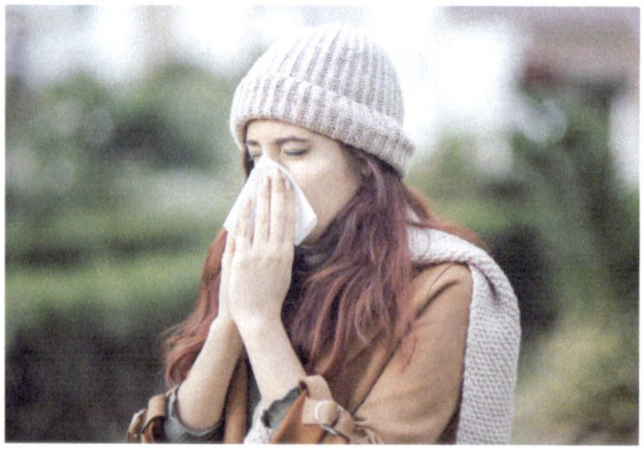

Figure 4.3. Infections represent a significant etiology of hemolytic anemias, often causing direct damage to red blood cells (RBCs) or indirectly triggering immune responses that compromise RBC integrity.

Source: https://cdn-prod.medicalnewstoday.com/content/images/articles/312/312508/aiha-can-happen-as-a-complication-of-an-infection-or-virus.jpg.

4.1.5. Drug-Induced Hemolytic Anemia

The etiology of drug-induced hemolytic anemia (DIIHA) is a complex interplay of drugs and the immune system, leading to the accidental lysis of RBCs. It is an infrequent but perilous disease that can be induced by a large number of medications, the most frequently encountered culprits being antibiotics, particularly the cephalosporins, and chemotherapy drugs. An instance involving dapagliflozin, an antidiabetic, highlighted the danger of severe hemolytic reactions, prompting its re-evaluation of safety among vulnerable populations (Lemack et al., 2025). Similarly, another report cited an instance where treatment with ceftriaxone for pyogenic meningitis resulted in catastrophic outcomes, such as intracranial hemorrhage, emphasizing the need for timely identification of DIIHA (Tomar et al., 2024). These reports illustrate the pressing need for close observation and early treatment of patients on high-risk drugs, as early diagnosis and treatment can radically alter prognosis and minimize morbidity from this disorder.

4.1.6. Mechanical Destruction of Red Blood Cells (RBCs)

Mechanical hemolysis of RBCs is responsible for a significant proportion of hemolytic anemias, where the membrane integrity of the erythrocyte is compromised through premature cell lysis. Turbulent blood flow, mechanical injury, and prosthetic heart valves are some of the causative agents for this form of hemolysis. The increased shear stress experienced by RBCs under these conditions can cause morphological alterations and lysis, resulting in the release of hemoglobin into the circulation. This is followed by compensatory mechanisms, including rapid phagocytosis by macrophages to counteract extracellular toxicity of hemoglobin. Notably, these erythrophagocytes not only destroy defective cells but also play a crucial role in modulating cell and inflammatory responses (To et al., 2018). A grasp of mechanical destruction dynamics is more accurate in the context of hemolytic anemias and provides insight into future targets of therapy aimed at reducing RBC lysis, as well as patient prognosis (To et al., 2018) (Figure 4.4).

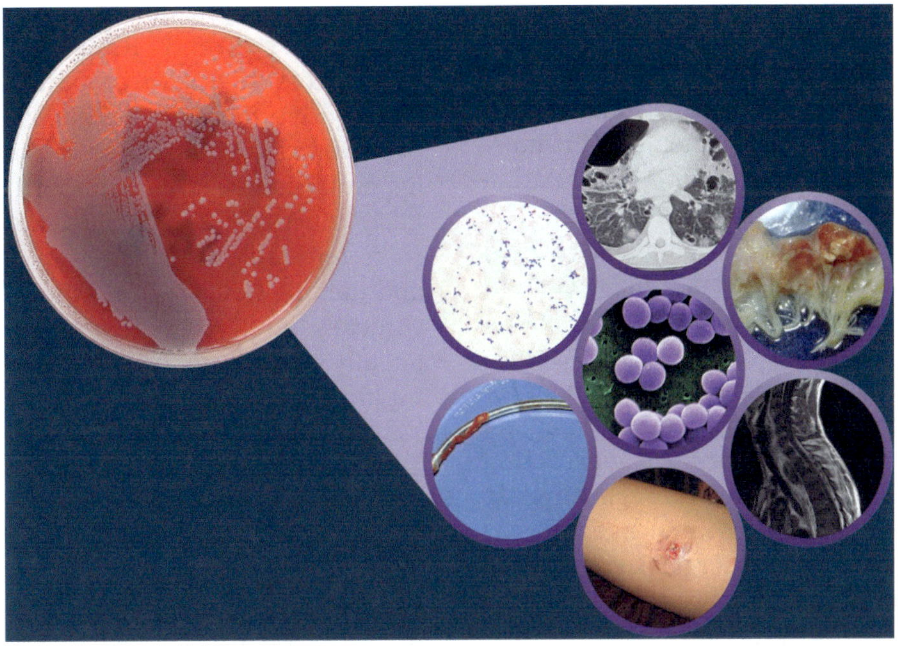

Figure 4.4. Mechanical destruction of red blood cells (RBCs) is a significant contributor to hemolytic anemias, wherein the integrity of the erythrocyte membrane is compromised, resulting in premature cell lysis.

Source: https://journals.asm.org/cms/asset/897bde9f-c463-485c-9c07-751e64608e3b/cmr.2015.28.issue-3.largecover.jpg.

4.1.7. Environmental Factors

Environmental factors play a significant role in the development and complications of hemolytic anemias, particularly due to toxic exposures and infection. For instance, bacteria in food, found in a wide variety of animal foods, have been established as primary environmental triggers of hemolytic states. Consumption of contaminated meat or milk products releases harmful bacteria such as Salmonella and E. coli into the body, triggering gastrointestinal symptoms that may lead to hemolytic anemia in susceptible individuals (Abebe et al., 2020). The drug-resistant forms of such foodborne pathogens are also an additional public health concern by hampering management interventions for infections that may lead to hemolysis (Abebe et al., 2020). Additionally, certain environmental toxins, such as heavy metals and chemicals, have been shown to interfere with erythropoiesis and provoke hemolysis, thereby affecting total hemoglobin content and RBC stability, ultimately leading to the clinical manifestation of hemolytic anemias.

4.1.8. Nutritional Deficiencies

Nutritional deficiencies are a significant reason why hemolytic anemias develop and appear because they weaken the body's ability to produce healthy RBCs. Critical nutrients, such as iron, folate, and vitamin B12, all play significant roles in erythropoiesis; without these, hemolysis will rise and RBC production will be inadequate. For instance, iron deficiency anemia is the most prevalent and illustrates the simple correlation of nutrition with hematological health. The Biomarkers of Nutrition for Development (BOND) program demonstrates that although current iron biomarkers are effective in quantifying iron nutrition, inflammation can render outcomes inaccurate and complicate the diagnosis of related disorders, such as hemolytic anemia (Lynch et al., 2018). Therefore, correcting such nutritional deficiencies through targeted dietary interventions is essential not only for preventing anemia but also for achieving overall health outcomes, which necessitates public health interventions in the form of nutritional education and access to the required nutrients (Figure 4.5).

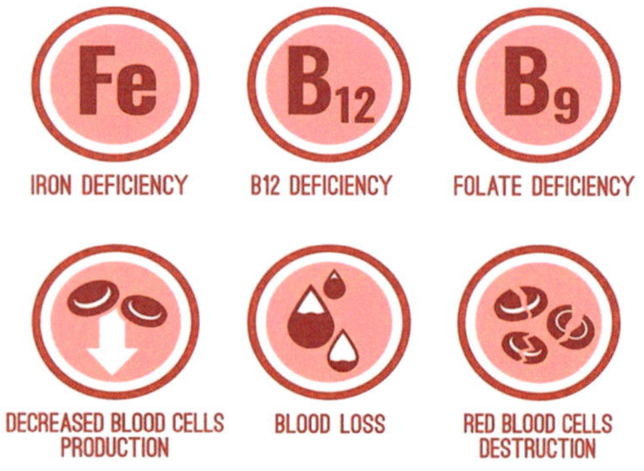

Figure 4.5. Nutritional deficiencies are a significant contributor to the onset and development of hemolytic anemias, as they impair the bodys ability to produce healthy red blood cells.

Source: https://d2jx2rerrg6sh3.cloudfront.net/image-handler/picture/2021/5/shutterstock_1155358696.jpg.

4.1.9. Hemolytic Disease of the Newborn

Hemolytic disease of the newborn (HDN) is a serious neonatal care problem, resulting from immune hemolysis due to maternal antibodies that destroy fetal RBCs. HDN primarily occurs due to Rh incompatibility, when an Rh-negative mother is pregnant with an Rh-positive baby, which can lead to severe anemia, hyperbilirubinemia, and newborn complications. Early diagnosis and management are critical since untreated HDN can result in kernicterus and lifelong neurological injury. Presentations clinically often present with jaundice, which usually occurs in the first 24 hours of life, highlighting the necessity of monitoring bilirubin and the need for phototherapy or exchange transfusion in cases of severity. It also encompasses ABO incompatibility cases, however less severe, which nevertheless require appropriate management. By understanding pathophysiology and the clinical importance of HDN, health professionals are capable of responding appropriately to its risks and improving neonatal outcomes (Debra et al., 2017; Joel, 2019).

4.2. Symptoms and Diagnosis

The clinical presentation of hemolytic anemias typically encompasses a varied assortment of symptoms that arise primarily from the increased destruction of RBCs. Fatigue, pallor, and jaundice are common signs resulting from low hemoglobin and elevated bilirubin levels, often associated with hemolysis. In certain types of hemolytic anemia, such as beta-thalassemia, patients may develop severe anemia, as well as splenomegaly and other systemic sequelae, due to iron overload resulting from chronic blood transfusions. Diagnosis is based on a combination of clinical examination and laboratory investigations, and tests such as complete blood count (CBC), reticulocyte count, and indirect bilirubin are of crucial significance. Besides, immunohematological analyses play a vital role in the case of diseases like AIHA, which involves the presence of autoantibodies that complicate standard diagnostic procedures (Elaroussi et al., 2025; Furmiga ISL, 2024). Early detection and accurate diagnosis are crucial for managing the numerous complications associated with these conditions.

4.2.1. Common Symptoms of Hemolytic Anemias

Hemolytic anemias exhibit a variety of symptoms that result directly from the premature destruction of RBCs. The most prevalent symptom is anemia, characterized by fatigue, pallor, and weakness due to decreased hemoglobin levels. Jaundice occurs in most patients and presents as yellow pigmentation of the skin and eyes, resulting from elevated bilirubin levels due to the breakdown of hemoglobin. In addition, splenomegaly may result as the spleen overcompensates to filter out the defective RBCs. In some cases, gallstones may develop as a consequence of increased bilirubin, resulting in cholecystitis (Holme et al., 2024). Moreover, AIHAs can present differently according to the etiology; for example, systemic lupus erythematosus can develop severe hematological complications necessitating prompt diagnosis and treatment (Osorio-Toro et al., 2023). Diagnosis of these symptoms is pivotal for effective management of the condition (Figure 4.6).

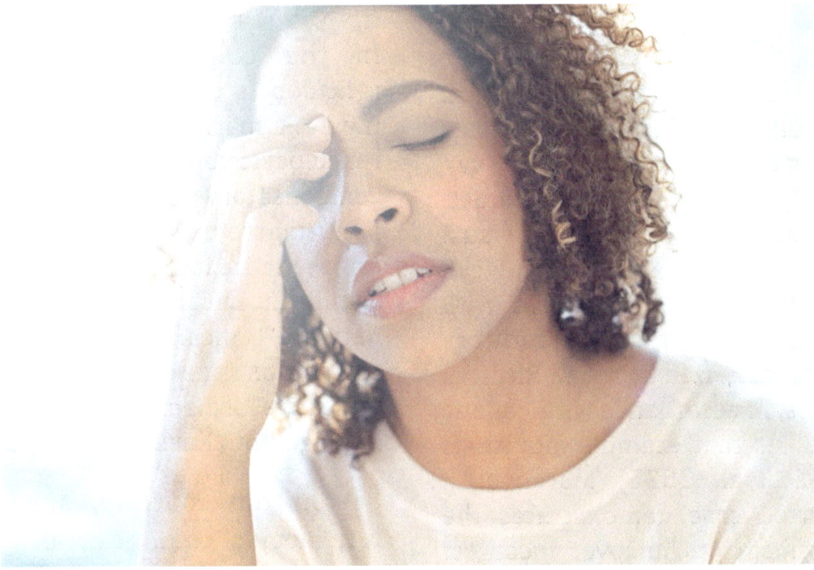

Figure 4.6. Hemolytic anemias present a variety of symptoms that directly result from the premature destruction of red blood cells.

Source: https://ucmscdn.healthgrades.com/7b/32/d0b7a8eb4fef829f047ca91d21a1/gettyimages-758312205-super.jpg.

4.2.2. Laboratory Tests for Diagnosis

Precise diagnosis of hemolytic anemias is based on a cascade of specific laboratory tests that provide hints to the underlying pathological processes. Initial tests include a CBC, which indicates decreased hemoglobin and abnormal RBC indices, essential for differentiating hemolytic anemia from other etiologies. Furthermore, reticulocyte counts are also crucial; increased reticulocyte production reflects a more vigorous marrow response to anemia and is usually present with hemolytic disease. Some studies can also incorporate the Coombs test to rule out autoimmune causes, and further examinations can reveal underlying infections, such as parvovirus, which has been reported in immunocompromised patients (Gartner et al., 1993). This virus leads to pronounced anemia, thus highlighting the importance of thorough diagnostic tests (Tuli et al., 2017). Lastly, the inclusion of these lab findings not only serves to confirm a diagnosis but also guides subsequent treatment plans, making them integral to the management of hemolytic anemias.

4.2.3. Role of Blood Smears

Blood smear examination is essential in hemolytic anemia diagnosis and management as a handy diagnostic tool for hematologists even in the scenario of novel molecular techniques. Traditional blood smears provide direct visual information about RBC morphology and can reveal characteristic changes associated with specific disorders. For instance, hereditary spherocytosis is characterized by round RBCs, as observed in smears, in accordance with genetic findings from studies that examine mutations such as SPTB (Li et al., 2025). Moreover, a thoroughly reported case demonstrates the power of blood smears to uncover incorrect prior diagnoses, highlighting their significant diagnostic value. Initial spherocytosis categorizations were disproven by thorough blood smear analysis, which instead identified target cells typical of an uncommon condition (Matzdorff et al., 2023). Therefore, blood smears remain an integral component of hematologic evaluation in patients, ensuring accurate diagnoses and guiding therapeutic management in hemolytic anemias (Figure 4.7).

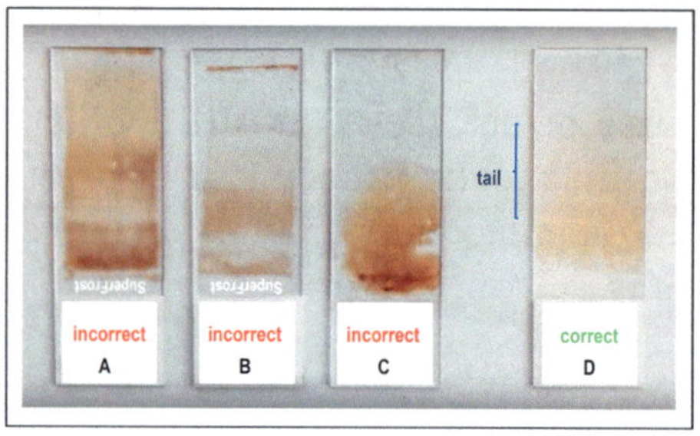

Figure 4.7. Traditional blood smears provide direct visual insights into red blood cell morphology, which can reveal characteristic changes associated with specific disorders.

Source: https://pub.mdpi-res.com/jcm/jcm-09-00539/article_deploy/html/images/jcm-09-00539-g001.png?1583574213.

4.2.4. Importance of Reticulocyte Count

In the context of hemolytic anemias, reticulocyte count is a significant indicator of the bone marrow's response to anemia. A high reticulocyte count generally indicates a standard compensatory mechanism, indicating that the bone marrow is actively producing RBCs to replace those lost due to hemolysis. This is most significant in conditions such as AIHA, in which patients typically have elevated reticulocyte counts alongside other hematological parameters indicative of hemolysis, such as bilirubin and hemoglobin (Karimah et al., 2025).

On the contrary, anemia with a low reticulocyte count can also be a cause for concern regarding an underlying marrow failure or an inappropriately elevated erythropoietic response, e.g., in extensive vitamin B12 deficiency, which may lead to peripheral pancytopenia and further obscure the clinical presentation (Labban et al., 2024). Thus, monitoring the reticulocyte count has a vital role to play in the diagnosis and management of hemolytic anemias.

4.2.5. Bilirubin Levels and Their Significance

Measurement of the level of bilirubin is an essential diagnostic tool in the interpretation of hemolytic anemias because it increases where there is enhanced RBC breakdown. Here, the liver's capability of conjugating and excreting bilirubin is normally overpowered and results in hyperbilirubinemia. This is especially relevant in patients with inherited hemolytic disease, where the incidence of conditions such as gallstones secondary to excess unconjugated bilirubin is significant (Abdullah et al., 2015). It is also essential to distinguish between the different types of hemolytic anemias, such as cold agglutinin disease, where laboratory tests can be misleading and diagnosis and treatment can be problematic (Aktaş et al., 2018). Accordingly, bilirubin level determinations not only reflect the severity of hemolysis but also influence management strategies and monitor resultant complications, with a focus on its significance in clinical evaluation of hemolytic anemias (Figure 4.8).

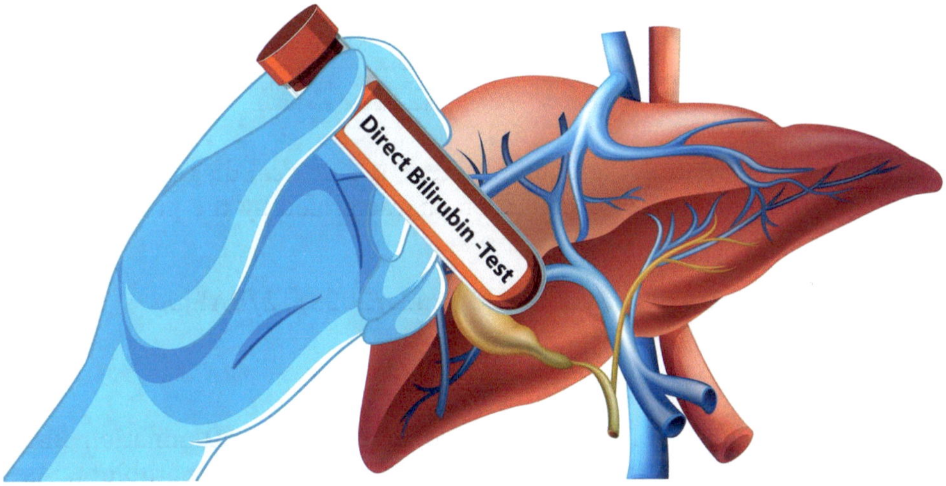

Figure 4.8. The measurement of bilirubin levels serves as a vital diagnostic tool in understanding hemolytic anemias, as elevated bilirubin indicates increased breakdown of red blood cells.

Source: https://mydiagnostics.in/cdn/shop/articles/img-1745900856135_262d3689-3099-4831-88e2-20675af0fd96_1200x.jpg?v=1745909399.

4.2.6. Coombs Test and Its Implications

The direct antiglobulin test, or the Coombs test, is a relevant diagnostic test for the diagnosis of AIHA, anemia characterized by the premature breakdown of RBCs. Not only does the test diagnose anemia, but it also detects autoantibodies against erythrocytes, which are used to assess underlying conditions such as malignancies or infections. This is particularly significant considering that AIHA can present in varying severity, from relatively mild illness to life-threatening anemia that complicates patient management (Fattizzo et al., 2020). Furthermore, the subtleties of AIHA diagnosis can be further complicated by factors such as the production of false positives by certain treatment drugs, like daratumumab, which complicates the clinical presentation for clinicians (Fattizzo et al., 2020). The challenge of diagnosing and treating AIHA, compared to specific diseases such as non-Hodgkin lymphoma (NHL), only serves to underscore the utility of the Coombs test in therapeutic decision-making and patient care (Figure 4.9).

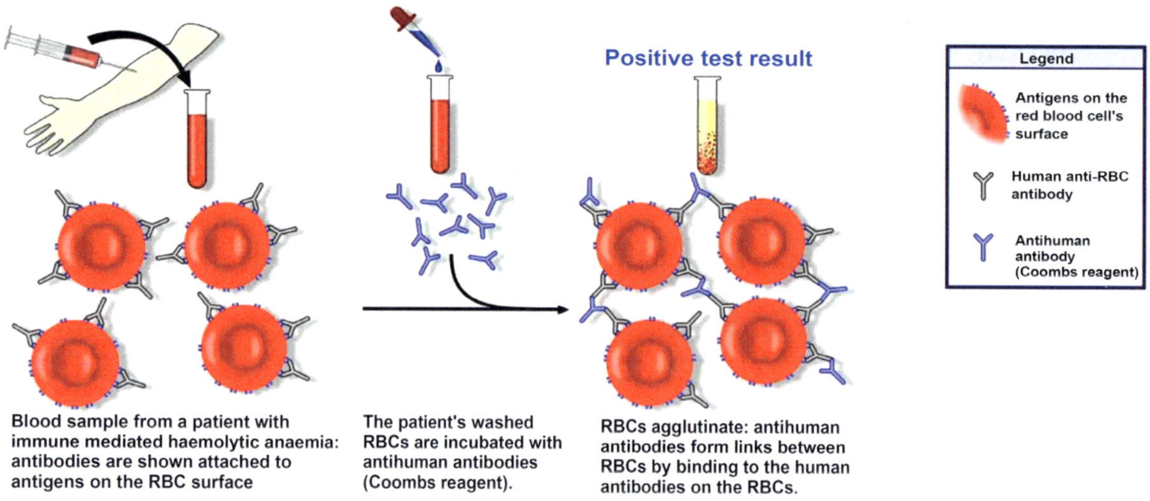

Figure 4.9. The Coombs test, or direct antiglobulin test, is a critical diagnostic tool for identifying autoimmune hemolytic anemia (AIHA), a condition characterized by the premature destruction of red blood cells.

Source: https://myhematology.com/wp-content/uploads/2023/12/DAT.jpg.

4.2.7. Bone Marrow Examination

Diagnosis of hemolytic anemias involves an extensive bone marrow examination since it provides critical information about erythropoiesis and the root cause of the pathology. As part of the procedure, bone marrow samples are analyzed to determine the normal functioning and cellular structure of hematopoietic cells, allowing for the identification of various types of anemia, such as bone marrow suppression or infiltration-based anemia. In hemolytic anemias, an elevated reticulocyte count may represent a compensatory attempt by the bone marrow in the wake of peripheral RBC destruction. The study may also provide clues to potential secondary causes, such as malignancies or autoimmune diseases, that can occur alongside hemolytic processes. Therefore, bone marrow examination is a valuable diagnostic tool through which physicians can formulate appropriate treatment strategies based on the individual patient's condition, particularly in the setting of the systemic findings of immune-related adverse events as defined by current guidelines (Elliott et al., 2020; Bryan et al., 2021).

4.2.8. Monitoring Disease Progression

Monitoring of disease activity in hemolytic anemias is crucial for optimizing treatment and improving patient outcomes. Physicians must monitor several biomarkers, including hemoglobin level, reticulocyte count, and indirect bilirubin level, which can indicate the severity and quality of hemolysis occurring. Non-invasive diagnostic methods, such as smartphone apps based on colorimetric detection, are increasingly becoming valuable tools to measure and identify changes in hemoglobin levels. As evidenced by the substantial healthcare costs associated with anemia, which totaled over $ 50 million from 2015 to 2020 in Brazil alone, the importance of effective monitoring techniques cannot be overstated. By facilitating early intervention, these monitoring tactics are capable of enhancing the management of hemolytic anemias, with the overall aim of reducing morbidity and mortality levels for the condition, as highlighted by Brill et al. (2009) and Abubakar et al. (2022) (Figure 4.10).

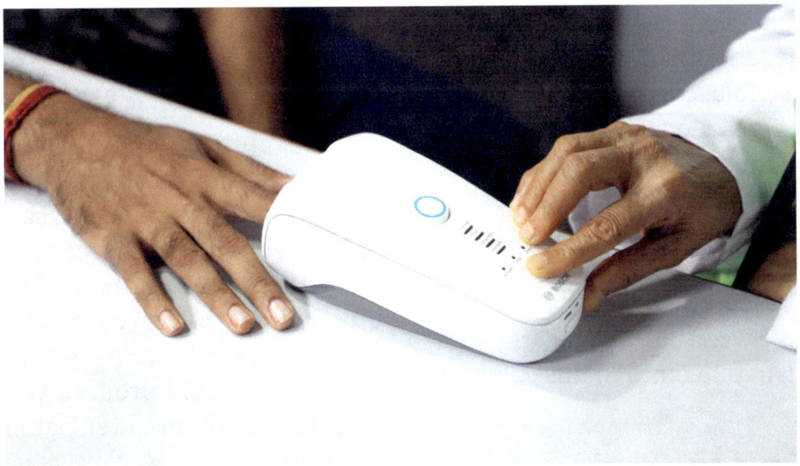

Figure 4.10. Non-invasive diagnostic approaches, such as smartphone applications utilizing colorimetric analysis, are emerging as practical tools to evaluate hemoglobin concentrations and monitor changes over time.

Source: https://www.bosch-presse.de/pressportal/zip?country=de&language=en&docId=223372.

4.3. Treatment and Management

Management of hemolytic anemias demands a multi-modal and individualized approach depending on the etiology and severity of the disease. Initial therapy is typically directed toward the principal cause of hemolysis, such as autoimmune mechanisms, congenital conditions, or other factors. In AIHA, corticosteroids are most commonly the first line of therapy; in severe cases, other options, such as immunosuppressants or splenectomy, can be employed to reduce hemolytic activity (Douglas et al., 2022). In hereditary disorders, such as SCD and β-thalassemia, new advances in therapy have involved new pharmacologic agents and gene therapy methodology. New agents, such as luspatercept and crizanlizumab, have revolutionized treatment practices, with the hope of more productive care and improved outcomes for patients (Cappellini et al., 2021). Continuing investigation will increasingly tend toward personalized treatment programs that respect individual patient variables and expressions of disease.

4.3.1. General Treatment Strategies

Effective control of hemolytic anemias requires a multi-faceted approach based on the etiology of the condition. Overall, therapeutic approaches begin with the diagnosis and management of the specific type of hemolytic anemia, e.g., autoimmune, genetic, or infectious etiologies. Supportive management is the cornerstone of therapy, such as blood transfusions in case of life-threatening anemia and intravenous immunoglobulin (IVIG) for autoimmune diseases. Furthermore, new treatment options are forthcoming, such as targeted biologic therapies to modulate immune processes or gene therapies to treat genetic abnormalities intrinsic to certain anemias (Iolascon et al., 2020). An inclusive model, as constructed by the European Hematology Association, emphasizes the value of standardized protocols in promoting effective treatment pathways for various hemolytic anemia presentations (Anagnou et al., 2021). Thus, continued research and collaboration among experts are crucial for optimizing care and improving patient outcomes in this complex field (Figure 4.11).

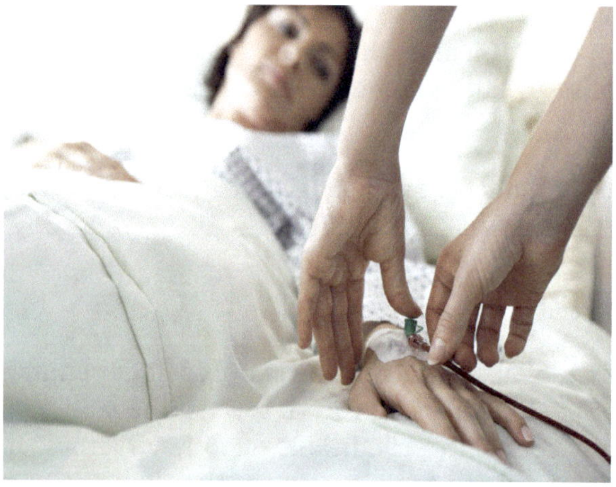

Figure 4.11. Supportive care is a cornerstone of treatment, encompassing measures such as blood transfusions to alleviate severe anemia and intravenous immunoglobulin (IVIG) for autoimmune cases.

Source: https://www.verywellhealth.com/thmb/pE2C7NYHcXD2vMM5trNg8WzjoH4=/1500x0/filters:no_upscale():max_bytes(150000):strip_icc()/GettyImages-77739876-566664b45f9b583dc39f30cb.jpg.

4.3.2. Use of Corticosteroids

Use of corticosteroids as a first-line treatment for AIHA is evidence of their role in immunomodulation, which is of special significance in light of the pathophysiology of these conditions. Corticosteroids are employed in warm AIHA, where autoantibodies act against RBCs, leading to their lysis. This first-line therapy will decrease hemolysis and improve patient outcomes, but should be referenced to have poor therapeutic response against cold agglutinin disease (CAD) (Kawamoto, 2024). Furthermore, prolonged corticosteroid therapy is hazardous and carries risks of great increased infection susceptibility, osteoporosis, and thromboembolism (Kawamoto, 2024). Accordingly, while corticosteroids are crucial in the management of temperature AIHA, clinicians should proceed with caution in their use, especially in older patients who may also have malignancies. This complexity, therefore, highlights the importance of a subtle approach in managing hemolytic anemias in balancing advantages versus possible adverse effects (Figure 4.12).

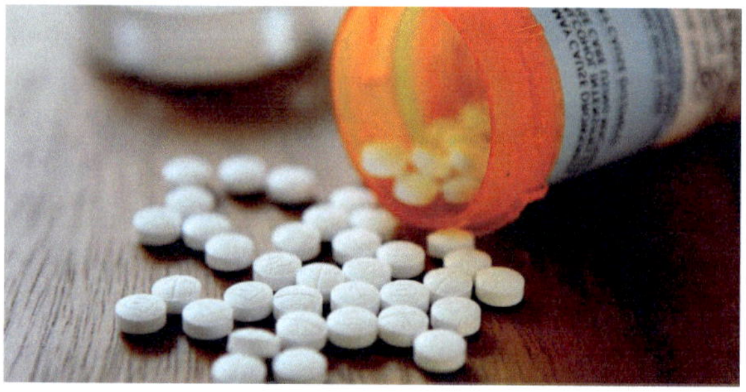

Figure 4.12. Corticosteroids are specifically employed in cases of warm AIHA, where autoantibodies target red blood cells, facilitating their destruction.

Source: https://medshadow.org/wp-content/uploads/2016/07/corticosteroids.jpg.

4.3.3. Blood Transfusions

Blood transfusion is a vital management

modality for hemolytic anemias, providing a crucial therapeutic maneuver in the case of severe RBC loss or dysfunction. In addition to its role in restoring the oxygen-carrying capacity of the blood to normal, transfusion is also used to treat the underlying cause of oxidative stress that exacerbates the symptoms of hemolytic disease. The complexity of blood transfusion is evident when considering the broad etiology of hemolytic anemias, particularly the need for adequate blood type matching to prevent adverse reactions. However, the recurrence of transfusions has complications with it, such as iron overload that can introduce more oxidative stress and organ damage (Dana et al., 2019). Along with this, patient treatment of rare inherited anemias is complicated and is all about the significance of guidelines that encompass treatment best practice, such as maternal and fetal outcomes during procedures (Iolascon et al., 2020). Though blood transfusions are an inseparable part of therapy, their application needs to be done carefully and with all the required knowledge.

4.3.4. Splenectomy and Its Indications

The operative procedure known as splenectomy, or removal of the spleen, holds substantial therapy in the management of several hemolytic anemias. The operation is particularly indicated for diseases associated with abnormal red cell breakdown, such as hereditary spherocytosis and AIHA. With the removal of the spleen, which plays a central role in blood purification and the elimination of faulty erythrocytes, splenectomy can enhance hemoglobin levels and alleviate symptoms of such diseases. It is important to note, however, that the procedure is not without risk; patients are at higher risk of overwhelming infection following splenectomy because of the immunoprotection function of the spleen (Ruggiero et al., 2018). Thus, preventive strategies, including vaccinations and antimicrobial prophylaxis, are crucial in mitigating these risks. These considerations underscore the need for selecting suitable candidates for splenectomy in the treatment of hemolytic anemia (Iolascon et al., 2020) (Figure 4.13).

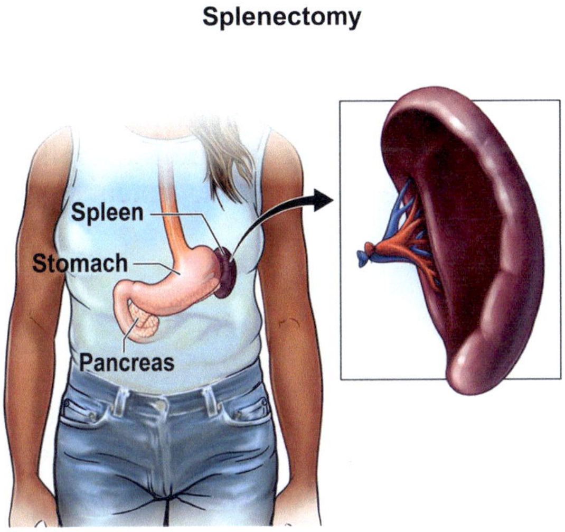

Figure 4.13. The surgical procedure known as splenectomy, defined as the removal of the spleen, holds significant therapeutic potential in the management of various hemolytic anemias.

Source: https://my.clevelandclinic.org/-/scassets/Images/org/health/articles/14614-splenectomy.jpg.

4.3.5. Management of Underlying Conditions

Adequate control of underlying conditions is important in the treatment of hemolytic anemias, which a myriad of precipitating factors can precipitate. Some examples include conditions such as complement-mediated thrombotic microangiopathies (CM-TMA), for which a multifaceted approach to therapy is necessary, encompassing not only symptomatic control but also the specific targeting of the underlying genetic or immunological dysregulation of the complement pathway (Musalem, 2025). Similarly, in cancer-related microangiopathic hemolytic anemia (CA-MAHA), the key strategy is strict management of the underlying malignancy, which is typically the underlying cause of anemia and associated issues (Shahd et al., 2024). By emphasizing the diagnosis and management of underlying conditions, clinicians can significantly enhance patient outcomes, thereby preventing the critical effects of hemolytic anemias and improving overall prognoses. This multistage strategy emphasizes the value of multidisciplinary treatment in the effective management of these complex syndromes.

4.3.6. Role of Immunosuppressive Therapy

The role of immunosuppressive therapy in the management of hemolytic anemias is pivotal, particularly when autoimmune mechanisms are involved in RBC destruction.

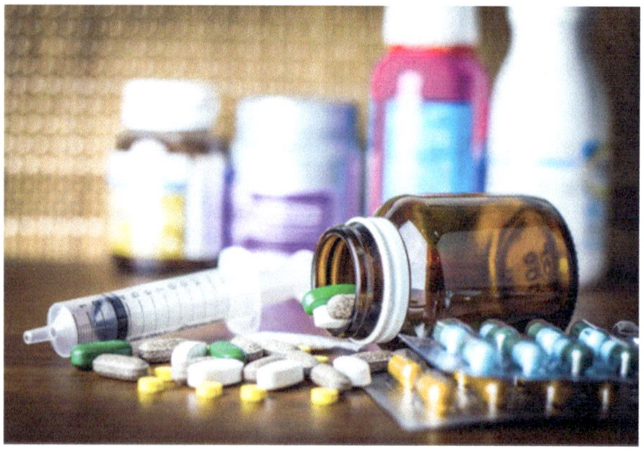

Figure 4.14. The role of immunosuppressive therapy in managing hemolytic anemias is pivotal, particularly in cases where autoimmune mechanisms drive red blood cell destruction.

Source: https://www.neoteryx.com/hs-fs/hubfs/shutterstock_544348294.jpg?width=500&height=334&name=shutterstock_544348294.jpg.

These therapies aim to prevent or minimize excessive immune responses that result in hemolysis, facilitating a return to erythropoiesis and normality in the patient. An example is the use of corticosteroids, whereby these can be administered to reduce inflammation and control immune activity. In cases of acute presentation, additional immunosuppression with agents targeting specific pathways would be required, particularly in those with a poor response to initial therapy. The existing guidelines suggest a multi-layered approach to managing immune-related adverse events, including early monitoring and dose adjustments based on severity (Bryan et al., 2021). Moreover, identifying potential thrombotic consequences is also required because syndromes like COVID-19-associated coagulopathy can complicate treatment plans (Iba et al., 2020). Lastly, tailored immunosuppressive therapy protocols are crucial to optimizing outcomes in patients with hemolytic anemias (Figure 4.14).

4.3.7. Nutritional Support and Supplementation

In the management of hemolytic anemias, nutritional support and supplementation play a dominant role in ensuring the best patient outcomes and symptomatic control. Appropriate nutrition is paramount, particularly because patients with hemolytic anemia may have increased nutritional needs secondary to the heightened turnover of RBCs and potential deficiencies. Interventions such as iron, folate, and vitamin B12 administration can significantly assist in maintaining erythropoiesis and mitigating the anemic effect. For example, in preterm populations with babies that require supplementation until breastfeeding is sufficient, studies have shown that some nutritional interventions influence overall well-being and growth profiles (Alexander et al., 2024). Furthermore, personalized nutritional monitoring and supplementation have also been shown to influence biochemical markers and overall well-being in various populations, including athletes who are subjected to unique physiological demands (Yu et al., 2024). Thus, the addition of specially designed nutritional measures becomes imperative for overall management of hemolytic anemias.

4.3.8. Patient Education and Support

Patient education and counseling are essential components of managing hemolytic anemias, as they enable patients to gain knowledge about their condition and take an active role in the treatment process. Patient education programs must focus on teaching patients about the nature of hemolytic anemias, including their presentations, complications, and treatment modalities.

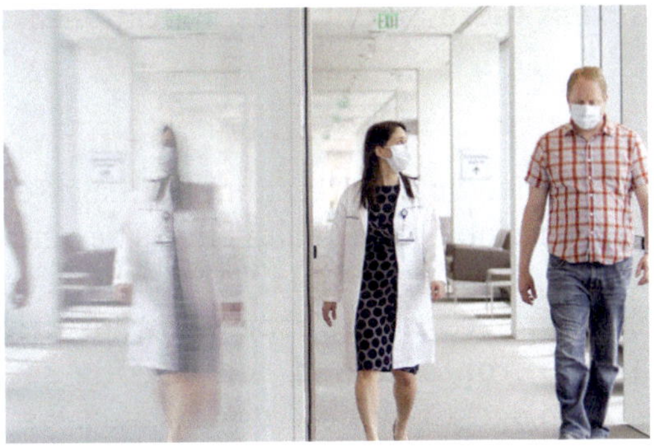

Figure 4.15. Patient education and support are crucial components in the management of hemolytic anemias, as they empower individuals to understand their condition and play an active role in treatment decisions.

Source: https://my.clevelandclinic.org/-/scassets/images/org/care-pages/cancer/benign-hematology-feature.jpg?w=640&q=75.

Effective communication enhances patient adherence to treatment protocols and fosters a supportive environment in which patients are encouraged to become increasingly engaged in controlling their health outcomes. Integrated care models, founded on teamwork between health professionals, have, as research indicates, been able to increase patient satisfaction and reduce hospital use among people with high needs (Adams et al., 2010). In addition, providing access to resources such as personalized educational materials and support groups can help patients navigate the challenges of hemolytic anemia and achieve better disease control and quality of life (To et al., 2018) (Figure 4.15).

4.4. Prognosis and Complications

The prognosis of hemolytic anemias is highly unpredictable, depending on the etiology and the immediate treatment implemented. Early diagnosis and effective management can prevent many potential complications, such as those caused by severe anemia, which may lead to cardiovascular compromise or organ failure due to inadequate tissue oxygenation. Especially, the disorders that are associated with severe hyper-eosinophilia, such as warm AIHA, underscore the fine points of management and prognostic condition, as demonstrated by difficulty experienced in cases that require intensive therapy (Brys et al., 2015). Furthermore, technological and innovative advances in hematology research continue to illuminate the pathophysiological mechanisms of such disorders, thereby optimizing clinical strategies to improve patient outcomes. The updated EHA Research Roadmap also emphasizes the importance of focused research into anemias and associated disorders, further underscoring the need for an evidence-based approach to prevention and treatment to achieve enhanced prognostic value (Anagnou et al., 2021).

4.4.1. Factors Influencing Prognosis

Prognosis in hemolytic anemias is influenced by a broad spectrum of variables that have considerable potential to impact patient outcomes. The etiology responsible for the anemia, patients' age, and their health status at the time of diagnosis are the primary determinants. For instance, AIHA in children typically has a fulminant course and a 10% mortality rate if it presents in the context of infections due to prolonged immunosuppression (Beretta et al., 2009). Furthermore, treatment modalities such as the creation of monoclonal antibodies, such as rituximab, not only enhance remission rates but also highlight ongoing clinical observation and supportive care during treatment (Allard et al., 2016). These evolving therapeutic strategies, alongside an appreciation of patient-specific factors, help to demonstrate the complexity of prognosis evaluation in hemolytic anemias, necessitating a holistic approach towards management and patient care (Figure 4.16).

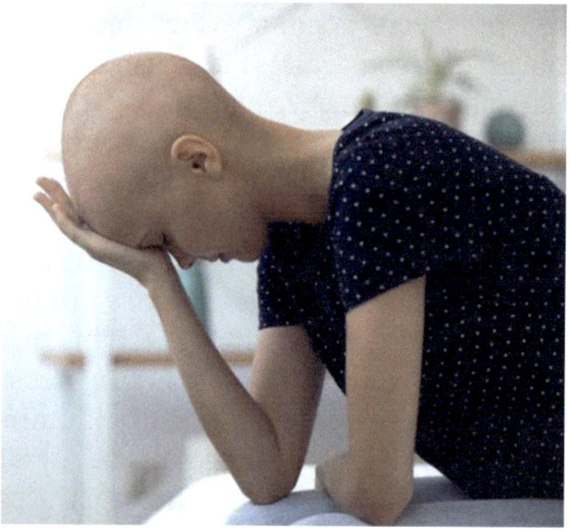

Figure 4.16. Key determinants include the underlying etiology of the anemia, the patients age, and their overall health status prior to diagnosis.

Source: https://zenonco-cf.zenonco.io/zen/website/images/uploads/CRF-scaled.jpg?format=auto&width=600.

4.4.2. Potential Complications of Hemolytic Anemias

The resultant complications of hemolytic anemias are multifaceted and can have significant impacts on patient mortality and morbidity. Patients with inherited conditions, such as Hereditary Spherocytosis (HS), may be at risk for chronic hemolysis, which can lead to gallstones and splenomegaly, particularly due to increased bilirubin production resulting from hemolysis (Toub et al., 2025). Age-related etiologies also play a significant role, e.g., elderly patients may have varied physiological presentation, including elevated blood pressure and biochemical markers that highlight renal and hepatic stress (Toub et al., 2025). In AIHA, complications can evolve acutely to intractable anemia, as seen in cases of intravascular hemolysis due to IgA antibodies. The subtle interaction between hemolytic effect and organ function requires close observation and control to prevent these potential complications.

4.4.3. Long-Term Health Effects

Chronic hemolytic anemias, namely β thalassemia, carry severe long-term health effects beyond the acute symptoms of anemia. Long-term red cell breakdown necessitates repeated transfusions, leading to iron overload and causing severe organ damage to critical organs such as the heart, liver, and endocrine glands. It causes a decline in physical and mental health, with chronic fatigue and late growth in children, and a decrease in the risk of skeletal deformity and fracture due to weakened bone strength. Furthermore, iron overload can lead to diabetes and cardiovascular diseases, and significantly impact overall quality of life (Lal et al., 2021). In addition, as treatment continues to evolve, deficits in transfusion care reflect the variable patient populations and their corresponding issues, highlighting the need for customized therapeutic approaches to mitigate such long-term consequences (Christopher et al., 2022). Intervention of such impacts on health is significant to improve patient outcomes and guide future health care approaches (Figure 4.17).

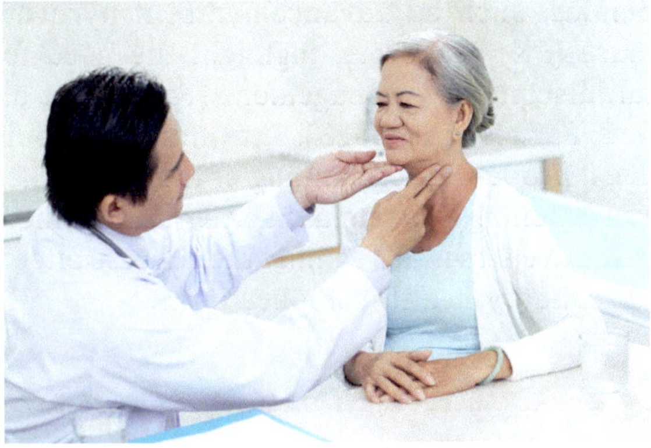

Figure 4.17. Chronic hemolytic anemias, such as β thalassemia, pose significant long-term health effects that extend beyond the immediate symptoms of anemia.

Source: https://cdn.drstemcellsthailand.com/wp-content/uploads/2025/01/image-55.png.

4.4.4. Quality of Life Considerations

Quality-of-life concerns are of utmost importance while contemplating the impact of hemolytic anemias, particularly in children. In hereditary spherocytosis (HS) or sickle cell disease (SCD) in children, surgery such as total or partial splenectomy has been found to result in significant hematologic benefits and improved outcomes in a clinical scenario, which is valuable for everyday functioning and overall well-being (Englum et al., 2020). Nevertheless, the benefits of such surgery must be weighed against potential complications, for instance, post-splenectomy sepsis risk, which may negatively affect the quality of life (Englum et al., 2020). Furthermore, neuropsychological dimensions of hemolytic anemias, particularly in SCD patients, refer to the role of intellectual functioning as one of the elements of quality of life. Studies have shown that nocturnal oxygen desaturations have a negative impact on cognitive functions, such as response speed and suppression, which may exacerbate issues in these individuals and suggest the need for comprehensive care strategies.

4.4.5. Psychological Impact on Patients

The psychological impact on patients with hemolytic anemia can indeed be substantial, both emotionally and in terms of overall well-being. Hemophilia patients become more depressed and anxious due to the nature of the illness's chronicity, as it may lead to uncertainty about the health outcomes and terror. These psychological problems are constantly augmented by the intricacies of the treatment and drug side effects, such as those observed with capecitabine, which induces non-immune hemolytic anemia, contributing to the emotional complexity of the patients as they seek to manage the disruptions of both their illness and its treatment (Hussain et al., 2022). Additionally, the social impact of suffering from a chronic illness can also result in feelings of isolation and stigma, further compounding the psychological burden. Management of such psychological morbidities is quite crucial in the integrated management of hemolytic anemias because they are well documented to highly impact the patient's compliance with therapy and overall quality of life (Tomasz et al., 2020).

4.4.6. Importance of Regular Follow-Up

The management of hemolytic anemias involves careful adherence to follow-up consultations, a critical component of therapeutic monitoring to assess patient response and adjust treatment protocols appropriately. Through follow-up consultations, clinicians can observe the effectiveness of ongoing therapy and detect any potential complications in their early stages. For instance, with the introduction of newer therapies, such as gene therapy or immunomodulator drugs, continuous monitoring ensures optimal results without risking potential side effects. Additionally, frequent evaluations enable personalized adjustments based on the patients' changing status, which is particularly crucial given the heterogeneity of hemolytic anemias. The European Hematology Association emphasizes the need for protocolized care plans, as rigorous follow-up has the potential to significantly enhance patient outcomes through optimally effective management (Bryan et al., 2021). The implementation of a robust follow-up mechanism is therefore crucial in addressing the complexities of hemolytic anemias and enhancing overall patient quality of life (Iolascon et al., 2021) (Figure 4.18).

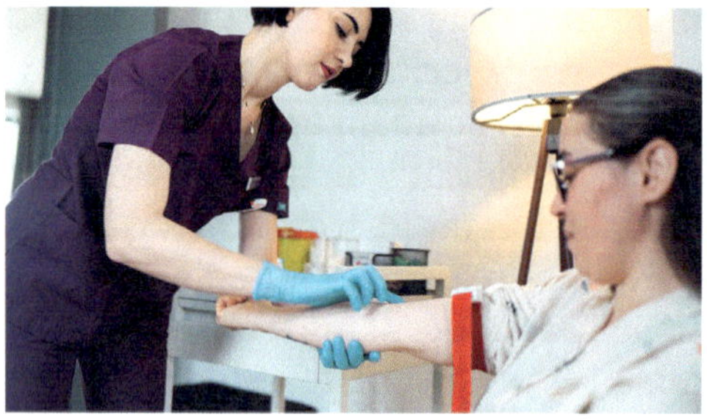

Figure 4.18. The management of hemolytic anemias necessitates the critical practice of regular follow-up appointments, which play an essential role in monitoring patient progress and adjusting treatment plans as needed.

Source: https://media.post.rvohealth.io/wp-content/uploads/2024/07/female-and-nurse-blood-test-1296-728-header.jpg.

4.4.7. Risk of Secondary Conditions

Hemolytic anemias pose significant issues not only due to their primary impact on RBCs but also for the possible secondary ailments that may develop. In the case of people with diseases like AIHA, the complexity of treatment options can complicate care and lead to additional health complications. The anemia itself can further exacerbate these secondary complications, as decreased oxygen delivery potentially has its effect on several organ systems and enhances the possibility of complications such as fatigue, cardiovascular stress, and even organ failure. In addition, emerging therapy approaches at targeting specific mechanisms in hemolytic anemias, such as advancements in pyruvate kinase (PK) activators, highlight the need for multidisciplinary management (Fattizzo et al., 2020; Bartels et al., 2023). The physician should have a proper understanding of the interlinked risks of hemolytic anemias in order to implement preventive strategies against the adverse effects of secondary health complications.

4.4.8. Advances in Treatment and Their Impact

The management of hemolytic anemias has evolved dramatically over the past few decades, primarily due to advances in treatment technologies and modalities that have significantly improved outcomes for patients.

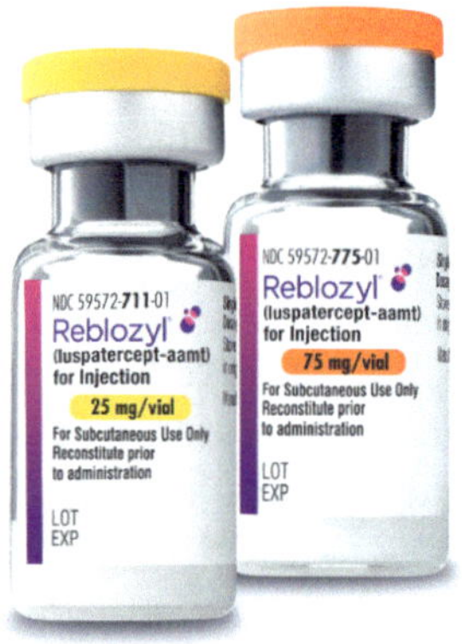

Figure 4.19. Reblozyl.

Source: https://www.reblozylpro.com/assets/buildeasy/us-commercial/reblozyl-hcp/en/images/reblozyl_1L_dosing_admin_hero_vials.png.web.540.960.png.

Central to such advances are new therapeutic modalities, such as gene therapy and targeted therapy, designed to treat the fundamental genetic defects responsible for diseases like β-thalassemia and others. For instance, drugs like Reblozyl (luspatercept-aamt), which increase red cell production, represent a significant innovation in clinical practice strategies, allowing patients to achieve a better quality of life with enhanced hemoglobin levels (Iolascon et al., 2021). Second, advancements in creating overall transfusion protocols based on precise research and coordination between academic institutions have optimized transfusion practices in order to meet its best possible outcomes. These developments not only enhance patient outcomes but also reduce long-term transfusion complications, such as iron overload, thereby highlighting the revolutionary nature of modern treatment modalities in the therapy of hemolytic anemias (Lal et al., 2021) (Figure 4.19).

4.4.9. Case Studies Illustrating Outcomes

The case study research provides thought-provoking insights into the various outcomes that characterize hemolytic anemias, highlighting the complexities involved in such cases. In a recent publication, for instance, it was reported that multifocal chorangiomatosis in a neonate had disastrous results, pointing out how this rare placental malformation led to widespread umbilical vein thrombosis, acute hemolytic anemia, and eventually a dire neonatal prognosis (Carlucci et al., 2020). Equally, retrospective studies of different types of anemia illustrate that specifically designed treatment protocols can provide dramatic improvements, with certain examples achieving complete remission in aplastic anemia through comprehensive treatment regimens (Zhu, 2020). Such instances highlight the importance of personalized medicine and demonstrate how distinct presentations of hemolytic anemias lead to varied patient outcomes. These instances collectively highlight the importance of ongoing research aimed at enhancing understanding and management strategies for hemolytic anemias, to mitigate negative health consequences.

A CLOSER LOOK

ANTIPHOSPHOLIPID ANTIBODY SYNDROME

Antiphospholipid Antibody Syndrome (APS) is a disease of the immune system in which the immune system mistakenly creates antibodies against normal proteins present in blood, phospholipids, and associated proteins. The antibodies make the formation of blood clots in veins and arteries likely to cause serious outcomes such as deep vein thrombosis (DVT), stroke, or PE.

APS also causes recurrent miscarriages, stillbirths, or other pregnancy complications due to inadequate blood supply to the placenta. The syndrome exists alone (primary APS) or as a component of another autoimmune disorder like systemic lupus erythematosus (SLE) (secondary APS).

Diagnosis is established through blood tests to detect some antiphospholipid antibodies, i.e., lupus anticoagulant, anticardiolipin antibodies, and anti-β2 glycoprotein I antibodies, which are usually performed on two occasions with a more than 12-week' interval. Treatment focuses on preventing blood clots, usually with long-term use of anticoagulants like warfarin or heparin, especially during high-risk situations like surgery or pregnancy.

SUMMARY

Hemolytic anemias are a heterogeneous series of disorders due to the abnormal premature destruction of RBCs, leading to significant clinical presentations and variable etiologic causes. The knowledge of these conditions is also considerably enhanced by biochemical tests, which yield information regarding the specific types of hemolytic anemias and treatment options. For instance, inherited spherocytosis as described by Toub et al. (2025) highlights the necessity of tailored diagnostic procedures focused on correcting genetic variation between populations, especially for regions like Saudi Arabia. Furthermore, the association of glutamate-cysteine ligase deficiency with hemolysis illustrates the intricate relationships of genetic mutations and clinical presentations, such as those reported in chronic hemolytic anemia case series, associated with neurological symptoms, as described by Al-Hatou et al. (2024). With such multi-faceted approaches, clinicians can more effectively treat the intricacies involved in hemolytic anemias and improve patient outcomes with targeted interventions.

A general overview of hemolytic anemias outlines several key features that contribute to the pathophysiology and treatment of this disease. Emerging research highlights the role of PK in sustaining RBC life, as PK deficiency has the potential to significantly decrease RBC life, leading to hemolytic anemias, a condition that is the subject of detailed explanation in recent research (Bartels et al., 2023). Also, some cases illustrate the complexities of hemolytic disorders, for instance, how therapy and metabolic complications converge in the case of G6PD-deficient patients. For example, a remarkable case illustrated that rasburicase-induced methemoglobinemia occurred in a patient with presumptive G6PD deficiency, and intravenous ascorbic acid was needed to treat the condition accordingly (Birhiray et al., 2016). Collectively, these results reflect the complexity of hemolytic anemias and ongoing study into therapeutic strategies to maximize patient outcomes.

REFERENCES

1. Abdullah, U. Y., Jassim, H. M., Baig, A. A., Khorsheed, R. M., Al-Khayat, A. M. H., Sulong, A. F., Abed, N. F., & Yassin, W. A. (2015). GALLSTONES IN PATIENTS WITH INHERITED HEMOLYTIC DISEASES. International Journal of Pharmacy and Pharmaceutical Sciences, 7(7), 9–15. http://irep.iium.edu.my/50805/Abebe, E., Gugsa, G., & Ahmed, M. (2020). Review on major food-borne zoonotic bacterial pathogens. Journal of Tropical Medicine, 2020, 1–19. https://doi.org/10.1155/2020/4674235 (accessed on 12th June 2025).
2. Abubakar, O., Carrilho, E., Chachá, S. G. F., et al. (2022). Mobile health (mHealth) and advances in noninvasive diagnosis of anemia: An overview. https://core.ac.uk/download/492971599.pdf (accessed on 12th June 2025).
3. Adams, J., Bardsley, M., Lewis, R., et al. (2010). Evaluation of UK integrated care pilots: Research protocol. https://core.ac.uk/download/pdf/8458425.pdf (accessed on 12th June 2025).
4. Aga Khan University Hospital, Karachi. (2021). LABRAD: Vol 46, Issue 4–October 2021. https://core.ac.uk/download/482026963.pdf (accessed on 12th June 2025).
5. Aktaş, G., Atak, B. M., Duman, T. T., et al. (2018). A rare non-hemolytic case of idiopathic cold agglutinin disease. https://core.ac.uk/download/539818653.pdf (accessed on 12th June 2025).
6. Al Toub, F. A., Asseri, A. H. O., Baig, M. R., Almalki, N. A. R., & Anwar, F. (2025). Crosstalk: Biochemical signatures and clinical implications in rare hereditary hemolytic anemias (hereditary spherocytosis). Current Pharmaceutical Design. https://www.semanticscholar.org/paper/72623c181ec9102ffb14643017a3426c109771ca (accessed on 12th June 2025).
7. Al-Hatou, M., Safan, A., Atta, M. A., & Siddiqi, M. (2024). Clinical and biochemical analysis of glutamate-cysteine ligase deficiency presented with late-onset spinocerebellar ataxia and hemolytic anemia. Molecular Sindonology, 15, 432–436. https://www.semanticscholar.org/paper/dff74d1fe8dfffd9b685382977d8365a17ca82f4 (accessed on 12th June 2025).
8. Alarcón-Segovia, D., & Sánchez-Guerrero, J. (2020). Primary antiphospholipid syndrome. Frontiers Research Topics. https://doi.org/10.3389/978-2-88966-108-4 (accessed on 12th June 2025).
9. Alexander, T., Asadi, S., Meyer, M., Harding, J. E., Jiang, Y., Alsweiler, J., Muelbert, M., et al. (2024). Nutritional support for moderate-to-late-preterm infants–A randomized trial. The New England Journal of Medicine, 390(16), 1493–1504. https://www.semanticscholar.org/paper/4e676695d99b8f8d621c7d4fb1ecf9c3d99738f9 (accessed on 12th June 2025).
10. Allard, S., Anagnou, N., Andolfo, I., et al. (2016). The European Hematology Association roadmap for European hematology research: A consensus document. https://core.ac.uk/download/79516495.pdf (accessed on 12th June 2025).
11. Anagnou, N. P., Andolfo, I., Barcellini, W., et al. (2021). The EHA research roadmap: Anemias. https://core.ac.uk/download/478721871.pdf (accessed on 12th June 2025).
12. Bao, E. L., Cheng, A., & Sankaran, V. G. (2019). The genetics of human hematopoiesis and its disruption in disease. EMBO Molecular Medicine, 11. https://doi.org/10.15252/emmm.201910316 (accessed on 12th June 2025).
13. Bartels, M., de Wilde, J. R. A., Glenthøj, A., et al. (2023). Activation of pyruvate kinase as therapeutic option for rare hemolytic anemias: Shedding new light on an old enzyme. https://core.ac.uk/download/588752678.pdf (accessed on 12th June 2025).

14. Beretta, C., Biagi, E., Foti, G., et al. (2009). Prolonged extracorporeal membrane oxygenation therapy for severe acute respiratory distress syndrome in a child affected by rituximab-resistant autoimmune hemolytic anemia: A case report. https://core.ac.uk/download/pdf/8318206.pdf (accessed on 12th June 2025).

15. Birhiray, R., Reeves, D. J., & Saum, L. (2016). Ascorbic acid for the treatment of rasburicase-induced methemoglobinemia in the setting of acute renal failure. https://core.ac.uk/download/62438655.pdf (accessed on 12th June 2025).

16. Blackall, D. P., & Dolatshahi, L. (2022). Autoimmune hemolytic anemia in children: Laboratory investigation, disease associations, and treatment strategies. Journal of Pediatric Hematology/Oncology, 44, 71–78. https://doi.org/10.1097/mph.0000000000002438 (accessed on 12th June 2025).

17. Bousfiha, A., Jeddane, L., Picard, C., Al–Herz, W., Ailal, F., Chatila, T. A., Cunningham-Rundles, C., et al. (2020). Human inborn errors of immunity: 2019 update of the IUIS phenotypical classification. Journal of Clinical Immunology, 40, 66–81. https://doi.org/10.1007/s10875-020-00758-x (accessed on 12th June 2025).

18. Brill, J. (2009). Anemia. https://core.ac.uk/download/62772179.pdf (accessed on 12th June 2025).

19. Brys, A. K., Sheth, M. R., Sohn, D. D., et al. (2015). Diagnostic and therapeutic considerations in idiopathic hyper eosinophilia with warm autoimmune hemolytic anemia. https://core.ac.uk/download/323075654.pdf (accessed on 12th June 2025).

20. Camaschella, C., Nai, A., & Silvestri, L. (2020). Iron metabolism and iron disorders revisited in the hepcidin era. Hematological, 105, 260–272. https://doi.org/10.3324/haematol.2019.232124 (accessed on 12th June 2025).

21. Cappellini, M. D., Marcon, A., Fattizzo, B., & Motta, I. (2021). Innovative treatments for rare anemias. Hemisphere, 5, e576–e576. https://doi.org/10.1097/hs9.0000000000000576 (accessed on 12th June 2025).

22. Carlucci, S., Stabile, G., Catagini, S., Borghi, C., Scutiero, G., Morano, D., & Greco, P. (2020). Fetal disseminated intravascular coagulopathy, hydrops and massive umbilical vein thrombosis consequence of a rare placental condition: Multifocal chorangiomatosis. The Journal of Maternal-Fetal & Neonatal Medicine, 35, 4009–4013. https://doi.org/10.1080/14767058.2020.1843154 (accessed on 12th June 2025).

23. Cherif, H., Cai, Q., Crivera, C., Leon, A., Rahman, I., Leval, A., Noel, W., et al. (2024). Overall survival and treatment patterns among patients with warm autoimmune hemolytic anemia in Sweden: A nationwide population-based study. European Journal of Hematology, 114, 129–138. https://www.semanticscholar.org/paper/105823a003fca5dd8d4a50a8c6df4e3463aedfa6 (accessed on 12th June 2025).

24. Crouser, E. D., Maier, L. A., Wilson, K. C., Bonham, C. A., Morgenthau, A. S., Patterson, K., Abston, E., et al. (2020). Diagnosis and detection of sarcoidosis: An official American Thoracic Society clinical practice guideline. American Journal of Respiratory and Critical Care Medicine, 201, e26–e51. https://doi.org/10.1164/rccm.202002-0251st (accessed on 12th June 2025).

25. Dana, M., & Fibach, E. (2019). Red blood cells as redox modulators in hemolytic anemia. https://core.ac.uk/download/322441264.pdf (accessed on 12th June 2025).

26. de Boer, E. C. W., Mulder, F. V. M., Neri, S., Wiskerke-van Stuijvenberg, M., Arts, J. J. G., Tol, S., Beuger, B. M., et al. (2025). Vesiculation as potential novel pathogenic mechanism in autoimmune hemolytic anemia. Transfusion. https://www.semanticscholar.org/paper/bf036b457efe36017e513f7d1040d66d6afd1baa (accessed on 12th June 2025).

27. Elaroussi, I., Mougui, A., & Bouchti, I. E. (2025). Tophaceous gout in a patient with beta thalassemia: A case report. Scholars Journal of Medical Case Reports. https://www.semanticscholar.org/paper/1b6a102be5b00fcf9f8b737e07c0f977d295a5b1 (accessed on 12th June 2025).

28. Englum, B. R., Hall, B. J., Reiter, A. J., et al. (2020). Long-term hematologic and clinical outcomes of splenectomy in children with hereditary spherocytosis and sickle cell disease. https://deepblue.lib.umich.edu/bitstream/2027.42/155920/2/pbc28290_am.pdf (accessed on 12th June 2025).

29. Fattizzo, B., & Barcellini, W. (2015). Clinical applications of hemolytic markers in the differential diagnosis and management of hemolytic anemia. https://core.ac.uk/download/333585364.pdf (accessed on 12th June 2025).

30. Furmiga, I. S. L. (2024). Diagnostic laboratorial das anemias hemolytic autoimmune. Absoulute Review. https://www.semanticscholar.org/paper/650d9fbd233b20ccab47d3b595a9c1138c5a82dc (accessed on 12th June 2025).

31. Garrahy, I., & Rahimian, S. (2024). Autoimmune hemolytic anemia: A rare presentation of mantle cell lymphoma. https://core.ac.uk/download/617991901.pdf (accessed on 12th June 2025).

32. Gartner, J. C., Green, M., McLoughlin, L., et al. (1993). Parvovirus B19 infection in pediatric transplant patients. https://core.ac.uk/download/12205038.pdf (accessed on 12th June 2025).

33. Guzik, T. J., Mohiddin, S., Dimarco, A., Patel, V., Savvatis, K., Marelli-Berg, F. M., Madhur, M. S., et al. (2020). COVID-19 and the cardiovascular system: Implications for risk assessment, diagnosis, and treatment options. Cardiovascular Research, 116, 1666–1687. https://doi.org/10.1093/cvr/cvaa106 (accessed on 12th June 2025).

34. Holme, S., van Wijk, R., Rasmussen, A. Ø., Petersen, J., & Glenthøj, A. (2024). Glucose phosphate isomerase deficiency demasked by whole-genome sequencing: A case report. Journal of Medical Case Reports, 18. https://www.semanticscholar.org/paper/20815fef2673011ac0430e250dd7ce122ca1171f (accessed on 12th June 2025).

35. Humar, R., Schaer, D. J., & Vallelian, F. (2022). Erythrophagocytosis in hemolytic anemia, wound healing, and cancer. https://www.zora.uzh.ch/id/eprint/221246/1/ZORA_pdf.pdf (accessed on 12th June 2025).

36. Hussain, H., Fadel, A., Guardiola, V., & Rodríguez, S. (2022). A rare case of non-immune hemolytic anemia in a stage IV breast cancer patient treated with capecitabine. Cureus. https://doi.org/10.7759/cureus.24921 (accessed on 12th June 2025).

37. Iba, T., Levy, J. H., Connors, J. M., Warkentin, T. E., Thachil, J., & Levi, M. (2020). The unique characteristics of COVID-19 coagulopathy. Critical Care, 24. https://doi.org/10.1186/s13054-020-03077-0 (accessed on 12th June 2025).

38. Iolascon, A., Rivella, S., Anagnou, N. P., Camaschella, C., Swinkels, D. W., Muckenthaler, M. U., Porto, G., et al. (2021). The EHA research roadmap: Anemias. HemaSphere, 5, e607–e607.

https://doi.org/10.1097/hs9.0000000000000607 (accessed on 12th June 2025).

39. Iolascon, A., Taher, A. T., Gulbis, B., Matar, C. F., Bencaiova, G. A., Forni, G., Tamary, H., et al. (2020). Recommendations for pregnancy in rare inherited anemias. https://core.ac.uk/download/373375214.pdf (accessed on 12th June 2025).

40. Kaplan, J. A. (2019). Leukemia in children. Pediatrics in Review, 40, 319–331. https://doi.org/10.1542/pir.2018-0192 (accessed on 12th June 2025).

41. Karimah, K., Rofinda, Z. D., Husni, R., Sari, D., & Chicamy, Y. A. (2025). The clinical significance of DAT positivity: A comparative analysis of IgG, C3d, and IgG/C3d-positive patients. Bio Scientia Medicina: Journal of Biomedicine and Translational Research. https://www.semanticscholar.org/paper/5784443c93d3656291d0bb7b29701a4266f70723 (accessed on 12th June 2025).

42. Kawamoto, S. (2024). [Current recommendations for the diagnosis and treatment of autoimmune hemolytic anemia based on etiology and pathology]. [Rinsho Ketsueki] The Japanese Journal of Clinical Hematology, 65(9), 892–901. https://www.semanticscholar.org/paper/b87968ef7e3655c1bd517b883cb0cb3e2f79ea57 (accessed on 12th June 2025).

43. Labban, H., Begum, F., Paracha, A., John, V., & Islam, M. (2024). Hemolytic anemia and pancytopenia secondary to vitamin B12 deficiency: Evaluation and clinical significance. Cureus, 16(3), e57286. https://www.semanticscholar.org/paper/482c1bbf415a0174b5a2f4c4de9e35536fbcfbfe (accessed on 12th June 2025).

44. Lal, A., Wong, T. E., Keel, S., Pagano, M. B., Chung, J., Kamdar, A., Rao, L., et al. (2021). The transfusion management of beta thalassemia in the United States. Transfusion, 61, 3027–3039. https://doi.org/10.1111/trf.16640 (accessed on 12th June 2025).

45. Lemack, B., Kupovics, G., & Kumar, R. (2025). Drug-induced immune hemolytic anemia following dapagliflozin administration: A case report. Cureus, 17. https://www.semanticscholar.org/paper/3749041eaca054ef52c4c13a8f6df606f660990b (accessed on 12th June 2025).

46. Li, X., Zhang, T., Li, X., Wang, L., Li, Q., Liu, Q., He, C., et al. (2025). Identification of a novel SPTB gene splicing mutation in hereditary spherocytosis: A case report and diagnostic insights. Frontiers in Genetics, 15. https://www.semanticscholar.org/paper/cd58884af54f5e9ab1dc9026e53676daa14ad095 (accessed on 12th June 2025).

47. Lynch, S., Pfeiffer, C. M., Georgieff, M., Brittenham, G. M., Fairweather-Tait, S. J., Hurrell, R. F., McArdle, H. J., et al. (2018). Biomarkers of Nutrition for Development (BOND)—Iron review. Journal of Nutrition, 148, 1001S–1067S. https://doi.org/10.1093/jn/nxx036 (accessed on 12th June 2025).

48. Matzdorff, A., Wojciechowski, A., Zyluk-Gadowska, P., Baluken, F., & Meier, A. (2023). A patient with target cells and hyperkalemia–or why hematologists should still be able to 'fly by sight.' Blood. https://www.semanticscholar.org/paper/1cab8548ab74bb88d0eef1e8a83ca704218a9f3f (accessed on 12th June 2025).

49. Murray, C. J. L., Ikuta, K. S., Sharara, F., Swetschinski, L. R., Robles Aguilar, G., Gray, A. P., Han, C., et al. (2022). Global burden of bacterial antimicrobial resistance in 2019: A systematic analysis. The Lancet, 399, 629–655. https://doi.org/10.1016/s0140-6736(21)02724-0 (accessed on 12th June 2025).

50. Musalem, P. (2025). Ten tips for managing complement-mediated thrombotic microangiopathies (formerly atypical hemolytic uremic syndrome): Narrative review. BMC Nephrology, 26.

https://www.semanticscholar.org/paper/85d72f4c33a9384bf23ed454422d4beba337ff3d (accessed on 12th June 2025).

51. Natsheh, S. T., Abu Ihlayel, T., Qasrawi, R., Alsalah, Q. A., Hammouri, A. G., Zughayyer, A., & Arafat, H. (2024). Microangiopathic hemolytic anemia as a paraneoplastic syndrome in a patient with metastatic gastric cancer. Clinical Medicine Insights: Case Reports, 17. https://www.semanticscholar.org/paper/1b51ca2fdb96deb2f2856aa651993787874aec93 (accessed on 12th June 2025).

52. Osorio-Toro, L. M., Quintana-Ospina, J., Melo-Burbano, L. Á., Ruiz-Jiménez, P. A., Daza-Arana, J. E., Rivas-Tafurt, G. P., & Izquierdo-Loaiza, J. H. (2023). Autoimmune hemolytic anemia caused by cold agglutinin antibodies in systemic lupus erythematosus—a rare association: Case report. Journal of Blood Medicine, 14, 507–511. https://www.semanticscholar.org/paper/2c8ab9512191a06fcc3c79bcef680ed9ba103610 (accessed on 12th June 2025).

53. Pan, D. H., & Rivas, Y. (2017). Jaundice: Newborn to age 2 months. Pediatrics in Review, 38, 499–510. https://doi.org/10.1542/pir.2015-0132 (accessed on 12th June 2025).

54. Phillips, J., & Henderson, A. C. (2018). Hemolytic anemia: Evaluation and differential diagnosis. PubMed, 98, 354–361. (accessed on 12th June 2025).

55. Ram, S. (2021). Neuropsychological Implications of Nocturnal Hypoxemia in Sickle Cell Disease. https://core.ac.uk/download/516462269.pdf (accessed on 12th June 2025).

56. Ruggiero, A., Rizzo, D., Nanni, L., Catalano, M., Mauriz, P., & Coccia, P. (2018). Can partial splenectomy preserve humoral immunity in pediatric patients? Risks and benefits of partial splenectomy. https://core.ac.uk/download/212468153.pdf (accessed on 12th June 2025).

57. Schneider, B. J., Naidoo, J., Santomasso, B., Lacchetti, C., Adkins, S., Anadkat, M. J., Atkins, M. B., et al. (2021). Management of immune-related adverse events in patients treated with immune checkpoint inhibitor therapy: ASCO guideline update. Journal of Clinical Oncology, 39, 4073–4126. https://doi.org/10.1200/jco.21.01440 (accessed on 12th June 2025).

58. To, M., Villatoro, V., et al. (2018). A Laboratory Guide to Clinical Hematology. https://core.ac.uk/download/622361655.pdf (accessed on 12th June 2025).

59. Tomar, A., Venkatesan, S., & Khajuria, S. P. (2024). Sometimes treatment kills: Ceftriaxone-induced hemolytic anemia in a case of pyogenic meningitis. Medical Journal of Dr. D.Y. Patil Vidyapeeth. https://www.semanticscholar.org/paper/95a38b0c56a83c2664ec0a45332fd8210922770f (accessed on 12th June 2025).

60. Tuli, A., & Yenilmez, E. D. (2017). Laboratory approach to anemia. https://core.ac.uk/download/322432622.pdf (accessed on 12th June 2025).

61. Tvedt, T. H. A., Steien, E., Øvrebø, B., Haaverstad, R., Hobbs, W. E., Wardęcki, M., Tjønnfjord, G. E., et al. (2021). Sutimlimab, an investigational C1s inhibitor, effectively prevents exacerbation of hemolytic anemia in a patient with cold agglutinin disease undergoing major surgery. American Journal of Hematology, 97. https://doi.org/10.1002/ajh.26409 (accessed on 12th June 2025).

62. Yu, L., & Cheng, L. (2024). Enhancing performance through biochemical monitoring and nutritional support in female weightlifters during pre-competition weight reduction: A randomized trial. Journal of the International Society of Sports Nutrition, 21. https://www.semanticscholar.org/paper/cb56c135655ce4acea5b48973bbcd4a24e1ac57c (accessed on 12th June 2025).

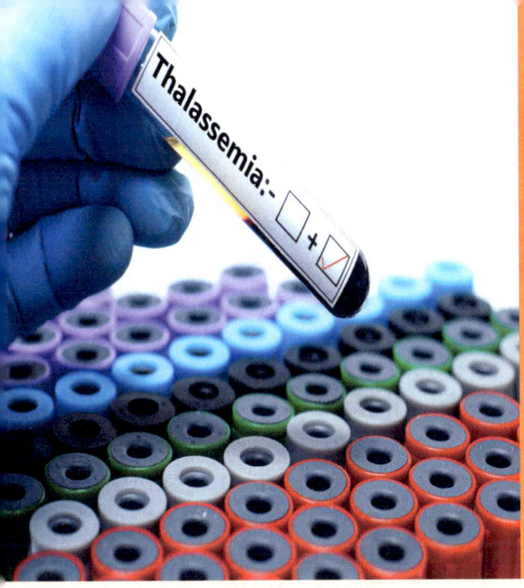

Chapter 5

HEMOGLOBINOPATHIES AND THALASSEMIAS

Contents

Introduction......107
5.1. Types of Hemoglobinopathies......108
5.2. Pathophysiology of Hemoglobin Disorders......112
5.3. Diagnosis and Screening......117
5.4. Management and Treatment......120
Summary......126
References......127

Introduction

Hemoglobinopathies and thalassemia's are a widespread public health issue throughout the world, particularly in populations where malaria is or was endemic. The genetic diseases that involve the structure and synthesis of hemoglobin are increasingly common because they confer a selective advantage in malaria-endemic regions, such as Africa, Asia, and the Mediterranean. With the rise in the worldwide tendency of globalization and migration, most of these patients have been transferred increasingly in various European countries, thus making it more challenging to provide health care. The demographic migration increases the demand for well-organized channels of diagnosis as well as appropriate guidelines for such diseases. Current research suggests that such a program can enhance patient outcomes, particularly in light of the rise in comorbidities, such as those experienced during the COVID-19 pandemic, which can exacerbate health issues for hemoglobinopathy patients (Franceschi et al., 2019; Alkindi et al., 2020). Education and enhancing diagnostic methods are therefore important to ensuring personalized medicine and solving such medical complexities.

5.1. Types of Hemoglobinopathies

Awareness of hemoglobinopathies is essential for formulating proper diagnosis and management strategies. The hemoglobinopathies are typically characterized by sickle cell disease and thalassemias as structural or functional hemoglobin alteration. Sickle cell disease (SCD) results from a mutation in the beta-globin gene, with the synthesis of aberrant hemoglobin S, whereas thalassemia results from interference in globin chain synthesis, with beta-thalassemia and alpha-thalassemia being described subtypes. In one such Indian critical research study, 47 hemoglobinopathies were detected, the most prevalent of which was beta-thalassemia trait, reflecting its prevalence among targeted groups (Bhargava et al., 2016). Transfusion-dependent patients of thalassemia major are also susceptible to acquiring severe complications due to secondary illnesses like COVID-19, which aggravate their anemia and lead to poor outcomes (Alkindi et al., 2020). Detection of such conditions in the initial stage is crucial to sustain preventive measures and enhance patient care.

5.1.1. Sickle Cell Disease (SCD)

SCD, the prevalent hemoglobinopathy, results from anomalous hemoglobin synthesis, which alters the morphology of the red cells to a rigid, sickle shape. The abnormal trait is responsible for an entire range of complications, including vaso-occlusive crisis, hemolytic anemia, and infections. SCD is prevalent with a very high incidence, especially notable in nations which have historically been plagued by malaria, where sickle cell carriers survived selectively (Franceschi et al., 2019). Global migration over the past decades has resulted in a more acute occurrence of SCD cases among most nations, including Europe, where numerous demographic requirements are addressed by the health systems (Eleftheriou et al., 2019). The present medical community emphasizes the extreme need for advanced diagnosis and specific treatment approaches to adequately address this long-standing illness and improve the quality of life in SCD patients (Figure 5.1).

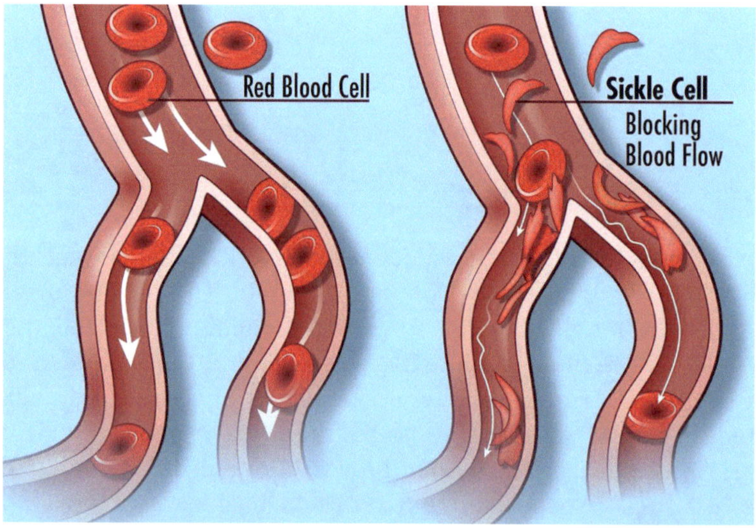

Figure 5.1. Sickle cell disease (SCD).

Source: https://metrohealthhmo.com/wp-content/uploads/2019/07/Sickle-Cell-Disease.jpg.

5.1.2. Hemoglobin C Disease

Hemoglobin C Disease (HbC) is a significant hemoglobinopathy due to a mutation of the gene that codes for the beta-globin subunit of hemoglobin, in which an abnormal hemoglobin, HbC, is produced. It is found in West Africans and their derivatives extensively, but can also be seen with variable clinical presentation in other individuals. HbC can present in combination with other hemoglobinopathies such as SCD and, hence, its diagnosis and treatment become complicated. Clinical presentation of HbC is mild anemia and splenomegaly but the disease is generally less severe compared to other hemoglobinopathies. However, the role of genetic versus environmental selection on its prevalence remains uninvestigated. For instance, studies in areas with malaria indicate that genetic disparity like HbC provides some selective advantage against malaria, consistent with findings in other hemoglobin diseases. This evidence highlights the potential of population genetics in targeted healthcare planning, as noted by organizations such as the Thalassemia International Federation (Aye et al., 2005; Angastiniotis et al., 2022).

5.1.3. Hemoglobin E Disease

Hemoglobin E Disease, which is a prevalent hemoglobinopathy that is predominantly located in Southeast Asia and India, is a health issue among the general category of hemoglobinopathies and thalassemias. It occurs due to substitution of glutamic acid at position 26 of the β-globin chain with lysine and is caused by an autosomal dominant single-nucleotide mutation. The condition is usually seen in association with other hemoglobin defects, and this causes variation in presentation like mild anemia and splenomegaly. Diagnosis is usually carried out with the use of high-performance liquid chromatography (HPLC), which has also been important to correctly diagnose not only Hemoglobin E Disease but other hemoglobinopathies that are frequently seen among the populations affected because research in India has established (Bhargava et al., 2016). Increased migration and population globalization patterns account for the global relevance of Hemoglobin E Disease, necessitating improved diagnostic channels and interventions in treating the disease as reported in existing literature (Franceschi et al., 2019) (Figure 5.2).

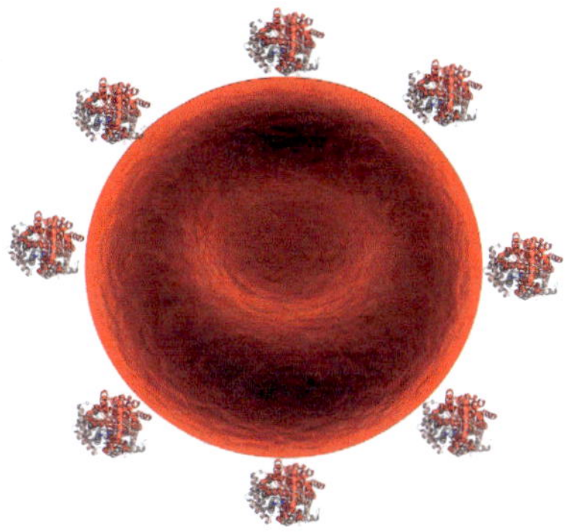

Figure 5.2. Hemoglobin E disease.

Source: https://cdn.storymd.com/optimized/lAW4OyPuno/original.jpg.

5.1.4. Hemoglobin D Disease

Hemoglobin D Disease is a beta-globin gene mutation variant hemoglobinopathy that leads to the production of Hemoglobin D (HbD) instead of normal adult hemoglobin (HbA). Although typically milder than other hemoglobinopathies, such as sickle cell anemia, Hemoglobin D Disease may manifest clinically in various ways, particularly in individuals who have co-inherited it with other disease-causing hemoglobins, like Hemoglobin S or E. In nations such as Myanmar, where Hemoglobin E is the predominant hemoglobin, prevalence rates of the disease among different types of hemoglobins reveal enormous racial differences, highlighting the complex interaction between disease expression and genetics (Aye et al., 2005). Furthermore, patients with Hemoglobin D Disease are also not immune to complications; anemia and vaso-occlusive crises like in sickle cell anemia may be present, which is why proper screening and management practices are necessary (Alrjjal et al., 2015).

5.1.5. Hemoglobin H Disease

Hemoglobin H Disease (Hb H disease) is a severe form of alpha-thalassemia in which three out of four genes are deleted and there is an interruption of globin chain synthesis. The interruption results in the formation of abnormal hemoglobin, specifically Hemoglobin H, which is a less efficient oxygen transport molecule than normal hemoglobin. Hb H disease patients show a variety of variable presentations from moderate to severe hemolytic anemia, splenomegaly, and increased vulnerability to infections, given the significance of hemoglobinopathies like sickle cell anemia (Alrjjal et al., 2015). In addition, Hb H disease management also involves the same challenges that thalassemia patients worldwide experience, and therefore requires access to specialized care and tailored treatment plans, which organizations like the Thalassemia International Federation (Angastiniotis et al., 2022) are lobbying for. Through ongoing research and diplomacy, the treatment and management of the condition can be significantly improved (Figure 5.3).

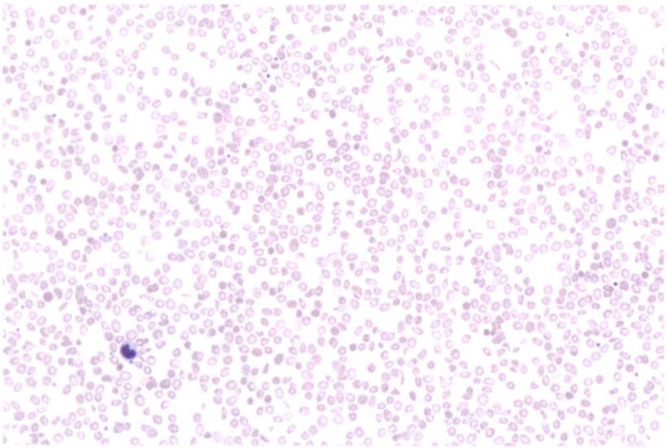

Figure 5.3. Hemoglobin H disease (Hb H disease).

Source: https://www.learnhaem.com/wp-content/uploads/2020/02/HbH-disease-1.jpg.

5.1.6. Thalassemia Major

Thalassemia Major, also known as major β-thalassemia, is a severe condition with gross clinical manifestations, presenting primarily with severe anemia and frequent blood transfusions. The disease arises as a result of mutations that inhibit the production of beta globin chains, leading to ineffective erythropoiesis and other hematologic disorders. As observed in a study involving 1400 reproductive-age Indian women, thalassemia diagnosis in anemic subjects also plays a crucial role in appropriate management (Bhargava et al., 2016). The patients, if left untreated, can have growth retardation, skeletal changes, and iron overload organ damage due to frequent transfusions. The global thalassemia prevalence is indicative of the need for comprehensive diagnosis and screening, especially in malaria-endemic regions where hemoglobinopathies are prevalent (Franceschi et al., 2019). Thalassemia Major management therefore calls for intervention of focused prevention, early detection, and individualized treatment regimens.

5.1.7. Thalassemia Minor

Thalassemia Minor, or the β-thalassemia trait, refers to the existence of a hemoglobin gene defect during the process of production. The disorder has asymptomatic or mildly symptomatic carriers who may be confused with healthy individuals because they do not have detectable anemia. Although apparently harmless, Thalassemia Minor is significant in β-thalassemia epidemiology, particularly in populations where malaria was once endemic, such as the majority of Africa, Asia, and the Mediterranean. Diagnosis of Thalassemia Minor is required for patient care as well as public health planning. High-performance liquid chromatography (HPLC) is an effective diagnostic method that enhances the diagnosis of such cases, as seen in recent studies estimating hemoglobinopathies in heterogeneously distributed populations (Bhargava et al., 2016).

The rising globalization and migration trends underscore the need for robust screening methods to manage and understand these inherited disorders effectively (Franceschi et al., 2019) (Figure 5.4).

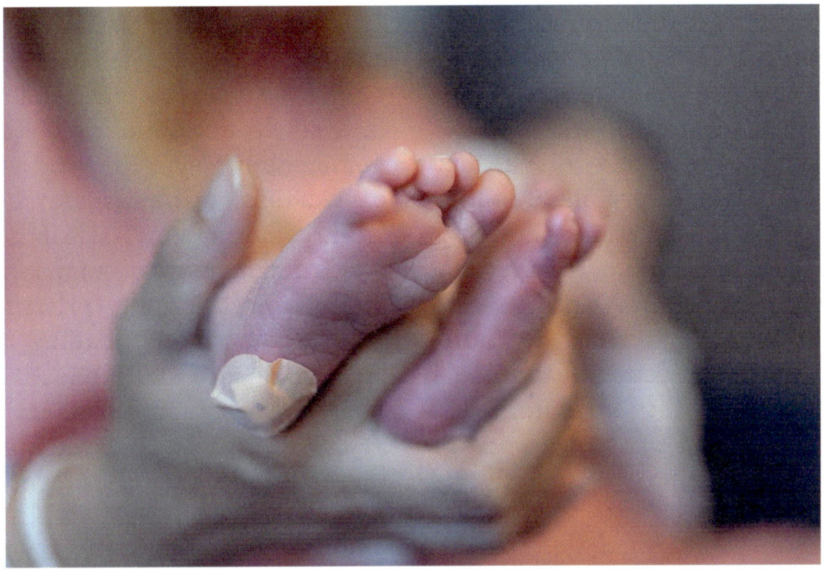

Figure 5.4. Thalassemia minor.

Source: https://www.verywellhealth.com/thmb/UhG7Y23XCsiUFaN285TgYBiuiTg=/1500x0/filters:no_upscale():max_bytes(150000):strip_icc()/GettyImages-1311343098-f02bff04786a4e11848e4f816fb861b9.jpg.

5.1.8. Compound Hemoglobinopathies

Compound hemoglobinopathies are a complex subcategory of genetic disorders with the coinheritance of two or more abnormal hemoglobin variants, leading to the expression of a wide range of clinical manifestations. They are particularly common in SCD and thalassemia high-endemic areas, which are critical public health problems. For instance, β-thalassemia and HbE have been recognized in studies as two of the most prevalent compound heterozygous conditions, each with varied complications when isolated. β-thalassemia trait and HbE β-thalassemia were found to be highly prevalent, according to a study conducted by Apollo Hospitals, indicating the importance of implementing wide-scale screening programs to promptly identify and address these conditions (Chandrashekar et al., 2011). Moreover, genetic disorder screening in high-risk groups, such as the Sindhi population, can be of significant value in terms of inherited hemolytic disorders and can offer appropriate genetic counseling and preventive treatment to diminish the burden of such disorders (Balgir et al., 2010).

5.1.9. Rare Hemoglobin Variants

The broad spectrum of hemoglobinopathies includes not only such widely reported conditions as alpha and beta thalassemia but also rare hemoglobin variants that can complicate both diagnosis and management. While less frequent, such variants can significantly affect patients' conditions, yielding atypical hematological findings. Detection of such atypical variants is significant, particularly in thalassemia and other hemoglobinopathies-prevalent regions. In 1400 rural Indian women, high-performance liquid chromatography was used for screening certain hemoglobinopathies and detecting cases of both rare and common variants, including beta-thalassemia Trait (Bhargava et al., 2016). Additionally, advances in molecular diagnostic procedures hold tremendous promise for the prenatal identification of such variants, thereby enhancing preventive measures and offering better management in the clinical setting (Tuli et al., 2018). This overall knowledge of rare hemoglobin variants is the secret to optimal patient management in the treatment of hemoglobinopathy (Figure 5.5).

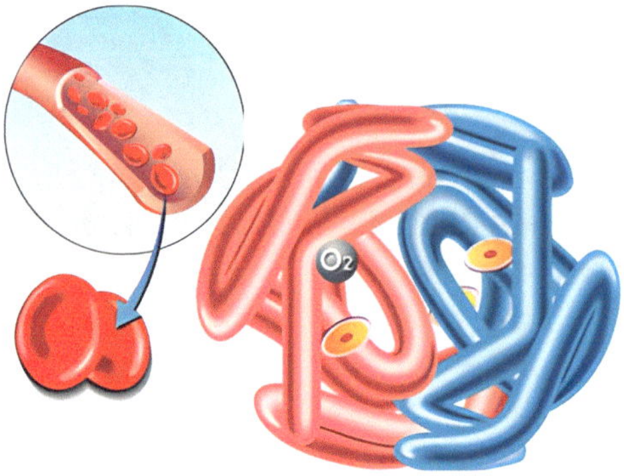

Figure 5.5. The vast spectrum of hemoglobinopathies includes not only prominent disorders such as alpha and beta thalassemia but also rare hemoglobin variants that can complicate diagnosis and management.

Source: https://images.medindia.net/health-images/1200_1000/hemoglobinopathy.jpg.

5.2. Pathophysiology of Hemoglobin Disorders

The hemoglobin disease pathophysiology, i.e., hemoglobinopathies and thalassemias, is centered upon the intricate molecular mechanism causing inadequate function of hemoglobin. The diseases are largely genetic in nature and result from mutations in the globin gene, causing aberrant hemoglobin structures and ineffective oxygen transport. SCD is just one of the diseases that result from a mutation in a single nucleotide with the production of hemoglobin S, which polymerizes under low oxygen tension and causes red cells to adopt the sickle conformation. These induce vaso-occlusive crises and hemolytic anemia. Thalassemias also result from the faulty production of alpha or beta globin chains, leading to a hemoglobin level imbalance and ineffective erythropoiesis. There are geographical associations, particularly in the context of endemic malaria regions, as there is a selection advantage in certain groups. As such, understanding their pathophysiology on an integrated basis is required for effective diagnosis, therapy, and the development of targeted therapies (Eleftheriou et al., 2019; Franceschi et al., 2019).

5.2.1. Mechanism of Hemoglobin Synthesis

Hemoglobin production is a complex biochemical process essential for oxygen transport in the body, and it is a concerted expression of globin genes. Hemoglobin consists predominantly of four polypeptide chains—two alpha chains and two beta chains—coded for by genes in separate chromosomes. Production begins in bone marrow erythroid precursors where various transcription factors and RNA polymerase regulate globin gene transcription. Following post-transcription, the mRNA is translated into polypeptide chains that are subsequently assembled to form functional hemoglobin tetramers. Disruption of this well-controlled process may lead to hemoglobinopathies and thalassemias in which either the quantity or the quality of hemoglobin is impaired. In regions of high malaria transmission, such as parts of Africa and Asia, hemoglobin gene mutations have conferred some protection against malaria, thus raising the prevalence of inherited diseases such as SCD and thalassemia (Bhargava et al., 2016; Franceschi et al., 2019) (Figure 5.6).

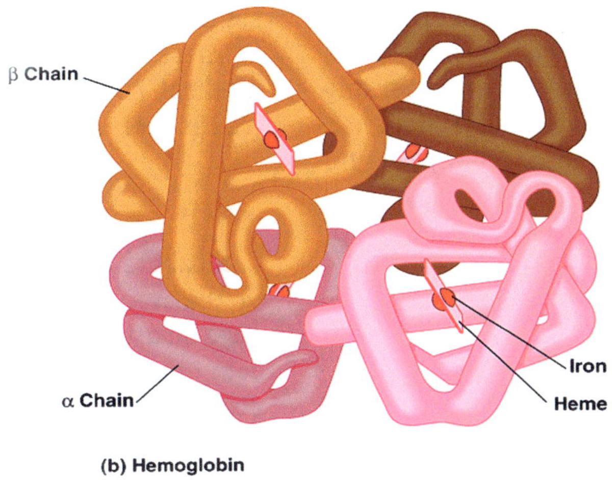

Figure 5.6. Hemoglobin is primarily composed of four polypeptide chains—two alpha and two beta chains—encoded by genes located on different chromosomes.

Source: https://themedicalbiochemistrypage.org/wp-content/uploads/2020/04/hemoglobin-1200x912.jpg.

5.2.2. Genetic Mutations Involved

Genetic mutations of the hemoglobinopathies and thalassemias are primarily due to mutations in the globin genes responsible for the production of hemoglobin. Both α-thalassemia and β-thalassemia are thalassemias due to certain mutations of the α-globin and β-globin chains, respectively. These can decrease the production of viable hemoglobin considerably, leading to severe anemia and, if undiagnosed, a potential death, particularly during early childhood (Tuli et al., 2018). Thalassemias are prevalent in certain parts of the world, such as South Asia, where population dynamics influence genetic traits (Al-Matary et al., 2017). Molecular diagnostic tests have become the primary tool for detecting these mutations, ensuring appropriate prenatal diagnosis and carrier testing. These developments not only enhance the frequency of early detection but also enable reproductive planning, thus lessening the impact of such genetic illnesses on public health.

5.2.3. Impact on Red Blood Cell Morphology

The impact on red blood cell (RBC) structure caused by thalassemias and hemoglobinopathies is notable and complex, with a large number of structural defects identified in erythrocytes. In particular, conditions such as β-thalassemia may result in the production of microcytic and hypochromic cells, which are indicative of interrupted hemoglobin synthesis and a consequent impaired capacity to supply oxygen. The RBC malformation is not only a biochemical abnormality but also clinically significant to the individuals involved. These are typically manifested as anemia and weakness. For example, the Sindhi community study presented a case of β-thalassemia major characterized by significant microcytic changes in RBC morphology, accompanied by mild anemia secondary to double heterozygosity for Hb D/β-thalassemia (Balgir et al., 2010). Additionally, morphological changes management remains a complex and multidisciplinary issue, according to the Thalassemia International Federation guidelines (Angastiniotis et al., 2022) (Figure 5.7).

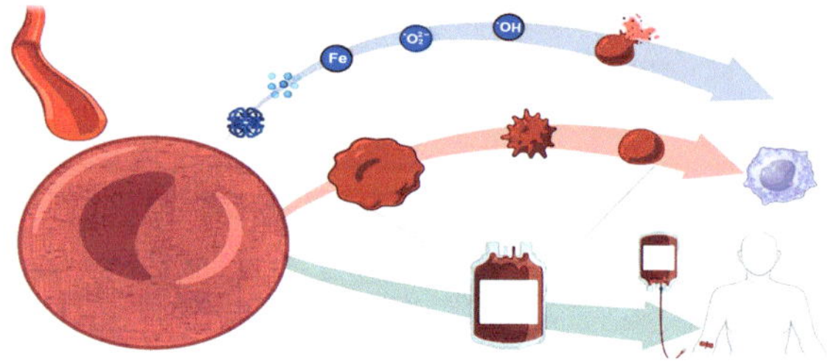

Figure 5.7. The impact of hemoglobinopathies and thalassemia's on red blood cell morphology is profound and multifaceted, leading to various structural abnormalities in erythrocytes.

Source: https://pub.mdpi-res.com/metabolites/metabolites-13-00793/article_deploy/html/images/metabolites-13-00793-ag.png?1690256922.

5.2.4. Effects on Oxygen Transport

SCD and beta-thalassemia are hemoglobinopathies that can significantly derange the ability of the blood to transport oxygen, leading to the imposition of significant physiological stress on the affected patient. With SCD, the sickling of red blood cells by the abnormal hemoglobin obstructs vessels, preventing oxygen delivery to tissues. This decreased efficiency of oxygen delivery has the potential to lead to pain crises and vulnerability to organ damage. The same applies to beta-thalassemia, which results from the absence of hemoglobin synthesis, leading to anemia and a decrease in oxygen-carrying capacity. Overall, such diseases not only lose the body's ability to supply adequate oxygenation but also render one vulnerable to many complications. Furthermore, research has shown that populations, including some of the Indian tribes, carry a large incidence of these hemoglobinopathies that make their medical condition complicated and medical treatments unavailable (Balgir et al., 2011).

5.2.5. Consequences of Hemolysis

Clinical presentations of hemolysis are manifest in thalassemias and hemoglobinopathies and have an attendant range of clinical pictures and complications. Red cell premature destruction occurs due to hemolysis, which eventually leads to anemia characterized by symptoms such as tiredness, pallor, and tachycardia. In patients with β-thalassemia, as recent studies have indicated, ongoing hemolysis exacerbates the anemic condition, and hence timely diagnosis and management are critical to prevent severe health conditions (Bhargava et al., 2016).

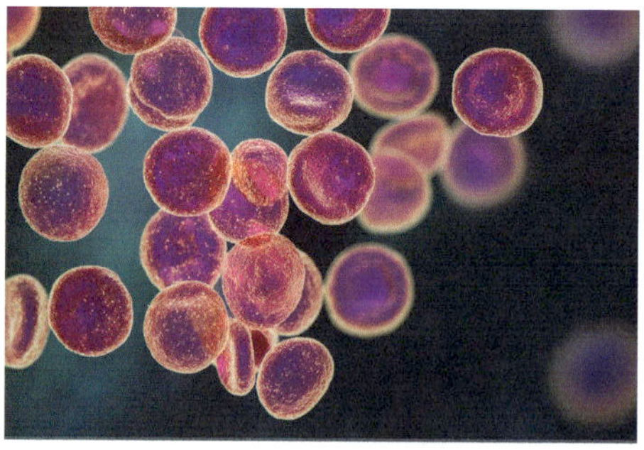

Figure 5.8. Hemolysis results in the premature destruction of red blood cells, which in turn precipitates anemia, often characterized by fatigue, pallor, and increased heart rate.

Source: https://mdsearchlight.com/wp-content/uploads/2024/11/27376-1729618185736.png.

Additionally, the progressive hemolysis of hemoglobin leads to free heme entering the circulation, thereby aggravating other systemic conditions, such as iron overload, and ultimately causing the destruction of vital organs. These areas underscore the need for intensive screening and intervention measures, particularly among risk groups such as refugees, who may have underlying, undiagnosed pre-existing hemoglobinopathies. Optimal management and outcome for patients hence rests in an understanding of consequences of hemolysis (Figure 5.8).

5.2.6. Complications of Chronic Anemia

Chronic anemia, particularly of the thalassemias and hemoglobinopathies, can lead to an amazingly diverse range of complications having a significant impact on the welfare of patients. For instance, patients with sickle cell anemia typically experience recurrent pain crisis events caused by occlusion of small-caliber vessels by morphologically aberrant RBCs. This occlusion of the vasculature may lead to infarction and ischemia of the tissue. It may lead to dysfunction of the organs, such as the liver, spleen, and kidneys, and may result in fatal complications like sequestration crisis. Furthermore, their ongoing hemolysis is likely to exacerbate anemia, further destabilizing health and patient stability, as in cases where aggravations also occur with infection, e.g., COVID-19, thereby augmenting the clinical severity of chronic anemia (Alkindi et al., 2020). In addition, cognitive dysfunction and brain injury could also be caused by recurrent ischemic insult, as the effect of distant chronic anemia over its immediate hematologic effects (Alrjjal et al., 2015).

5.2.7. Role of Iron Metabolism

Iron metabolism plays a significant role in the pathophysiology of thalassemias and hemoglobinopathies because iron is an essential part of hemoglobin, the protein used for the transport of oxygen in blood. Dyserythropoiesis due to beta thalassemia and other etiologies results in inefficient red blood cell production, accompanied by a compensatory mechanism that causes disproportionate iron absorption from the gut and subsequent iron overload.

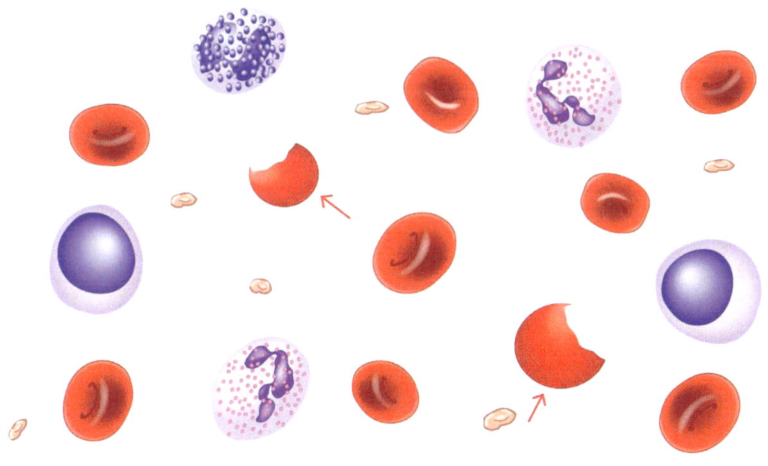

Figure 5.9. Iron metabolism plays a crucial role in the pathophysiology of hemoglobinopathies and thalassemia's, as iron is an essential component of hemoglobin, which is responsible for oxygen transport in the bloodstream.

Source: https://myhematology.com/wp-content/uploads/2024/03/Bite-cells.jpg.

This excess iron can cause extensive tissue damage in most organs with several organs, significantly aggravating the clinical presentation of these patients. Understanding iron metabolisms role in these conditions brings the treatment into perspective, as proper treatment can reduce the complications of excess iron. The recent progress in clinical science emphasizes the importance of iron monitoring and chelation therapy as a standard procedure for maximizing health gains in inherited disease subjects (Costa et al., 2020) (Figure 5.9).

5.2.8. Interaction with Other Diseases

Hemoglobinopathies, particularly thalassemias, tend to cross-react with other hematological disorders that aggravate clinical syndromes and therapeutic approaches. For instance, Hb Grey Lynn's association with α+-thalassemia, reported in a recent article, indicates how the presence of variant hemoglobins plays a role in determining the severity of anemia expressed by patients. A Thai female patient presenting with mild anemia exhibited unexpected hematological features due to the interaction between these two mutations, which resulted in increased mean corpuscular volume in systemic circulation despite reduced Hb levels (Fucharoen et al., 2014). Furthermore, hemolysis kinetics in thalassemia will exaggerate or diminish features of concomitant diseases, such as hereditary spherocytosis. The Hemoglobin release test has confirmed that α-thalassemia may result in augmented hemoglobin release from erythrocytes, which may affect the clinical presentation of such interactions and further complicate the disease's treatment (Gao et al., 2015). Detection of such interactions is crucial for successful treatment and optimal patient outcomes.

5.2.9. Cellular and Molecular Consequences

The cellular and molecular manifestations of thalassemias and hemoglobinopathies are profound and include damage to oxygen-carrying as well as an extensive range of clinical findings.

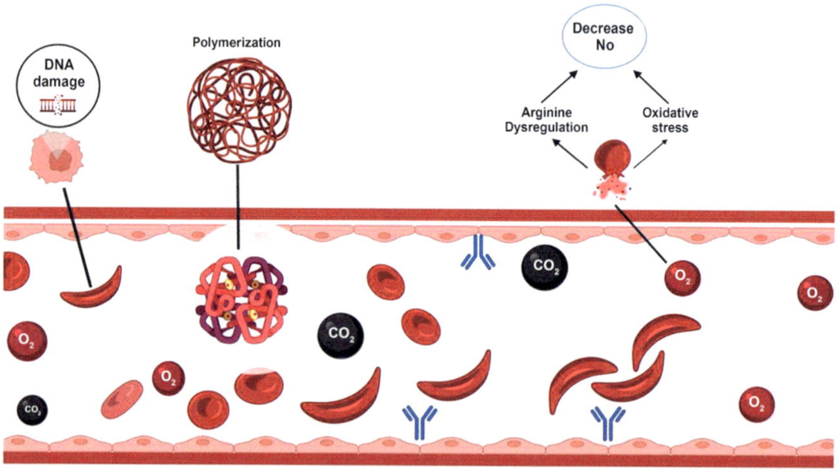

Figure 5.10. The cellular and molecular consequences of hemoglobinopathies and thalassemia's are profound, affecting oxygen transport and leading to a spectrum of clinical manifestations.

Source: https://media.springernature.com/lw1200/springer-static/image/art%3A10.1186%2Fs43088-023-00373-w/MediaObjects/43088_2023_373_Fig2_HTML.png.

The disease pathophysiology is a consequence of the disruption of globin chain production, secondary to gene mutations that either alter the structure of hemoglobin or its production. Most significantly, thalassemias are caused by defective globin chain production, most frequently with mutations of hemoglobin controlling genes, resulting in ineffective erythropoiesis and hemolytic anemia. Beta thalassemia, perhaps the most prevalent form of thalassemia worldwide, affects millions of newborns annually. These conditions not only tax the healthcare system but also necessitate lifelong management solutions to alleviate their burden, thereby making ongoing research into diagnosis and treatment measures even more critical. Current studies have shed light on the complexity of these conditions' pathogenesis and their respective cellular conversions, which are still core in the construction of treatment regimens (Attri et al., 2023) (Figure 5.10).

5.3. Diagnosis and Screening

The screening and diagnosis of hemoglobinopathies, which include the thalassemias, require an integrated approach to effective prevention and management of the conditions. Techniques such as HPLC are now an essential part of confirmatory diagnosis of the hemoglobin disorder spectrum, as observed in research among 1,400 rural Indian women of reproductive age, where several instances of thalassemia trait and other hemoglobinopathies were diagnosed with detailed hematological tests (Bhargava et al., 2016). In addition, prenatal screening is also gaining significance as a key component of preventive healthcare so that high-risk pregnancies can be tackled at an early stage. Noninvasive methods of prenatal diagnosis, like cell-free fetal DNA analysis from maternal blood, are a vital step since these bypass the procedural issues of invasive tests traditionally employed for prenatal diagnosis (Tuli et al., 2018). In general, these methods affirm the benefit of systematic screening programs in avoiding morbidity due to hemoglobinopathies and thalassemia.

5.3.1. Clinical Presentation and Symptoms

The clinical presentation of SCD and the thalassemia, or hemoglobinopathies, is a spectrum of expression, ranging from mild to severe and varied in presentation. Patients have evidence of secondary anemia of ineffective erythropoiesis or increased hemolysis, including jaundice, pallor, and fatigue.

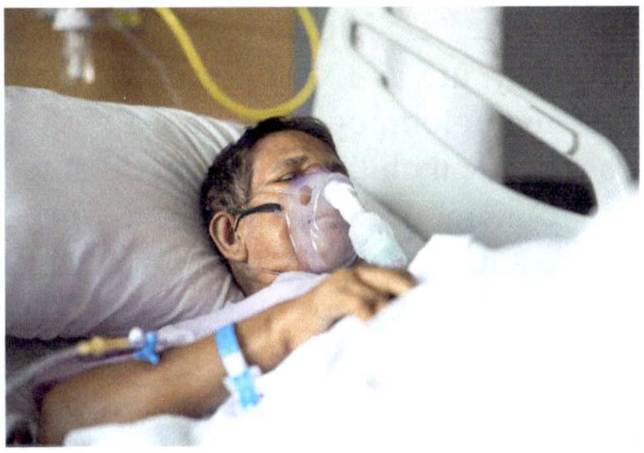

Figure 5.11. The clinical presentation of hemoglobinopathies, including thalassemia's and sickle cell disease (SCD), is characterized by a spectrum of symptoms that vary in severity and manifestation.

Source: https://www.hematologyadvisor.com/wp-content/uploads/sites/14/2021/01/ventilator_G_623185666.jpg.

In SCD, vaso-occlusive crises lead to acute pain episodes, a typical presentation that can be the cause of extreme morbidity and compromised quality of life. Moreover, complications such as pneumonia and acute chest syndrome further complicate treatment in these patients, as evidenced by research in which it was revealed that 70% of symptomatic

COVID-19 patients were hospital-admitted, which speaks volumes for the severity of the effect of co-morbid infections on their health status (Alkindi et al., 2020). Recurrent ischemic attacks can also cause cumulative damage to organs, such as the lungs, liver, and spleen, and exacerbate the clinical status (Alrjjal et al., 2015) (Figure 5.11).

5.3.2. Laboratory Tests for Diagnosis

Diagnosis of hemoglobinopathies, including the thalassemias, is primarily based on a variety of laboratory tests for the determination of hemoglobin structure and function. Abnormalities in RBC morphology can be detected through complete blood counts (CBCs) and peripheral blood smears. More sophisticated techniques like hemoglobin electrophoresis are subsequently utilized to differentiate among various hemoglobinopathies based on their electrophoretic mobility. In addition, molecular diagnostic methods have reached a very high level, too, and precise α- and β-thalassemia-related mutations can be identified through PCR and next-generation sequencing technologies. Due to the impact of such a diagnosis on patient management, e.g., the requirement for blood transfusion or potential prenatal therapy, the correct laboratory protocols must be applied. Thus, the integration of both noninvasive and invasive methods, e.g., those utilizing cell-free fetal DNA (cfDNA), is of foremost importance in genotypic diagnosis and improved treatment outcomes (Tuli et al., 2018; Alkindi et al., 2020).

5.3.3. Hemoglobin Electrophoresis

Hemoglobin electrophoresis is an essential diagnostic test used in the diagnosis of hemoglobinopathies, particularly in the differentiation of the different forms of thalassemia. In this technique, the different hemoglobin variants, based on charge and size, are separated, enabling the detection of abnormal hemoglobin patterns. In research conducted in thalassemia-endemic regions, such as India, high-performance liquid chromatography has been found to be a highly effective method, which is more sensitive in diagnosing both β-thalassemia trait and other hemoglobinopathies (Bhargava et al., 2016). Since thalassemias, if not treated, may result in severe anemia and other related health complications, proper and early diagnosis by methods like hemoglobin electrophoresis is required for effective treatment and preventive measures (Tuli et al., 2018). The application of this technique not only ensures accurate diagnosis but also supports effective and good screening techniques, thereby enhancing patient outcomes (Figure 5.12).

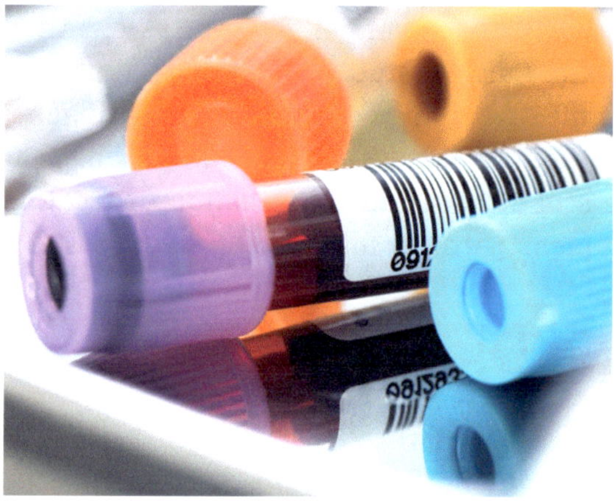

Figure 5.12. Hemoglobin electrophoresis serves as a pivotal diagnostic tool in the investigation of hemoglobinopathies, particularly in differentiating various types of thalassemia's.

Source: https://www.ucsfbenioffchildrens.org/-/media/project/ucsf/ucsf-bch/images/medical-tests/hero/hemoglobin-electrophoresis-708x556-2x.jpg?rev=4903911970a546e89ad36c513dbe8d72.

5.3.4. Genetic Testing Methods

Genetic testing technologies play a crucial role in the treatment of hemoglobinopathies and thalassemias through early diagnosis and treatment. Technological advancements in molecular diagnosis technologies, particularly those involving polymerase chain reaction (PCR) and high-throughput methods, have significantly enhanced the ability to genotype these disorders. According to (Tuli et al., 2018), prenatal diagnosis previously relied on invasive procedures but now encompasses noninvasive ones such as maternal blood sample cell-free DNA (cfDNA), in a move that helps eliminate fetal loss associated with invasive procedures. Additionally, previous attempts as cited by (Cooper et al., 1977) show screening and education in public health measures for hemoglobin disorder control. These interventions are not only crucial in identifying high-risk individuals but also vital in developing prevention strategies, such as carrier screening and genetic counseling, thereby improving health outcomes for these populations worldwide.

5.3.5. Newborn Screening Programs

Neonatal screening schemes are a valuable resource for the early detection of hemoglobinopathies and thalassemias, allowing early treatment that can significantly enhance the health outcome in affected infants. Early detection of diseases such as SCD at birth enables health workers to set up preventative procedures and intervention programs that can reduce complications of such diseases, such as anemia and organ damage, in cases where they have not been treated and, therefore, avoid severe health crises. However, the effectiveness of such screening programs in low- and middle-income countries is eroded by a wide array of challenges, ranging from inadequate infrastructure to a lack of access to genetic services (Anwar et al., 2021). These barriers highlight the need for tailored solutions to integrate newborn screening into overall public health programs in a manner that enables all newborns, within their respective geographical or socio-economic contexts, to access the necessary tests for optimal health management (Figure 5.13).

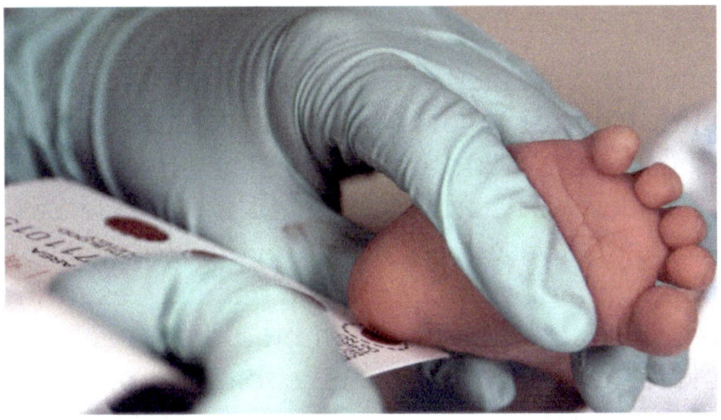

Figure 5.13. Newborn screening programs play a critical role in the early detection of hemoglobinopathies and thalassemia's, allowing for timely intervention that can significantly improve health outcomes for affected infants.

Source: https://upload.wikimedia.org/wikipedia/commons/1/16/Phenylketonuria_testing.jpg.

5.3.6. Importance of Family History

Family history is relevant in hemoglobinopathies and thalassemias as it provides valuable information on genetic predispositions that will influence disease management and treatment. A good family history enables clinicians to identify individuals at risk for conditions such as beta thalassemia, which is prevalent in certain populations worldwide. The significance of this genetic linkage is evident in the fact that thousands of infants are born annually with beta thalassemia, necessitating well-informed clinical practice based on family patterns of inheritance. Furthermore, the European Hematology Association maintains that comprehensive research involving genetic variables is crucial because understanding family patterns can lead to enhanced diagnostics and treatment modalities (Allard et al., 2016). Thus, comprehending the value of family history not only assists in early diagnosis but also allows for targeted interventions that respond to patients' unique genetic profiles, essentially enhancing health outcomes.

5.3.7. Role of Imaging Studies

Imaging tests play a critical role in the diagnosis and treatment of hemoglobinopathies and thalassemia's and deliver critical information regarding the complications of these diseases. MRI and ultrasound are some of the technologies applied in determining organ damage resulting from excess iron, a common consequence of frequent blood transfusions in patients with conditions such as beta thalassemia. MRI, particularly, can offer a non-invasive measurement of myocardial iron load, and thus permit early intervention before irreversible damage occurs. Furthermore, imaging tests are helpful in providing valuable information regarding skeletal deformity and assessing splenic size and function, which are often compromised in these patients. As recognized in recent reviews, the fusion of imaging modalities with clinical evaluation not only enhances the understanding of the disease process but also informs therapeutic decision-making, thereby improving patient outcomes (Alkindi et al., 2020) (Figure 5.14).

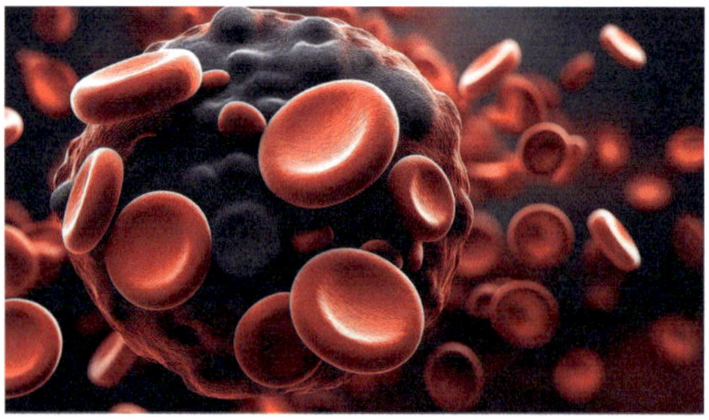

Figure 5.14. Techniques such as magnetic resonance imaging (MRI) and ultrasound are instrumental in evaluating organ damage caused by iron overload, a common consequence of frequent blood transfusions in patients with conditions like beta thalassemia.

Source: https://images.prismic.io/sterlings-hospitals/aBn93fIqRLdaB52k_Untitleddesign-8-.png?auto=format,compress.

5.3.8. Challenges in Diagnosis

Hemoglobinopathies and thalassemia diagnosis come with significant challenges that complicate effective management and treatment. The conditions are not only common but also genetically heterogeneous in their expression, often leading to misdiagnosis or delayed diagnosis in affected individuals. For instance, increasing globalization and migration lead to a multi-ethnic patient population in nations such as Europe, where guidelines for appropriate diagnostic procedures are highly sought after due to the heterogeneous patient populations affected by these diseases (Franceschi et al., 2019). Furthermore, limited access to advanced genetic screening techniques, especially in Third World nations, makes early detection of diseases like β-thalassemia and G6PD deficiency challenging. In India, for example, community screening for genetic disorders is limited, contributing to the burden placed on susceptible populations (Balgir et al., 2010). Overall, these difficulties underscore the importance of standardized diagnostic procedures and enhanced healthcare efforts in promoting early detection and intervention.

5.4. Management and Treatment

Effective management and treatment of thalassemias and hemoglobinopathies demand a holistic, multi-dimensional approach in dealing with individual patient needs. Management strategies typically involve regular monitoring and patient education about the disorder, which is crucial for early identification and intervention. Genetic screening is particularly crucial in high-prevalence population groups such as conditions β-thalassemia, as has been established by population studies in India's Sindhi population, wherein a prevalence of β-thalassemia trait was 20.5% (Balgir et al., 2010). This practice enables healthcare providers to offer genetic advice and preventive strategies to high-risk families, thereby mitigating the overall burden of such inherited disorders. Moreover, novel therapeutic advancements, such as the development of new medications and the establishment of diagnostic guidelines, should be integrated to enhance patient survival and outcomes (Franceschi et al., 2019). By establishing an integrated management system, the healthcare system can better manage the complexity of hemoglobinopathies and thalassemias.

5.4.1. Supportive Care Strategies

Supportive care interventions are the backbone of hemoglobinopathy and thalassemia care, catering to the multifaceted needs of patients.

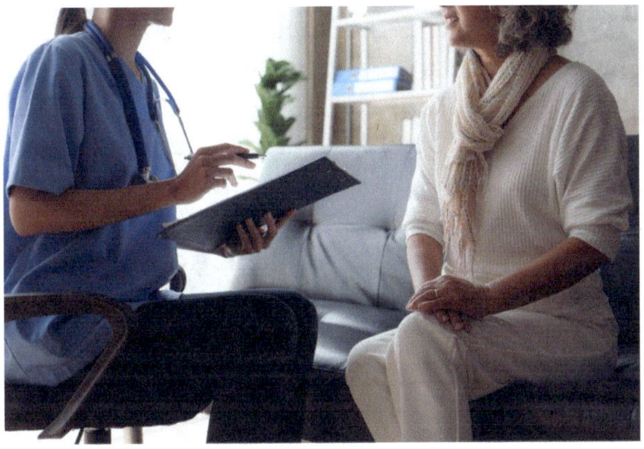

Figure 5.15. Patient education is crucial for fostering adherence to treatment protocols and empowering patients to manage their health effectively.

Source: https://aihcp.net/main/wp-content/uploads/2024/02/Depositphotos_622838168_S-1-1.jpg.

These interventions include regular blood transfusions, iron chelation treatment, and prevention of associated complications such as infection and organ damage. Regular transfusions are essential to maintain hemoglobin levels and alleviate symptoms of anemia, while iron chelation therapy averts secondary iron overload, a common complication of recurrent transfusions. In addition, customized patient education is very important in promoting treatment adherence and empowering patients to effectively manage their health. Recent progress in hematology, as illustrated in current clinical trials, holds promise for improving the quality of life and life expectancy of patients with these conditions (Eleftheriou et al., 2019; Franceschi et al., 2019). Finally, a combination approach utilizing all of these supportive care strategies coupled with newer therapeutic strategies is needed to advance overall outcomes in thalassemia and hemoglobinopathy patients (Figure 5.15).

5.4.2. Blood Transfusion Therapy

Blood transfusion therapy is essential in the management of hemoglobinopathies and thalassemia's and overall improves patient outcomes. Especially, patients with conditions such as beta thalassemia rely on regular transfusions to maintain their hemoglobin requirements and alleviate symptoms of anemia-related disease. These transfusions not only enhance quality of life but also decrease disease complications, such as infection risk due to immune incompetence. The risks of transfusions, particularly those related to transfusion-transmitted infections, underscore the need for stringent safety measures in clinical practice. Advances in new screening techniques in recent years have significantly reduced the incidence of these infections, although the challenges are primarily faced by those with compromised immune systems due to their underlying condition. Therefore, the fine points of blood transfusion therapy become essential for optimizing treatment regimens and delivering comprehensive care to patients with hemoglobinopathies and thalassemia (Girolamo et al., 2009).

5.4.3. Iron Chelation Therapy

Iron chelation therapy is one of the treatments for hemoglobinopathies, particularly beta-thalassemia, due to the complications associated with excessive iron overload resulting from repeated blood transfusions. Although transfusion is required to improve anemia and quality of life, it carries a risk of causing secondary complications such as iron overload-caused organ injury, which poses serious health complications for the patients.

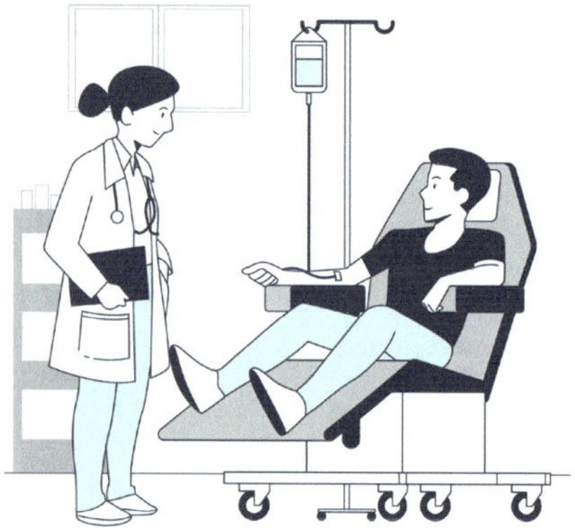

Figure 5.16. The management of hemoglobinopathies, particularly beta-thalassemia, often necessitates iron chelation therapy due to the risks associated with excessive iron accumulation from repeated blood transfusions.

Source: https://www.vtitan.com/ATP.png.

It is revealed that optimal iron chelation not only minimizes such risks but also enhances patients' prognosis and quality of life, particularly in regions where available medical treatment is prevalent, as elucidated by the Thalassemia International Federation (TIF) in their recent guidelines (Angastiniotis et al., 2022). Furthermore, the increasing migration of thalassemia-affected individuals to other countries necessitates the development of standardized care protocols, such as iron chelation protocols tailored to various patient groups (Franceschi et al., 2019). Fulfilling these demands through consistent care and treatment models is essential for achieving improved outcomes in affected individuals (Figure 5.16).

5.4.4. Bone Marrow Transplantation (BMT)

Bone marrow transplantation (BMT) is seen as a principal therapeutic option for patients with hemoglobinopathies, most notably thalassemia major, who are likely to benefit insufficiently from conventional therapies. Not only does the procedure offer the potential for a real cure, but it also significantly enhances patient quality of life, at least in regions where access to comprehensive care remains suboptimal. For instance, the International Federation of Thalassemia has emphasized the importance of equitable care and the development of clinical pathways, thereby highlighting the significance of specialized centers in managing such complex cases (Angastiniotis et al., 2022). The increasing prevalence of hemoglobinopathies, particularly in multiethnic populations due to global migration, underscores the importance of good therapies like BMT that can counter the unique challenges posed by these diseases (Franceschi et al., 2019). Lastly, advancements in transplantation techniques, combined with concerted efforts in healthcare, bring optimism to improved long-term outcomes in such patients.

5.4.5. Gene Therapy Advancements

Gene therapy innovations hold revolutionary potential for treating hemoglobinopathies and thalassemias with prospects for genetic disorders long deemed untreatable otherwise. Recent advances have underscored the pivotal contribution of gene editing technologies, such as CRISPR-Cas9, which enables precise modifications to the faulty globin genes that cause these conditions. These technological advancements have not only enhanced the knowledge regarding the genetic etiology of thalassemia but have also provided an entry for novel therapeutic modalities, enhancing the efficacy of existing interventions. The prognosis for patients has been transformed due to ongoing research, including the development of targeted therapies that can potentially cure thalassemia, as illustrated by progress in hematopoietic cell transplantation and novel gene delivery methods. As outlined in recent literature, such developments have the potential to redefine the outcomes of patients, making thalassemia no longer a lifelong condition, but rather an eradicable disease (Angelucci et al., 2021; Attri et al., 2023) (Figure 5.17).

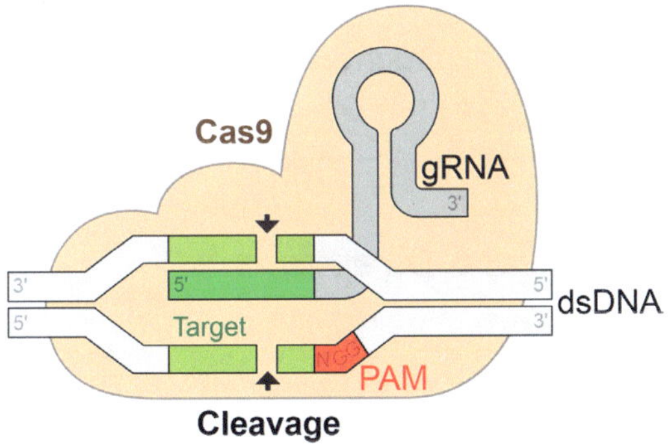

Figure 5.17. Gene editing techniques, such as CRISPR-Cas9, which enable precise alterations to the faulty globin genes responsible for these conditions.

Source: https://upload.wikimedia.org/wikipedia/commons/5/57/GRNA-Cas9.svg.

5.4.6. Pharmacological Treatments

Pharmacotherapy is the cornerstone in the management of hemoglobinopathies and thalassemia, playing a pivotal role in patient survival. It is performed to alleviate symptoms, prevent complications, and improve the quality of life for patients. One such milestone is the use of hydroxyurea, which increases fetal hemoglobin and reduces vaso-occlusive crisis events in SCD, marking a significant therapeutic management breakthrough. Additionally, iron chelation therapy is a crucial treatment for individuals with chronic blood transfusions, as it inhibits iron overload, a priority in thalassemia management. Such diseases require intense investigation so that further developments can be made to the existing pharmacological treatments and new treatment methods can be developed. With increasing understanding of the pathophysiology of these diseases, it will open up the door for the development of target therapies that act against the root cause of hemoglobinopathies and thalassemia more efficiently (Musgrove et al., 2015; Costa FF et al., 2020).

5.4.7. Nutritional Management

Nutrition is a primary issue in the treatment of thalassemias and hemoglobinopathies, and particularly the reversal of anemia's impact, which is common to the two disorders. Promising methods involve the administration of substances used for the incorporation into hemoglobin production and the generation of red blood cells in general. Iron and folic acid supplements, for instance, form the core of pregnancy anemia prevention, a condition that matters in that pregnant women are especially susceptible to anemia due to increased nutritional requirements (Adam et al., 2016). In addition, the European Hematology Association notes that individually adapted nutrition interventions can optimize the efficacy of therapeutic treatment, accelerating the course and outcome in most blood disorders, including thalassemia (Anagnou et al., 2021).

By focusing on a generalized nutritional intervention involving dietary supplementation and support, health care providers are able to exert a significant influence on the treatment and management of hemoglobinopathies and consequently improve the quality of life of the patients (Figure 5.18).

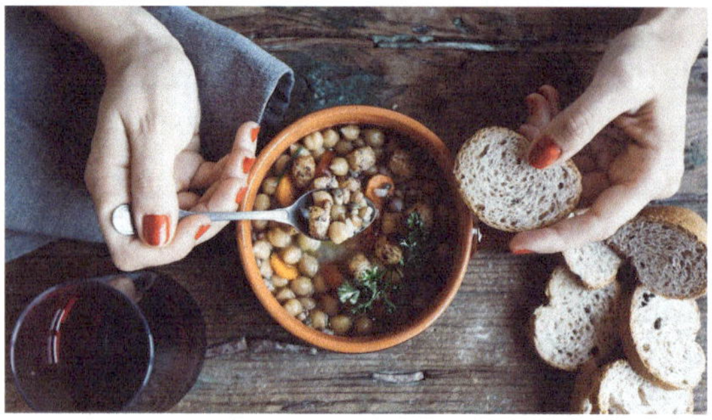

Figure 5.18. Iron and folic acid supplements form the bedrock of anemia prevention during pregnancy, a significant concern given that pregnant women are particularly susceptible to anemia due to increased nutritional demands

Source: https://i0.wp.com/post.healthline.com/wp-content/uploads/2019/06/Beans_Hands_1296x728-header-1296x728.jpg?w=1155&h=1528.

5.4.8. Psychological Support for Patients

Psychological management is also part of hemoglobinopathy management, particularly thalassemia's. It has a significant impact on determining the patient's outcomes. With the chronic lifetime of diseases such as transfusion-dependent thalassemia (TDT), alongside medical treatment, there must be ongoing psychological and emotional support. The patient must deal with many concerns, including worry about the timing of treatments, stigmatization, and psychosocial implications of having a chronic disease. Organizations like the Thalassemia International Federation (TIF) draw attention to the fact that such psychosocial issues need to be treated in addition to clinical management, in the form of education and lobbying so that patients are given access to such counseling support systems, which play a crucial role in enhancing their quality of life. In addition, TIFs guidelines also emphasize the intervention by multidisciplinary teams in specific regard to such psychological problems so that care to the patient is holistic and does not overlook the emotional loads that are involved with the care of chronic disease (Alassaf et al., 2022; Angastiniotis et al., 2022) (Figure 5.19).

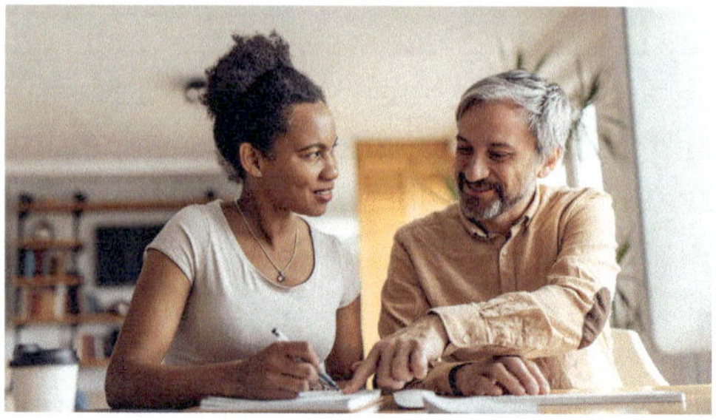

Figure 5.19. In the management of hemoglobinopathies, particularly thalassemia's, the provision of psychological support is an essential component that greatly influences patient outcomes.

Source: https://patientbetter.com/wp-content/uploads/2023/08/1920-x-1080-Patient-Education-and-Self-Management.jpg.

5.4.9. Future Directions in Treatment

Thalassemia and hemoglobinopathy management is on the cusp of breakthrough revolutions in blood transfusion and hematological practice, driven by new mechanisms. The developments in science and technology in recent years highlight the use of evidence-based practice for maximizing the management of such disorders and patient safety, as well as treatment efficacy. According to recent literature, the general enhancement of methodology development, standardization, and quality control holds promise for optimized therapeutic interventions in hemoglobinopathies, as innovative studies explore the intersection of diet, exercise, and patient education within comprehensive treatment regimens. For instance, studies have shown that consolidated treatments can indeed enhance patient outcomes, suggesting that integration is necessary in clinical practice.

A CLOSER LOOK

HIGH-PERFORMANCE LIQUID CHROMATOGRAPHY (HPLC)

HPLC is a precise and high-strength separation, identification, and quantitation method of components in a liquid sample. It entails the passage of the sample through a column packed with a solid material (stationary phase) under the influence of a liquid solvent (mobile phase). Different components in the sample pass through the column at different speeds based on the interaction between the components and the stationary phase; therefore, the mode of separation. HPLC finds widespread use in pharmaceuticals, clinical diagnostics, food safety, and environmental analysis due to its accuracy, sensitivity, and versatility.

SUMMARY

The long-term disease burden of hemoglobinopathies, particularly thalassemias, underscores the importance of proper screening and accurate diagnosis among patients. The application of advanced diagnostic techniques, such as HPLC, can sufficiently enhance the identification of many hemoglobinopathies, facilitating early and appropriate intervention is evident from research, which indicated a high burden of anemia and hemoglobinopathies in some groups, targeted interventions through antenatal screening need to be conducted to halt the associated morbidity (Bhargava et al., 2016). Additionally, even as innovations in dog models may offer clues toward hemoglobin structure, the conflicting findings require caution in extrapolating them to human diseases (Kritsepi-Konstantinou et al., 2019). Ultimately, increasing awareness and improving diagnostic abilities are steps back to reducing the impact of these genetic conditions, providing better health to individuals who are vulnerable to hemoglobinopathies and thalassemias.

A literature review of thalassemia and hemoglobinopathies highlights the complexity of the diseases as well as the ongoing challenges posed by their treatment. Beta-thalassemia, particularly its TDT, necessitates a lifetime of treatment and management by specialized healthcare teams, highlighting the need for a multidisciplinary approach to address the disease (Angastiniotis et al., 2022). Technological improvements in diagnostics and treatments have advantageously affected patients; however, inequalities in access to treatment still exist critically, particularly between high-prevalence and low-incidence areas where health systems are not capable of responding to migrant groups' needs (Alassaf et al., 2022). The TIF plays a critical role in resolving disparities in access to medical care and has established comprehensive clinical practice guidelines, the latest of which came out in 2021, for appropriate management alternatives for TDT patients. The report not only directs clinical interventions but also helps raise awareness and initiate research, addressing the medical and psychosocial dimensions of care.

REFERENCES

1. Adam, I., & Ali, A. A. (2016). Anemia during pregnancy. In InTech eBooks. https://doi.org/10.5772/63211Alassaf, A., Angastiniotis, M., Angastiniotis, M., Angelucci, E., Aydinok, Y., Bou-Fakhredin, R. R., Brunetta, L., et al. (2022). 2021 Thalassemia International Federation guidelines for the management of transfusion-dependent thalassemia. https://core.ac.uk/download/614062765.pdf (accessed on 12th June 2025).
2. Aljaaly, E. A. M. (2012). Factors affecting nutritional status and eating behaviors of adolescent girls in Saudi Arabia. https://core.ac.uk/download/16238776.pdf (accessed on 12th June 2025).
3. Alkindi, S., Alyaarubi, S., Banchev, A., Campisi, R., et al. (2020). Preliminary data on COVID-19 in patients with hemoglobinopathies: A multicenter ICET-A study. https://core.ac.uk/download/390052235.pdf (accessed on 12th June 2025).
4. Allard, S., Anagnou, N., Andolfo, I., Andrau, M., et al. (2016). The European Hematology Association roadmap for European hematology research: A consensus document. https://core.ac.uk/download/43718574.pdf (accessed on 12th June 2025).
5. Al-Matary, A., Allen, A., Islam, A., Koren, A., O'Donnell, A., Panja, A., Premawardhena, A., et al. (2017). Thalassemias in South Asia: Clinical lessons learnt from Bangladesh. https://core.ac.uk/download/322326228.pdf (accessed on 12th June 2025).
6. Alrjjal, K., Alwakeel, A., Darwish, A., El-Ashry, H., et al. (2015). Sickle cell disease (SCD). https://core.ac.uk/download/322425389.pdf (accessed on 12th June 2025).
7. Anagnou, N. P., Andolfo, I., Barcellini, W., Camaschella, C., et al. (2021). The EHA research roadmap: Anemias. https://core.ac.uk/download/478721871.pdf (accessed on 12th June 2025).
8. Angelucci, E., & Giannoni, L. (2021). Current and future therapies for β-thalassemia: A review article. https://core.ac.uk/download/589958541.pdf (accessed on 12th June 2025).
9. Anwar, S., Chakraborty, S., Hosen, M. J., Miah, M., et al. (2021). Genetic counseling in the context of Bangladesh: Current scenario, challenges, and a framework for genetic service implementation. https://core.ac.uk/download/416394774.pdf (accessed on 12th June 2025).
10. Attri, K., Sharma, K., Sharma, L., Kaur, N., Ronald William, N., Rathi, S., Yadav, S., et al. (2023). A review on current status of blood disorder: Thalassemia and its treatment. https://core.ac.uk/download/588567546.pdf (accessed on 12th June 2025).
11. Aye, K. S., Lwin, A. A., Okada, S., Oo, M. M., et al. (2005). Hemoglobin E prevalence in malaria-endemic villages in Myanmar. https://core.ac.uk/download/12548694.pdf (accessed on 12th June 2025).
12. Balgir, R. S. (2010). Inherited hemolytic disorders with high occurrence of β-thalassemia in Sindhi community of Jabalpur town in Madhya Pradesh, India. https://core.ac.uk/download/pdf/87430.pdf (accessed on 12th June 2025).
13. Balgir, R. S. (2011). Genetic disease burden, nutrition and determinants of tribal health care in Chhattisgarh State of Central-East India: A status paper. https://core.ac.uk/download/pdf/332892.pdf (accessed on 12th June 2025).
14. Bhargava, S., Jain, P., Kumar, V., Sen, D., et al. (2016). Prevalence of haemoglobinopathies in

anemic females. https://core.ac.uk/download/539909930.pdf (accessed on 12th June 2025).

15. Chandrashekar, V., & Soni, M. (2011). Hemoglobin disorders in South India. https://core.ac.uk/download/pdf/8632857.pdf (accessed on 12th June 2025).
16. Cooper, F. N., & Scott, R. B. (1977). The Virginia Sickle Cell Anemia Awareness Program: Education, screening, and counseling. https://core.ac.uk/download/51294858.pdf (accessed on 12th June 2025).
17. Costa, F. F., & Sonati, M. D. (2020). The genetics of blood disorders: Hereditary hemoglobinopathies. https://core.ac.uk/download/357336244.pdf (accessed on 12th June 2025).
18. De Franceschi, L., de Montalembert, M., Cappellini, M. D., Eleftheriou, A., et al. (2019). EHA research roadmap on hemoglobinopathies and thalassemia: An update. https://core.ac.uk/download/289261511.pdf (accessed on 12th June 2025).
19. Di Girolamo, A., Ricerca, B. M., & Rund, D. (2009). Infections in thalassemia and hemoglobinopathies: Focus on therapy-related complications. https://core.ac.uk/download/pdf/8522729.pdf (accessed on 12th June 2025).
20. Eleftheriou, A., Iolascon, A., Taher, A., Rees, D., De Franceschi, L., de Montalembert, M., Muckenthaler, M., et al. (2019). EHA research roadmap on hemoglobinopathies and thalassemia: An update. https://core.ac.uk/download/268913099.pdf (accessed on 12th June 2025).
21. Fucharoen, G., Singha, K., & Fucharoen, S. (2014). Interaction of hemoglobin Grey Lynn (Vientiane) with a non-deletional α+-thalassemia in an adult Thai proband. https://core.ac.uk/download/19544937.pdf (accessed on 12th June 2025).
22. Gao, L., He, Q., Jia, G., Ma, Y., et al. (2015). Comparative study of the amount of re-released hemoglobin from α-thalassemia and hereditary spherocytosis erythrocytes. https://core.ac.uk/download/322425517.pdf (accessed on 12th June 2025).
23. Kritsepi-Konstantinou, M., Mylonakis, M., Oikonomidis, I., Tsouloufi, T., et al. (2019). Capillary hemoglobin electrophoresis of healthy and anemic dogs: Quantification, validation, and reference intervals of hemoglobin fractions. https://core.ac.uk/download/322483238.pdf (accessed on 12th June 2025).
24. Musgrove, L. E. (2015). Transition Together: A Study of Pediatric Patients with Sickle Cell Disease as They Transition to Adult Health Care. https://core.ac.uk/download/33562243.pdf (accessed on 12th June 2025).
25. Tuli, A., & Yenilmez, E. D. (2018). Invasive and noninvasive approaches in prenatal diagnosis of thalassemia's. https://core.ac.uk/download/322436249.pdf (accessed on 12th June 2025).

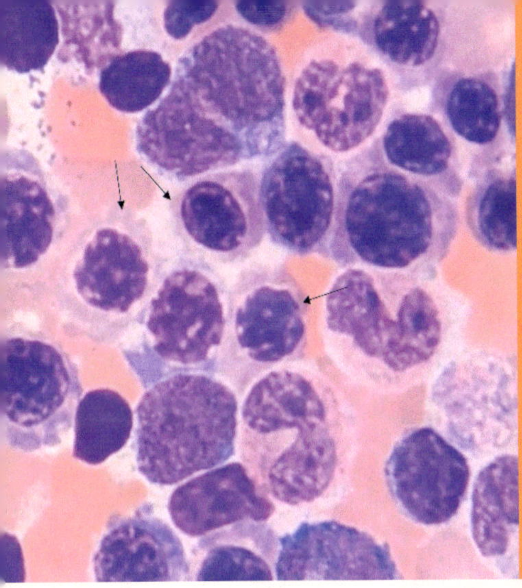

Chapter 6

MEGALOBLASTIC AND APLASTIC ANEMIAS

Contents

Introduction....129

6.1. Megaloblastic Anemia....130

6.2. Aplastic Anemia....134

6.3. Current Research and Advances....139

Summary....145

References....146

Introduction

It is essential to understand the intricacies of megaloblastic and aplastic anemias, including their underlying mechanisms, clinical significance, and treatment. Megaloblastic anemia, a condition often associated with vitamin B12 or folate deficiency, interferes with DNA synthesis, leading to ineffective erythropoiesis and the production of abnormally large red blood cells (RBCs). Conversely, aplastic anemia results from the bone marrow's inability to produce sufficient blood cells as a consequence of various reasons, including autoimmune conditions or exposure to certain drugs. Importantly, drug-induced hematologic disorders are problematic, with certain medications having the ability to induce a variety of syndromes, including aplastic and megaloblastic anemias (Billet et al., 2009; Hospital AKU et al., 2018). This chapter will discuss the etiology, pathophysiology, and treatment of the anemias in question, noting their differences as well as the potential overlap in their clinical presentation. By examining these, we aim to gain a deeper understanding of these applicable hematologic conditions (Figure 6.1).

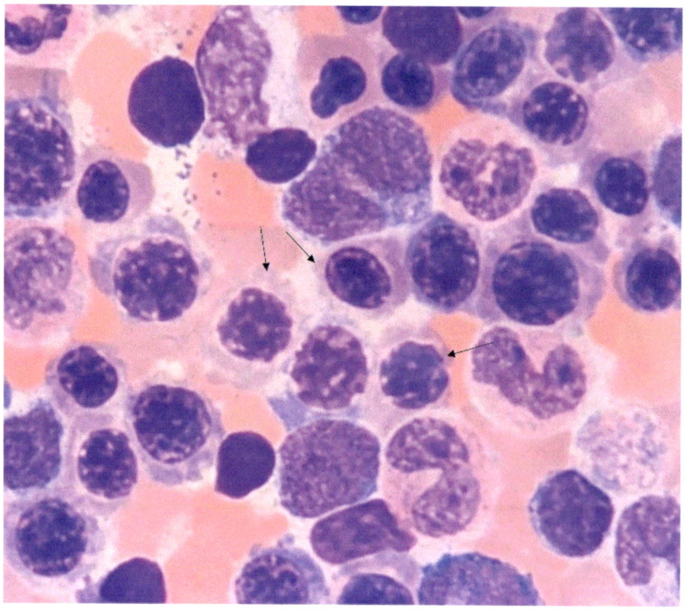

Figure 6.1. Megaloblastic anemia, commonly attributed to deficiencies in vitamin B12 or folate, disrupts DNA synthesis, leading to ineffective erythropoiesis and the production of abnormally large red blood cells.

Source: https://www.pathologyoutlines.com/imgau/bonemarrowmegaloblasticanemiateruyafeldsteinbhardwaj09.jpg.

6.1. Megaloblastic Anemia

Megaloblastic anemia is a special form of anemia characterized by the production of abnormally large RBCs, or megaloblasts, due to a deficiency of either vitamin B12 or folate. These deficiencies disrupt DNA synthesis, resulting in ineffective erythropoiesis that ultimately leads to the suppression of functional RBC production. As emphasized in recent literature, the multifactorial pathogenesis of anemia highlights the importance of understanding its underlying causes, particularly nutritional deficiencies prevalent in various groups, which are potent causes of megaloblastic anemia (Camila et al., 2019). Moreover, distinguishing megaloblastic anemia from other forms, such as congenital dyserythropoietic anemias (CDAs), is crucial for accurate diagnosis and management (Gambale et al., 2015). Proper identification of the cause and implementation of proper treatment modalities are essential to prevent the adverse health consequences associated with megaloblastic anemia, including neurologic dysfunction and overall decline in quality of life.

6.1.1. Definition and Characteristics

Megaloblastic and aplastic anemias are two distinct but clinically significant subtypes of anemia characterized by distinct underlying pathologies. Megaloblastic anemia is essentially characterized by the impaired synthesis of DNA, leading to the production of abnormally large and ineffective RBCs due to a deficiency of either vitamin B12 or folate. This results in characteristic morphological changes under blood smears, i.e., macrocytic erythrocytes and hypersegmented neutrophils. On the other hand, aplastic anemia is defined by the inability of bone marrow to produce sufficient blood cells, which can be caused by autoimmune diseases, toxic exposures, or congenital diseases (Iolascon et al., 2020). This etiology of the anemias often involves a double mechanism with both hematopoietic stem cell (HSC) failure and environmental toxin exposure complicating the clinical picture. It is essential to understand these definitions and features for the appropriate management and treatment of both megaloblastic and aplastic anemias, as both disorders require quite different therapies (Hospital AKU et al., 2018) (Figure 6.2).

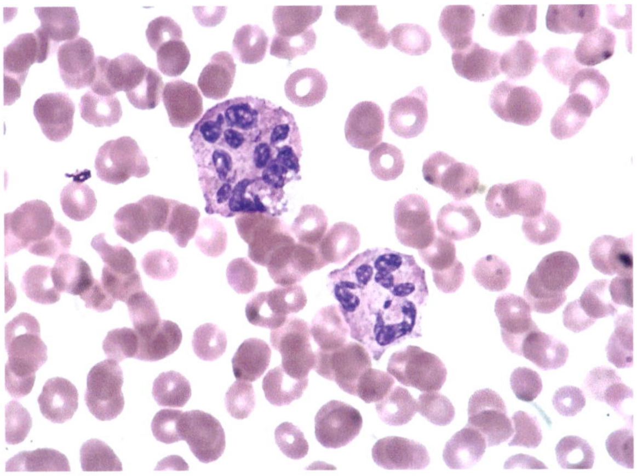

Figure 6.2. Hypersegmented neutrophils.

Source: https://upload.wikimedia.org/wikipedia/commons/6/6b/Hypersegmented_Neutrophils_%2836831145373%29.jpg.

6.1.2. Causes of Megaloblastic Anemia

The majority of megaloblastic anemia is caused by deficiencies in folate and vitamin B12, which are required for normal RBC formation. It results in the production of abnormally large and nonfunctional RBCs, and this causes symptoms such as pallor and fatigue. Research has indicated that severe cobalamin deficiency is prevalent, particularly within certain populations, and was found in 81% of patients with megaloblastic anemia to be very low in vitamin B12 (Gupta et al., 2012). Folate deficiency, however, was not found to be prevalent and affected a negligible subset of patients, indicating that cobalamin deficiency would be a more significant concern in the majority of clinical practices (Imchen et al., 2019). Additionally, dietary causes, such as suboptimal intake and absorption, contribute to the risk of such deficiency, in agreement with findings that identify megaloblastic anemia as a significant cause of pancytopenia among populations. Correction of such deficiencies through dietary supplementation is crucial for controlling and preventing the condition.

6.1.3. Role of Vitamin B12 Deficiency

Vitamin B12 deficiency is the central mechanism of megaloblastic anemia, a condition characterized by the production of large, abnormally shaped red blood cells resulting from impaired DNA synthesis. The nutrient plays a vital role in the production of normal red blood cells, and its deficiency can lead to macrocytic anemia, which is characterized clinically by fatigue, pallor, and weakness. In cases such as those experienced by celiac disease patients, cobalamin serum levels were found to be significantly lower compared to controls in normal individuals, showing an evident correlation between vitamin B12 deficiency and altered RBC morphology, including megaloblastic changes (Bugti et al., 2018). Etiologies of such deficiency range from dietary insufficiency to malabsorption disorders as in some gastroenterological diseases. Therefore, early treatment and diagnosis—most commonly with vitamin replacement—are essential in reversing the hematological abnormalities and avoiding possible systemic consequences (Ayodele et al., 2017) (Figure 6.3).

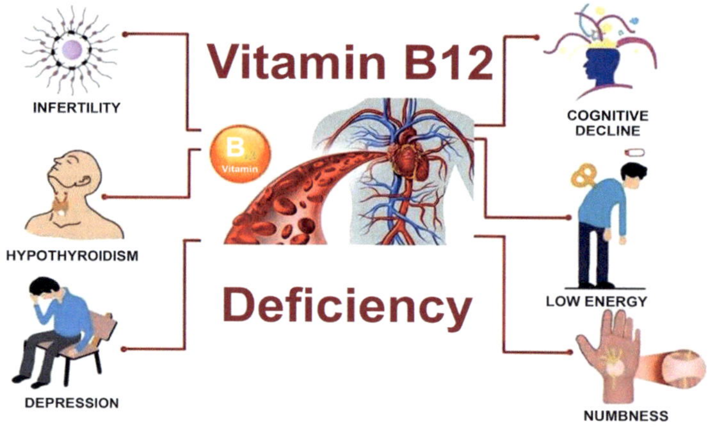

Figure 6.3. Vitamin B12 deficiency plays a critical role in the pathophysiology of megaloblastic anemia, a condition characterized by large, abnormal red blood cells resulting from impaired DNA synthesis.

Source: https://healthjade.net/wp-content/uploads/2023/01/vitamin-b12-deficiency.jpg.

6.1.4. Role of Folate Deficiency

Folate deficiency emerges as a key feature of megaloblastic anemia pathophysiology, where the interference with DNA synthesis leads to the production of abnormally large RBCs. Malnutrition, particularly in susceptible groups that rely on staple crops lacking sufficient quantities of micronutrients, is most frequently associated with folate deficiency. The condition of hidden hunger indicates the prevalence of deficiency diseases, such as vitamin and mineral deficiencies, including folate, among over two billion individuals worldwide (Strobbe et al., 2018). Furthermore, certain medical surgeries, such as Roux-en-Y gastric bypass surgery, tend to cause a range of nutritional deficiencies, including folate deficiency, which complicates the clinical presentation of postoperative anemia (Wright et al., 2014). Because folate plays a central role in DNA synthesis and cell division, its deficiency not only aggravates megaloblastic anemia but also indicates the importance of comprehensive nutritional screening in high-risk populations to avoid adverse health effects.

6.1.5. Pathophysiology of Megaloblastic Anemia

Megaloblastic anemia is characterized by the impaired formation of DNA, which is necessary for healthy cell division. This deficiency most commonly occurs due to a lack of vitamin B12 or folate, which are vital nutrients that participate in nucleotide synthesis. Because of this deficiency, hematopoietic progenitor cells in the bone marrow fail to develop into mature cells, thus forming megaloblasts—large, immature, and dysfunctional RBCs. This abnormality not only causes ineffective erythropoiesis but also results in an increased mean corpuscular volume (MCV) of RBCs, a characteristic of megaloblastic anemia. The occurrence of such megaloblasts is also accompanied by increased levels of homocysteine and methylmalonic acid, which are markers that indicate deranged metabolic pathways shared by both vitamin B12 and folate deficiency (To et al., 2018). These imbalances underscore the complex pathophysiology of megaloblastic anemia, which necessitates targeted clinical interventions to address these nutritional deficiencies (Nandhini et al., 2016) (Figure 6.4).

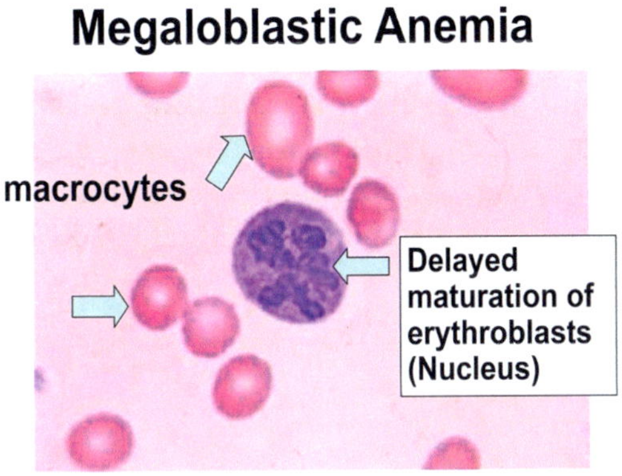

Figure 6.4. Production of megaloblasts.

Source: https://drsujatasingh.com/Drsujata_Admin/postimages/f0b12bce647e88cb02e55113445154ea.jpg.

6.1.6. Symptoms and Clinical Manifestations

The laboratory and clinical presentation of megaloblastic anemia typically demonstrates intrinsic abnormalities in vitamin B12 or folate, which produce characteristic hematologic derangements. Macrocytic RBCs are typically present in the patient, which are quantified as elevated MCV values that are important for diagnosis (Gupta et al., 2016). The presenting symptoms are typically characterized by pallor, palpitations, and fatigue, along with neurological presentations such as peripheral neuropathy resulting from the demyelination process associated with vitamin B12 deficiency. Ocular presentations are also evident, highlighting the systemic nature of the disease; retinal hemorrhage and cotton-wool spots are frequently observed in patients with blood dyscrasias and therefore require careful ophthalmic evaluation (Suhasini et al., 2017). An understanding of these clinical manifestations not only aids in the diagnosis of megaloblastic anemia but also underscores the need for early intervention to prevent some of the complications of the disease.

6.1.7. Diagnostic Methods

Diagnostic methods are crucial in establishing the etiology of megaloblastic and aplastic anemias, with bone marrow examination being the primary investigative method. Bone marrow aspiration (BMA) and trephine biopsy are supporting investigations that provide essential cytological and histological data regarding hematological disorders. Studies indicate that BMA is generally sufficient for diagnosing megaloblastic anemia, the most prevalent type of such disorders, and nutritional anemias in general (Akhter et al., 2018). Such methods enable clinicians to diagnose numerous hematologic disorders by allowing them to examine cellular morphology and bone marrow architecture (Anem et al., 2017).

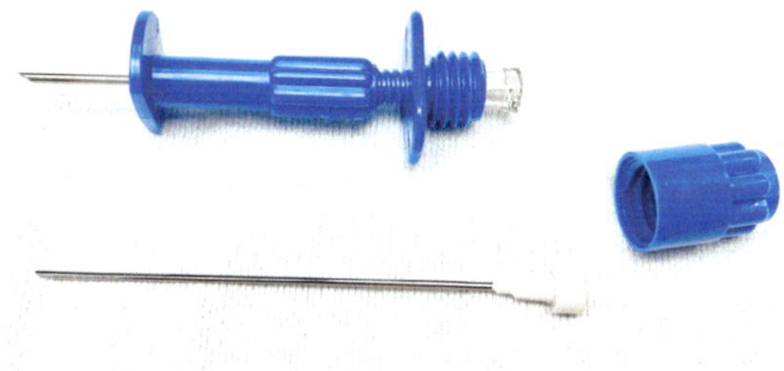

Figure 6.5. Bone marrow aspiration (BMA) and trephine biopsy are complementary techniques that provide critical cytological and histological insights into hematological disorders.

Source: https://todaysveterinarypractice.com/wp-content/uploads/sites/4/2023/06/HuIntile_TVPJulAug23_BoneMarrowAspiration_FigC.png.

With these anemias' non-specific symptoms, proper utilization of the said diagnostic procedures plays a vital role in initial identification and subsequent treatment planning. Moreover, information derived from these tests can play a significant role in management strategies employed with affected individuals, especially emphasizing the need for high-quality diagnostic procedures in the field of hematology (Figure 6.5).

6.1.8. Treatment Options

Effective management of aplastic and megaloblastic anemias is case-dependent, based on treatment modalities that are tailored to the etiology of these conditions. For megaloblastic anemia, whose causes are most often deficiency of vitamin B12 or folate, supplementation of both nutrients is indicated (which may involve dietary modification or intramuscular therapy to address malabsorption issues) (Kucera et al., 2014). Conversely, aplastic anemia, which is failure of the bone marrow, can be treated with immunosuppressive therapy or HSC transplantation, depending on the disease severity and etiology (Bogun et al., 2015). Additionally, supportive therapies like blood transfusions can alleviate symptoms and improve the patient's quality of life until effective treatments become available. Overall, an integrated strategy specifically for the specific kind of anemia is crucial in achieving maximum patient outcomes and moving forward with management practices in the clinical setting.

6.1.9. Complications Associated with Megaloblastic Anemia

Megaloblastic anemia, characterized by the presence of megaloblasts in the bone marrow, has a propensity to result in severe complications if left untreated. Among the most dangerous complications is pancytopenia, which is the reduction of RBCs, white blood cells (WBCs), and platelets, leading to symptoms such as tiredness, enhanced predisposition to infections, and bleeding disturbances. The most common reason for pancytopenia was found in a study to be megaloblastic anemia, emphasizing the necessity for early diagnosis and treatment to prevent adverse consequences (Mansuri et al., 2017). Patients may also present with neurological signs, including neuropathy and mental alteration, because of vitamin B12 deficiency. Moreover, the etiology of megaloblastic anemia in itself, particularly dietary deficiencies or malabsorptive syndromes, can complicate general health and therapy and thereby a comprehensive clinical evaluation needs to be done to minimize risks and enhance management strategies (Wankhede et al., 2017) (Figure 6.6).

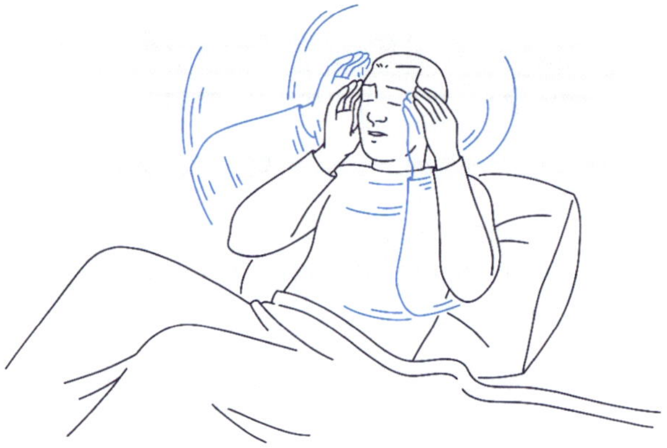

Figure 6.6: Health Pancytopenia.

Source: https://www.health.com/thmb/nSjxwzLaO7YVs9wTzVMNq1Fukqc=/4000x0/filters:no_upscale():max_bytes(150000):strip_icc()/Health-pancytopenia-overview-7107210-final-ec9f44e4c2874a758099552c0469abe0.jpg.

6.2. Aplastic Anemia

Aplastic anemia is a rare yet serious hematologic disease characterized by the bone marrow's inability to produce sufficient blood cells, resulting in deficiencies of red blood cells, white blood cells, and platelets. Aplastic anemia can be caused by many different etiologies, including autoimmune reactions, toxic chemical exposure, or certain viral infections, ultimately leading to bone marrow failure. The clinical presentations of aplastic anemia can be considerable, ranging from fatigue and pallor to increased susceptibility to infection and bleeding, highlighting the crucial role that the manufacture of blood cells plays in maintaining homeostasis. Consequently, because of the complexity of diagnosis as well as treatment of aplastic anemia, medical professionals are required to be exceptionally well-versed in aplastic anemia's implications and treatment. As underscored in recent learning materials for healthcare professionals, understanding the complexities of such disorders is crucial for effective intervention and patient management (Kucera et al., 2014; Bogun et al., 2015) (Figure 6.6).

6.2.1. Definition and Characteristics

Anemias constitute a heterogeneous collection of disorders characterized by a decrease in either the number or the functional capacity of RBCs, which play a significant part in the delivery of oxygen throughout the body. Of these, aplastic and megaloblastic anemias are of specific clinical significance due to their differing causes and presentations.

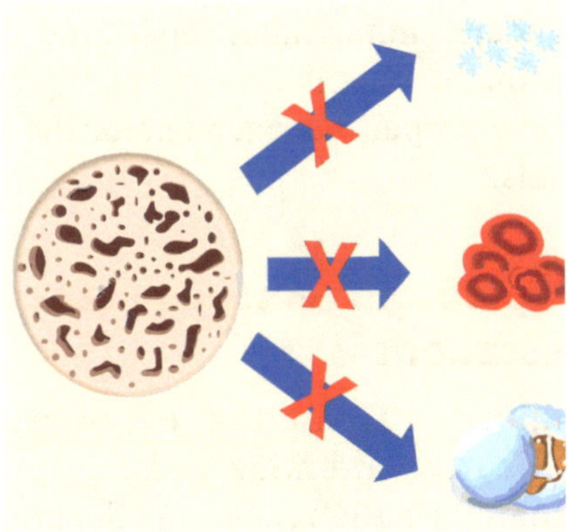

Figure 6.7. Aplastic anemia is marked by the bone marrows failure to produce adequate blood cells due to autoimmune destruction, exposure to toxins, or genetic predispositions.

Source: https://knyamed.com/cdn/shop/files/aplastic-anemia-vs-hemolytic-anemia-2560x1000.jpg?v=1718167403&width=1600.

Megaloblastic anemia results primarily from defective DNA synthesis, typically secondary to deficiencies in vitamins B12 or folate, leading to the production of incredibly large, immature RBCs (megaloblasts) in the bone marrow. In contrast, aplastic anemia is defined by the inability of the bone marrow to produce adequate blood cells due to autoimmune destruction, toxin exposure, or genetic predisposition (Iolascon et al., 2020). The identification of the conditions' features is pivotal to successful diagnosis and management, as attested by ongoing controversies surrounding the value of recognizing rare inherited anemias in extended clinical contexts (Hospital AKU et al., 2018) (Figure 6.7).

6.2.2. Causes of Aplastic Anemia

Aplastic anemia is a severe form of bone marrow failure caused by a wide range of causative agents that disrupt hematopoiesis. Drug exposure is one of the leading causes, and it is capable of inducing toxicities that lead to aplastic anemia through the damage of the HSCs in the marrow. This procedure identifies the magnitude of drug-induced hematologic syndromes, as testified by the literature that outlines many iatrogenic drugs linked to cytopenias, including aplastic anemia (Billet et al., 2009). Additionally, autoimmune illnesses can be a major contributor to this disorder, where the bodys immune system mistakenly destroys and kills its bone marrow cells. This complexity is also evident in many studies that examine the interaction between blood dyscrasias and other systemic disorders, emphasizing the interrelatedness of different hematological conditions (Suhasini et al., 2017). These complicated aetiologies are essential to understand in order to guarantee early diagnosis and effective treatment of aplastic anemia.

6.2.3. Role of Bone Marrow Failure

Bone marrow failure (BMF) plays a pivotal role in the pathogenesis of megaloblastic and aplastic anemias, underscoring the delicate balance between hematologic health and hematopoietic cell production. In megaloblastic anemia, ineffective hematopoiesis under these conditions usually arises from deficiencies of essential nutrients such as vitamin B12 and folate that elicit failure in proper RBC production and, thereby, form a build-up of immature precursors. Conversely, aplastic anemia presents because of an extensive reduction of the HSCs within the bone marrow, such as that with STAT1 gain-of-function mutations, presenting with extreme pancytopenia and hypo-cellularity of the bone marrow (Solimando et al., 2023).

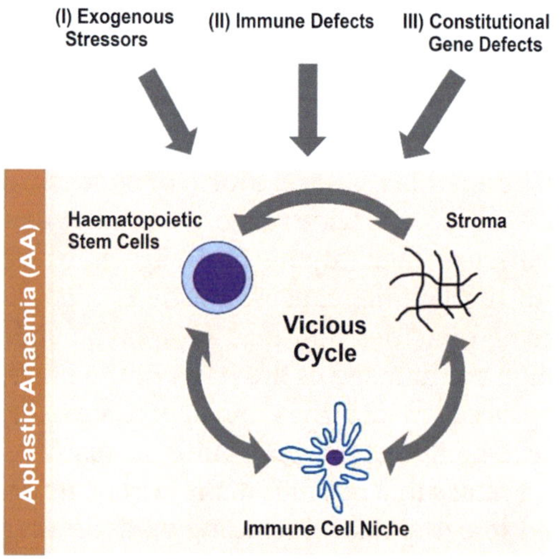

Figure 6.8. Bone marrow failure (BMF) plays a crucial role in the pathology of both megaloblastic and aplastic anemias, highlighting the intricate relationship between hematopoietic cell production and hematological health.

Source: https://www.mdpi.com/ijms/ijms-23-11765/article_deploy/html/images/ijms-23-11765-g002.png.

These conditions emphasize the necessity of understanding the etiology of BMF, as therapies like androgen therapy, although less frequent today, may still be therapeutically beneficial when traditional treatment methods are ineffective (Nassani et al., 2023). The failure of the bone marrow hence forms a key role in the diagnosis as well as treatment of these anemias (Figure 6.8).

6.2.4. Genetic Factors Contributing to Aplastic Anemia

Aplastic anemia, a severe syndrome of bone marrow failure, is most often caused by a genetic abnormality that disrupts normal hematopoiesis. Immune-related genetic mutations play a significant role in the pathogenesis of the disease. For instance, Fanconi anemia and dyskeratosis congenita, inherited disorders, exhibit a high predisposition to aplastic anemia, emphasizing the contribution of genetic abnormality to bone marrow function. Current studies have shown that these genetic mutations can increase the risk of susceptibility to harm from external factors, such as harmful chemicals or radiation, thereby exacerbating hematological decline. Moreover, the complex interaction between gene predispositions and external stressors can provoke immune-mediated mechanisms, resulting in the loss of bone marrow cells (Lahr et al., 2017), which ultimately leads to the clinical presentation of aplastic anemia. Hence, understanding these genetic mechanisms is exceptionally crucial for developing targeted therapy and proper management for the affected individuals.

6.2.5. Symptoms and Clinical Manifestations

The clinical presentation of aplastic and megaloblastic anemias often provides significant information regarding the underlying pathologies. Metabolic anemia is typically associated with a variety of symptoms like fatigue, pallor, and breathlessness, all of which are sequelae of the ineffective erythrocyte production. Additionally, there may be neurological features secondary to vitamin B12 deficiency in the form of peripheral neuropathy and mental disturbances. Among the notable features of some blood dyscrasias is eye involvement; one study highlighted that 41% of patients exhibited retinopathy, with hemorrhages within the retina being exceedingly prevalent (Suhasini et al., 2017). Aplastic anemia, on the other hand, presents with even more severe symptoms, including profound fatigue, increased susceptibility to infection, and easy bruising due to thrombocytopenia. Clinical tests, such as complete blood counts (CBCs) and reticulocyte counts, are crucial in distinguishing these anemias and initiating appropriate treatment regimens (Gupta et al., 2016) (Figure 6.9).

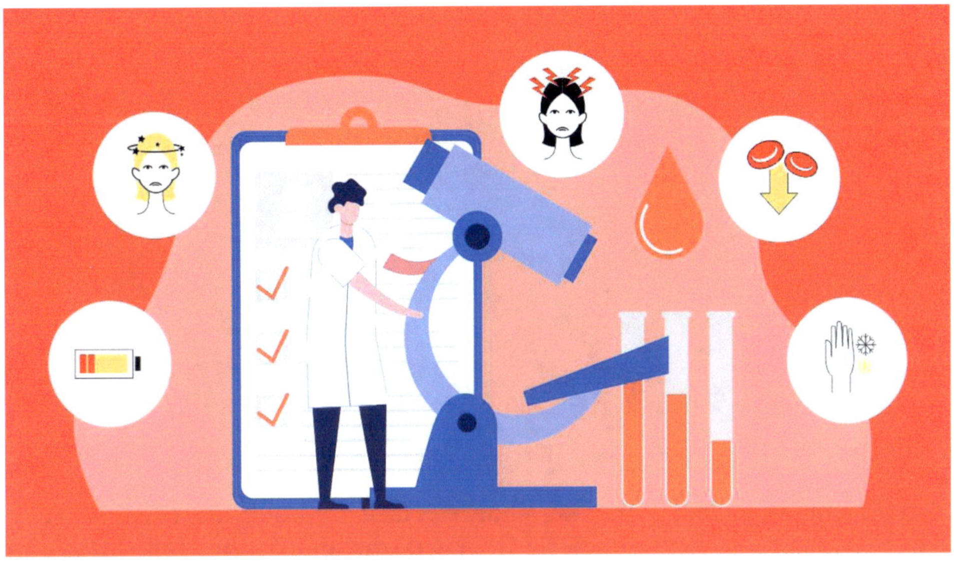

Figure 6.9. Patients suffering from megaloblastic anemia typically present with symptoms such as fatigue, pallor, and shortness of breath, which stem from the ineffective production of erythrocytes.

Source: https://blogs.fitpage.in/wp-content/uploads/2021/07/Article_1-13.jpg.

6.2.6. Diagnostic Methods

Precise diagnostic methods are crucial in differentiating megaloblastic anemia from aplastic anemia, as these two disorders could present similarly. Clinically, the test often begins with a CBC to assess hemoglobin, reticulocyte levels, and mean corpuscular volume, which are relevant to determine the existence of macrocytes for the diagnosis of megaloblastic anemia. Staining of bone marrow aspirates with reticulin is a valuable tool for differentiating among various benign hematologic disorders, including aplastic anemia (Shabbir et al., 2024). Secondly, physicians must also consider vitamin B12 and folate levels, given that their deficiency is a common cause of megaloblastic anemia (Cherepanova et al., 2024). The multifactorial etiology of these diseases places great value on thorough laboratory testing and clinical acumen, which enables accurate diagnosis and good management specifically tailored to each unique type of anemia.

6.2.7. Treatment Options

Treatment of megaloblastic and aplastic anemias depends on the underlying cause of each condition. For megaloblastic anemia, which is typically caused by a deficiency of vitamin B12 or folate, supplementing the missing nutrient is necessary. Not only is this treatment successful in alleviating symptoms, but it also helps ensure that RBCs are produced correctly, thereby preventing the long-term complications of anemia. In contrast, aplastic anemia, a bone marrow failure syndrome, can be cured with the use of immunosuppressive therapy or hematopoietic stem cell transplantation (HSCT), depending on the individual's health. The former seeks to suppress the immune process that may harm the bone marrow, whereas the latter is a more direct, though potentially dangerous, method of replacing the defective marrow with normal stem cells. Continuing education is also required for medical staff to understand these myriad treatment modalities (Kucera et al., 2014; Bogun et al., 2015) (Figure 6.10).

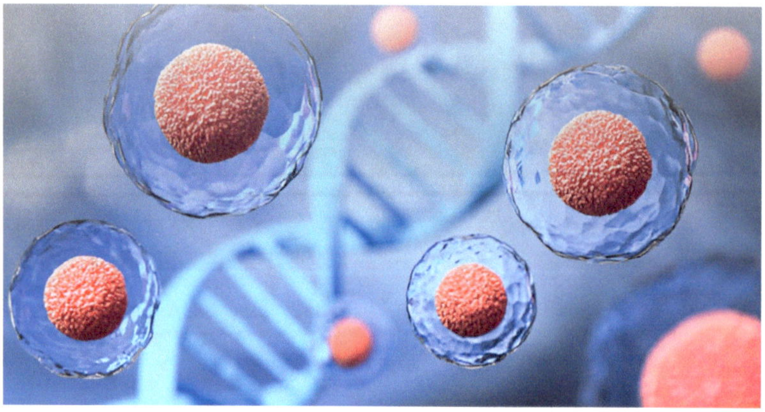

Figure 6.10. Treatment for aplastic anemia, characterized by bone marrow failure, may involve immunosuppressive therapy or hematopoietic stem cell transplantation, depending on the severity of the patient's condition.

Source: https://conquest.health/wp-content/uploads/2025/02/The-state-of-the-art-in-the-treatment-of-severe-aplastic-anemia.webp.

6.2.8. Prognosis and Long-Term Outcomes

The prognosis and long-term outcome for megaloblastic and aplastic anemias can be highly variable based on the etiology and therapeutic interventions used. Megaloblastic anemia, typically secondary to vitamin B12 or folate deficiency, normally responds well to supplementation with improvement of hematological results and minimal complications if diagnosed early. Prolonged severe deficiency will lead to irreversible neurological damage, so adequate long-term management programs must be initiated. On the other hand, aplastic anemia complicated by bone marrow failure is more serious; its prognosis will depend heavily on the age of the patient, etiology, and response to treatment protocols, such as immunosuppressive therapy or HSCT. Notably, new evidence suggests that drug-induced disease can produce a range of hematologic syndromes to complicate patient prognosis. Hence, awareness and vigilance in diagnosing and treating such syndromes are necessary to achieve optimal long-term survival and health rates (Billet et al., 2009; Iolascon et al., 2020).

6.2.9. Complications Associated with Aplastic Anemia

Aplastic anemia, which is the failure of HSCs to produce enough blood cells, is plagued by a range of complications that have serious consequences for the patient's health. Of most concern is the infection risk resulting from the dramatic reduction in WBC counts, thus compromising the immune system. Moreover, patients may suffer from severe anemia, which can lead to fatigue, pallor, and even cardiac issues, as the body is unable to supply tissues with sufficient oxygen. The relationship between substance abuse and aplastic anemia is curious in that alcohol and drug abuse worsen hematologic abnormalities, exposing the patient to more critical complications (Raka et al., 2020). This interaction highlights the complexity of managing aplastic anemia in various patient groups. In addition, as anemia is a prevalent condition among the global population, it is essential to understand the spectrum of causes of anemia, both genetic and nutritional, to develop sufficient interventions (Camila et al., 2019) (Figure 6.11).

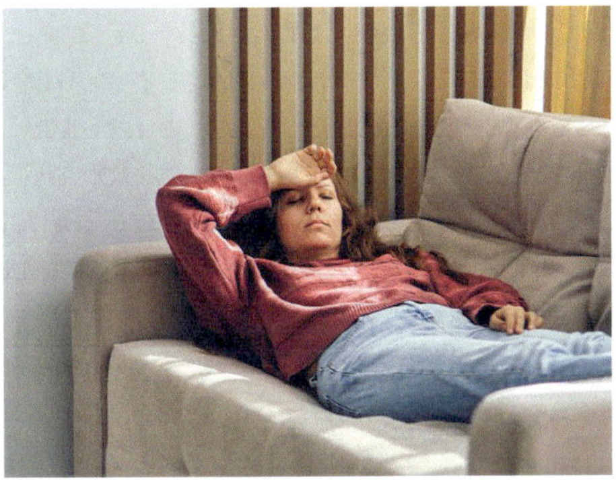

Figure 6.11. Patients may experience severe anemia, leading to fatigue, pallor, and even heart complications as the body struggles to deliver sufficient oxygen to tissues.

Source: https://media.post.rvohealth.io/wp-content/uploads/2025/03/hemorrhoids-and-anemia-thumb.jpg.

6.3. Current Research and Advances

There have been significant recent advances in the pathogenesis of megaloblastic and aplastic anemias, particularly concerning their etiology and treatment. Current research points towards the heterogeneity of these disorders, and a variety of drug-induced reasons being accountable for hematologic perturbation. As underscored by Billet et al. (2009), drug-induced syndromes can present in a range of forms, such as megaloblastic anemia and aplastic anemia, and necessitate awareness of the iatrogenic risk among healthcare providers. Furthermore, increased knowledge about the rare congenital anemias has led to more evidence on how to treat them, particularly in special populations like pregnant women. The guidelines established by (Iolascon et al., 2020) represent a crucial step in the development of standardized therapeutic interventions for patients. Cumulatively, such development represents a promise towards development of better diagnostic procedures and maximization of the results of treatment in such patients with complex anemias.

6.3.1. Recent Studies on Megaloblastic Anemia

Current studies on megaloblastic anemia have highlighted the multifaceted and complex nature of the condition, as well as its association with other hematological disorders and the impact of pharmacological interventions. The discussion on drug-induced hematologic syndromes also highlights that megaloblastic anemia can be induced by certain drugs, which produce toxicities that disrupt normal hematopoiesis, which is a reflection of the broad range of drug actions in this regard (Billet et al., 2009). Furthermore, recent research has emphasized the ocular presentation that typically precedes blood dyscrasias, such as megaloblastic anemia, and concluded that the likelihood of retinal changes can be used as diagnostic indicators of hidden hematologic pathology (Suhasini et al., 2017). This example highlights the importance of thorough patient assessment, which involves integrating both ocular and hematologic assessments within the clinic. By studying drug interactions and eye complications, more recent studies have elucidated further the complexity of megaloblastic anemia, favoring a more complete understanding of its etiology and potential therapeutic possibilities (Figure 6.12).

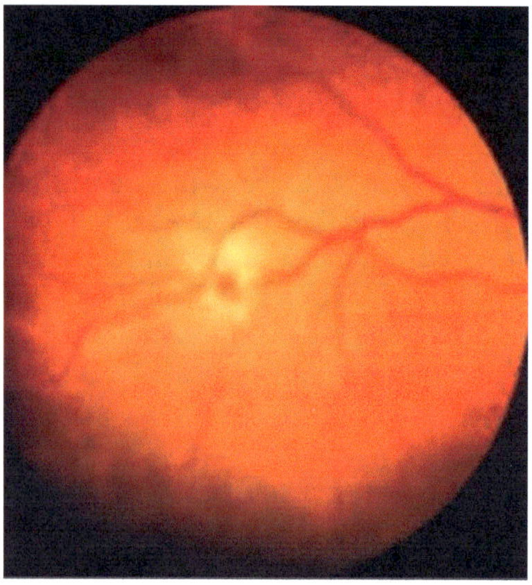

Figure 6.12. Ocular manifestations that often accompany blood dyscrasias.

Source: https://entokey.com/wp-content/uploads/2016/07/DA1-DB3-DC1-C18-FF5.gif.

6.3.2. Recent Studies on Aplastic Anemia

Recent studies on aplastic anemia have significantly advanced the knowledge of its pathophysiology and therapy. Aplastic anemia is characterized by the inability of the bone marrow to produce adequate blood cells, resulting in acute anemia, leukopenia, and thrombocytopenia. Recent studies have recognized the multifactorial etiology of the disease, which can be influenced by genetic susceptibilities, environmental exposures, and immune-mediated mechanisms. One notably important discovery was the identification of personalized biomarkers that could signal how patients would respond to treatment, allowing for the development of personalized therapeutic regimens. The literature also points to immunosuppressive therapy and HSCT as curative regimens. New evidence has demonstrated that the pathogenesis of anemia, including aplastic anemia, varies significantly within and between populations and geographical regions, with an increasing need for personalized intervention techniques (Hakami, 2021; Camila et al., 2019). These findings open the door for ensuing research in attempting to improve patient outcomes in aplastic anemia victims

6.3.3. Advances in Diagnostic Techniques

New diagnostic tools in the past few years have significantly enhanced the diagnosis and management of aplastic and megaloblastic anemias. With the inclusion of molecular genetics and high-throughput sequencing technologies, clinicians are currently able to diagnose inherited anemia forms more accurately, which in the past were difficult to separate from standard types. For instance, it is now achievable with hematology-guided genetic panels to detect rare genetic mutations with conditions like Diamond-Blackfan Anemia and CDAs. In addition, techniques such as liquid biopsy and sophisticated imaging modalities provide valuable information regarding the bone marrow microenvironment, which aids in the evaluation of aplastic anemia and myelodysplastic syndromes. Moreover, the development of evidence- and consensus-based guidelines promotes standardized approaches in diagnostic processes to ensure that clinicians are adequately trained in managing these conditions, particularly in complex cases with maternal and fetal outcomes (Hospital AKU et al., 2018; Iolascon et al., 2020). The convergence of these innovations leads to a deeper understanding of anemia and its diverse manifestations (Figure 6.13).

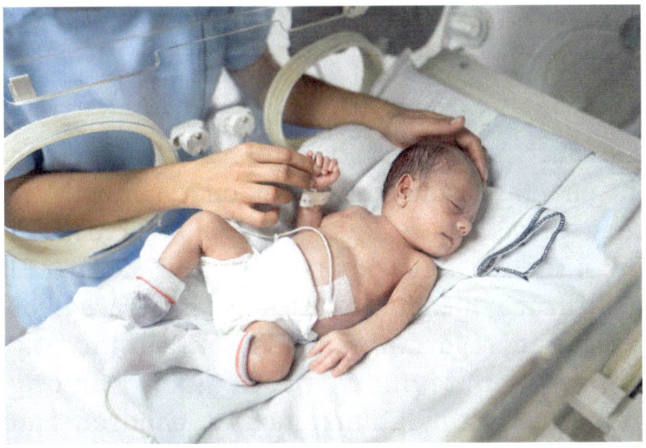

Figure 6.13. Diamond-blackfan anemia.

Source: https://www.health.com/thmb/JqT17m7pBtjHEQxgvwK-CtmBL4I=/7952x0/filters:no_upscale():max_bytes(150000):strip_icc()/diamondblackfananemia-GettyImages-956193216-69f3e97392b841719870e09a0d442b91.jpg.

6.3.4. Innovations in Treatment Options

Advances in the treatment of megaloblastic and aplastic anemia have revolutionized patient management, significantly improving clinical outcomes. For instance, the use of micronutrient-guided strategies indicates a trend toward more tailored treatment approaches, enabling clinicians to address specific nutritional deficiencies underlying anemia. Such sophisticated practice is in alignment with emerging research that is indicative of the fact that micronutrient deficiencies will negatively impact health, particularly within restricted resource environments like Ghana, where dietary practice has been evolving to counteract the same (Qubty et al., 2022). Coupled with this, sophisticated models of retrieving relevant health information have enhanced patient education by informing patients of the measures required for management, thereby improving self-management processes (Russell et al., 2020). These advances not only improve treatment but also equip patients with tools to better understand and manage their diseases, marking a significant leap forward in the battle against such anemia.

6.3.5. Genetic Research and Implications

The significance of genetic discoveries in the pathogenesis of megaloblastic and aplastic anemias is enormous, as they provide the causative mechanisms that lead to these disorders. Current developments in genetic profiling have provided insights into how mutations and deficiencies in specific genes, particularly those involved in DNA metabolism, are linked to the pathogenesis of megaloblastic anemia.

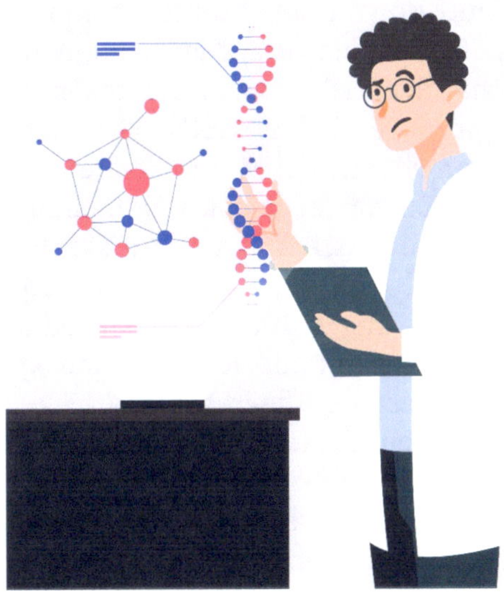

Figure 6.14. Advancements in genetic profiling have revealed how mutations and deficiencies in specific genes, such as those involved in DNA metabolism, are linked to the pathogenesis of megaloblastic anemia.

Source: https://sequencing.com/sites/default/files/wysiwyg/283026/what_diseases_can_be_detected_through_genetic_testing.jpg.

For instance, the role of folate and vitamin B12 metabolism is critical because deficiency leads to ineffective erythropoiesis and megaloblastic change in RBCs (To et al., 2018). Aplastic anemia, on the other hand, is more likely to be caused by genetic predisposition, which disrupts hematopoiesis normally, and can be aggravated by environmental or drug exposure. Intriguingly, drugs can induce a range of hematologic syndromes, including aplastic anemia and megaloblastic anemia, through different mechanisms (Billet et al., 2009). Thus, genetic data not only explain the pathogenesis of these anemias but also enable us to make informed decisions about therapeutic intervention and prevention (Figure 6.14).

6.3.6. Role of Nutrition in Prevention

Adequate nutrition is a significantelement in the avoidance of megaloblastic and aplastic anemias, diseases that seriously complicate the body's ability to produce healthy RBCs. The dietary deficiency of vitamins B12 and folate is the principal reason for megaloblastic anemia, as these vitamins are essential for DNA synthesis and proper cell division. Supplementation of these vitamins along with a well-balanced diet that includes whole grains, legumes, and leafy greens can effectively decrease the risk for this type of anemia. Moreover, an awareness of nutritional imbalances plays an essential role in the treatment of aplastic anemia, where the bone marrow fails to produce sufficient blood cells.

As observed, nutritional interventions not only enhance the general well-being but also address the complexities in connection with anemia etiology (Camila et al., 2019; Cotoraci et al., 2021). By addressing nutrition as a form of prevention, we can encourage better outcomes and reduce the prevalence of such disabling diseases.

6.3.7. Patient Education and Awareness

Effective education and sensitization of the patient are critical pillars in managing megaloblastic and aplastic anemias, recognizing that these conditions are primarily caused by nutritional deficiencies and inadequate healthcare measures. Patient and caregiver education regarding anemia can significantly improve outcomes, particularly among vulnerable populations such as children and pregnant women. Evidence suggests that anemia has a significant impact on physical and cognitive growth in infants, particularly in cases of iron deficiency, underscoring the need for targeted educational campaigns (Thakur et al., 2024).

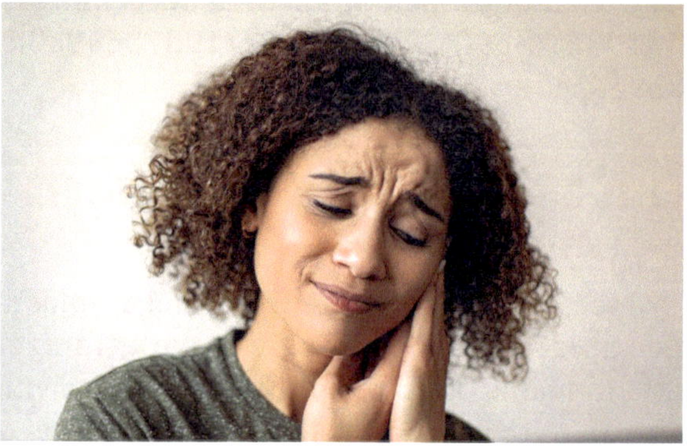

Figure 6.15. Effective patient education and awareness are crucial components in managing megaloblastic and aplastic anemias, as these conditions often arise from nutritional deficiencies and lack of appropriate healthcare practices.

Source: https://cdn-prod.medicalnewstoday.com/content/images/articles/188/188770/a-woman-experiencing-tinnitus-due-to-nutritional-deficiency-anemia.jpg.

Furthermore, studies in Enugu, Nigeria, indicated inadequate practices and limited knowledge regarding childhood anemia among children's mothers, showing that even where there is awareness, it may not be translated to prevention action (Akubueze et al., 2023).

Enhancing patient education programs regarding food needs, exclusive breastfeeding, and hygiene habits could lead to a positive shift in health behavior, ultimately decreasing the incidence of these anemias (Figure 6.15).

6.3.8. Future Directions in Research

With an increasingly better understanding of aplastic and megaloblastic anemias, upcoming studies must concentrate on multidimensional approaches that connect nutritional, genetic, and environmental factors. For instance, while decreased serum folate levels have been used extensively as a marker for folate deficiency, studies highlight that decreased levels can be misleading in cases of vitamin B12 deficiency or hemolytic diseases, particularly in impoverished regions, leading to an underestimation of tissue folate deficiency (Antony et al., 2017). Thus, there is a requirement to enhance diagnostic criteria for identifying at-risk populations more precisely. Furthermore, the growing burden of hemolytic anemia in middle- and low-income countries underscores the need for simpler examination panels that can efficiently classify underlying causes, as evidenced by recent literature demonstrating the efficacy of simple examinations in detecting various types of hemolysis (Vishnuprathap et al., 2016). Combined, these advancements give insight into the path towards targeted interventions and health policies for addressing the complexities of these anemias.

6.3.9. Collaboration Between Healthcare Providers

Practical multidisciplinary cooperation among health practitioners is essential in the treatment of chronic diseases such as megaloblastic and aplastic anemias. Interdisciplinary management of these conditions requires the integration of hematologists, primary care physicians, and expert nurses to ensure effective patient management. Because diagnostic mistakes are perilous, the implementation of computerized diagnostic decision support systems could enhance clinical judgment and reduce diagnostic errors, benefiting differential diagnosis and ultimately improving treatment outcomes (Bridges et al., 2022). Additionally, the establishment of a collaborative environment enables healthcare professionals to collaborate, utilizing one another's expertise to interpret the complexity involved in such anemias. Through facilitated open communication and collaboration, providers can formulate specialized treatment plans that target the complex issues of patients. Ultimately, such a partnership not only enhances diagnostic precision but also enables more effective control of megaloblastic and aplastic anemias, resulting in improved patient outcomes and experiences (Figure 6.16).

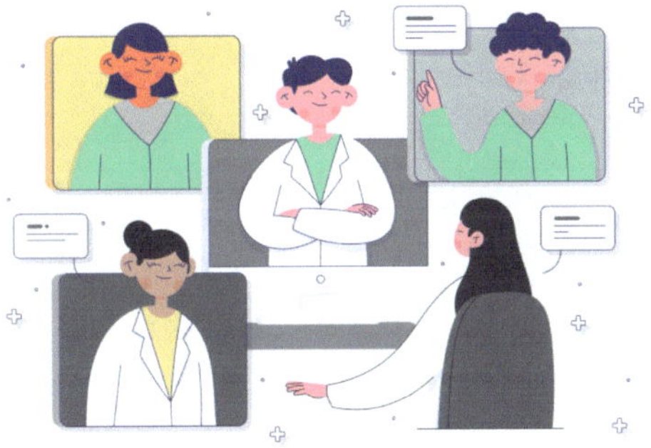

Figure 6.16. Fostering a collaborative environment enables healthcare professionals to engage in shared problem-solving, drawing on each other's expertise to navigate the intricacies of these anemias.

Source: https://www.culturemonkey.io/employee-engagement/content/images/2024/04/7-common-challenges-for-collaboration-in-health-care.png.

A CLOSER LOOK

CONGENITAL DYSERYTHROPOIETIC ANEMIAS (CDAS)

Congenital Dyserythropoietic Anemias (CDAs) are a group of rare genetic anemias due to ineffective erythropoiesis and dysplastic development of the RBC precursors within the bone marrow. It causes chronic anemia, typically coupled with hepatosplenomegaly, jaundice, and iron overload even without the use of routine blood transfusions.

CDAs are categorized into several forms (CDA I, II, III, etc.), based on genetic mutations and certain characteristics visible under the microscope in bone marrow tissue. CDA II, the most frequent of these, for example, is a result of mutations in the SEC23B gene.

Diagnosis involves blood tests, bone marrow examination, and genetic testing. Treatment varies depending on severity and type but may include blood transfusions, iron chelation therapy, and in some cases, BMT. Regular monitoring is essential to manage complications such as iron overload and organ damage.

SUMMARY

The studies of megaloblastic and aplastic anemias provide critical data regarding their clinical presentation and etiologic determinants, above all, their role in pancytopenia. As is clear from more recent studies, megaloblastic anemia has been demonstrated to be a significant etiology of the hematologic condition, with findings indicating its prevalence of 18.7% to 35% among various populations (Singh et al., 2017; Gamit et al., 2017). These facts underscore the importance of increasing clinician awareness of the prevalence of megaloblastic anemia, particularly in regions where deficiencies are prevalent. In addition, the similarity between megaloblastic and aplastic anemias underscores the need for comprehensive diagnostic examinations, such as bone marrow tests, to account for the complexity of these conditions. By gaining a better understanding of their etiology and occurrence, healthcare providers can more effectively tailor treatment plans and improve patient outcomes among affected groups.

Briefly, the key points about megaloblastic and aplastic anemias highlight the multifactorial and complex nature of these two diseases. Megaloblastic anemia is typically characterized by abnormal DNA synthesis, most commonly due to deficiency of vitamin B12 or folate, leading to the production of immature but oversized RBCs. In contrast, aplastic anemia refers to failure of the HSCs such that all forms of blood cells are lacking and this may result from genetic reasons or insult. These various though related disorders should be well understood because treatment strategies are quite different; megaloblastic anemia will be reversed with vitamin replacement and aplastic anemia may demand immunosuppression or stem cell transplant. This fine detail highlights the importance of proper diagnostic procedures and corresponding therapeutic interventions in managing these hematological disorders (Field et al., 1958; Ezzibdeh et al., 2016).

REFERENCES

1. Aga Khan University Hospital, Karachi. (2018). LABRAD: Vol 44, Issue 2–September 2018. https://core.ac.uk/download/286085026.pdf (accessed on 12th June 2025).
2. Khan, S. P., Geelani, S., Akhter, S., Bhat, S., Hussain, S., Manzoor, F., Rasool, J., & Khan, F. P. (2018). Bone marrow aspiration in haematological disorders: study at a tertiary care centre. International Journal of Research in Medical Sciences, 6(7), 2361. https://doi.org/10.18203/2320-6012.ijrms20182817Akubueze, D., & Omale, J. J. (2023). Knowledge, attitude and practices of mothers attending primary healthcare facilities in South-east Nigeria towards prevention of childhood anemia. International Journal of Innovative Research and Development. https://doi.org/10.24940/ijird/2023/v12/i9/sep23011 (accessed on 12th June 2025).
3. Anem, V., Atla, B. L., & Dasari, A. (2017). Prospective study of bone marrow in hematological disorders. https://core.ac.uk/download/539912932.pdf (accessed on 12th June 2025).
4. Antony, A. C. (2017). Evidence for potential underestimation of clinical folate deficiency in resource-limited countries using blood tests. https://core.ac.uk/download/157829010.pdf (accessed on 12th June 2025).
5. Ayodele, O. J. (2017). Megaloblastic anemia. https://core.ac.uk/download/322432314.pdf (accessed on 12th June 2025).
6. Billet, S. N., Chmielewski, L., & Mintzer, D. M. (2009). Drug-induced hematologic syndromes. https://core.ac.uk/download/pdf/8349513.pdf (accessed on 12th June 2025).
7. Bogun, L., Bychkova, O., Lysenko, N., Makienko, I., et al. (2015). Anemias. https://core.ac.uk/download/46595382.pdf (accessed on 12th June 2025).
8. Bolaños-Meade, J., Jacobsohn, D., Anders, V., Higman, M., Chen, A. R., Phelps, M., & Vogelsang, G. (2005). Pentostatin in steroid-refractory chronic graft-versus-host disease. Blood, 106, 1805–1805. https://www.semanticscholar.org/paper/714b837b3519caecab54bad2f40b8a69a88538c5 (accessed on 12th June 2025).
9. Bridges, J. (2022). Evaluation, validation & implementation of a computerized diagnostic decision support system in primary practice. https://core.ac.uk/download/572713498.pdf (accessed on 12th June 2025).
10. Bugti, S. (2018). Serum cobalamin levels and red blood cell morphology among celiac disease patients. https://core.ac.uk/download/551320455.pdf (accessed on 12th June 2025).
11. Chaparro, C. M., & Suchdev, P. S. (2019). Anemia epidemiology, pathophysiology, and etiology in low- and middle-income countries. Annals of the New York Academy of Sciences, 1450, 15–31. https://doi.org/10.1111/nyas.14092 (accessed on 12th June 2025).
12. Cherepanova, V. V., Sidnev, G. V., Konyshkina, T. M., Borisov, V. I., & Moiseenko, N. (2024). Diagnostic errors and treatment of anemia caused by vitamin B12 deficiency. Onomatology. https://www.semanticscholar.org/paper/516f1474bca287d23588626a6e5516a16b31d8cd (accessed on 12th June 2025).
13. Cotoraci, C., Ciceu, A., Sasu, A., & Hermenean, A. (2021). Natural antioxidants in anemia treatment. International Journal of Molecular Sciences, 22, 1883–1883. https://doi.org/10.3390/ijms22041883 (accessed on 12th June 2025).

14. Ezzibdeh, R. (2016). Biochemical characterization of C15ORF41: A novel nuclease. https://core.ac.uk/download/346541235.pdf (accessed on 12th June 2025).

15. Field, M. (1958). Hemosiderosis and hemochromatosis: A study of the pathophysiology of iron overload. https://open.bu.edu/bitstream/2144/32849/1/Field_Michael_1958_web.pdf (accessed on 12th June 2025).

16. Fisher, K. D., & Talbot, J. M. (2025). Research opportunities in loss of red blood cell mass in space flight. https://core.ac.uk/download/pdf/42845286.pdf (accessed on 12th June 2025).

17. Fisher, M. (2007). Anemia in PEDs. https://core.ac.uk/download/62771891.pdf (accessed on 12th June 2025).

18. Gambale, A., Iolascon, A., Andolfo, I., & Russo, R. (2015). Diagnosis and management of congenital dyserythropoietic anemias. Expert Review of Hematology, 9, 283–296. https://doi.org/10.1586/17474086.2016.1131608 (accessed on 12th June 2025).

19. Gamit, B., Gheewala, S., Patel, R. D., Shah, H., et al. (2017). Bone marrow examination in cases of pancytopenia. https://core.ac.uk/download/543134922.pdf (accessed on 12th June 2025).

20. Gupta, N., Premkumar, M., Singh, T., Velpandian, M., et al. (2012). Cobalamin and folic acid status in relation to the etiopathogenesis of pancytopenia in adults at a tertiary care center in North India. https://core.ac.uk/download/pdf/8707649.pdf (accessed on 12th June 2025).

21. Gupta, V., Kannan, A., Rai, M., Tilak, V., et al. (2016). Evaluation of clinical, biochemical and hematological parameters in macrocytic anemia. https://core.ac.uk/download/539913903.pdf (accessed on 12th June 2025).

22. Hakami, T. (2021). Neuropharmacology of antiseizure drugs. Neuropsychopharmacology Reports, 41, 336–351. https://doi.org/10.1002/npr2.12196 (accessed on 12th June 2025).

23. Imchen, N. (2019). Pancytopenia: Clinical and etiological profile in tertiary care hospital. https://core.ac.uk/download/235670868.pdf (accessed on 12th June 2025).

24. Iolascon, A., Taher, A. T., Gulbis, B., Matar, C. F., Bencaiova, G. A., Forni, G., Tamary, H., et al. (2020). Recommendations for pregnancy in rare inherited anemias. https://core.ac.uk/download/373375214.pdf (accessed on 12th June 2025).

25. Jain, R., George, A. A. B., & Narnoli, S. (2020). Hematological changes in alcohol and substance use disorders–An overview. International Archives of Substance Abuse and Rehabilitation, 2. https://doi.org/10.23937/2690-263x/1710006 (accessed on 12th June 2025).

26. Kelk, P., Fasth, A., Holgerson, P. L., & Sjöström, M. (2023). Successful complete oral rehabilitation of a patient with osteopetrosis with extensive pre-treatments, bone grafts, dental implants and fixed bridges: A multidisciplinary case report. BMC Oral Health, 23. https://www.semanticscholar.org/paper/2fada4cc099814f487e2e3899a27d884cc0480b1 (accessed on 12th June 2025).

27. Kucera, A., Smith, B., & Tsu, L. V. (2014). Anemia and the role of the pharmacist. https://core.ac.uk/download/215741022.pdf (accessed on 12th June 2025).

28. Lahr, M. M., & Rivera, F. (2017). New evidence suggesting a dissociated etiology for cribra orbitalia and porotic hyperostosis. https://core.ac.uk/download/84588577.pdf (accessed on 12th June 2025).

29. Mansuri, B., & Thekdi, K. P. (2017). A prospective study among cases of the pancytopenia on the basis of clinic-hematological analysis and bone marrow aspiration. https://core.ac.uk/download/539910417.pdf (accessed on 12th June 2025).

30. Muneer, M. (2022). To determine the common causes leading to pancytopenia in patients presenting to tertiary care hospital, Lahore. Pakistan Journal of Medical & Health Sciences, 16, 283–285. https://doi.org/10.53350/pjmhs22163283 (accessed on 12th June 2025).

31. Nandhini, J. G. (2016). A study of the etiology, contributory factors and correlation of the clinical and laboratory profiles of anemia in elderly patients presenting at a tertiary hospital in rural South India. https://core.ac.uk/download/235655176.pdf (accessed on 12th June 2025).

32. Nassani, M., Fakih, R., Passweg, J., Cesaro, S., Alzahrani, H., Alahmari, A., Bonfim, C., et al. (2023). The role of androgen therapy in acquired aplastic anemia and other bone marrow failure syndromes. Frontiers in Oncology, 13. https://www.semanticscholar.org/paper/ef2e619886e43f7865ef91f12f0ecdf6db7e41f8 (accessed on 12th June 2025).

33. Olcay, L., & Yetgin, S. (2016). Disorders mimicking myelodysplastic syndrome and difficulties in its diagnosis. https://core.ac.uk/download/322427721.pdf (accessed on 12th June 2025).

34. Prakash, M. M. (2018). Clinic-hematological study in pancytopenia patients presenting to tertiary care hospital. https://core.ac.uk/download/235668815.pdf (accessed on 12th June 2025).

35. Qubty, L. A. (2022). A two-day virtual workshop on the micronutrient-directed nutrition-focused physical exam for Ghanaian nutrition professionals: Examining perceived self-efficacy and innovation. https://core.ac.uk/download/541292941.pdf (accessed on 12th June 2025).

36. Regis, M. D. (2017). Pancytopenia: A clinico-haematological evaluation and correlation with bone marrow examination. https://core.ac.uk/download/327695851.pdf (accessed on 12th June 2025).

37. Russell, M. (2020). Analysis of information value chains for gout self-care management. https://core.ac.uk/download/346141354.pdf (accessed on 12th June 2025).

38. Safiri, S., Kolahi, A. A., Noori, M., Nejadghaderi, S. A., Karamzad, N., Bragazzi, N. L., Sullman, M. J. M., et al. (2021). Burden of anemia and its underlying causes in 204 countries and territories, 1990–2019: Results from the Global Burden of Disease Study 2019. Journal of Hematology & Oncology, 14. https://doi.org/10.1186/s13045-021-01202-2 (accessed on 12th June 2025).

39. Shabbir, Y., Hameed, A., Chaudhry, R., Ahmad, Q. A., Waseem, U., & Hameed, S. (2024). Diagnostic significance and association of reticulin fibrosis in benign hematologic disorders. Pakistan Journal of Health Sciences. https://www.semanticscholar.org/paper/ec61dbbe329b14f777e6e56aa140608db9a09c59 (accessed on 12th June 2025).

40. Singh, S. P., Singh, M., & Singh, V. (2017). Pancytopenia: Etiologies and manifestation in eastern India. https://core.ac.uk/download/539911736.pdf (accessed on 12th June 2025).

41. Solimando, A. G., Desantis, V., Palumbo, C., Marasco, C., Pappagallo, F., Montagnani, M., Ingravallo, G., et al. (2023). STAT1 overexpression triggers aplastic anemia: A pilot study unravelling novel pathogenetic insights in bone marrow failure. Clinical and Experimental Medicine, 23, 2687–2694. https://www.semanticscholar.org/paper/13f635d61c9da0d3b27feb805ebfdb79b0d4a217 (accessed on 12th June 2025).

42. Strobbe, S., & Van Der Straeten, D. (2018). Toward eradication of B-vitamin deficiencies: Considerations for crop biofortification. https://core.ac.uk/download/158346323.pdf (accessed on 12th June 2025).

43. Suhasini, S. (2017). Ocular manifestations of blood dyscrasias. https://core.ac.uk/download/288215952.pdf (accessed on 12th June 2025).

44. Thakur, H., Tiwari, A. K., Kumar, A., Mishra, P. K., & Kumar, U. (2024). Impact of anemia in development of infants: A review. Acta Scientific Microbiology. https://doi.org/10.31080/asmi.2024.07.1345 (accessed on 12th June 2025).

45. To, M., Villatoro, V., et al. (2018). A Laboratory Guide to Clinical Hematology. https://core.ac.uk/download/622361655.pdf (accessed on 12th June 2025).

46. Vishnuprathap, D. (2016). Typing of hemolytic anemias: Role of basic diagnostic screening panel. https://core.ac.uk/download/235668092.pdf (accessed on 12th June 2025).

47. Wankhede, N., & Rajput, Y. (2017). A rare case report: Pregnancy with pancytopenia. https://core.ac.uk/download/543136497.pdf (accessed on 12th June 2025).

48. Wright, B. N. (2014). Iron nutriture following Roux-en-Y gastric bypass surgery. https://core.ac.uk/download/77955417.pdf (accessed on 12th June 2025).

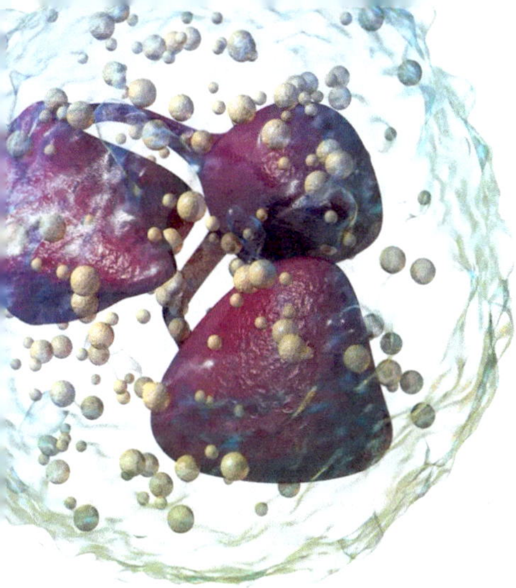

Chapter 7

DISORDERS OF LEUKOCYTES

Contents

Introduction....151
7.1. Types of Leukocytes....152
7.2. Common Disorders of Leukocytes....156
7.3. Diagnosis of Leukocyte Disorders....159
7.4. Treatment and Management of Leukocyte Disorders....163
Summary....170
References....171

Introduction

The study of leukocyte disorders is crucial, as white blood cells (WBCs) play a vital role in the immune system, which safeguards the body against infection and disease. Together, they constitute part of the innate and adaptive immunity, with neutrophils, lymphocytes, and monocytes being the various types with varied roles in immune surveillance and response. Leukocyte disorders can manifest as either a decreased immune response, such as leukopenia, or hyperactivity, including leukemias and autoimmune disorders. Understanding these disorders requires a balanced approach of knowing the cellular and molecular mechanisms but also considering the greater issues of patient well-being and treatment outcome. The clinical and pathological consequences of such disorders are better understood through enhanced research techniques, which also highlight the need for targeted treatment and interventions aimed at restoring immunological homeostasis (Voet et al., 2019; Daniel et al., 2020).

7.1. Types of Leukocytes

The immune system is supported by various types of leukocytes that perform functions essential for maintaining health and preventing disorders. Leukocytes are primarily categorized as agranulocytes and granulocytes. Lymphocytes, which play a vital role in adaptive immunity and consist of T cells and B cells, and monocytes, which mature , are essential for phagocytosis and antigen presentation, and are examples of agranulocytes. Granulocytes, on the other hand, comprise neutrophils, eosinophils, and basophils that have roles in the innate immune response. Neutrophils are particularly significant in neutralizing infections caused by bacteria and inflammation, while eosinophils play a role in neutralizing parasitic infections and allergic responses. Leukocyte diversity contributes to the significance of all leukocytes in immune function. Current research has revealed the implications of leukocyte behavior-modulating genetic variants, which have intricate mechanisms that can influence susceptibility to infection and inflammatory diseases (Cifuentes et al., 2024). Moreover, technological advancements such as PGD+HLA typing reveal the intersection of technology and immune disease (Eker et al., 2025) (Figure 7.1).

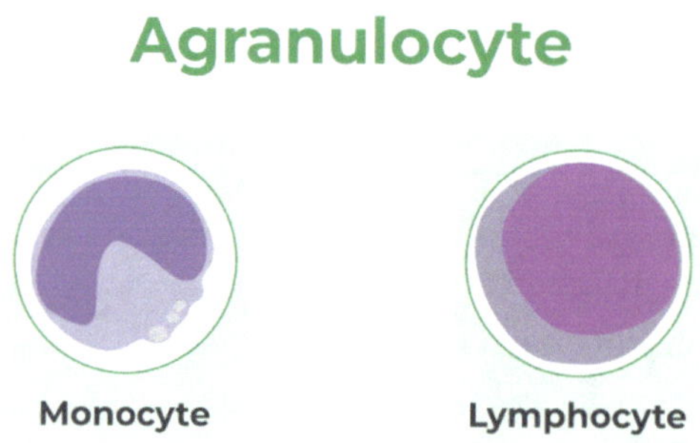

Figure 7.1. Agranulocytes.

Source: https://media.geeksforgeeks.org/wp-content/uploads/20230227173645/Agranulocyte.png.

7.1.1. Overview of Leukocyte Classification

In the intricate area of immunology, leukocyte categorization is a milestone in comprehending various disorders related to these essential WBCs. Leukocytes are generally classified into two main categories: granulocytes and agranulocytes, which comprise various types of cells that play significant roles in immune responses. Granulocytes, which include neutrophils, eosinophils, and basophils, are characterized by the presence of cytoplasmic granules that are responsible for inflammation and allergic responses. Agranulocytes contain an increase in lymphocytes and monocytes, which are fundamental to adaptive immunity and chronic inflammation. The emergence of advanced classification systems, the upcoming 5th edition of the World Health Organization (WHO) Classification of Hematolymphoid Tumors, emphasizes complex appreciation of leukocyte disorders by highlighting therapeutic and prognostic biomarkers within a genetically enlightened framework (Joseph et al., 2022). Determining these groups can assist in the diagnosis and development of targeted treatment for leukocyte-related disorders, which remain pertinent in clinical practice (Daniel et al., 2020).

7.1.2. Neutrophils: Function and Significance

Neutrophils are essential components of the body's immune system, primarily responsible for detecting and eliminating invading pathogens. Renowned for its rapid response to infection, neutrophilic granulocytes are the most prevalent type of leukocytes, constituting approximately 60-70% of all circulating WBCs. Their significance is particularly underscored in clinical settings, where abnormalities such as elevated neutrophil counts can indicate systemic inflammation, as evidenced in studies comparing diseased and healthy cows, where lame cows displayed a higher neutrophil percentage and increased stress markers, indicating a physiological response to infection (Aggarwal et al., 2014).

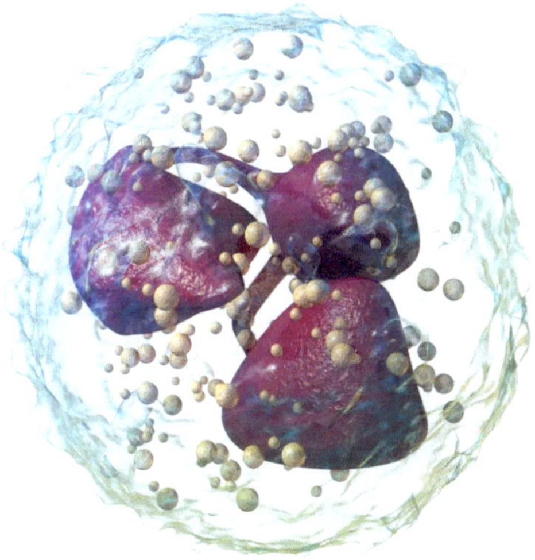

Figure 7.2. Neutrophils serve as essential components of the immune system, primarily tasked with identifying and eliminating pathogens.

Source: https://biologynotesonline.com/wp-content/uploads/2024/04/image-1696.png.

Furthermore, therapies such as the provision of granulocyte-colony stimulating factor have been demonstrated to have the capability to significantly elevate circulating numbers of neutrophils, therefore potentially to enhance health outcomes during periods of stress, such as at calving (Pascottini et al., 2018). This underlines the role of neutrophils not only in immediate immune defense but also in broad systemic effects on health (Figure 7.2).

7.1.3. Lymphocytes: Types and Roles

Lymphocytes, the central component of the immune system, come in three broad categories: B cells, T cells, and natural killer (NK) cells, each playing a distinct role in immune responses. B cells are predominantly specialized in producing antibodies that kill pathogens, while T cells are composed of helper T cells, which coordinate immune responses, and cytotoxic T cells, which kill infected cells. NK cells, on the other hand, target and kill virally infected cells or cancer cells without prior sensitization. The proper functioning of these lymphocytes is especially crucial in understanding leukocyte disorders, as their dysregulation may be responsible for autoimmune diseases, immunodeficiency, or neoplasia. For instance, the complex interaction between innate and adaptive immunity, through mechanisms like the discharge of cytokines, is critical in infections like multiple sclerosis, where inflammatory responses lead to neurological damage, indicating the relevance of lymphocytes in such cases (Hristova et al., 2015; Adams et al., 2018).

7.1.4. Monocytes: Characteristics and Functions

Monocytes, being a part of the leukocyte lineage, possess distinctive characteristics and varied roles that influence many disorders, including inflammatory and autoimmune diseases. Originating from the bone marrow, these large, phagocytic mononuclear cells are also capable of further differentiation into dendritic cells or macrophages, and thus play a crucial role in innate immunity. Functional-wise, monocytes can respond rapidly to infection or tissue injury by the production of pro-inflammatory cytokines, which also regulate adaptive immunity through the activation of T cells and B cells (Vivek, 2024). Dysregulation of monocyte function in pathological conditions has the potential to exacerbate diseases such as Non-specific Orbital Inflammation (NSOI), as they are implicated in leukocyte-mediated immunity and the coordination of immune cell infiltration into inflamed tissues (Wu et al., 2024). Understanding the properties and functions of monocytes is crucial for interpreting the complications of leukocyte disorders (Figure 7.3).

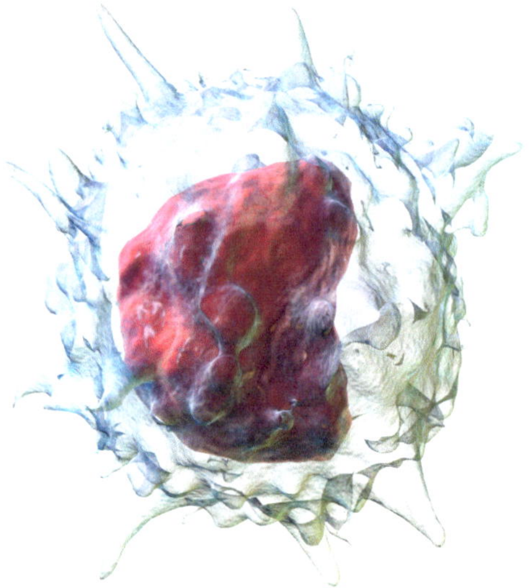

Figure 7.3. Monocytes, a critical component of the leukocyte family, exhibit unique characteristics and multifaceted functions that influence various disorders, including inflammatory and autoimmune diseases.

Source: https://upload.wikimedia.org/wikipedia/commons/8/84/Blausen_0649_Monocyte_%28crop%29.pngs.

7.1.5. Eosinophils: Role in Allergic Reactions

In allergic reactions, eosinophils are key effectors and mediators that play crucial roles in the pathophysiology of numerous hypersensitivity reactions. The activation and accumulation of cells in tissues lead to the production of pro-inflammatory mediators, such as cytokines, chemokines, and cytotoxic granules, which have the ability to augment tissue damage and contribute to the symptomatic manifestations of asthma and rhinitis. Notably, eosinophils also interact with other immune cells in partnership through adhesion molecules to facilitate their migration into infected tissue and promote the inflammatory process (Bruce, 2020). This is essential for eosinophil recruitment in allergic disease, thereby emphasizing their bivalent nature as defenders against parasitic infections as well as participants in allergic disease. Dysregulation of eosinophilic activity can potentially lead to severe allergic reactions, highlighting their critical role in leukocyte disorders (Qin et al., 2020).

7.1.6. Basophils: Functions in Inflammation

Basophils play a specialized role in the inflammatory response, a critical process in the majority of leukocyte disorders, particularly during allergic reactions and inflammation. As effector cells, basophils release chemicals such as histamine and heparin, which facilitate vascular permeability and the accumulation of other immune cells at the site of inflammation. This is vital in triggering and sustaining inflammatory signals, as revealed through basophil interactions with cytokines and adhesion molecules that enhance their migratory activity (Bruce, 2020). Furthermore, basophils also participate in the regulation of Th2 responses through the release of cytokines, such as IL-4, which can exacerbate allergy disorders, presenting them as bivalent effectors of both protective immunity and hypersensitivity (Zhao et al., 2021). Understanding these functions sheds light on the complex interaction between innate and adaptive immunity, with a focus on the significance of basophils in the disease pathology of leukocyte-associated diseases (Figure 7.4).

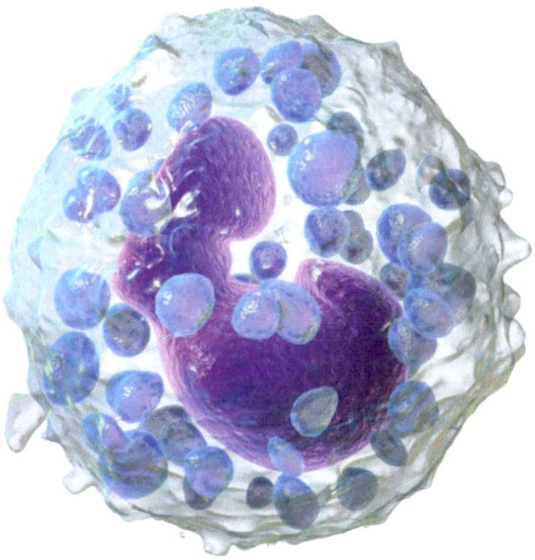

Figure 7.4. Basophils.

Source: https://upload.wikimedia.org/wikipedia/commons/f/fe/Blausen_0077_Basophil_%28crop%29.png.

7.1.7. Natural Killer Cells: Importance in Immune Response

NK cells play a crucial role in the immune response because they function as the first line of defense against viruses and tumor cells, thereby maintaining general immune homeostasis. NK cells possess the innate capacity to recognize and kill infected cells without prior sensitization, making them unique among all other leukocytes, such as T cells. Their activation is strongly linked to the dynamic nature of the decidual immune microenvironment, particularly during pregnancy, where decidual NK cells contribute to the remodeling of uteroplacental spiral arteries that is essential to successful implantation and placentation (Staff et al., 2020). NK cell dysfunction or deficiency can result in a variety of disorders with adverse consequences such as preeclampsia and fetal growth restriction (Tilg et al., 2020). It is therefore essential to investigate the mechanisms that govern NK cell function for predicting immune disorders and optimizing therapeutic approaches in reproductive medicine and cancer immunotherapy.

7.1.8. Dendritic Cells: Role in Antigen Presentation

Within the intricate immune network, dendritic cells (DCs) play a pivotal role in antigen presentation, bridging innate and adaptive immunity. These professional antigen-presenting cells are highly efficient in capturing, processing, and presenting antigens to T cells, thereby initiating adaptive immune responses that are indispensable against infections and tumors.

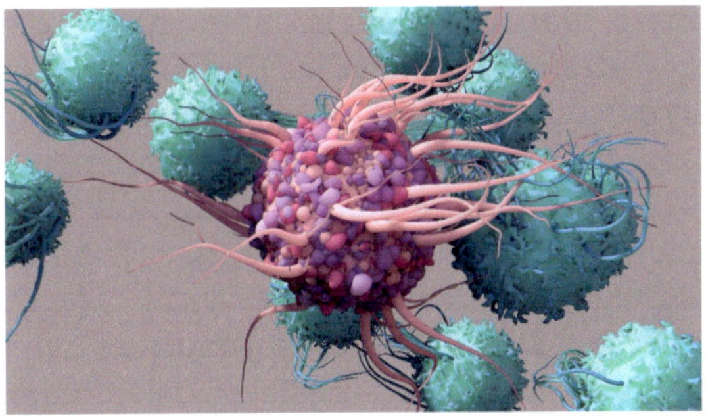

Figure 7.5. Dendritic cells.

Source: https://d2jx2rerrg6sh3.cloudfront.net/images/Article_Images/ImageForArticle_1354_16623535606785338.jpg.

Dendritic cells possess a remarkable capacity to change their phenotype in response to diverse stimuli, including cytokines and signals from various pathogens, a feature that mirrors their diverse range of functions (Fernando et al., 2014). Their role becomes particularly crucial in maintaining immune homeostasis; disruption in this role can lead to autoimmune diseases, allergies, and chronic inflammation. Additionally, research indicates that communication between dendritic cells and gut microbiota significantly affects their antigen-presenting activity, connecting microbial health to immune responses within the body. It is critical to grasp the complex functions of DCs to design specific therapies for leukocyte-related diseases (Cohen et al., 2019) (Figure 7.5).

7.2. Common Disorders of Leukocytes

The leukocyte disorders are a group of diseases that significantly impact the effectiveness of the immune systems. The most common among these are leukopenia, which is characterized by below-normal leukocyte levels, and leukocytosis, which is characterized by above-normal leukocyte levels. Both are due to many etiologies, including infections, bone marrow disorders, or autoimmune diseases. For instance, in the pandemic environment of COVID-19, patients exhibited striking alterations in leukocyte counts, reflecting the critical role of immune response against viral infection (Shi et al., 2020). A second condition, which is characterized by dysregulated inflammatory cytokine production, such as interleukin-36, is associated with conditions such as psoriasis and leads to increased leukocyte infiltration and inflammation (Satveer et al., 2017). Understanding these disorders not only allows for the diagnosis and management of the underlying illness but also points to the delicate balance required to maintain practical immune function.

7.2.1. Leukopenia: Definition and Causes

Leukopenia, or a reduced WBC count, is a key disorder within the overall category of leukocyte-related disorders. Leukopenia can be caused by many reasons, such as disorders in the bone marrow, autoimmune diseases, or infections that interfere with the immune system's function. More specifically, congenital immunodeficiency errors, as highlighted by the recent typology of such conditions, can lead to significant leukopenia due to impairment in leukocyte production and control (Stuart et al., 2020). Furthermore, under certain circumstances, like for transplant recipients, leukopenia can occur due to the immunosuppressive drugs administered to prevent organ rejection, aggravating susceptibility to opportunistic infections in patients (Fishman, 2017). Knowledge of these underlying etiologies is crucial for successful diagnosis and management, as they have direct implications for therapeutic modalities and improved patient outcomes in numerous clinical settings. Understanding the complex nature of leukopenia is crucial for advancing our knowledge of leukocyte disorders (Figure 7.6).

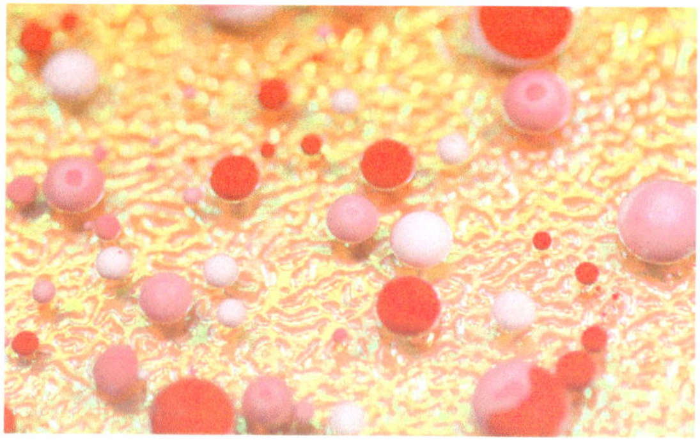

Figure 7.6. Leukopenia.

Source: https://www.metropolisindia.com/upgrade/blog/upload/2023/08/Leukopenia.webp.

7.2.2. Leukocytosis: Definition and Causes

Leukocytosis, as popularly defined as an increase in the WBC count in the bloodstream, is a significant indicator of underlying medical conditions and inflammation. Leukocytosis is caused by many reasons, including infection, stress, inflammation, and even more serious conditions such as leukemia or myeloproliferative neoplasms (MPNs). The body's natural immunity triggers leukocyte production and mobilization in situations such as acute infection, where neutrophils typically increase, or chronic inflammatory disease, leading to an increase in monocytes and lymphocytes (Tabas et al., 2017). Furthermore, leukocytosis can also occur due to physiological stressors like exercise, trauma, or psychological stress, which characterizes its intricate nature as a response to benign as well as pathological stimuli (Allan et al., 2016). Determining the underlying causes is crucial for effective diagnosis and management of associated disorders, thereby aiding in informed clinical decision-making and treatment approaches.

7.2.3. Lymphoma: Types and Implications

Lymphoma, a lymphocytic cancer, is a well-characterized group of leukocyte disorders that are largely understood in terms of two main categories: Hodgkin lymphoma (HL) and non-Hodgkin lymphoma (NHL). Both have distinct biological behaviors and therapeutic considerations that may hold significant implications for patient care. The presence of Reed-Sternberg cells traditionally characterizes HL and has a more predictable clinical course and better prognosis than NHL. In contrast, NHL is a heterogeneous collection of diseases with highly variable aggressiveness and reaction to treatment. The constant improvement in hematology research, as indicated in the EHA Roadmap, highlights the requirement for targeted therapies and improved early detection methods, particularly in NHL, in which the patient stratification based on prognosis is of extreme significance (Allard et al., 2016). Further, the role of immune dysregulation and inflammation within the lymphoma tumor microenvironment is evidence of the complex interaction between leukocyte function and cancer (Marković et al., 2022) (Figure 7.7).

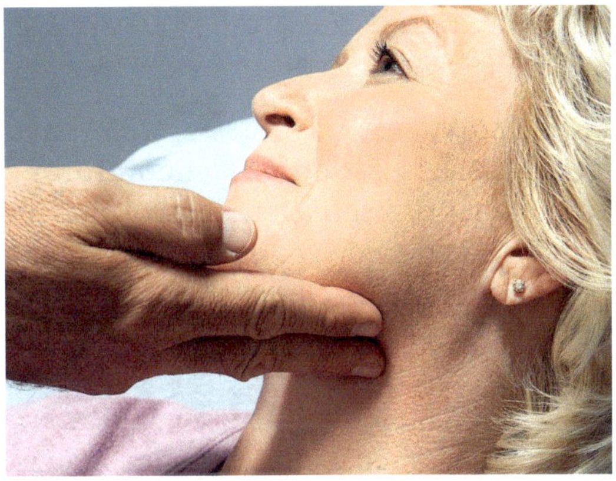

Figure 7.7. Lymphoma.

Source: https://media.post.rvohealth.io/wp-content/uploads/2020/09/lymphoma-symptoms_thumb.jpg.

7.2.4. Leukemia: Types and Symptoms

Leukemia, a malignant disease characterized by the overproduction of defective WBCs, falls into several categories, primarily acute and chronic, and each of these subcategories is based on the cell lineage. The two most frequent acute types are acute myeloid leukemia (AML) and acute lymphoblastic leukemia (ALL), distinguished by an aggressive course of disease and an early appearance of symptoms like fatigue, fever, and susceptibility to infection. In contrast, chronic lymphocytic leukemia (CLL) and chronic myeloid leukemia (CML) typically progress slowly with presentations of lymphadenopathy and splenomegaly (Diseas DOGAMC et al., 2021). Notably, secondary acute myeloid leukemia (s-AML) normally arises from pre-existing hematological conditions like myelodysplastic syndromes (MDSs), demonstrating a characteristic clinical presentation with signs of poor prognosis like advanced age and cytogenetic aberrations (Ovilla et al., 2019). Knowledge of these categories and symptoms is crucial for efficient diagnosis and treatment in the management of leukocyte disorders.

7.2.5. Myelodysplastic Syndromes: Overview

Myelodysplastic syndromes (MDS) are a heterogeneous group of hematological disorders that are characterized by ineffective hematopoiesis and an increased risk of progression to AML. The syndromes typically occur due to genetic mutations and chromosomal abnormalities that interfere with normal blood cell development, leading to the manifestations of anemia, leukopenia, and thrombocytopenia. Interestingly, a high percentage of secondary acute myeloid leukemia is secondary to MDS, and studies have indicated that 58.2% of s-AML cases might have started in such syndromes, as evidenced by the clinical data collected from Latin American centers (Ovilla et al., 2019). Diagnosis primarily depends on peripheral blood morphology, cytogenetic analysis, and mutational profiling, i.e., the detection of specific leukocyte markers (Iland et al., 2006). Consequently, MDS is quite a therapeutic challenge due to its multifactorial pathophysiology and the need for individualized therapeutic approaches to manage its diverse clinical presentations (Figure 7.8).

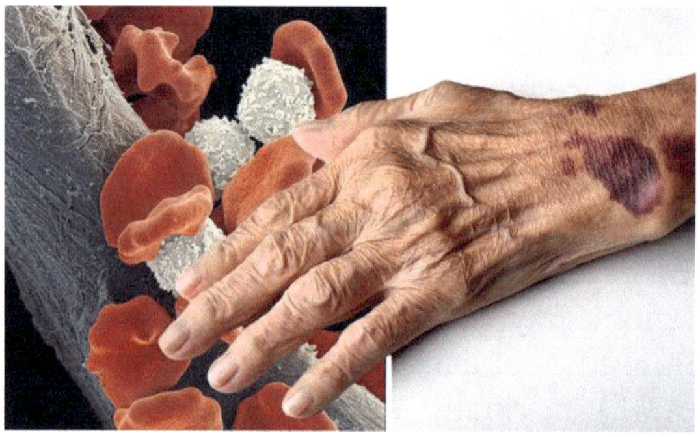

Figure 7.8. Myelodysplastic syndromes (MDS).

Source: https://cms.leapcure.com/mds_71d3888fa4.jpg.

7.2.6. Aplastic Anemia: Causes and Effects

Aplastic anemia is a critical leukocyte disease characterized by the failure of the bone marrow to produce sufficient blood cells, resulting in pancytopenia. The etiology of such a disease can be multifactorial, e.g., autoimmune responses, toxins, and genetic predispositions. Patient presentation can include congenital amegakaryocytic thrombocytopenia, an inherited condition that disrupts megakaryocyte maturation, which subsequently evolves into aplastic anemia during childhood. Surprisingly, THPO gene mutations have also been identified as one of the primary causes of this development, with a great effect on platelet production (Sundd et al., 2018). The signs of aplastic anemia include weakness, heightened risk of infection, and hemorrhage due to the compromised leukocyte and platelet levels. The complexity of its pathogenesis underscores the need for tailored therapeutic approaches, which can include immunosuppressive therapy or hematopoietic stem cell transplant (Pecci et al., 2017), underscoring the need for further sophisticated research in this field.

7.2.7. Autoimmune Disorders Affecting Leukocytes

The relationship between autoimmune conditions and leukocytes is multifaceted, highlighting the complexity of the immune response and its regulation. Autoimmune diseases often involve the improper activation of leukocytes, resulting in tissue damage and inflammation. For instance, studies have shown that female premutation carriers of alleles in the FMR1 gene exhibit an abnormal immune profile, characterized by reduced cytokine production upon stimulation, which is believed to render them susceptible to autoimmune disorders (Ashwood et al., 2014). In addition, the relationship between chronic inflammation and hypoxia also provides potential for aggravating leukocyte dysfunction, as chronic inflammation has the ability to induce pathways that augment leukocyte recruitment and proliferation, ultimately leading to chronic tissue damage and impaired cellular repair mechanisms (Carnevale et al., 2015). These are observations critical to appreciating the systemic aspect of autoimmune diseases and the need for specific therapies aimed at restoring immune equilibrium in affected individuals (Figure 7.9).

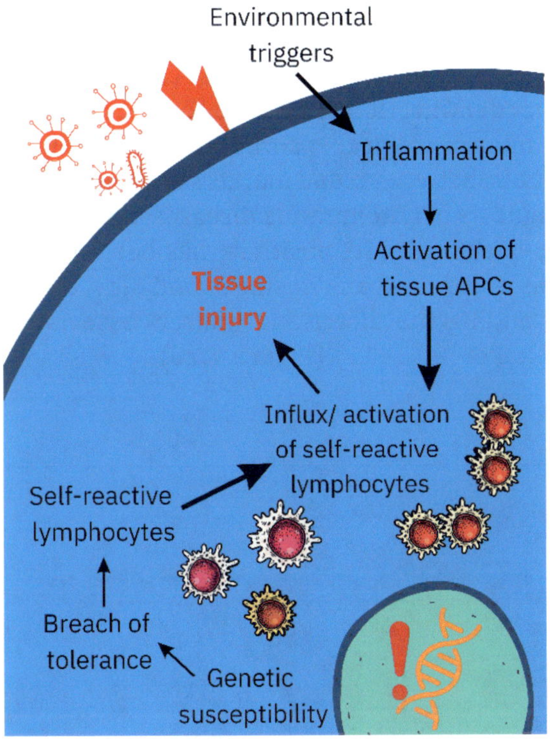

Figure 7.9. Autoimmune diseases often involve the aberrant activation of leukocytes, leading to tissue damage and chronic inflammation.

Source: https://www.biosynth.com/uploads/Blog/Autoimmune%20blog/Autoimmune%20disease.png.

7.2.8. Infections Leading to Leukocyte Disorders

Infections are capable of having a significant impact on leukocyte function and integrity and yield disorders that include qualitative or quantitative WBC abnormalities. For instance, certain viral infections and specific bacterial infections elicit an exaggerated immune response, leading to leukocyte disorders that can be either qualitative or quantitative. One such glaring example is Chédiak-Higashi syndrome (CHS), in which infection leads to the formation of giant inclusion bodies in leukocytes, rendering them non-functional and compromising the body's defense against infections (Saiz-Sierra et al., 2024). Also, diabetic patients with diabetes mellitus become hyperglycemia-sensitive to infections due to functional alterations in leukocytes, particularly those caused by hyperglycemia, which can compromise leukocyte function as well as cause urinary infections (Rajagukguk et al., 2023). These examples illustrate the close association between infectious organisms and leukocyte disorders, highlighting the importance of diligent observation and control in managing covert infections that complicate leukocyte dysfunction.

7.3. Diagnosis of Leukocyte Disorders

Diagnosis of leukocyte disorders is a critical component of understanding many immune dysfunctions and is often reliant upon the coming together of clinical evaluation and advanced laboratory investigation. Such disorders, ranging from leukocyte adhesion deficiencies to catastrophic dermatologic reactions such as Stevens–Johnson syndrome and toxic epidermal necrolysis, present peculiar challenges. For instance, early diagnosis of SJS/TEN can be challenging due to its non-specific presentation, and identification of valid biomarkers for patient assessment and management thus becomes essential (Hasegawa et al., 2024). Similarly, others, such as Leukocyte Adhesion Deficiency type I (LAD-I), need special laboratory tests, such as flow cytometry, to detect leukocyte abnormalities in markers such as CD18 and CD11 (Nadakuduti et al., 2023). The integration of molecular diagnostics and immunophenotyping not only facilitates an accurate diagnosis but also augments the possibility of developing tailored therapeutic approaches, which is crucial in improving patient outcomes for leukocyte disorders.

7.3.1. Importance of Blood Tests in Diagnosis

The role of blood tests in diagnosing leukocyte disorders cannot be overstated, as they provide significant information regarding the integrity and functionality of the immune system. Through testing various parameters in the blood, healthcare providers are capable of identifying abnormalities in leukocyte numbers and direction, which usually indicate underlying diseases such as infections, immune system disorders, and cancers. For instance, the identification of specific gene coexpression modules in blood leukocytes was linked to various neurobiological disorders, establishing the significance of these tests in identifying complex correlations between blood markers and neurological health (Battle et al., 2018). Furthermore, during the diagnosis of autoimmune diseases, the presence of HLA-B27 can be highly influential while concluding. Specifically, its positivity has been noted to be associated with an increased risk for diseases such as uveitis and ankylosing spondylitis, thereby establishing the importance of blood tests in understanding the direct and indirect associations between leukocyte disorders and systemic diseases (Cox et al., 2011) (Figure 7.10).

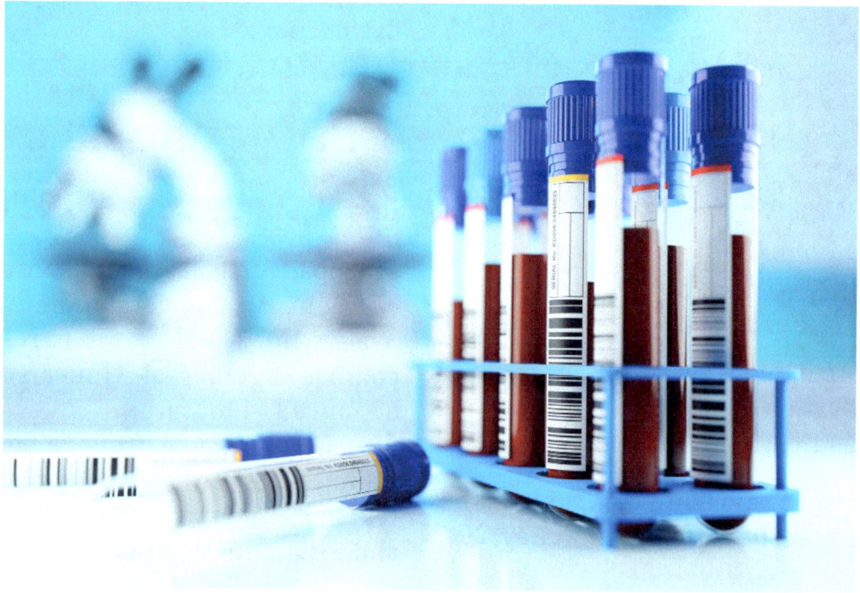

Figure 7.10. The role of blood tests in diagnosing disorders of leukocytes cannot be overstated, as these diagnostic tools provide critical insights into the functionality and health of the immune system.

Source: https://labs.selfdecode.com/app/uploads/2020/05/Labs-for-Immune-Health.jpg.

7.3.2. Complete Blood Count (CBC): Overview

The Complete Blood Count (CBC) is a staple of diagnostic techniques in evaluating hematologic health, particularly in the context of leukocyte disorders. The total blood test assays cellular elements like red blood cells, WBCs, and platelets, and provides valuable information on the immune function of the body and the body's general state of being. A CBC is also informative regarding leukocyte abnormalities, such as increased WBC counts that reflect infections or inflammation, or decreased counts that indicate potential bone marrow dysfunction or immunosuppression. Surprisingly, sex-related differences also make it challenging to interpret CBC results; research has shown that females have more robust immune profiles, thus affecting susceptibility and progression of disease, as seen in recent analyses for biological implications (Gadi et al. 2020). Therefore, the improved understanding of such nuances assists clinicians in designing useful, beneficial therapeutic interventions for leukocyte disorders (Gervin et al., 2019).

7.3.3. Bone Marrow Biopsy: Procedure and Significance

Bone marrow biopsy is a crucial diagnostic procedure that provides significant information about various leukocyte disorders, particularly hematological malignancies and other bone marrow pathologies. During the procedure, a needle is inserted into the bone, usually the iliac crest, to aspirate a sample of the bone marrow. This sample is then screened for morphologic cell abnormalities and leukocyte counts that can identify conditions such as leukemia or MDSs. This process is not only for diagnosis, but also crucial for treatment and prognosis, directing therapy based on individual patient requirements. Besides, the interaction between recipient and donor leukocytes following bone marrow transplantation (BMT) shows its importance, as low donor leukocyte chimerism levels impact long-term graft success, as well as tolerance to the transplanted organs, indicating the interconnectedness of leukocyte dynamics in disease and health (AJ et al., 1995; Abu-Elmagd et al., 1995) (Figure 7.11).

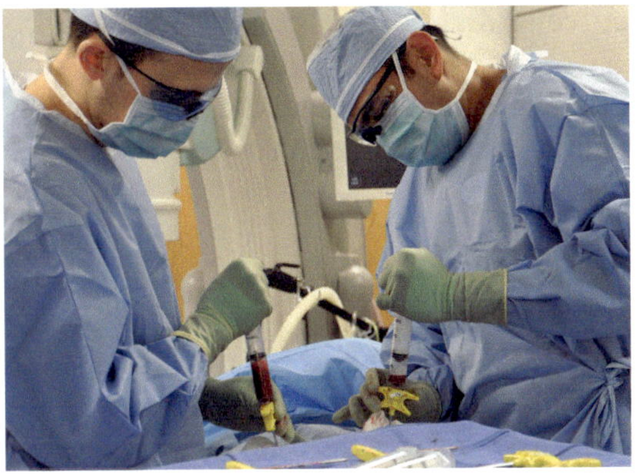

Figure 7.11. The bone marrow biopsy is a critical diagnostic procedure that provides essential insights into various disorders of leukocytes, particularly those related to hematological malignancies and other bone marrow pathologies.

Source: https://www.drnaveenanvekar.com/Uploads/Services/Bone%20marrow%20biopsy.png.

7.3.4. Flow Cytometry: Role in Diagnosis

The role of flow cytometry in the diagnosis of leukocyte disorders has been of particular interest because it can provide detailed immunophenotyping and functional studies of blood cells. Flow cytometry facilitates the early assessment of discrete populations of leukocytes, helping identify leukemic or lymphomatous-associated abnormalities. Flow cytometry, in turn, can analyze glycoprotein expressions and detect leukocyte–platelet aggregates that are important in diagnosing inherited and acquired dysfunctions in platelets. The advantage of flow cytometry is its sensitivity to low cell numbers and its requirement for a minimal volume of blood (Chih-Shen et al., 2022). Additionally, as the World Health Organization keeps developing its classification of hematolymphoid tumors, flow cytometry is at the forefront of identifying therapeutically actionable biomarkers in leukemias, determining its position at the center of current diagnostic approaches (Joseph et al., 2022). Thus, flow cytometry is a strictly essential element in the complex network of leukocyte disorder diagnosis.

7.3.5. Genetic Testing: Applications in Leukocyte Disorders

Genetic testing plays a critical role in the diagnosis and treatment of leukocyte disorders, significantly enhancing our understanding of several hematological diseases. By measuring levels of gene expression that affect leukocyte functioning, scientists can identify genetic differences leading to immunological deficiency or malignancy, and thus provide proper treatment alternatives.

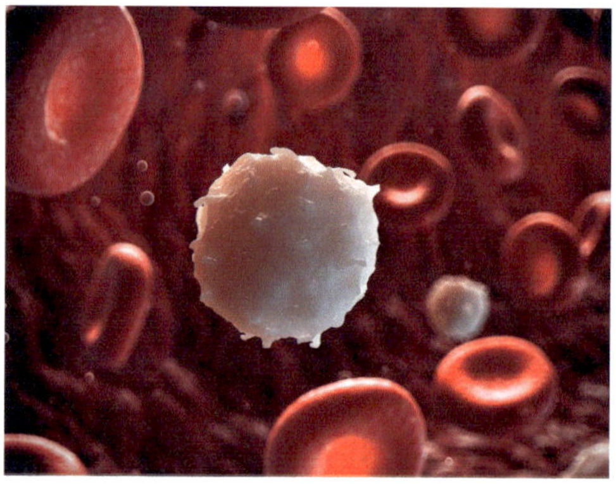

Figure 7.12. Genetic testing plays a crucial role in the diagnosis and management of leukocyte disorders, significantly enhancing our understanding of various hematological conditions.

Source: https://www.verywellhealth.com/thmb/9dTI_DKeZzYb97W53J2y3rSZV5Q=/1500x0/filters:no_upscale():max_bytes(150000):strip_icc()/GettyImages-535642077-8ce9c7448baf40fb896c246b7f4a47a9.jpgs.

For instance, studies have shown that genetic variation in blood leukocyte expression is linked to neurobiological features, which are essential in the case of diseases such as autism spectrum disorder (ASD) (Battle et al., 2018). Furthermore, the identification of stability and reliability of gene expression profiles over time can aid in understanding the mechanisms of leukocyte disorders, thereby highlighting the application of genetic testing in the clinical setting (Craig et al., 2009). Lastly, these breakthroughs underline the potential of genetic testing not only to diagnose but also to illuminate the complex biological processes of leukocyte-associated conditions (Figure 7.12).

7.3.6. Imaging Studies: When They Are Used

Imaging studies play a crucial role in the diagnosis and treatment of leukocyte disorders, particularly when other methods are ineffective. Imaging studies, such as magnetic resonance imaging (MRI) and positron emission tomography (PET), are employed to visualize leukocyte function and distribution disorders. For instance, leukocyte blood abnormalities can be linked to neurological conditions, for example, in the study that revealed a significant association between leukocyte gene expression and neuroimaging responses in ASD (Battle et al., 2018). Furthermore, imaging studies extend beyond diagnosis; they enable tracking of therapeutic response and disease progression in leukocyte disorders. Liquid biopsies in cancer research investigate circulating tumor products that can signal leukocyte activity, a point that necessitates the identification of significant biomarkers to inform treatment and relapse diagnosis (Calborean et al., 2018). Imaging studies are a substantial resource in both investigating and treating leukocyte-related illnesses.

7.3.7. Clinical Symptoms and Their Relevance

Understanding of the clinical presentation of leukocyte disorders is paramount to prevent misdiagnosis and improper management of the disorders. Symptoms usually present as a direct consequence of dysregulation in the function of leukocytes, and the resultant clinical presentation varies from frequent infections, chronic inflammation, or malignancy of the blood cells. For instance, the presence of chronic fever and weakness may indicate an underlying disease in leukocytes, and further investigation into causes such as leukocytosis or leukopenia is necessary. Moreover, a diagnostic criterion such as that found in current research, e.g., the Rome IV criteria, emphasizes the significance of symptom evaluation in pinpointing the underlying pathology and determining appropriate therapeutic interventions, e.g., techniques such as biofeedback therapy for related disorders (Park et al., 2024). As noted in the case of obstructive sleep apnea, variability in symptoms may impact the effectiveness of screening, underlining the need to develop more uniform criteria for better leukocyte disorder detection (Gauld et al., 2024) (Figure 7.13).

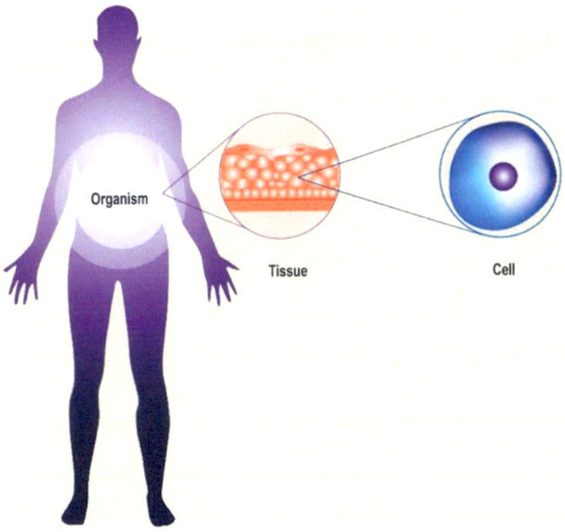

Figure 7.13. Symptoms often manifest as a result of dysregulation in leukocyte function, leading to various clinical presentations, including recurrent infections, chronic inflammation, or hematological malignancies.

Source: https://image.oaes.cc/357bd32f-956a-4957-b2d0-c8d12e6c49d0/3625.fig.1.jpg.

7.3.8. Differential Diagnosis: Importance and Methods

In the field of medical diagnosis, the process of differential diagnosis plays a significant role, particularly in cases involving leukocyte disorders. Accurate differentiation of various leukocyte conditions is crucial to provide appropriate treatment and management. For instance, genetic analysis can detect specific biomarkers differentiating between genetically equivalent disorders, such as early childhood schizophrenia and ASD, as revealed through varying quantities of ribosomal genes and telomere length in blood leukocytes (Ershova et al., 2025). Also, differential diagnosis effectively integrates thorough clinical examination and laboratory analysis that considers demographic factors, symptomology, and genetic susceptibility. It is worth noting the nuances of such disorders; hence, correct identification can avoid risks of misdiagnosis and guide proper therapeutic interventions. Such a guarded process is replicated in other specialties of medicine, where precise symptom evaluation reduces overlap between presentations of pathologies, thereby playing a critical role in diagnosis (Ogut, 2025).

7.4. Treatment and Management of Leukocyte Disorders

In the treatment and management of leukocyte disorders, a balanced strategy in the majority of situations is needed due to the complex interaction among the immune mechanisms involved. For diseases such as allergic disease and systemic lupus erythematosus (SLE), sharing a point of commonality regarding treatment strategies may prove beneficial. As observed, SLE patients exhibit increased sensitivity to allergic diseases, implying that therapies designed to modulate immune responses are likely to have cross-benefits. For instance, drugs used to treat allergic dermatitis are also expected to relieve symptoms of SLE (Jung et al., 2025). Additionally, diseases such as COPD necessitate an understanding of the roles of various leukocyte subpopulations, as neutrophils and eosinophils play crucial roles in inflammation and the loss of lung function (Lan et al., 2025). Thus, treatment strategies personalized to individual requirements via leukocyte profiling can enhance clinical outcomes, offering a promising avenue for effective treatment of such diseases.

7.4.1. Overview of Treatment Options

Leukocyte disorder treatment is variable and depends on the etiology and severity of the disease. It can be from conservative management, e.g., observation in mild disease, to intense treatment such as chemotherapy or stem cell transplant in more serious forms, particularly in MDS, where there is a high risk of transformation to acute leukemia (Orgueira et al., 2023). In addition, pathophysiologically targeted therapies are also increasingly in demand, as exemplified by the application of anti-inflammatory interventions for neuroinflammatory elements present in diseases, such as ASD with leukocyte dysfunction (Obodzinskaya et al., 2023). Understanding the biological processes involved allows clinicians to personalize treatment plans, integrating pharmacotherapy and support care to maximize patient outcomes and quality of life. This advanced strategy highlights the importance of personalized medicine in the treatment of leukocyte disorders (Figure 7.14).

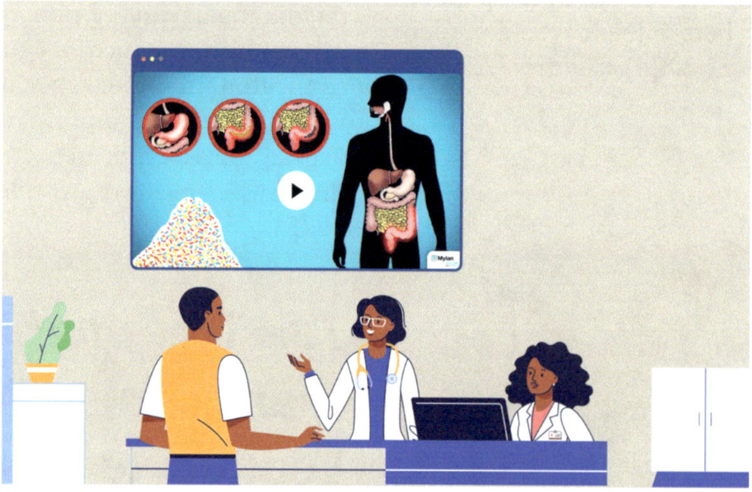

Figure 7.14. Understanding the biological mechanisms at play allows clinicians to optimize treatment plans, integrating pharmacological and supportive interventions to improve patient outcomes and quality of life effectively.

Source: https://explainvisually.co/wp-content/uploads/2024/06/grafika-do-artykulu-na-bloga-2024.07.03.png.

7.4.2. Chemotherapy: Role in Treating Leukemias

Chemotherapy is of primary significance in the treatment of leukemias, a group of conditions characterized by excessive leukocyte growth. Chemotherapy exploits the dividing cancer cells by trying to reduce the tumor burden and bring about remission. The effectiveness of chemotherapy also relies not only on the cytotoxic effect of chemotherapeutic agents but also on their capacity to induce inflammatory responses, which can further amplify anti-tumor action. For instance, chronic inflammation is the cause of treatment resistance, while acute inflammatory reactions can trigger immune responses by boosting dendritic cell maturation to facilitate more efficient antigen presentation (Zhao et al., 2021). Furthermore, the phenomenon of pyroptosis, that is a form of programmed cell death associated with innate immunity, has been a two-edged sword during cancer therapy, impacting the efficacy and the toxicity of chemotherapy (Yu et al., 2021). It is essential to comprehend these intricate interactions to optimize the therapeutic approach in treating leukemia.

7.4.3. Radiation Therapy: Applications and Effects

Radiation therapy has emerged as a key component in the management of various leukocyte disorders, particularly in neoplasms such as CLL, in which it targets and treats malignant leukocyte proliferation.

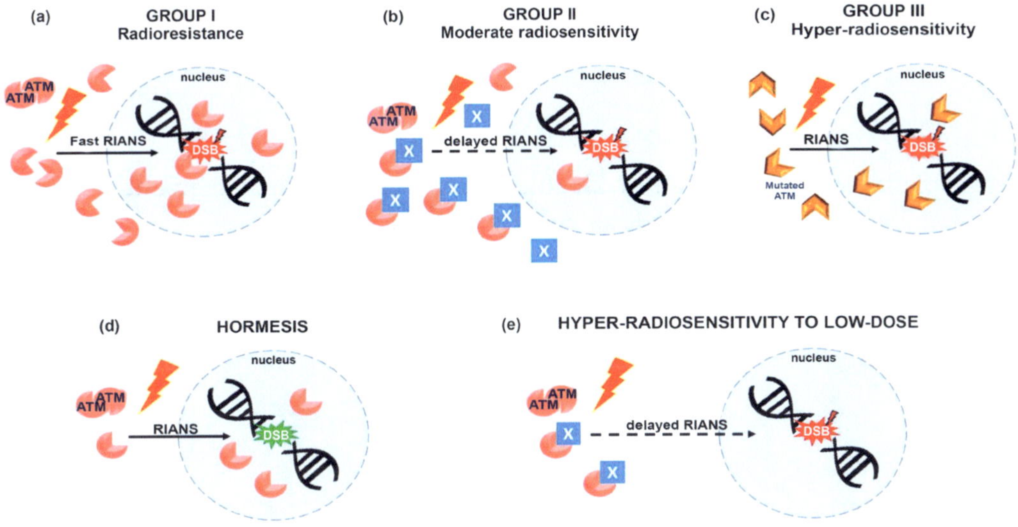

Figure 7.15. Radiation therapy has emerged as a pivotal component in the treatment of various leukocyte disorders, particularly in cancers such as chronic lymphocytic leukemia (CLL), where it addresses the abnormal proliferation of leukocytes.

Source: https://www.mdpi.com/cancers/cancers-15-01482/article_deploy/html/images/cancers-15-01482-g001.png.

Radiation therapy kills and destroys cancer cells by utilizing ionizing radiation, thus reducing tumor burden and improving survival in patients. However, radiation therapy usage comes with limitations, as collateral tissue damage to surrounding healthy tissues represents a severe limiting factor to patient recovery and quality of life. In direct response to these restrictions, current advancements in immunotherapy, such as chimeric antigen receptor (CAR) T-cell therapy, hold promise in selectively targeting tumor cells while leaving normal cells intact. Thus, the intercalation of radiation therapy with innovative treatments is a multi-dimensional strategy for leukocyte disorder management, a path towards greater therapeutic efficacy and patient well-being (Devi et al., 2019) (Figure 7.15).

7.4.4. Immunotherapy: Types and Effectiveness

The introduction of immunotherapy has revolutionized the treatment paradigm for various diseases, particularly those mediated by leukocytes, such as hematologic malignancies. This new form of therapy leverages the body's immune system to recognize and eliminate cancer cells, thereby significantly improving patient outcomes. Notably, immunotherapies include monoclonal antibodies, checkpoint inhibitors, and CAR T-cell therapy that are differentially effective against various cancers. For instance, checkpoint inhibitors have been effective in revealing tumor cells, enhancing anti-tumor immunity through modulation of the inflammatory environment, while CAR T-cell therapy presents a novel way of targeting specific leukocyte populations with enhanced specificity. The interaction between inflammation and cancer dynamics also renders the efficacy of treatments even more complicated in that chronic inflammation can both be tumorigenic and suppress therapeutic action (Zhao et al., 2021). These therapeutic approaches also emphasize the central role of leukocyte dysregulation in oncology, underscoring the necessity of an individualized approach to ensure optimal therapeutic effectiveness (Hou et al., 2022).

7.4.5. Stem Cell Transplantation: Procedure and Outcomes

Stem cell transplantation has been an invaluable treatment in the management of leukemias and other hematologic malignancies, as well as genetic disorders.

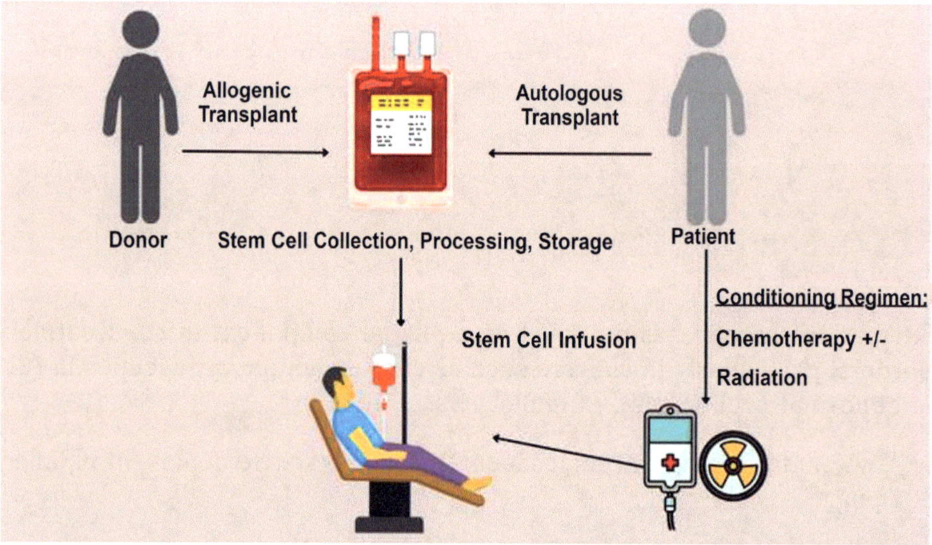

Figure 7.16. In treating disorders of leukocytes, stem cell transplantation has emerged as a pivotal procedure, particularly in addressing hematologic malignancies and genetic disorders.

Source: https://media.springernature.com/lw685/springer-static/image/art%3A10.1007%2Fs11864-024-01240-1/MediaObjects/11864_2024_1240_Fig1_HTML.png.

The procedure typically involves conditioning the patient through the use of chemotherapy or radiation to eliminate the defective cells, and subsequently transplanting hematopoietic stem cells (HSCs) sourced from peripheral blood, bone marrow, or umbilical cord blood. The outcome of such transplantations can be rewarding, with a potential cure achieved through the recovery of normal bone marrow function, as in mucopolysaccharidosis type I (MPS-I), where transplantation at an early age greatly increases enzyme activity and improves indicators of disease (Oikawa et al., 2017). Furthermore, the efficiency of stem cell collection and its correlation with successful transplantation outcome emphasize the optimization of methods for enhancing stem cell yield, particularly from healthy and even leukemic donors (Ding et al., 2020). This complex treatment highlights the critical importance of stem cell transplantation in treating leukocyte disorders (Figure 7.16).

7.4.6. Supportive Care: Importance in Management

The management of leukocyte disorders, particularly in hematologic malignancy, needs an effective supportive care system to maximize patient outcomes and quality of life. Supportive care includes a multidimensional approach that takes into account the physical, psychological, and social aspects of patients being treated. For example, in head and neck squamous cell carcinoma (HNSCC), which is found frequently due to risk factors like tobacco smoking and HPV, individually targeted supportive interventions can improve side effects of intensive treatments like chemoradiotherapy and result in improved pain control and nutritional support (Daniel et al., 2020). Additionally, hematopoietic cell transplant (HCT) requires precise supportive treatment to manage complications like graft-versus-host disease (GVHD) and to facilitate recovery of immune function following transplant (Saad et al., 2020). Hence, having complete supportive treatment protocols is key to enhancing the effectiveness of treatment and upholding patient well-being when leukocyte disorders are present.

7.4.7. Lifestyle Modifications: Role in Recovery

The role of lifestyle modification in healing from leukocyte disease is increasingly being seen as fundamental to the holistic management of health. The use of diet interventions, engaging in regular exercise, and managing stress through mindfulness interventions can all support overall immune function and directly impact leukocyte behavior and health. For instance, a diet rich in antioxidants can help combat oxidative stress, which is responsible for telomere shortening and cellular senescence (Erusalimsky et al., 2020).

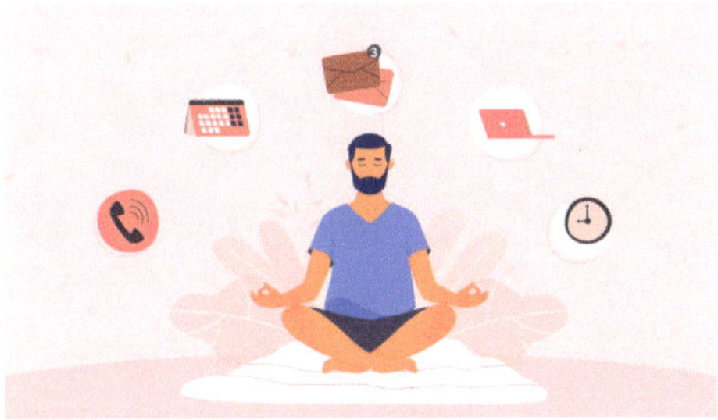

Figure 7.17. Adopting nutritional strategies, engaging in regular physical activity, and minimizing stress through mindfulness practices can promote overall immune function, directly impacting leukocyte behavior and health.

Source: https://saffron4health.com/wp-content/uploads/2024/06/13-2.pngs.

The cellular aging process has the potential to contribute to immune dysfunction, leading to chronic inflammation, a condition often associated with leukocyte disorders. Furthermore, lifestyle changes to mitigate chronic hypoxia—a common characteristic of many disorders—can also help reduce undue leukocyte activation and inflammation, thereby facilitating an improved environment for recovery (Carnevale et al., 2015). Therefore, the inclusion of lifestyle interventions must be accorded top priority as part of an overall treatment plan to restore immune homeostasis and enhance long-term clinical outcomes in patients with leukocyte disorders (Figure 7.17).

7.4.8. Emerging Therapies: Current Research Trends

With expanding research in leukocyte disorders, new treatments are increasingly focused on attacking the pathophysiologic pathways of the illness with novel and innovative approaches. Of special interest is the regulation of matrix metalloproteinases (MMPs) and their tissue inhibitors (TIMPs), whose pivotal roles in extracellular matrix remodeling and cell phenotype are critical. MMPs dysregulation, such as MMP-2 and MMP-9, correlates with chronic degenerative disease, and this underscores their therapeutic target value in leukocyte-associated disorders (Griselda et al., 2020). Further advances in the pathophysiology of disease-related conditions, like ischemic stroke, have spurred drug development to maximize neurological recovery while controlling the leukocytes contribution to inflammation and tissue damage (Kuriakose et al., 2020). Through these new approaches, the face of research is shifting toward a greater understanding of leukocyte function, paving the way to successful therapies that address the systemic and localized manifestations of such disease.

A CLOSER LOOK

ADAPTIVE IMMUNITY

Adaptive immunity is a key aspect of the immune system that provides long-term and targeted protection against infections. In contrast to innate immunity, which produces a quick but generalized response, adaptive immunity offers a slower response but is specific in its response to particular antigens and builds immunological memory.

- It involves two main types of lymphocytes:
- B cells, which produce antibodies that neutralize pathogens or mark them for destruction.
- T cells, which either help other immune cells (helper T cells) or directly kill infected cells (cytotoxic T cells).

When the body encounters a pathogen, it "remembers" it, and future responses are faster and more potent—this is the basis of vaccination. Flexibility of immunity is of great importance in long-term protection from infection and is necessary in the identification and response to foreign substances but under normal circumstances disregarding cells of the body.

SUMMARY

The complexity of leukocyte disorders underscores the critical need for further research and improved clinical approaches. Through the investigation of genetic causes associated with these disorders, researchers have identified significant loci that contribute to conditions such as autoimmune diseases and certain leukemias, as summarized in recent studies examining genetic correlations among different populations. Secondarily, the comorbidity of leukocyte disorders with mental diseases and skin conditions, as evidenced by the prevalence of psychiatric morbidity in individuals with illnesses such as psoriasis, demonstrates complicated health associations demanding multidisciplinary treatment. To meet these challenges, not only should genetic investigation and validation progress, particularly through system-wide meta-analyses like those regarding suicide attempts, but also healthcare provision systems must be enhanced to bridge existing gaps in patient treatment (Docherty et al., 2023; Torres et al., 2023). Ultimately, coordination among various disciplines is necessary to improve patient outcomes and address the long-term consequences of leukocyte disorders.

WBCs or leukocytes are the essential constituents of the immune system and play a significant role in innate as well as adaptive immunity. Their functional heterogeneity enables them to function effectively against diverse pathogens, injury, and inflammation, which are critical processes in maintaining homeostasis. Dysregulation of leukocyte function can lead to a multitude of diseases, reflecting their dual role in both disease and health. For instance, in obesity, there is chronic low-grade inflammation that is leukocyte-mediated, ultimately resulting in complications like insulin resistance and metabolic syndrome. This dysfunction is not limited to metabolic disorders; alterations in leukocyte populations are also responsible for pregnancy complications. Maternal obesity has been observed to result in unsuccessful utero-placental establishment due to alterations in leukocyte function (St-Germain et al., 2020). In concert, understanding leukocyte function and its dysfunctions is central to creating specific therapies that restore immune homeostasis and promote healthy outcomes (Tilg et al., 2020).

REFERENCES

1. Abu-Elmagd, K., Demetris, J., Fontes, P., Fung, J., et al. (1995). The current status of hepatic transplantation at the University of Pittsburgh. https://core.ac.uk/download/12205275.pdf (accessed on 12th June 2025).
2. Plantone, D., Inglese, M., Salvetti, M., & Koudriavtseva, T. (2019). A perspective of coagulation dysfunction in multiple sclerosis and in experimental allergic encephalomyelitis. Frontiers in Neurology, 9. https://doi.org/10.3389/fneur.2018.01175Aggarwal, A., Almeida, M., Alsemgeest, E., Apple, F., Arya, D., Earley, B., et al. (2014). Differences in leukocyte profile, gene expression, and metabolite status of dairy cows with or without sole ulcers. https://core.ac.uk/download/45656534.pdf (accessed on 12th June 2025).
3. Ahakoud, M., Belghiti, H. D., Ihlal, H., & Bouguenouch, L. (2023). A mosaic PIK3CA mutation in a Moroccan female: Exploring the diagnostic challenges of PIK3CA-related overgrowth spectrum. Cureus, 15. https://www.semanticscholar.org/paper/b86c27aa8c06c14e72561ce84478ae7f6b1c5540 (accessed on 12th June 2025).
4. Allard, S., Anagnou, N., Andolfo, I., Andrau, M., et al. (2016). The European Hematology Association Roadmap for European Hematology Research: A consensus document. https://core.ac.uk/download/79516495.pdf (accessed on 12th June 2025).
5. Ashwood, P., Berman, R. F., Careaga, M., Hagerman, R., et al. (2014). Immune dysregulation as a cause of autoinflammation in fragile X premutation carriers: Link between FMRI CGG repeat number and decreased cytokine responses. https://core.ac.uk/download/323071233.pdf (accessed on 12th June 2025).
6. Battle, A., Krishnan, A., Perry, A., Schroeder, A., Sugathan, A., Venter, A., Willsey, A. J., et al. (2018). Large-scale associations between the leukocyte transcriptome and BOLD responses to speech differ in autism early language outcome subtypes. https://core.ac.uk/download/323064141.pdf (accessed on 12th June 2025).
7. Bochner, B. S. (2020). Adhesion Molecules in Allergic Disease. https://doi.org/10.1201/9781003067603 (accessed on 12th June 2025).
8. Cabral-Pacheco, G. A., Garza-Veloz, I., Castruita-De la Rosa, C., Ramirez-Acuña, J. M., Perez-Romero, B. A., Guerrero-Rodriguez, J. F., Martínez-Avila, N., et al. (2020). The roles of matrix metalloproteinases and their inhibitors in human diseases. International Journal of Molecular Sciences, 21, 9739. https://doi.org/10.3390/ijms21249739 (accessed on 12th June 2025).
9. Calborean, V., Miscoci, A., Pirvu, C. D., Pădureanu, V., et al. (2018). The importance of circulating tumor products as "liquid biopsies" in colorectal cancer. https://core.ac.uk/download/216808108.pdf (accessed on 12th June 2025).
10. Carnevale, I., De Santis, E., Limana, F., Perrone, M., et al. (2015). One special question to start with: Can HIF/NFkB be a target in inflammation? https://core.ac.uk/download/54248898.pdf (accessed on 12th June 2025).
11. Cohen, L., Cho, J. H., Gevers, D., & Chu, H. (2019). Genetic factors and the intestinal microbiome guide development of microbe-based therapies for inflammatory bowel diseases. Gastroenterology, 156, 2174–2189. https://doi.org/10.1053/j.gastro.2019.03.017 (accessed on 12th June 2025).
12. Corsini, A., Perticarini, L., Palermi, S., Bettinsoli, P., & Marchini, A. (2025). Re-evaluating

platelet-rich plasma dosing strategies in sports medicine: The role of the "10 billion platelet dose" in optimizing therapeutic outcomes—A narrative review. Journal of Clinical Medicine, 14. https://www.semanticscholar.org/paper/dcfa3ae59ad98230ab70810f0a6cd5fa561db324 (accessed on 12th June 2025).

13. Cox, C. L., Evans, P., Gibbons, H., Titmus, M., et al. (2011). HLA-B27 positivity: Associated health implications. https://core.ac.uk/download/9983108.pdf (accessed on 12th June 2025).
14. Craig, I. W., Fernandes, C., Meaburn, E. L., Plomin, R., et al. (2009). Assessing individual differences in genome-wide gene expression in human whole blood: Reliability over four hours and stability over 10 months. https://core.ac.uk/download/11305773.pdf (accessed on 12th June 2025).
15. Demetris, A. J., Lu, L., Murase, N., Starzl, T. E., et al. (1995). The changing immunology of organ transplantation. https://core.ac.uk/download/12205241.pdf (accessed on 12th June 2025).
16. Devi, P., Brindha, R., & Raghunathan, K. (2019). Chimeric antigen receptor for chronic lymphocytic leukemia–A review. https://core.ac.uk/download/477855067.pdf (accessed on 12th June 2025).
17. Ding, M. (2020). Applications of statistical methods studying the impact of mobilization regimes on the total collection yield of hematologic stem cell. https://core.ac.uk/download/515469525.pdf (accessed on 12th June 2025).
18. Docherty, A., Mullins, N., Ashley-Koch, A. E., Qin, X. J., Coleman, J. R. I., Shabalin, A., Kang, J., et al. (2023). GWAS meta-analysis of suicide attempt: Identification of 12 genome-wide significant loci and implication of genetic risks for specific health factors. The American Journal of Psychiatry, 180(10), 723–738. https://www.semanticscholar.org/paper/e2af2e2393a481739871006e584dd931898c7fe3 (accessed on 12th June 2025).
19. Eker, I., Özdemir, H. N. Ç., Yılmaz, F., Yeşilipek, A., Küpesiz, A., Uygun, V., Karasu, G., et al. (2025). Navigating hope and complexity: Turkish parents' experiences with savior siblings. Turkish Journal of Hematology, 42, 47–55. https://www.semanticscholar.org/paper/897cec67995080772635c88c18a7a5c878f243c0 (accessed on 12th June 2025).
20. Ershova, E., Chudakova, Y. M., Veiko, N., Martynov, A. V., Kostyuk, S., Kostyuk, S. V., Nikitina, S., et al. (2025). Variation in the content of three tandem repeats (ribosomal, satellite III and telomeric) in the DNA of blood leukocytes of children with mental disorders, as a potential marker for the differential diagnosis of childhood schizophrenia and autism spectrum disorders. Psychiatry (Moscow) (Psikhiatriya). https://www.semanticscholar.org/paper/3588d9b9dce7a2ca534f0f4ee525114ec2e6d9e2 (accessed on 12th June 2025).
21. Erusalimsky, J. (2020). Oxidative stress, telomeres and cellular senescence: What non-drug interventions might break the link? https://core.ac.uk/download/287586288.pdf (accessed on 12th June 2025).
22. Fishman, J. A. (2017). Infection in organ transplantation. American Journal of Transplantation, 17, 856–879. https://doi.org/10.1111/ajt.14208 (accessed on 12th June 2025).
23. Gadi, N., Wu, S., Spihlman, A. P., & Moulton, V. R. (2020). What's sex got to do with COVID-19? Gender-based differences in the host immune response to coronaviruses. Frontiers in Immunology, 11. https://doi.org/10.3389/fimmu.2020.02147 (accessed on 12th June 2025).
24. Gauld, C., Baillieul, S., Martin, V. P., Richaud, A., Lopez, R., Pelou, M., Abi-Saab, P., et al. (2024).

Symptom content analysis of OSA questionnaires: Time to identify and improve relevance of diversity of OSA symptoms? Journal of Clinical Sleep Medicine. https://www.semanticscholar.org/paper/d17a38ffaa4c8e566ec7db84eeba883d89315ea1 (accessed on 12th June 2025).

25. Gervin, K., Salas, L. A., Bakulski, K. M., van Zelm, M. C., Koestler, D. C., Wiencke, J. K., Duijts, L., et al. (2019). Systematic evaluation and validation of reference and library selection methods for deconvolution of cord blood DNA methylation data. Clinical Epigenetics, 11. https://doi.org/10.1186/s13148-019-0717-y (accessed on 12th June 2025).

26. Gomez Cifuentes, E. A., De Matteis, R., Udomjarumanee, P., Genes and Health Queen Mary University of London, Munroe, P. B., & Dalli, J. (2024). LGR6 frameshift variant abrogates receptor expression on select leukocyte subsets and associates with viral infections. Blood. https://www.semanticscholar.org/paper/212be31c4c0d9bdbaeb53d9cedd55e461fb795af (accessed on 12th June 2025).

27. Hasegawa, A., & Abe, R. (2024). Stevens–Johnson syndrome and toxic epidermal necrolysis: Updates in pathophysiology and management. Chinese Medical Journal, 137, 2294–2307. https://www.semanticscholar.org/paper/5688c13a77a5b926bb1b5d045d952c6a8c633d32 (accessed on 12th June 2025).

28. Hou, K., Wu, Z. X., Chen, X. Y., Wang, J. Q., Zhang, D., Xiao, C., Zhu, D., et al. (2022). Microbiota in health and diseases. Signal Transduction and Targeted Therapy, 7. https://doi.org/10.1038/s41392-022-00974-4 (accessed on 12th June 2025).

29. Hristova, M., & Rocha-Ferreira, E. (2015). Antimicrobial peptides and complement in neonatal hypoxia-ischemia induced brain damage. https://core.ac.uk/download/29413591.pdf (accessed on 12th June 2025).

30. Iland, H., Hertzberg, M., & Marlton, P. (2006). Myeloid Leukemia: Methods and Protocols. https://www.semanticscholar.org/paper/5ed9f60a39e60de38d13b9249e57999f87887b24 (accessed on 12th June 2025).

31. Johnson, D. E., Burtness, B., Leemans, C. R., Lui, V. W. Y., Bauman, J. E., & Grandis, J. R. (2020). Head and neck squamous cell carcinoma. Nature Reviews Disease Primers, 6. https://doi.org/10.1038/s41572-020-00224-3 (accessed on 12th June 2025).

32. Jung, H., Ali, S. M., Khianey, R., & Mikdashi, J. (2025). Allergic disorders and systemic lupus erythematosus: Common pathogenesis and caveats in management. Allergies. https://www.semanticscholar.org/paper/3d961bc05c108d2242744ea61b4995e188e771af (accessed on 12th June 2025).

33. Khoury, J. D., Solary, É., Abla, O., Akkari, Y., Alaggio, R., Apperley, J. F., Bejar, R., et al. (2022). The 5th edition of the World Health Organization classification of hematolymphoid tumors: Myeloid and histiocytic/dendritic neoplasms. Leukemia, 36, 1703–1719. https://doi.org/10.1038/s41375-022-01613-1 (accessed on 12th June 2025).

34. Kuriakose, D., & Xiao, Z. C. (2020). Pathophysiology and treatment of stroke: Present status and future perspectives. International Journal of Molecular Sciences, 21, 7609. https://doi.org/10.3390/ijms21207609 (accessed on 12th June 2025).

35. Lan, C., Yang, M. C., Su, W. L., Huang, K. L., Lin, C. C., Huang, Y. C., Huang, C. Y., et al. (2025). Unraveling the immune landscape of chronic obstructive pulmonary disease: Insights into inflammatory cell subtypes, pathogenesis, and treatment strategies. International Journal of Molecular Sciences, 26. https://www.semanticscholar.org/paper/

cf325796b7c3b551fdaecf324b0d63cbb81435ea (accessed on 12th June 2025).

36. Mahil, S. K., Catapano, M., Di Meglio, P., Dand, N., Ahlfors, H., Carr, I., Smith, C., et al. (2017). An analysis of IL-36 signature genes and individuals with IL1RL2 knockout mutations validates IL-36 as a psoriasis therapeutic target. Science Translational Medicine, 9. https://doi.org/10.1126/scitranslmed.aan2514 (accessed on 12th June 2025).

37. Marković, D., Maslovarić, I., Čokić, V., Đikić, M., et al. (2022). Neutrophil death in myeloproliferative neoplasms: Shedding more light on neutrophils as a pathogenic link to chronic inflammation. https://core.ac.uk/download/492750914.pdf (accessed on 12th June 2025).

38. Martínez, F. O., & Gordon, S. (2014). The M1 and M2 paradigm of macrophage activation: Time for reassessment. F1000Prime Reports, 6. https://doi.org/10.12703/p6-13 (accessed on 12th June 2025).

39. Mosquera Orgueira, A., Pérez Encinas, M. P., Diaz Varela, N. D., Mora, E., Díaz-Beyá, M., Montoro, M. J., Pomares, H., et al. (2023). Machine learning improves risk stratification in myelodysplastic neoplasms: An analysis of the Spanish group of myelodysplastic syndromes. Hemisphere, 7. https://www.semanticscholar.org/paper/5b8bf1295b9090a80e9a9b67e3a02b5f8ac13413 (accessed on 12th June 2025).

40. Nadakuditi, D., Cheni, G., Sekuri, S. L., & Katuri, K. K. (2023). Periodontal management of leukocyte adhesion deficiency type-I with photodynamic therapy–A case report. Journal of Clinical and Diagnostic Research. https://www.semanticscholar.org/paper/febd81235aca996cc8bce619eb2af9ab67a817cb (accessed on 12th June 2025).

41. Nair, V. V. (2024). Biomarkers associated with temporomandibular disorders: Current status and prospective paths. The Journal of Prosthetic and Implant Dentistry. https://www.semanticscholar.org/paper/1360488fcc982bbaeb6af4ac0cde2028c5403777 (accessed on 12th June 2025).

42. Novoa-Bolivar, E. M., Ros, J. A., Pérez-Fernández, S., Campillo, J. A., López-Hernández, R., González-López, R., Ruiz-Lorente, I., et al. (2025). Diagnostic utility of bronchoalveolar lavage flow cytometric leukocyte profiling in interstitial lung disease and infection. Biomolecules, 15. https://www.semanticscholar.org/paper/61109d38008c3d4d965eb939da0e8dd2867c50f6 (accessed on 12th June 2025).

43. Obodzinskaya, T., Generalov, V. O., Sadykov, T. R., Aleksandrenkova, A., Larionov, G. V., & Niculina, L. V. (2023). Neuroinflammation process as a key etiopathogenetic factor in the evolution of autism spectrum disorders in child patients. Psikhiatriya. https://www.semanticscholar.org/paper/56ae0529b70b518f5b5bdb33b5937b2006f5ba44 (accessed on 12th June 2025).

44. Ogut, E. (2025). Anatomical variability, morphofunctional characteristics, and clinical relevance of accessory ossicles of the back: Implications for spinal pathophysiology and differential diagnosis. Journal of Orthopedic Surgery and Research, 20. https://www.semanticscholar.org/paper/eed6ee293f636179ac5ddc260a73e25384117b70 (accessed on 12th June 2025).

45. Oikawa, A., Pievani, A., Scaradavou, A., Willing, A. E., Sacchetti, B., Davenport, C., et al. (2017). Neonatal umbilical cord blood transplantation halts skeletal disease progression in the murine model of MPS-I. https://core.ac.uk/download/127587389.pdf (accessed on 12th June 2025).

46. Ovilla, R., Crisp, R., Baez-Islas, P., Arbelbide, J., Grille, S., Díaz, L., Idrobo, H., et al. (2019). Secondary acute myeloid leukemia: Demographic, physio pathogenic, clinical and therapeutic

comparative study. Blood. https://www.semanticscholar.org/paper/7801756596fd91c5f012a588d1bbc060534997ad (accessed on 12th June 2025).

47. Park, C. J., Jones, M. P., Prott, G., Sequeira, C., & Malcolm, A. (2024). Rome IV functional defecation disorder: Time for a change in symptom criteria for improved clinical relevance? The American Journal of Gastroenterology. https://www.semanticscholar.org/paper/2eb449927065328db299fcf4413c033887845718 (accessed on 12th June 2025).

48. Pascottini, B., Carrier, J., LeBlanc, S. J., Van Schyndel, R., et al. (2018). The effect of pegbovigrastim on circulating neutrophil count in dairy cattle: A randomized controlled trial. https://core.ac.uk/download/237010954.pdf (accessed on 12th June 2025).

49. Pecci, A., Ragab, I., Bozzi, V., De Rocco, D., Barozzi, S., Giangregorio, T., Ali, H. A., et al. (2017). Thrombopoietin mutation in congenital a megakaryocytic thrombocytopenia treatable with romiplostim. EMBO Molecular Medicine, 10, 63–75. https://doi.org/10.15252/emmm.201708168 (accessed on 12th June 2025).

50. Pezhman, L., Tahrani, A. A., & Chimen, M. (2021). Dysregulation of leukocyte trafficking in type 2 diabetes: Mechanisms and potential therapeutic avenues. Frontiers in Cell and Developmental Biology, 9. https://doi.org/10.3389/fcell.2021.624184 (accessed on 12th June 2025).

51. Qin, C., Zhou, L. Q., Hu, Z., Zhang, S., Yang, S., Yu, T., Xie, C., et al. (2020). Dysregulation of immune response in patients with coronavirus 2019 (COVID-19) in Wuhan, China. Clinical Infectious Diseases, 71, 762–768. https://doi.org/10.1093/cid/ciaa248 (accessed on 12th June 2025).

52. Rajagukguk, T., Rajagukguk, D. L., & Aritonang, E. (2023). Description of urine sediment in diabetes mellites patients at Bunda Thamrin Hospital Medan in 2023. Journal Analis Laboratorium Medik. https://www.semanticscholar.org/paper/aa889ae03673f4c7be20a862e3ae78fc1214ad94 (accessed on 12th June 2025).

53. Saad, A., de Lima, M., Anand, S., Bhatt, V. R., Bookout, R., Chen, G., Couriel, D. R., et al. (2020). Hematopoietic cell transplantation, version 2.2020, NCCN clinical practice guidelines in oncology. Journal of the National Comprehensive Cancer Network, 18, 599–634. https://doi.org/10.6004/jnccn.2020.0021 (accessed on 12th June 2025).

54. Saiz-Sierra, L., Marull Arnall, A., Nieto-Moragas, J., Deulofeu, M., Jiménez Romero, O., Mademont, I., Obón Ferrer, M., et al. (2024). Detection of giant cytoplasmic inclusions in a pediatric patient with recurrent infections: A case report. Advances in Laboratory Medicine, 5, 221–225. https://www.semanticscholar.org/paper/77726f86a325573068a66eac4a57cac903c8477e (accessed on 12th June 2025).

55. Shen, C. L., & Wu, Y. F. (2022). Flow cytometry for evaluating platelet immunophenotyping and function in patients with thrombocytopenia. Tzu Chi Medical Journal, 34, 381–387. https://doi.org/10.4103/tcmj.tcmj_117_22 (accessed on 12th June 2025).

56. Shi, S., Qin, M., Shen, B., Cai, Y., Liu, T., Yang, F., Gong, W., et al. (2020). Association of cardiac injury with mortality in hospitalized patients with COVID-19 in Wuhan, China. JAMA Cardiology, 5, 802–802. https://doi.org/10.1001/jamacardio.2020.0950 (accessed on 12th June 2025).

57. Silva, G., de Oliveira Silva, M. S., Nascimento, D., Lima Silva, E., Gouvêa, F. F. F., de França Lopes, L. G., Araújo, A. V., et al. (2021). Nitric oxide as a central molecule in hypertension: Focus on the vasorelaxant activity of new nitric oxide donors. Biology, 10, 1041. https://

doi.org/10.3390/biology10101041 (accessed on 12th June 2025).

58. St-Germain, L. E., Castellana, B., Baltayeva, J., & Beristain, A. G. (2020). Maternal obesity and the uterine immune cell landscape: The shaping role of inflammation. International Journal of Molecular Sciences, 21, 3776. https://doi.org/10.3390/ijms21113776 (accessed on 12th June 2025).
59. Staff, A. C., Fjeldstad, H. E., Fosheim, I. K., Moe, K., Turowski, G., Johnsen, G. M., Alnæs-Katjavivi, P., et al. (2020). Failure of physiological transformation and spiral artery arthrosis: Their roles in preeclampsia. American Journal of Obstetrics and Gynecology, 226, S895–S906. https://doi.org/10.1016/j.ajog.2020.09.026 (accessed on 12th June 2025).
60. Sundd, P., Gladwin, M. T., & Novelli, E. M. (2018). Pathophysiology of sickle cell disease. Annual Review of Pathology: Mechanisms of Disease, 14, 263–292. https://doi.org/10.1146/annurev-pathmechdis-012418-012838 (accessed on 12th June 2025).
61. Szczerbal, I., & Świtoński, M. (2020). Genetic disorders of sex development in cats: An update. Animal Reproduction Science, 216, 106353. https://doi.org/10.1016/j.anireprosci.2020.106353 (accessed on 12th June 2025).
62. Tabas, I., & Lichtman, A. H. (2017). Monocyte-macrophages and T cells in atherosclerosis. Immunity, 47, 621–634. https://doi.org/10.1016/j.immuni.2017.09.008 (accessed on 12th June 2025).
63. Tangye, S. G., Al–Herz, W., Bousfiha, A., Chatila, T. A., Cunningham-Rundles, C., Etzioni, A., Franco, J. L., et al. (2020). Human inborn errors of immunity: 2019 update on the classification from the International Union of Immunological Societies Expert Committee. Journal of Clinical Immunology, 40, 24–64. https://doi.org/10.1007/s10875-019-00737-x (accessed on 12th June 2025).
64. Tilg, H., Adolph, T. E., & Moschen, A. R. (2020). Multiple parallel hits hypothesis in nonalcoholic fatty liver disease: Revisited after a decade. Hepatology, 73, 833–842. https://doi.org/10.1002/hep.31518 (accessed on 12th June 2025).
65. Torres, T., Filipe, P., Menezes Brandão, F., Figueiredo, A., Pinto Soares, A., Sousa Basto, A., Rebelo, C., et al. (2023). Epidemiology of psoriasis in Portugal: A population-based study. Acta Medica Portuguesa. https://www.semanticscholar.org/paper/2212b929e6450009dba9de42612fb8b74f852eb1 (accessed on 12th June 2025).
66. Tunkel, A. R., Hasbun, R., Bhimraj, A., Byers, K., Kaplan, S. L., Scheld, W. M., van de Beek, D., et al. (2016). 2017 Infectious Diseases Society of America's Clinical Practice Guidelines for Healthcare-Associated Ventriculitis and Meningitis. Clinical Infectious Diseases, 64, e34–e65. https://doi.org/10.1093/cid/ciw861 (accessed on 12th June 2025).
67. Voet, S., Srinivasan, S., Lamkanfi, M., & Loo, G. (2019). Inflammasomes in neuroinflammatory and neurodegenerative diseases. EMBO Molecular Medicine, 11. https://doi.org/10.15252/emmm.201810248 (accessed on 12th June 2025).
68. Wu, Z., Xu, J., Hu, Y., Peng, X., Zhang, Z., Yao, X., & Peng, Q. (2024). The roles of IRF8 in nonspecific orbital inflammation: An integrated analysis by bioinformatics and machine learning. Journal of Ophthalmic Inflammation and Infection, 14. https://www.semanticscholar.org/paper/8548d1408cae05487c3942cf5f1d3be5c5107666 (accessed on 12th June 2025).
69. Yu, P., Zhang, X., Liu, N., Tang, L., Peng, C., & Chen, X. (2021). Proptosis: Mechanisms and

diseases. Signal Transduction and Targeted Therapy, 6. https://doi.org/10.1038/s41392-021-00507-5 (accessed on 12th June 2025).

70. Zhao, H., Wu, L., Yan, G., Chen, Y., Zhou, M., Wu, Y., & Li, Y. (2021). Inflammation and tumor progression: Signaling pathways and targeted intervention. Signal Transduction and Targeted Therapy, 6. https://doi.org/10.1038/s41392-021-00658-5 (accessed on 12th June 2025).

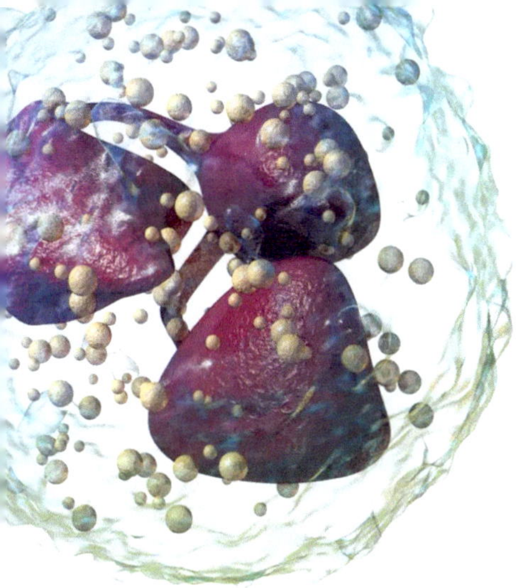

Chapter 8

PLATELET DISORDERS

Contents

Introduction....179

8.1. Types of Platelet Disorders....180

8.2. Pathophysiology of Platelet Disorders....184

8.3. Diagnosis of Platelet Disorders....189

8.4. Treatment and Management of Platelet Disorders....194

Summary....199

References....200

Introduction

Platelet disorder study is a significant branch of hematology, highlighting the need to understand the complexities of platelet function and regulation. Platelets are integral hemostatic particles, playing a protective role against bleeding and facilitating wound healing; thus, their dysfunction has profound clinical implications. Alterations in platelet production, activation, or survival can result in a spectrum of conditions, ranging from thrombocytopenia to thrombocytopathy, underscoring the importance of accurate diagnosis and therapeutic strategies. Recent advances have renewed interest in platelet disorders, particularly the therapeutic potential of targeted therapies. For instance, recent advances in radionuclide therapy illustrate a move towards more targeted action with reduced damage to normal tissues. With our enhanced understanding, there is a growing need to classify and manage these disorders effectively, thereby improving patient outcomes and optimizing treatment protocols (Aquilina et al., 2008; Akin et al., 2011) (Figure 8.1).

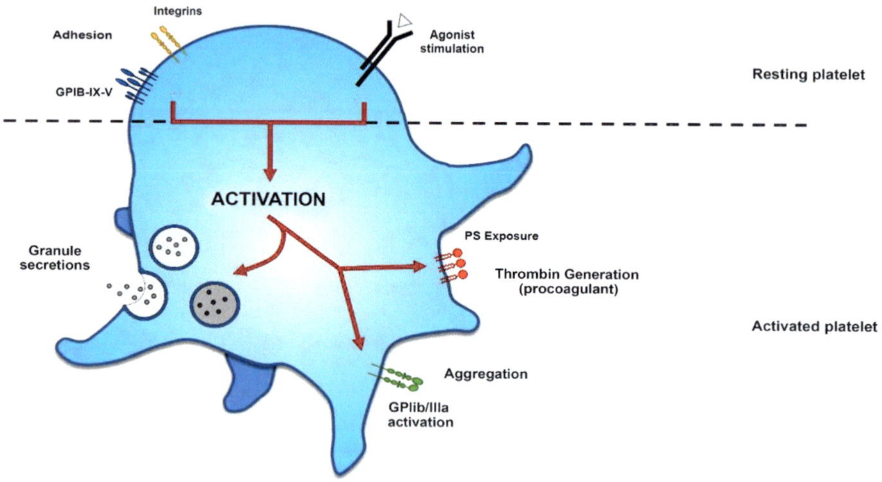

Figure 8.1. Anomalies in platelet production, activation, or survival can lead to a spectrum of conditions, from thrombocytopenia to thrombocytopathy, highlighting the importance of accurate diagnosis and treatment modalities.

Source: https://www.mdpi.com/jcm/jcm-10-00894/article_deploy/html/images/jcm-10-00894-g001.png.

8.1. Types of Platelet Disorders

It is highly essential to know the various types of platelet disorders so that they can be diagnosed and treated to cure hematological diseases. The majority of platelet disorders are either quantitative or qualitative disorders. Quantitative disorders such as thrombocytopenia are a deficiency in the number of plates, and this may occur due to numerous reasons such as low production in the bone marrow or excessive destruction in the circulation. Contrarily, qualitative disorders such as Glanzmann's thrombasthenia present normal platelet counts but impaired function, leading to abnormal response to clotting. Balancing the clinical significance of these differences, the evolving field of treatment approaches has come under scrutiny in recent studies, not only to emphasize the effectiveness of platelet-rich plasma (PRP) treatments for chosen ailments but also the diversity of results based on preparation methods and patient responsiveness (Shahbaz et al., 2024). In addition, the development of artificial intelligence for blood smear analysis could be pivotal in identifying and classifying these disorders correctly (Perumal et al., 2024).

8.1.1. Thrombocytopenia: Definition and Causes

Thrombocytopenia, characterized by a platelet count of fewer than 150,000 per microliter of blood, is a significant condition within the group of platelet disorders. The falling number of platelets can be caused by numerous etiologies, including decreased production within the bone marrow, increased destruction of the platelets, or sequestration of the platelets within the spleen. Bone marrow diseases, such as leukemia or aplastic anemia, can significantly alter platelet production, while systemic illnesses like immune thrombocytopenic purpura (ITP) lead to increased platelet destruction due to autoimmune mechanisms. Systemic illness, particularly cirrhosis of the liver, contributes to coagulopathies, which enhance bleeding susceptibility in patients. Inherited advanced liver disease is associated with multifactorial clotting abnormalities, making awareness of these associations crucial in clinical practice (Bacalbașa et al., 2019). In addition, prolonged bleeding tendencies during dental treatment underscore the necessity for careful assessment of patients with acquired coagulopathy to ensure that treatment protocols are congruent with the inherent pathophysiologic processes (Barber et al., 2003) (Figure 8.2).

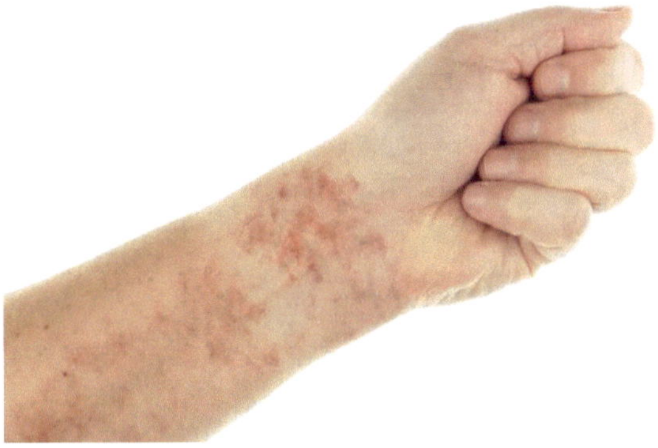

Figure 8.2. Thrombocytopenia.

Source: https://drkarthikrengaraj.com/wp-content/uploads/sites/18/2024/09/Immune-Thrombocytopenia-ITP.jpg.

8.1.2. Thrombocytopathy: Definition and Mechanisms

Thrombocytopathy is a group of platelet diseases characterized by impaired platelet function, in the absence of normal platelet number and structure. The abnormalities are caused by either inherited or acquired conditions that lead to impaired hemostasis and a bleeding tendency. Pathogenic processes most commonly refer to defects in platelet activation, aggregation, or granule release that inhibit the physiological response to vascular injury. Mutations of the key proteins in the platelet activation pathways, such as glycoproteins and integrins, are typically responsible for hereditary thrombocytopathies. Acquired abnormalities also might result from drugs, systemic disease, or environmental poisons that disrupt normal platelet function. For instance, thrombotic thrombocytopenic purpura (TTP) illustrates how altered platelet function can lead to severe clinical manifestations, including ischemic strokes and thrombotic events, underscoring the importance of understanding mechanisms of thrombocytopathy in effective disease management (Breum et al., 2023; Biso et al., 2023).

8.1.3. Inherited Platelet Disorders

Inherited platelet disorders (IPDs) constitute a heterogeneous group of conditions resulting from the effects of genetic mutations on platelet formation and function. The diagnostic difficulties of IPDs underscore the role played by innovative genomic technologies, such as high-throughput sequencing (HTS), in revolutionizing the rates of diagnosis. For instance, in a clinical study of 2,396 thrombotic and bleeding patients, molecular diagnosis was achieved in nearly half of them, indicating the importance of genetic testing in the clinic (Downes et al., 2019). Further studies on candidate genes have revealed numerous defects in platelet function, with evidence of intricate genetic pathways underlying such disorders, particularly those involving Gi signaling and secretion defects. These genetic underpinnings are helpful as they not only facilitate diagnosis but also provide insight into personalized treatment protocols for those affected, thereby improving patient outcomes for inherited platelet disorders (Figure 8.3).

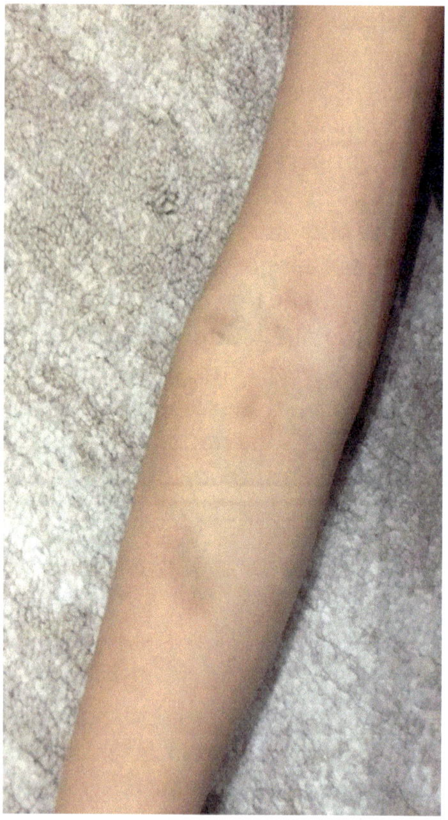

Figure 8.3. Inherited platelet disorders (IPDs).

Source: https://assets.cureus.com/uploads/figure/file/166370/article_river_64f904b02c4c11eba4b1f9c0b8e63a3d-Figure-1.png.

8.1.4. Acquired Platelet Disorders

Acquired Platelet Disorders are a significant category of hemostatic disorders involving the dysfunction or deficiency of platelets, typically initiated by an underlying condition rather than a genetic etiology. The disorders are caused by various etiologies like autoimmune diseases, drug action, or infection, and lead to a multifactorial interaction that renders their diagnosis and management difficult. For instance, patients with diseases such as systemic lupus erythematosus can produce antibodies that inhibit platelet function and disrupt normal blood clotting. Moreover, their diagnosis always begins with a full blood count (CBC) that identifies platelet abnormalities in both quantity and morphology (Chalmers et al., 2009). Knowledge of the complex mechanisms that govern acquired disorders not only improves diagnostic accuracy but also guides therapeutic interventions, i.e., treating the causative factors or adjusting current medications. Lastly, increased patient awareness is necessary to improve patient outcomes and prevent severe complications (Franchini et al., 2017).

8.1.5. Immune Thrombocytopenic Purpura (ITP)

ITP is an intricate platelet disorder characterized by an unusually low platelet count resulting from enhanced platelet destruction and reduced platelet production.

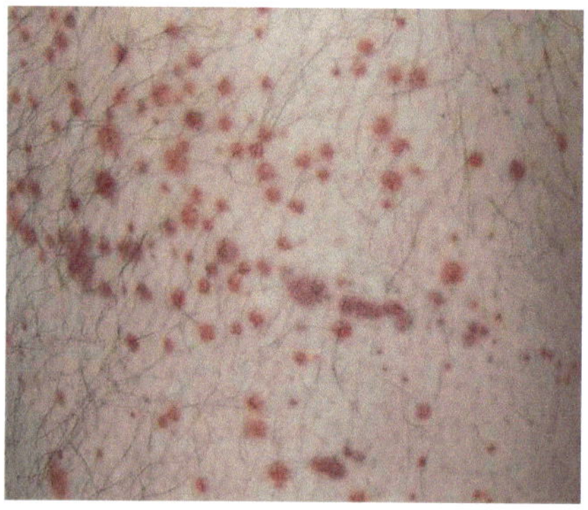

Figure 8.4. Immune thrombocytopenic purpura (ITP) represents a complex platelet disorder characterized by a markedly low platelet count, resulting from both accelerated destruction and inadequate production of platelets.

Source: https://upload.wikimedia.org/wikipedia/commons/thumb/9/92/Purpura.jpg/640px-Purpura.jpg.

Central to this is the production of autoantibodies directed against platelet glycoproteins, which are harmful to platelet survival in circulation (Amadori et al., 2008). In addition, various immune modulation mechanisms have been identified to account for the complexity of these disorders. Traditional treatment modalities in ITP generally focus on immunosuppression or splenectomy to decrease platelet utilization. Recent advances have involved the addition of new thrombopoietic medications, such as AMG 531 and eltrombopag, which stimulate the production of platelets in refractory patients who do not respond to conventional therapy (Amadori et al., 2008). This evolving therapeutic landscape not only underlines the significance of understanding ITP's mechanistic foundation but also puts in sharp relief the need for individualized treatment regimens in managing this multifactorial illness (Figure 8.4).

8.1.6. Thrombotic Thrombocytopenic Purpura (TTP)

TTP is a potentially life-threatening platelet disorder that is characterized by a pentad of clinical manifestations: microangiopathic hemolytic anemia, thrombocytopenia, neurological dysfunction, renal failure, and fever. TTP results from a severe deficiency of the von Willebrand factor-cleaving protease ADAMTS13, which causes abnormal multimerization of large von Willebrand factor multimers, leading to the widespread formation of microthrombi. Clinically, TTP presents with altered mental status, which is a distinguishing characteristic from other similar conditions, such as hemolytic uremic syndrome and ITP (Megan et al., 2024). The urgency in diagnosis of TTP comes from its potential for rapid clinical deterioration and high mortality if left untreated. Apart from that, the severity of the clinical presentation can be overwhelming to healthcare providers; thus, proper social histories and laboratory investigations are crucial in the early identification of TTP (Perez et al., 2024). Effective and timely intervention can greatly reduce morbidity and mortality due to the serious condition.

8.1.7. Bernard-Soulier Syndrome

Bernard-Soulier Syndrome (BSS) is a rare congenital platelet disorder that has glycoprotein (GP) Ib/IX/V deficiency and defective platelet adhesion to the vascular wall. It is an autosomal recessive condition and is also characterized by the presence of large platelets, or macrothrombocytes, which can be observed in laboratory investigations as well. Clinically, patients with BSS are typically admitted with severe to moderate bleeding disorders, such as mucocutaneous bleeding, and it can be quite morbid. Treatment options are limited, despite this, and options may include platelet transfusions, particularly in cases of excessive bleeding, similar to those used for other platelet disorders, such as immune thrombocytopenia (Cooper et al., 2019). Moreover, an understanding of the molecular pathology of BSS would be essential because it would facilitate the use of targeted therapies and outcomes within a multidisciplinary model of care, as has been the experience in other syndromes, such as Glanzmann thrombasthenia (Botero et al., 2020) (Figure 8.5).

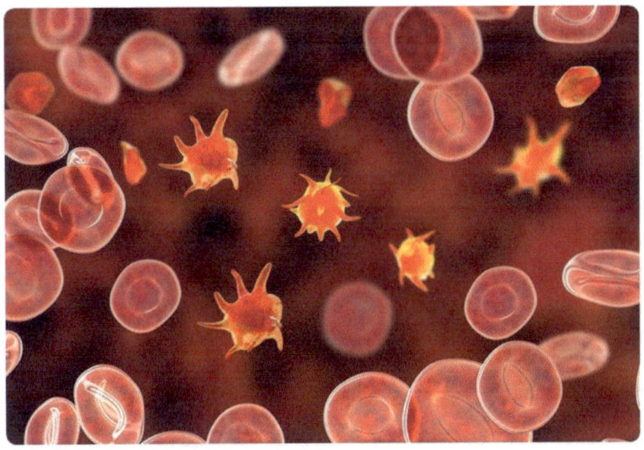

Figure 8.5. Bernard-soulier syndrome (BSS).

Source: https://d2jx2rerrg6sh3.cloudfront.net/image-handler/picture/2021/12/shutterstock_2012190989.jpg.

8.1.8. Glanzmann Thrombasthenia

Glanzmann Thrombasthenia (GT) is a major inherited disorder of platelet function characterized by a deficiency of glycoprotein IIb/IIIa, a crucial component for platelet aggregation. This defect results in a characteristic bleeding tendency that can heavily impact the quality of life in patients, especially in females and girls who present with heavy menstrual bleeding (HMB) as the main symptom. Notably, GT poses substantial obstetrical challenges, as the risk of postpartum hemorrhage (PPH) is markedly heightened during pregnancy and delivery, with studies indicating that 63% of affected pregnancies result in PPH, necessitating platelet and red blood cell (RBC) transfusions to manage bleeding crises (Obeng-Tuudah et al., 2025). Furthermore, the complex management of HMB and PPH in GT requires a multidisciplinary approach, incorporating a combination of hormonal therapies and hemostatic agents such as recombinant factor VIIa to mitigate complications and reduce the potential for alloimmunization during platelet transfusions (Althaus et al., 2024).

8.1.9. Essential Thrombocythemia

Essential Thrombocythemia (ET) is a myeloproliferative neoplasm (MPN) involving overproduction of platelets, usually as a result of mutation in genes like JAK2, CALR, or MPL. ET can cause serious complications, and the most common cause of morbidity and mortality in ET patients is thrombosis. The pathophysiology leading to thrombotic risk is multi-factorial, not only including increased platelet counts but also the existence of qualitative abnormalities that increase their reactivity and aggregation. In recent studies, cytokines produced by both clonal and non-clonal cells have been shown to lead to a chronic state of inflammation, thereby worsening thrombotic tendencies in ET patients (Heller et al., 2019). Moreover, these patients exhibit unique risk factors for splanchnic vein thrombosis (SVT), suggesting specific interactions between activated blood cells and endothelial environments that warrant further investigation (How et al., 2016). Understanding these mechanisms is crucial for developing targeted therapeutic strategies to manage ET and mitigate thrombotic risks (Figure 8.6).

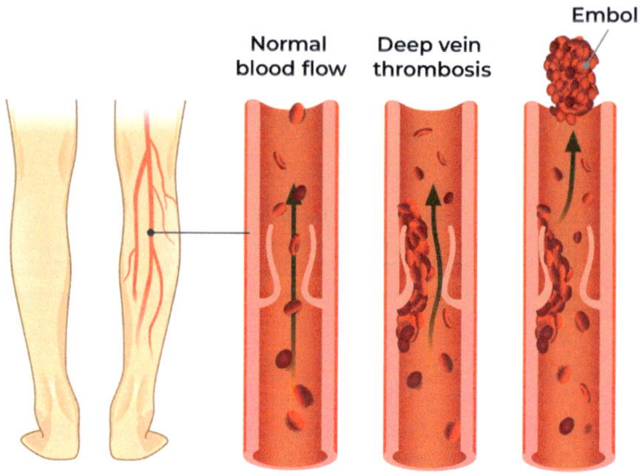

Figure 8.6. Essential thrombocythemia (ET).

Source: https://leukeemia.ee/wp-content/uploads/2022/05/verevool_eng-12.png.

8.2. Pathophysiology of Platelet Disorders

One of the key facets of understanding the pathophysiology of platelet disorders is examining the study of MPNs, which are renowned for their significant role in prothrombotic states, such as SVT. Clinical presentation of MPN-related SVT is multifold, shaped by risk factors such as younger age, female gender, and genetic predispositions, particularly the JAK2 V617F mutation. Such observations suggest the presence of an underlying process that differs from the mechanisms of arterial or deep venous thrombosis (DVT) typically, and therefore, the disease processes involved here are more complex. Furthermore, the interaction between activated blood cells and the unique endothelial milieu of the splanchnic circulation can facilitate thrombosis formation in susceptible patients, justifying further investigation into the molecular kinetics of platelet behavior and thrombus formation in MPNs (Estes et al., 1962; How et al., 2016).

8.2.1. Role of Bone Marrow in Platelet Production

The bone marrow is also essential in the production of platelets, as it serves as the primary location for thrombopoiesis—the process by which platelets are produced from megakaryocytes.

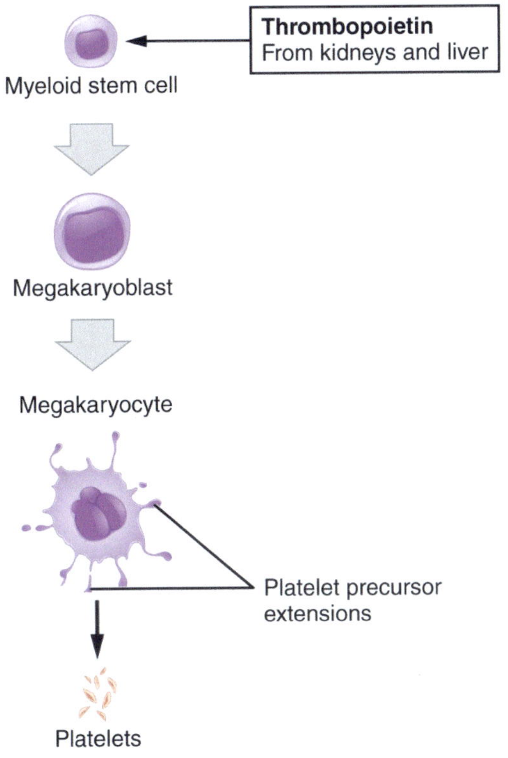

Figure 8.7. The bone marrow plays a crucial role in the production of platelets, acting as the primary site for thrombopoiesis—the process through which platelets are generated from megakaryocytes.

Source: https://upload.wikimedia.org/wikipedia/commons/8/84/1908_Platelet_Development.jpg.

These platelets mature and fragment in a special manner, where they discharge platelets directly into the bloodstream. This function is strictly regulated through thrombopoietin (TPO), a hormone synthesized mainly by the liver and kidneys, that regulates megakaryocyte growth and development. Even when bone marrow function is compromised, as in various platelet disorders, it may lead to insufficient platelet counts, resulting in a thrombocytopenic state and an increased risk of bleeding. Moreover, the dysregulation of the TPO-MPL signaling pathway can exacerbate these conditions, revealing a complex interplay between hormonal regulation and marrow health in maintaining adequate platelet levels (Ian et al., 2021). Understanding these mechanisms is vital for developing targeted therapies to manage platelet-related diseases in clinical practice, which can enhance patient outcomes (Patrick et al., 2020) (Figure 8.7).

8.2.2. Mechanisms of Platelet Activation

Elucidation of the mechanisms of platelet activation is crucial for clarifying various platelet disorders, particularly dysregulated hemostatic responses. Platelet activation begins with receptor-mediated interactions with agonists, including collagen, thrombin, and adenosine diphosphate (ADP), which trigger a cascade of intracellular signaling events. One key signaling pathway involves the stimulation of phospholipase C, resulting in an increase in inositol trisphosphate (IP3) and diacylglycerol (DAG) levels, which facilitates calcium release and platelet granule secretion. These signal events also amplify the expression of activation markers, such as P-selectin, on the platelet surface, which helps the platelet interact with other cells and advances the process of thrombus formation. Recent reports, including those detailing vaccine-induced thrombocytopenia, have highlighted the complexity of platelet activation mechanisms, revealing an immune-mediated pathway in which antibodies target platelet factor 4, leading to severe thrombocytopenia and thrombotic events (Sangli et al., 2021; Eun-Lee et al., 2021). These insights highlight the need for ongoing research to develop targeted therapies for platelet-related disorders.

8.2.3. Genetic Mutations and Their Effects

These mutations deeply influence different platelet disorders, which occur mostly in their function in defective proteins that are integral to hemostasis. For example, von Willebrand disease (VWD) results from mutations in the gene that codes for von Willebrand factor (vWF). This factor plays a critical role in the adhesion of platelets. The disorder is autosomal and results in varying degrees of susceptibility to bleeding, establishing the need for proper genotypic analysis to recognize the specific variant that contributes to VWD (Blanco et al., 2017). Furthermore, MPNs, characterized by mutations such as JAK2 V617F, can predispose individuals to thrombotic events like SVT, highlighting the interplay between genetic factors and environmental influences in disease manifestation (How et al., 2016). These examples illustrate how genetic mutations not only serve as a key indicator of platelet dysfunction but also direct treatments, underlining the necessity of molecular knowledge in effective treatment (Figure 8.8).

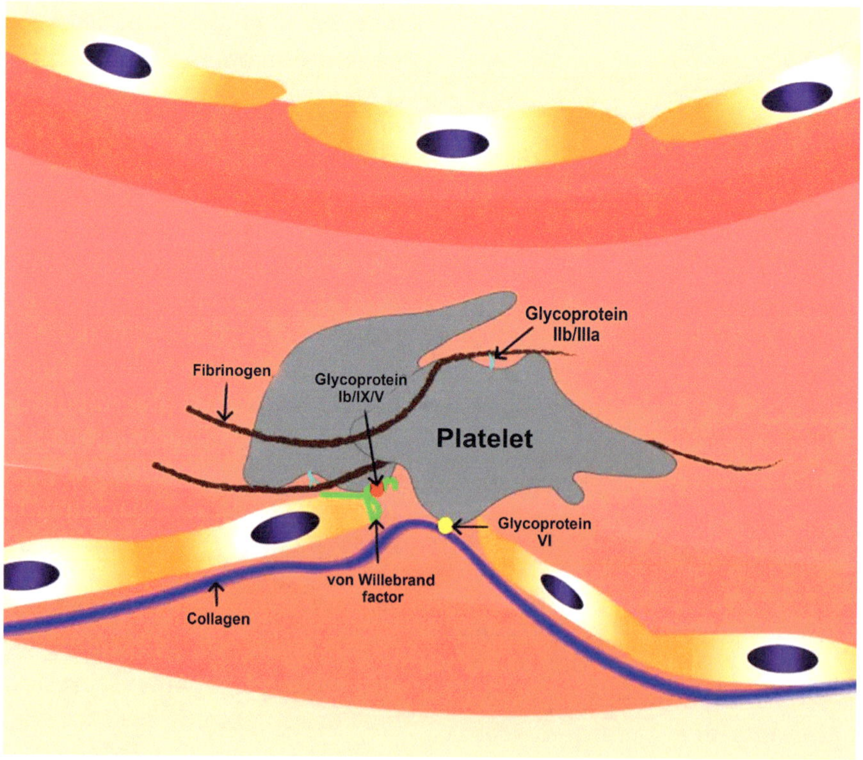

Figure 8.8. von Willebrand disease (VWD) arises from mutations affecting the von Willebrand factor (VWF), crucial for platelet adhesion.

Source: https://myhematology.com/wp-content/uploads/2023/10/vWF.png.

8.2.4. Immune System Involvement

The immune response plays a crucial role in the pathophysiology of platelet disorders, particularly through its effects on coagulation pathways. In multiple sclerosis (MS), for instance, the activation of resident innate immune cells, such as microglia, is accompanied by the deposition of thrombin and fibrinogen, which can further amplify neuronal injury and inflammation, reflecting the dual role of the immune system in disease induction and tissue damage (Adams et al., 2018). Furthermore, in infectious diseases such as Chagas disease, the protozoan Trypanosoma cruzi induces severe thrombocytopenia, attributed to the action of its virulence factor, trans-sialidase. This enzyme alters the sialic acid content on platelets, accelerating their clearance from circulation and linking immune responses directly to platelet dysfunction (Campetella et al., 2005). Thus, the relationship between the immune system and platelet disorders is complex, underscoring the need for targeted therapeutic strategies that consider both hematological and immunological factors in managing these conditions.

8.2.5. Environmental Factors Influencing Platelet Function

The interaction of environmental components and platelet function is important in the study of platelet disorders. Some of the elements that could have a significant effect on platelet activation and aggregation processes, which ultimately influence hemostatic responses, include temperature, pH, and shear stress. For instance, increased shear stress, commonly experienced under conditions of turbulent blood flow, may stimulate platelet activation, thus predisposing to thrombotic events. Recently, it has also been established that oxidative stress impairs platelet bioenergetics, leading to dysregulated function and an increased incidence of disorders such as thrombocytopenia and thrombocytosis.

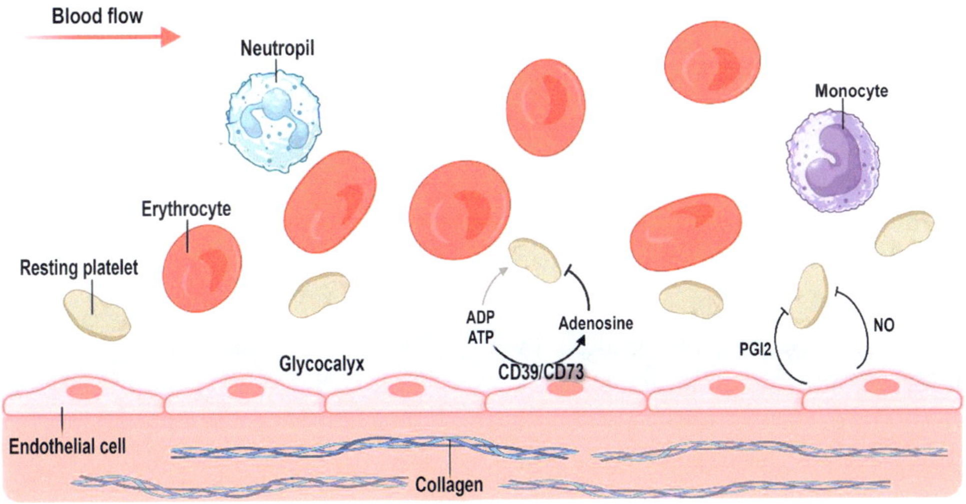

Figure 8.9. The interplay between environmental factors and platelet function is crucial in understanding platelet disorders.

Source: https://www.mdpi.com/ijms/ijms-24-14724/article_deploy/html/images/ijms-24-14724-g001.png.

The involvement of mitochondrial health is particularly noteworthy, because malfunctioning mitochondria have been associated with a number of defects in platelet function and the overall viability of platelets, which underscores the necessity to investigate further how environmental stressors impact mitochondrial dynamics in platelets (Zhang et al., 2024). In this regard, uncovering these environmental determinants is crucial for developing targeted therapeutic interventions and improving clinical outcomes in patients with platelet disorders (Sumbalová et al., 2024) (Figure 8.9).

8.2.6. Interaction with Other Blood Components

The interaction of platelets with other blood components is pivotal in understanding platelet disorders and their associated complications. In chronic MPN, for instance, the balance between thrombosis and hemorrhage is often disrupted, highlighting the intricate interplay among platelets, leukocytes, and erythrocytes. Increased cytokine levels not only exacerbate the inflammatory condition but also promote platelet activation, which leads to heterotypic aggregation with leukocytes —a process crucial in thromboinflammatory events associated with MPN. This results in a paradox where the patient exhibits both thrombotic and bleeding tendencies, highlighting the intricate role of platelets beyond conventional hemostasis (Heller et al., 2019).

In addition, erythrocytes are known to express numerous adhesion molecules that facilitate their interaction with activated platelets, potentially affecting coagulation processes and inflammation (Oliveira et al., 2010). Such interactions highlight the importance of developing a comprehensive understanding of platelet disorders within the frame of complex blood component interactions.

8.2.7. Role of Cytokines in Platelet Disorders

The intricate relationship between cytokines and platelet disorders is pivotal in understanding both the pathophysiology and potential therapeutic targets for various hematologic conditions. Cytokines, as signaling molecules in the immune system, play a significant role in regulating platelet production and activation. For example, inflammatory cytokines such as interleukin-6 and tumor necrosis factor-alpha have been observed to increase the release of platelets from the bone marrow and activate their release, potentially aggravating thrombotic complications in diseases like essential thrombocythemia. In addition, certain chemokines present may be used as biomarkers to distinguish between diverse pathologies of platelet disorders, where high levels might reflect underlying inflammation contributing to disease progression. This reinforces the need for continual investigation into how cytokines are mediated and work, especially in relation to their dual ability to induce both inflammation and thrombosis, as identified in inflammatory markers analysis and their clinical application (Cavanagh et al., 2018; Cammisotto et al., 2017) (Figure 8.10).

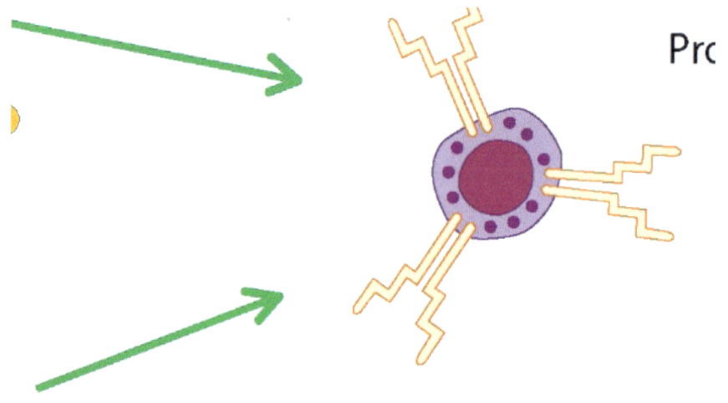

Figure 8.10. Cytokines, as signaling molecules in the immune system, significantly influence platelet production and activation.

Source: https://www.dental-update.co.uk/media/3f2momz2/denu-2017-44-8-753_f05.jpg.

8.2.8. Impact of Chronic Diseases on Platelet Function

Chronic diseases significantly alter platelet function, leading to an increased risk of bleeding and thrombotic events, thus complicating the management of patients with coagulopathies. For instance, liver diseases such as cirrhosis disrupt the delicate balance of hemostasis, as they impair the synthesis of clotting factors and lead to platelet dysfunction through various mechanisms, including alterations in platelet reactivity and survival (Bacalbașa et al., 2019). These complications are further compounded by systemic conditions that can diminish the effectiveness of anticoagulant therapies, leading to adverse outcomes during surgical interventions and invasive procedures (Barber et al., 2003). Additionally, the inability of medical professionals to accurately assess bleeding risks in patients with these chronic conditions often leads to suboptimal treatment decisions. Therefore, it is essential to understand the complex effect of chronic diseases on platelet function for the development of specific therapeutic interventions that counteract the danger of platelet disorders in those populations.

8.2.9. Diagnostic Markers in Platelet Disorders

The identification of diagnostic markers in platelet disorders is essential for accurate disease classification and effective treatment planning. Platelet pathologies, which can range from thrombocytopenia to qualitative defects, necessitate nuanced diagnostic strategies that often incorporate biomarkers. Recent studies have highlighted the importance of evaluating circulating protein biomarkers that reflect various pathophysiological mechanisms involved in platelet dysfunction, including oxidative stress and vascular inflammation. These biomarkers not only assist in risk stratification of patients but also optimize clinical decision-making by providing insight into their cardiovascular risk profile, which is significant for diseases such as acute coronary syndrome. Diabetic patients, in particular, gain much from early intervention (Heeschen et al., 2005). Consequently, a comprehensive understanding of these diagnostic markers could lead to targeted therapies that improve patient outcomes, potentially reducing the incidence of severe complications associated with these disorders (Balzo et al., 2016) (Figure 8.11).

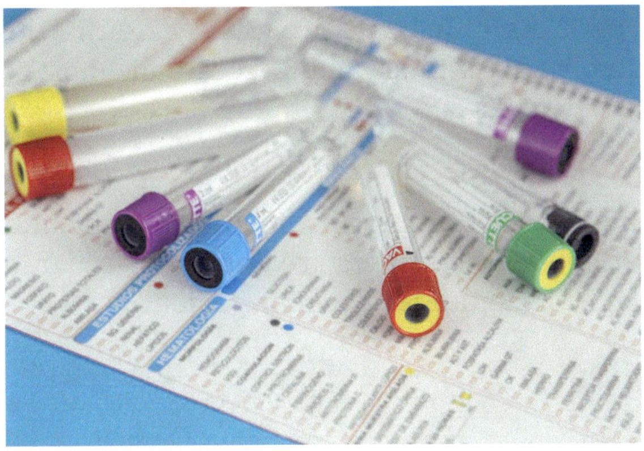

Figure 8.11. Diagnostic markers in platelet disorders.

Source: https://www.roswellpark.org/sites/default/files/styles/1600x800/public/2020-06/adobestock_216855468.jpeg?itok=FOvbVXfL.

8.3. Diagnosis of Platelet Disorders

Accurate diagnosis of platelet disorders is crucial for effective management and treatment, as the symptoms can vary widely and mimic those of other medical conditions. The diagnostic process typically begins with a thorough clinical history and physical examination, followed by laboratory tests to evaluate platelet function and number. Key assays may include platelet count, morphology, and function tests to assess aggregation and secretion responses. For instance, VWD, the most common autosomal bleeding disorder, requires specific assays such as VWF:Ag and VWF:RCo to ascertain the presence and function of vWF, as well as genotypic analysis to evaluate inherited variants (Blanco et al., 2017). Additionally, conditions such as mitochondrial neurogastrointestinal encephalomyopathy (MNGIE) underscore the complexity of differential diagnosis in platelet disorders, where patients frequently encounter diagnostic delays due to overlapping symptoms with other diseases (Bax et al., 2020). Thus, a multidisciplinary approach is essential for establishing a timely and accurate diagnosis.

8.3.1. Clinical Symptoms and Signs

The clinical symptoms and signs associated with platelet disorders are critical for accurate diagnosis and effective management.

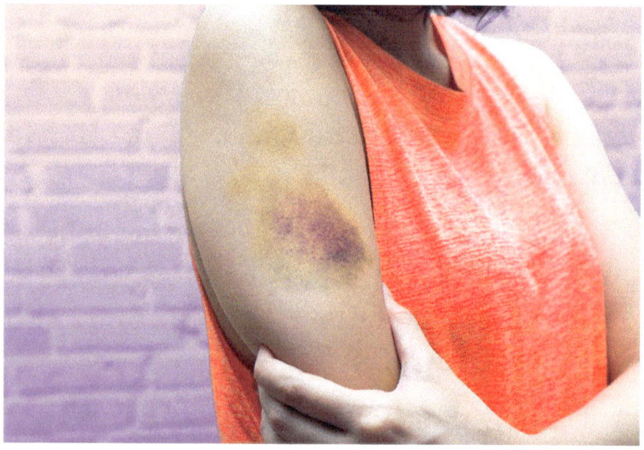

Figure 8.12. Patients experiencing abnormal bleeding patterns, such as easy bruising or prolonged bleeding from minor cuts, often present with symptoms indicative of underlying platelet dysfunction.

Source: https://www.health.com/thmb/qZhv7pR4NsmUukvILTmKbTOsriA=/2000x0/filters:no_upscale():max_bytes(150000):strip_icc()/bruise-GettyImages-1059076258-25904d34b90544e7bc58bd6d1ec4d47f.jpg.

Patients experiencing abnormal bleeding patterns, such as easy bruising or prolonged bleeding from minor cuts, often present with symptoms indicative of underlying platelet dysfunction. These manifestations can arise from various conditions, ranging from inherited disorders to acquired syndromes, each posing unique challenges in clinical interpretation. For instance, abnormalities in mast cells may affect platelet function, leading to a spectrum of clinical presentations, as noted in research on mast cell activation syndromes (MCAS) (Akin et al., 2011). Additionally, secondary headaches during significant medical scenarios like pregnancy may also represent an emergent symptom of severe conditions linked to platelet disorders, such as eclampsia or stroke (Negro et al., 2017). Hence, recognizing these clinical signs is paramount for initiating timely interventions and avoiding severe complications in affected individuals (Figure 8.12).

8.3.2. Laboratory Tests for Platelet Count

It is essential to comprehend the laboratory investigations of platelet count in the diagnosis and treatment of various platelet disorders. The complete blood count or the full blood count, which is a basic test carried out in hospital and general practitioner settings, presents crucial information regarding a patient's hematologic status. This test enables clinicians to efficiently examine not only platelet count but also other blood components, making differential diagnosis easier (Chalmers et al., 2009). In case of detection of abnormality, further investigations with coagulation screen and blood film report can be conducted to identify underlying pathology. Additionally, some patient groups, such as liver cirrhosis patients, typically come with complex clotting disorders and thus need comprehensive hemostatic examinations before surgery (Bacalbașa et al., 2019). Therefore, an inclusive laboratory test strategy is crucial for developing the most effective management and treatment strategies in patients with platelet disorders.

8.3.3. Platelet Function Tests

The evaluation of platelet function is critical for diagnosing various platelet disorders, including Glanzmann's thrombasthenia (GT), which is characterized by normal platelet counts but impaired aggregation responses to physiological agonists. Platelet function tests are instrumental in identifying such disorders, providing insights into the underlying mechanisms of platelet dysfunction. These tests can reveal qualitative abnormalities, such as those caused by mutations in the genes encoding GPIIb or GPIIIa, leading to a heterogeneous genetic landscape that complicates diagnosis (Ethayathulla et al., 2008). Accurate assessment is vital not only for understanding the specific disorder but also for determining appropriate treatment strategies. Furthermore, advancements in molecular testing technologies enhance the ability to correlate genotype with phenotype, underscoring the importance of these evaluations in clinical practice. In light of ongoing research, the role of platelet function tests remains pivotal for guiding therapeutic decisions in individuals with diverse platelet disorders, including GT (Wahab et al., 2020) (Figure 8.13).

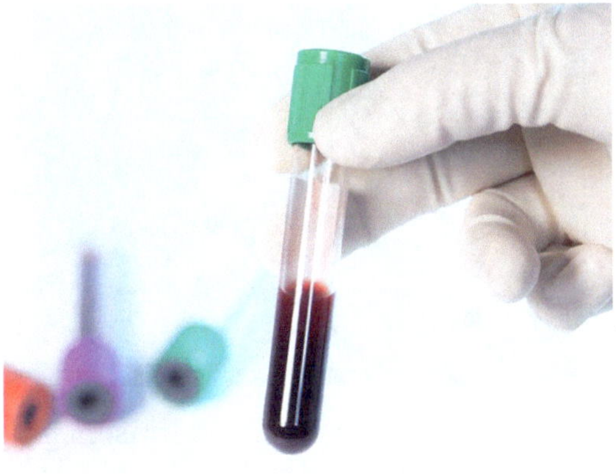

Figure 8.13. Platelet function tests.

Source: https://media.post.rvohealth.io/wp-content/uploads/2020/08/PVPV157-Platelet_Aggregation_Test-732x549-Thumbnail-1-732x549.jpg.

8.3.4. Bone Marrow Biopsy

Bone marrow biopsy is of pivotal importance in the diagnosis of numerous platelet disorders, providing information on the etiopathogenic conditions underlying platelet production and function. In particular, a bone marrow biopsy allows for the examination of bone marrow morphology, cellularity, and the presence of pathologic processes, such as myelodysplastic syndromes (MDSs), that may cause thrombocytopenia.

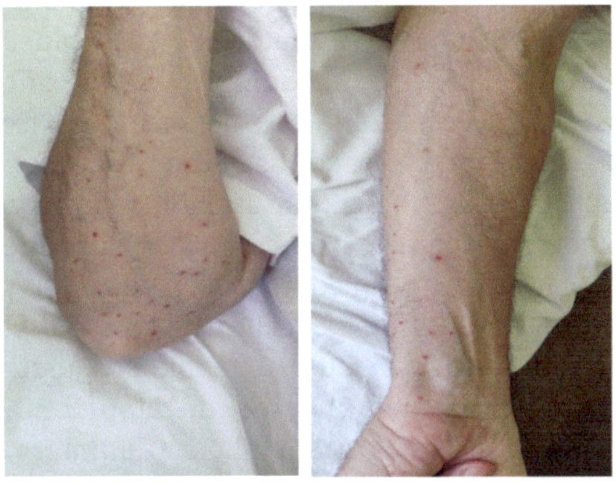

Figure 8.14. Conditions like immune thrombocytopenic purpura (ITP) can sometimes present with thrombocytopenia linked to malignancies, making a biopsy essential for ruling out neoplastic processes and ensuring appropriate management.

Source: https://www.mdpi.com/life/life-12-00077/article_deploy/html/images/life-12-00077-g001.png.

In cases of anemia in HIV/AIDS patients, for instance, a bone marrow biopsy may assist in discriminating between anemia of chronic disease (ACD) and other etiologies, as documented in the observation that the majority of anemic patients present with multifactorial etiologies, with significant treatment implications (Banerjee et al., 2012). Besides, disorders like ITP can sometimes be related to thrombocytopenia due to malignancies, and thus, biopsy is required for neoplastic processes exclusion and appropriate treatment (Faraj et al., 2010). The bone marrow biopsy is an invaluable tool in the comprehensive evaluation of patients with platelet disorders.

8.3.5. Genetic Testing for Inherited Disorders

The integration of genetic testing into the diagnostic workup for inherited diseases, and indeed for platelet disorders, has completely altered the landscape of patient management. Enhanced technology now enables clinicians to identify specific gene mutations that cause a variety of disorders, including VWD, one of the most prevalent bleeding disorders resulting from deficiencies or dysfunctions of the VWF (Blanco et al., 2017). It will facilitate attending physicians in understanding the bleeding status of a patient better by conducting comprehensive genotypic analyses in addition to routine hematological tests, such as full blood counts and coagulation screens, thus enabling the development of appropriate management plans (Chalmers et al., 2009). Genetic diagnosis not only leads to better identification but also helps predict the pattern of inheritance of these disorders, thus providing great information for family planning and future interventions. Together, these developments make the demands clear enough for genetic testing to be integrated into general clinical practice for hereditary platelet disorders.

8.3.6. Imaging Studies in Diagnosis

Imaging tests are crucial for determining if a patient has a platelet disorder, particularly to rule out other potential causes of blood clots. Techniques such as ultrasonography and MRI are often employed to visualize vascular abnormalities or complications arising from these disorders. For instance, in cases where patients present with arterial ischemic strokes, imaging can reveal underlying pathologies such as moyamoya disease, which has been shown to increase the risk of clinical recurrence in affected children significantly (Ganesan et al., 2006).

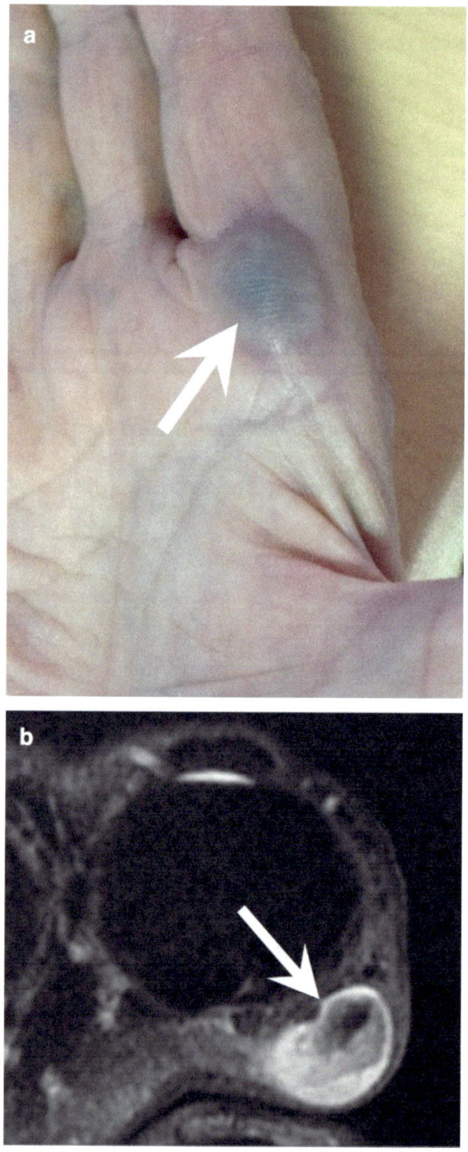

Figure 8.15. Techniques such as ultrasonography and magnetic resonance imaging (MRI) are often employed to visualize vascular abnormalities or complications arising from these disorders.

Source: https://media.springernature.com/lw1200/springer-static/image/art%3A10.1186%2Fs13244-020-00958-4/MediaObjects/13244_2020_958_Fig9_HTML.jpg.

Additionally, new neuroimaging techniques enable doctors to distinguish between reinfarctions that cause no symptoms and those that do, which supports the comprehensive care of patients. Furthermore, as seen in MNGIE, timely and accurate imaging can facilitate early diagnosis and intervention, thereby preventing the progression of irreversible conditions that encompass a wide range of systemic complications (Bax et al., 2020) (Figure 8.15).

8.3.7. Differential Diagnosis Considerations

When assessing platelet disorders, it is necessary to use differential diagnosis to help identify the real condition. Conditions such as MNGIE demonstrate the complexity of misdiagnosis, as patients with this disorder often present with symptoms that can mimic more common hematological issues, leading to diagnostic delays and inappropriate management strategies (Bax et al., 2020). Similarly, mast cell activation syndromes (MCAS) may confound clinical presentations, with symptoms overlapping those of platelet disorders, necessitating a meticulous approach to differentiate between primary and secondary manifestations of mast cell activity (Akin et al., 2011). If diagnostic criteria are used correctly and clinical examinations are thorough, and doctors consider rare platelet diseases, it will be easier to understand and treat platelet disorders, thereby improving outcomes for patients. So, it is important to use differential diagnosis to understand the details of these complicated conditions.

8.3.8. Role of Hematologists in Diagnosis

It is essential for hematologists to diagnose platelet disorders since they have the knowledge and skills to assess blood components and spot unusual blood conditions. They utilize blood tests and other advanced diagnostic tools to examine the details of platelet-related diseases. Their ability to analyze indicators such as platelet counts and the ratios of neutrophils and lymphocytes contributes significantly to understanding systemic inflammation associated with these disorders (Gorbunova et al., 2024). Furthermore, emerging research highlights the correlation between platelet dynamics and neurological health, suggesting that platelets can serve as biomarkers for early diagnosis and monitoring disease progression (Cadoni et al., 2024). As hematologists refine their methods of diagnosis, they play a more significant role in developing therapies and enhancing outcomes for individuals with platelet disorders, underscoring their pivotal role in contemporary medicine (Figure 8.16).

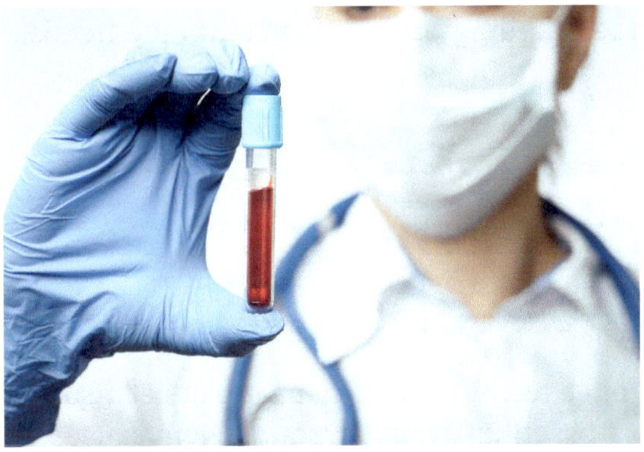

Figure 8.16. The role of hematologists in the diagnosis of platelet disorders is crucial, especially given their expertise in evaluating blood components and identifying hematological abnormalities.

Source: https://www.jeffersonhealth.org/content/dam/health2021/images/photos/stock/equipment/blood-hematology.jpg.

8.3.9. Challenges in Accurate Diagnosis

Diagnosing platelet disorders can be challenging due to the complexity of their causes. While advancements in biomarker identification have emerged, as highlighted in recent literature, the integration of multi-omics data—spanning genomics, proteomics, and metabolomics—remains necessary for a comprehensive understanding of these disorders (Argano et al., 2019). Using only one type of omics often provides a limited view of the complex ways in which molecules interact, which may result in incorrect or missed diagnoses. Furthermore, the variability in presentation among patients can obscure the identification of distinctive biomarkers that are critical for effective management (Lygirou et al., 2017). If healthcare providers do not fully understand these relationships, they may have difficulties in identifying platelet disorders, which could affect the optimal treatment plans. For this reason, making accurate diagnoses means joining different biological information and understanding each patient's unique needs.

8.4. Treatment and Management of Platelet Disorders

To effectively treat and manage platelet disorders, it is essential to understand their causes and how they manifest in different patients. For instance, in the treatment of neonatal patients experiencing platelet deficiencies, interventions such as platelet transfusions and Fresh-Frozen Plasma (FFP) are commonly employed, despite a lack of strict adherence to international guidelines. This variability in practice, largely due to limited robust evidence, can increase the risk of complications, particularly in vulnerable populations like neonates (Sokou et al., 2025). Furthermore, the management of conditions such as antineutrophil cytoplasmic antibody (ANCA)-associated vasculitis illustrates the complexity of immunothrombotic disorders where anti-platelet factor 4 (PF4) antibodies can trigger significant thrombotic events. Treatment strategies, including the use of intravenous immunoglobulin (IVIG), have shown promise in mitigating these complications, thus highlighting the importance of individualized patient management in achieving optimal outcomes (Remez-Gabay et al., 2025).

8.4.1. General Treatment Approaches

It is crucial to understand and implement effective treatment strategies for platelet disorders to improve patient outcomes. Treatment approaches typically differ and take into account the specific type of disorder, the frequency of bleeding attacks, and factors specific to the patient, such as age and gender. Various established techniques, including local hemostatic treatment and the application of tranexamic acid, have been proven beneficial in minimizing risk and managing symptoms in conditions such as inherited platelet disorders (IPDs).

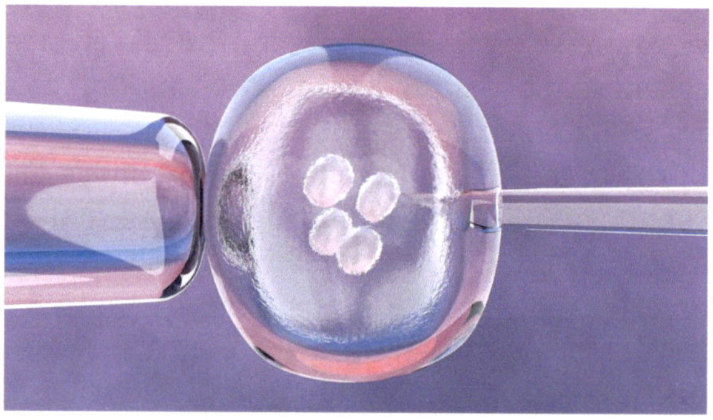

Figure 8.17. Hematopoietic stem cell therapy.

Source: https://assets.technologynetworks.com/production/dynamic/images/content/385564/organabio-launches-on-demand-gmp-compliant-hematopoietic-stem-cell-source-for-advanced-therapy-385564-960x540.jpg?cb=12767531.

Further, advances in treatment, such as HSCT, are also promising for curative therapy in some patients, highlighting individualized treatment regimens (Trushkina, 2024). Also, the awareness of inter-disciplinary collaboration among practitioners of health care has increased; this increases the better understanding and strategy that can be applied during treatment, especially concerning emotional and social determinants that will influence the experiences and recovery of patients, thereby making the need for innovative models during treatment arise (Trushkina, 2024) (Figure 8.17).

8.4.2. Medications for Thrombocytopenia

When the number of platelets is too low due to thrombocytopenia, doctors use treatments based on the underlying cause of the condition. In cases of ITP, traditional treatments include glucocorticoids and splenectomy. However, these have evolved with the introduction of newer agents, such as TPO-mimetics, notably romiplostim and eltrombopag, which have demonstrated efficacy in significantly raising platelet counts among refractory patients (Rice et al., 2009). Meanwhile, in hematologic malignancies like multiple myeloma (MM), bortezomib-based therapies are employed, albeit with the recognized risk of thrombocytopenia as a notable side effect (Lee et al., 2016). By using these drugs, patients can experience increased platelet counts and also enjoy reduced bleeding and improved outcomes, which represents a significant step forward in the treatment of thrombocytopenia.

8.4.3. Platelet Transfusions: Indications and Risks

Platelet transfusion is crucial in treating various platelet disorders, particularly for patients with hematologic malignancies, who often experience low platelet counts. Transfusion is mostly needed for both preventive and therapeutic reasons, since keeping hemostasis is crucial for these groups. Despite the existence of platelet transfusion guidelines that provide thresholds for intervention, their implementation remains inconsistent across clinical settings (Otrock et al., 2021). Since there are many ways to determine transfusion thresholds, it is essential to have standard methods that can adapt to changing situations in the clinic. Furthermore, this inconsistency highlights the potential risks associated with transfusions, including transfusion-related immunomodulation and allergic reactions, necessitating careful assessment and management strategies to mitigate adverse effects (Andreani et al., 2016). Taking into account the pros and cons of platelet transfusions is essential for the proper care of patients with platelet disorders (Figure 8.18).

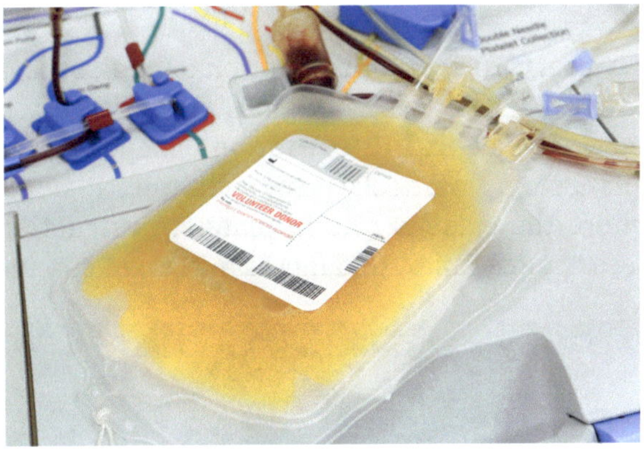

Figure 8.18. Platelet transfusions.

Source: https://stanfordbloodcenter.org/wp-content/uploads/2017/07/Platelets.jpg.

8.4.4. Immunosuppressive Therapy for ITP

Immunosuppressive therapy is a pivotal component in the management of ITP, particularly for patients who have not responded to first-line treatments such as corticosteroids or intravenous immunoglobulin. They are designed to regulate the immune system's response to platelets, thereby increasing their number and reducing the risk of bleeding. Rituximab and newer drugs such as azathioprine and mycophenolate mofetil have helped in keeping chronic cases in remission for an extended period. Specifically, thrombopoietin receptor agonists (TPO-RAs) are gaining traction as a second-line treatment, offering unique mechanisms that stimulate platelet production (Troiano et al., 2024). Furthermore, the management of ITP in specific populations, such as pregnant women, necessitates careful consideration of immunosuppressive therapy to balance maternal and fetal health outcomes (Dahiphale et al., 2024). Therefore, it remains crucial to employ personalized approaches in managing the challenges of ITP.

8.4.5. Surgical Options for Severe Cases

If conservative treatments for platelet disorders do not work well enough, surgery is often needed. Surgical interventions may involve splenectomy, particularly for conditions like ITP, where the spleens role in platelet destruction necessitates removal to increase platelet counts.

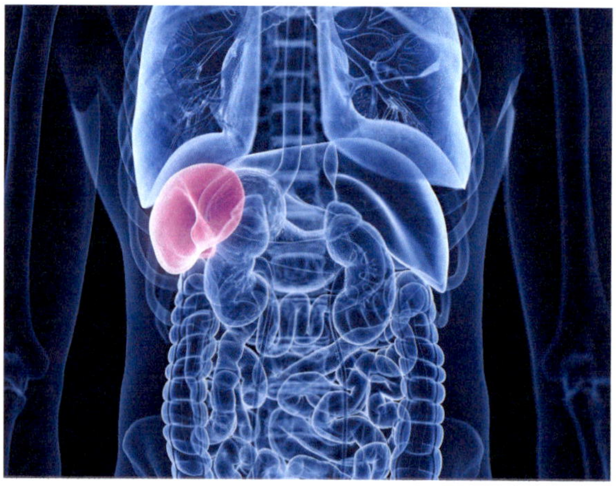

Figure 8.19. Surgical interventions may involve splenectomy, particularly for conditions like immune thrombocytopenic purpura (ITP), where the spleens role in platelet destruction necessitates removal to increase platelet counts.

Source: https://www.rarediseaseadvisor.com/wp-content/uploads/sites/25/2022/11/spleen_G_1190674609.jpg.

Other procedures, such as platelet transfusions or treatments to address the primary hematologic issues, may be used to help the body function normally and reduce complications associated with low platelet levels. Making the right choice about surgery involves weighing the potential benefits and risks, as it can significantly improve a patient's quality of life. As emphasized in the literature, a thorough review of existing guidelines is essential in optimizing surgical strategies for these patients, aiming to enhance overall treatment efficacy while minimizing resource use in clinical practice (Bossa et al., 2015) (Figure 8.19).

8.4.6. Lifestyle Modifications and Patient Education

Treatment of platelet disorders involves a combination of drug therapy, lifestyle modifications, and patient education. Knowing the illness of the individual is very important, as it allows for the formulation of more effective treatment strategies. For example, increased consumption of omega-3 fatty acids and antioxidants may be helpful for patients with thrombocytopenia or thrombocytopathy. Teaching the patients to exercise every day will improve their cardiovascular health, which in turn can improve the functioning of the platelets.

Good communication is important because explaining the condition to patients makes them feel accountable for their own care. Furthermore, the adoption of a personalized medicine approach, as detailed in recent literature, may best utilize these interventions by personalizing strategies to fit individual needs and circumstances, thereby optimizing overall patient adherence and satisfaction (Kitsiou et al., 2013; Borro et al., 2017).

8.4.7. Role of Support Groups and Counseling

Treatment of platelet disorders, such as Glanzmann thrombasthenia, involves both medical and psychosocial interventions that are best provided in support groups and counseling. Through these sites, the patients can discuss their conditions and feel less isolated because of their illnesses. Support groups help individuals understand their condition, feel supported, and develop more effective coping strategies. Counseling can also assist patients with the psychological effects of having a platelet disorder and help address issues, for example, in terms of pain management or emotional well-being. For example, there is evidence that an improved acceptance of pain is related to the quality of mental life, indicating the potential benefits that can be gained from acceptance-based approaches in support settings (Acharya et al., 2014). By integrating educational materials with psychosocial support, these interventions can lead to improved patient outcomes, ultimately resulting in a better quality of life for patients with platelet disorders (Bergmeier et al., 2020).

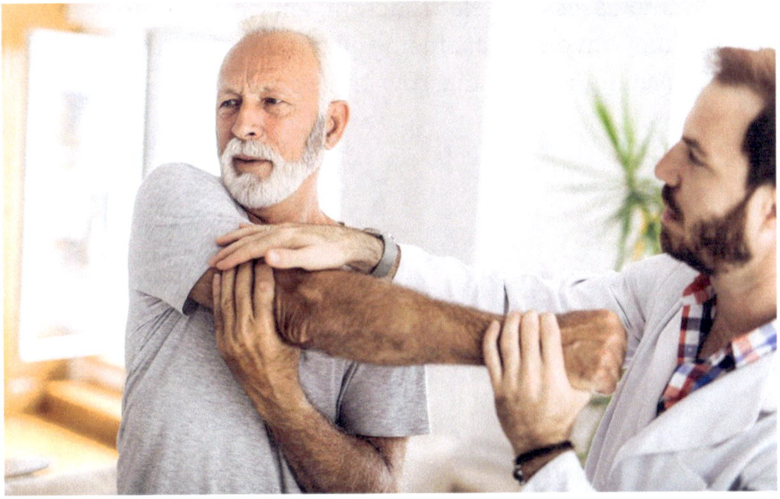

Figure 8.20. Counseling can address the psychological impacts of living with a platelet disorder, helping patients manage issues related to pain and emotional well-being.

Source: https://midamortho.com/wp-content/uploads/2024/09/man-during-physical-therapy.jpg.

8.4.8. Long-Term Management Strategies

To effectively manage treatment in the long term for patients with platelet disorders, the effects of these conditions on both the blood and overall health of the patient must be addressed. Treatment usually involves checking the platelet count and how they function, prescribing appropriate treatments that suit a given patient, and educating the patient on signs of bleeding or clotting. For example, patients with both cardiac and hematologic comorbidities might require careful examination of anticoagulation treatment to maximize safety and effectiveness in operations or interventional procedures (Goldhammer et al., 2016). Additionally, studies of low-frequency conditions, such as MNGIE, highlight the value of early diagnosis and changes in treatment, which can substantially enhance patient outcomes where platelet function is impaired (Bax et al., 2020). Moreover, when hematology and primary care physicians collaborate, the result can be better lives and longer,more prolonged survival for such patients.

A CLOSER LOOK

GLANZMANNS THROMBASTHENIA

Glanzmann's thrombasthenia is a rare disorder that results from a deficiency or abnormality in the platelet glycoprotein IIb/IIIa complex. This complex enables platelets to adhere to one another and coalesce to form a blood clot, thereby preventing blood from leaking away.

Platelet counts are normal in people who have Glanzmann's thrombasthenia, but their platelets don't stick together as they are supposed to, making them bleed for a long time, bruise with ease, get nosebleeds, and bleed excessively after an injury or surgery. Most cases of the disorder are caused by genes that are inherited in an autosomal recessive manner.

We perform blood tests to assess platelet function, and interventions focus on preventing and managing bleeding, which may involve transfusing platelets, administering antifibrinolytic drugs, or, in a few instances, performing a bone marrow transplant.

SUMMARY

After exploring platelet disorders, it becomes clear that they are not only strenuous for the patient but also for the healthcare system as a whole. As these disorders have many aspects, it is essential to study these causes and possible treatments in detail as well. A crucial aspect of effective management entails early recognition and control of complications, such as trauma leading to coagulopathy, as emphasized by evolving technology in treatment algorithms (Aquilina et al., 2009). The complexity of mast cell activation syndromes also sets the stage for the recognition of the role of accurate diagnosis and classification in therapeutic decision-making, emphasizing that not all disorders are straightforward (Akin et al., 2011). Therefore, research and close observation of patients are crucial for improving results and solving platelet disorders; perhaps better treatments can be achieved in the future.

All in all, looking into platelet disorders provides us with necessary information on their role in different health problems and treatments. Evidence suggests that the effectiveness of interventions such as platelet-rich plasma (PRP) is still under scrutiny, as demonstrated by a meta-analysis evaluating PRP for orthopaedic procedures, which concluded that its marginal effectiveness does not support widespread use (Cruciani et al., 2018). Further, the interrelation between psychosocial characteristics and platelet function identifies a significant way of explaining diseases. It has been found through research that stress can cause molecular alterations with immune signaling and platelet activation and thus contribute to the pathogenesis of cardiovascular illnesses and other disorders involving immune dysregulation (Benjamin et al., 2020). All these findings show that the disorders of platelets are complex and many things influence the symptoms as well as their method of treatment, so their research is far from over.

REFERENCES

1. Abd Wahab, M. B. A., Mahmood, S., Mohamad Rus, M. A., et al. (2020). Quality control improvement at Jana DCS Sdn. Bhd. https://core.ac.uk/download/12007130.pdf (accessed on 12th June 2025).
2. Elander, J. (2013). A review of evidence about behavioural and psychological aspects of chronic joint pain among people with haemophilia. Haemophilia, 20(2), 168–175. https://doi.org/10.1111/hae.12291Adams, A., Akassoglou, A., Akenami, F. O., Albright, A. V., et al. (2018). A perspective of coagulation dysfunction in multiple sclerosis and in experimental allergic encephalomyelitis. https://core.ac.uk/download/195777098.pdf (accessed on 12th June 2025).
3. Akin, C., Orfao, A., Alvarez-Twose, I., Arock, M., Arredondo, A. R., et al. (2011). Definitions, criteria and global classification of mast cell disorders with special reference to mast cell activation syndromes: A consensus proposal. https://core.ac.uk/download/16432570.pdf (accessed on 12th June 2025).
4. Althaus, K., Hoepner, G., Zieger, B., Prüller, F., Pavlova, A., Boeckelmann, D., Birschmann, I., et al. (2024). The diagnostic assessment of platelet function defects–Part 2: Update on platelet disorders. Hämostaseologie. https://www.semanticscholar.org/paper/7c4db1982abccf906596cd3ccb7c6286fc497b10 (accessed on 12th June 2025).
5. Amadori, S., Buccisano, F., Evangelista, M., Stasi, R., et al. (2008). Idiopathic thrombocytopenic purpura: Current concepts in pathophysiology and management. https://core.ac.uk/download/pdf/53824028.pdf (accessed on 12th June 2025).
6. Andreani, L., Antonioli, P., Basso, L., Biancofiore, G., et al. (2016). Recommendations for the implementation of a patient blood management programmed. Application to elective major orthopedic surgery in adults. https://core.ac.uk/download/54532470.pdf (accessed on 12th June 2025).
7. Aquilina, A., & Sciberras, S. C. (2009). The use of two novel techniques in the coagulopathic trauma patient in intensive care. https://core.ac.uk/download/46602240.pdf (accessed on 12th June 2025).
8. Aquilina, M. A. (2008). The expanding role of nuclear medicine in therapeutic strategies. https://core.ac.uk/download/46602172.pdf (accessed on 12th June 2025).
9. Argano, V., Balistreri, C. R., Giarratana, R. M., Lio, D., et al. (2019). On the road to accurate biomarkers for cardiometabolic diseases by integrating precision and gender medicine approaches. https://core.ac.uk/download/268910274.pdf (accessed on 12th June 2025).
10. Bacalbașa, N., Banu, P., Bălălău, C., Ghinghină, O., et al. (2019). The risk of bleeding and encephalopathy in surgical patients with liver cirrhosis. https://core.ac.uk/download/216811033.pdf (accessed on 12th June 2025).
11. Banerjee, A., Bhattacharyya, M., Ghosh, A., Ghosh, T., et al. (2012). Anemia in antiretroviral naïve HIV/AIDS patients: A study from Eastern India. https://core.ac.uk/download/pdf/13598709.pdf (accessed on 12th June 2025).
12. Barber, A., Lumb, A. B., Kaye, A. D., Turpie, A. G. G., Friedlander, A. H., Schafer, A. I., Ziffer, A. M., et al. (2003). Dental management considerations for the patient with an acquired coagulopathy.

Part 1: Coagulopathies from systemic disease. https://core.ac.uk/download/9348885.pdf (accessed on 12th June 2025).

13. Bargehr, C., Knöfler, R., & Streif, W. (2023). Treatment of inherited platelet disorders: Current status and future options. Hämostaseologie, 43, 261–270. https://www.semanticscholar.org/paper/f1d5ed6485958e12fd78a146bfa42e30af8ec8e3 (accessed on 12th June 2025).

14. Bax, B. E. (2020). Mitochondrial neurogastrointestinal encephalomyopathy: Approaches to diagnosis and treatment. https://core.ac.uk/download/287649788.pdf (accessed on 12th June 2025).

15. Benjamin, C., Coppola, G., Freimer, N. B., He, Y., et al. (2020). Immunosuppressive effect and global dysregulation of blood transcriptome in response to psychosocial stress in vervet monkeys (Chlorocebus sabaeus). https://core.ac.uk/download/323080367.pdf (accessed on 12th June 2025).

16. Bergmeier, W., Botero, J. P., Branchford, B. R., Bray, P. F., et al. (2020). Glanzmann thrombasthenia: Genetic basis and clinical correlates. https://core.ac.uk/download/322802267.pdf (accessed on 12th June 2025).

17. Biso, G. M. N., Reichman, N., Reddy, A., & Masoud, H. (2023). Abstract 160: Recurrent multi-territorial ischemic stroke as an initial presentation of thrombotic thrombocytopenic purpura. Stroke: Vascular and Interventional Neurology. https://www.semanticscholar.org/paper/047c348b5d9347703b200ea7f13f75de6308f3c3 (accessed on 12th June 2025).

18. Blanco, A. N., Kempfer, A. C., Lazzari, M. Á., Paiva Palomino, M., et al. (2017). Diagnosis of von Willebrand disease in Argentina: A single institution experience. https://core.ac.uk/download/159297861.pdf (accessed on 12th June 2025).

19. Borro, M., Di Sanzo, M., Fineschi, V., Frati, P., et al. (2017). Clinical applications of personalized medicine: A new paradigm and challenge. https://core.ac.uk/download/80315182.pdf (accessed on 12th June 2025).

20. Bossa, M., Brancaccio, P., Castagna, A., Chillemi, C., et al. (2015). I.S.Mu.L.T–Rotator cuff tears guidelines. https://core.ac.uk/download/53528697.pdf (accessed on 12th June 2025).

21. Breum, M. S., Munch, A., Gerds, T., & Martinussen, T. (2023). Estimation of separable direct and indirect effects in a continuous-time illness-death model. Lifetime Data Analysis, 30, 143–180. https://www.semanticscholar.org/paper/2d88cb14d69bcffa4b4729747219e241f0448df1 (accessed on 12th June 2025).

22. Cadoni, M. P. L., Coradduzza, D., Congiargiu, A., Sedda, S., Zinellu, A., Medici, S., Nivoli, A., et al. (2024). Platelet dynamics in neurodegenerative disorders: Investigating the role of platelets in neurological pathology. Journal of Clinical Medicine, 13. https://www.semanticscholar.org/paper/3b392c8673cc43c11014957f460dc63a14700f48 (accessed on 12th June 2025).

23. Cammisotto, V., Carnevale, R., Castellani, V., D'Amico, M., et al. (2017). Extra virgin olive oil and cardiovascular diseases: Benefits for human health. https://core.ac.uk/download/141695177.pdf (accessed on 12th June 2025).

24. Campetella, O., Leguizamon, M. S., Mucci, J., Rooijen, N., et al. (2005). The trans-sialidase from Trypanosoma cruzi induces thrombocytopenia during acute Chagas' disease by reducing the platelet sialic acid contents. https://core.ac.uk/download/pdf/15459329.pdf (accessed on 12th June 2025).

25. Cavanagh, J., Graham, G. J., Johnman, C., Krishnadas, R., et al. (2018). Chemokines in depression in health and in inflammatory illness: A systematic review and meta-analysis. https://core.ac.uk/download/96882057.pdf (accessed on 12th June 2025).

26. Chalmers, E. A., & Halsey, C. (2009). Hematological investigations in children. https://core.ac.uk/download/110273.pdf (accessed on 12th June 2025).

27. Cooper, N., & Ghanima, W. (2019). Immune thrombocytopenia. New England Journal of Medicine, 381, 945–955. https://doi.org/10.1056/nejmcp1810479

28. Cruciani, M., Franchini, M., Liumbruno, G. M., Marano, G., et al. (2018). Efficacy of platelet-rich plasma as conservative treatment in orthopedics: A systematic review and meta-analysis. https://core.ac.uk/download/188826282.pdf (accessed on 12th June 2025).

29. Dahiphale, S., Dewani, D. K. C., Agrawal, M., Dahiphale, J. M., Jyotsna, G., Saloni, & Desale, R. (2024). Navigating primary immune thrombocytopenia during pregnancy with management strategies and considerations: A comprehensive review. Cureus, 16. https://www.semanticscholar.org/paper/354a1e4a2e4999e72a5edfe96c54d334f9202381 (accessed on 12th June 2025).

30. Del Balzo, F., Duse, M., Nicita, F., Occasi, F., et al. (2016). Stroke and migraine: Is there a possible comorbidity? https://core.ac.uk/download/154947765.pdf (accessed on 12th June 2025).

31. Douglass, M. B., Yessin, O., Elengickal, J., Charpenter, S., & Campbell, C. H. (2024). Acquired thrombotic thrombocytopenic purpura (TTP) presenting with synthetic cannabinoid use. Cureus, 16. https://www.semanticscholar.org/paper/9d0e70f077fb5b29d94436e10ca060c09a1bbc5e (accessed on 12th June 2025).

32. Downes, K. (2019). Diagnostic high-throughput sequencing of 2,396 patients with bleeding, thrombotic and platelet disorders. https://core.ac.uk/download/200999594.pdf (accessed on 12th June 2025).

33. Estes, J. W. (1962). Modern concepts of the platelet in health and disease. https://open.bu.edu/bitstream/2144/26002/1/Estes_J.%20Worth_1962_web.pdf (accessed on 12th June 2025).

34. Ethayathulla, A., Yadav, B., Ahmad, F., Kannan, M., Kumar, R., Saxena, R., & Choudhry, V. (2008). Identification of 22 novel mutations in patients with Glanzmann's thrombasthenia. https://core.ac.uk/download/pdf/288086.pdf (accessed on 12th June 2025).

35. Faraj, H., Khasraw, M., & Sheikha, A. (2010). Thrombocytopenia in solid tumors. http://hdl.handle.net/10536/DRO/DU:30046484 (accessed on 12th June 2025).

36. Franchini, M., Liumbruno, G. M., Marano, G., Mengoli, C., et al. (2017). Inhibitors in patients with congenital bleeding disorders other than hemophilia. https://core.ac.uk/download/153367572.pdf (accessed on 12th June 2025).

37. Ganesan, V., Kirkham, F. J., Prengler, M., Wade, A., et al. (2006). Clinical and radiological recurrence after childhood arterial ischemic stroke. https://core.ac.uk/download/1677193.pdf (accessed on 12th June 2025).

38. Goldhammer, J. E., & Kohl, B. A. (2016). Coexisting cardiac and hematologic disorders. https://core.ac.uk/download/83049377.pdf (accessed on 12th June 2025).

39. Gorbunova, A. P., Rukavishnikov, G., Kasyanov, E., & Mazo, G. (2024). The role of hematological coefficients of systemic inflammation in the diagnosis and risk assessment of affective

disorders. V. M. Bekhterev Review of Psychiatry and Medical Psychology. https://www.semanticscholar.org/paper/1ddfdf75e23d2c2fd7fdc5615c28e720b01b1b26 (accessed on 12th June 2025).

40. Heeschen, C., James, S. K., Khaliq, A., Luttun, A., & Mak, K. H. (2005). Biomarkers in acute coronary syndromes and their role in diabetic patients. https://core.ac.uk/download/12175738.pdf (accessed on 12th June 2025).

41. Heller, P. G., & Marin Oyarzún, C. P. (2019). Platelets as mediators of thromboinflammation in chronic myeloproliferative neoplasms. https://core.ac.uk/download/323211431.pdf (accessed on 12th June 2025).

42. Hitchcock, I. S., Hafer, M., Sangkhae, V., & Tucker, J. A. (2021). The thrombopoietin receptor: Revisiting the master regulator of platelet production. Platelets, 32, 770–778. https://doi.org/10.1080/09537104.2021.1925102

43. How, J., Oh, S. T., & Zhou, A. (2016). Splanchnic vein thrombosis in myeloproliferative neoplasms: Pathophysiology and molecular mechanisms of disease. https://core.ac.uk/download/80495017.pdf (accessed on 12th June 2025).

44. Kharat, S., Mali, S., Korade, G., & Gaykar, R. (2024). Navigating neurodegenerative disorders: A comprehensive review of current and emerging therapies for neurodegenerative disorders. Journal of Neuroscience and Neurological Disorders. https://www.semanticscholar.org/paper/34e53f42d457a00e7829813ef4feaa18fdbc2228 (accessed on 12th June 2025).

45. Kitsiou, A., Caforio, A. L. P., Porta-Sanchez, A., Vahanian, A., Iung, B., Carrera, C., Szymanski, C., et al. (2013). ESC core curriculum for the general cardiologist (2013). https://core.ac.uk/download/55756305.pdf (accessed on 12th June 2025).

46. Lee, E. J., Cines, D. B., Gernsheimer, T., Kessler, C. M., Michel, M., Tarantino, M. D., Semple, J. W., et al. (2021). Thrombocytopenia following Pfizer and Moderna SARS-CoV-2 vaccination. American Journal of Hematology, 96, 534–537. https://doi.org/10.1002/ajh.26132

47. Lee, S. (2016). Efficacy and safety of bortezomib with dexamethasone regimen in elderly newly diagnosed multiple myeloma patients with co-morbidities. https://open.bu.edu/bitstream/2144/14373/9/Lee_bu_0017N_10435.pdf (accessed on 12th June 2025).

48. Lygirou, V., Mischak, H., Mokou, M., Vlahou, A., et al. (2017). Proteomics in cardiovascular disease: Recent progress and clinical implication and implementation. https://core.ac.uk/download/77600933.pdf (accessed on 12th June 2025).

49. Negro, A., Terrin, A., Raffaelli, B., Mitsikostas, D. D., Ornello, R., Khan, S., et al. (2017). Headache and pregnancy. A systematic review. https://core.ac.uk/download/153369041.pdf (accessed on 12th June 2025).

50. Northup, P. G., García-Pagán, J. C., García-Tsao, G., Intagliata, N. M., Superina, R., Roberts, L. N., Lisman, T., et al. (2020). Vascular liver disorders, portal vein thrombosis, and procedural bleeding in patients with liver disease: 2020 practice guidance by the American Association for the Study of Liver Diseases. Hepatology, 73, 366–413. https://doi.org/10.1002/hep.31646

51. Obeng-Tuudah, D., Tarawah, A., Ozkan, M., & Abdul-Kadir, R. (2025). Obstetric and gynecological challenges and outcomes in women and girls with Glanzmann's thrombasthenia. Hemophilia: The Official Journal of the World Federation of Hemophilia. https://www.semanticscholar.org/paper/c8ac3c299e39797f523d69b5e1d15ff2a9a8c34d (accessed on 12th June 2025).

52. Oliveira, S. de, & Saldanha, C. (2010). An overview about erythrocyte membrane. https://core.ac.uk/download/12426151.pdf (accessed on 12th June 2025).

53. Otrock, Z. K., & Yuan, S. (2021). Platelet transfusion: An update on indications and guidelines. https://core.ac.uk/download/524796557.pdf (accessed on 12th June 2025).

54. Perez Botero, J., Lee, K., Branchford, B. R., Bray, P. F., Freson, K., Lambert, M. P., Luo, M., et al. (2020). Glanzmann thrombasthenia: Genetic basis and clinical correlates. Hematological, 105, 888–894. https://doi.org/10.3324/haematol.2018.214239

55. Perez, E., Guevara, N., Smith, J., & Velasquez, R. (2024). Altered mental status in the setting of thrombotic thrombocytopenic purpura (TTP) and spontaneous coronary artery dissection (SCAD): A case report and literature review. Cureus, 16. https://www.semanticscholar.org/paper/7d974134ba320bf4cd534410b676ab17b9ceb92e (accessed on 12th June 2025).

56. Perumal, V., Narayanan, A. S., Parayil, S., Debnath, A., Kannan, B., & Bose, S. S. N. (2024). Hierarchical AI-powered digital white blood cell and platelet morphology analysis using multi-class classification. 2024 IEEE International Conference on Electronics, Computing and Communication Technologies (CONECCT). https://www.semanticscholar.org/paper/2815373428952d4c6ae04ea4bc93e806edbe88ef (accessed on 12th June 2025).

57. Remez-Gabay, L., Vdovich, O., Akria, L., & Kruzel-Davila, E. (2025). Case report: Anti-platelet factor 4-mediated immunothrombosis in a patient with ANCA vasculitis–a shared mechanism of NETosis. Frontiers in Immunology, 16. https://www.semanticscholar.org/paper/5b4039f26756a7ebd83bcec4532a4664de8b83e0 (accessed on 12th June 2025).

58. Rice, L. (2009). Treatment of immune thrombocytopenic purpura: Focus on entomophagy. https://core.ac.uk/download/pdf/8317863.pdf (accessed on 12th June 2025).

59. Samakkhiwitthayakhom, T. S. (2024). Advancements in Alzheimer's disease: Emerging therapies, lifestyle modifications, and early intervention strategies. International Journal of Current Science Research and Review. https://www.semanticscholar.org/paper/fbc7f2c9e77e6050205c24c35a24db9200893993 (accessed on 12th June 2025).

60. Sangli, S., Virani, A., Cheronis, N., Vannatter, B., Minich, C., Noronha, S., Bhagavatula, R., et al. (2021). Thrombosis with thrombocytopenia after the messenger RNA–1273 vaccine. Annals of Internal Medicine, 174, 1480–1482. https://doi.org/10.7326/l21-0244

61. Shahbaz, A., Alzarooni, A., Veeranagari, V. R., Patel, K., Mohammed, C., Kuruba, V., Rajkumar, N., et al. (2024). Efficacy of platelet-rich plasma intra-articular injections in hip and knee osteoarthritis. Cureus, 16. https://www.semanticscholar.org/paper/b6879bee0b82169921019ec0b323ddd5ba2a99bb (accessed on 12th June 2025).

62. Sokou, R., Gounari, E. A., Lianou, A., Tsantes, A., Piovani, D., Bonovas, S., Iacovidou, N., et al. (2025). Rethinking platelet and plasma transfusion strategies for neonates: Evidence, guidelines, and unanswered questions. Seminars in Thrombosis and Hemostasis. https://www.semanticscholar.org/paper/d032a55056893079daa00b0d8117cc20daa5a41d (accessed on 12th June 2025).

63. Sumbalová, Z., Rausová, Z., Kucharská, J., Šranko, P., Harbulák, P., Svitok, P., López-Lluch, G., et al. (2024). Platelet mitochondrial function and endogenous coenzyme Q10 levels could be used as markers of mitochondrial health in infertile men: A pilot study. International Journal of Molecular Sciences, 26. https://www.semanticscholar.org/paper/e8de9a63cf36a042dab34e9bd96dfc2a3d37333c (accessed on 12th June 2025).

64. Troiano, M., Giordano, C., Rossi, E., Scalzulli, P., Mettivier, L., D'Ambrosio, A., Mazzoni, D., et al. (2024). Treatment of chronic ITP with avatrombopag: A multicentric real-world experience. Blood. https://www.semanticscholar.org/paper/d7024a4e077c1df6c6074308e929381c89f69460 (accessed on 12th June 2025).

65. Trushkina, S. V. (2024). A multidisciplinary approach to the diagnosis, treatment and prevention of developmental disorders of children in the first years of life. Autism and Developmental Disorders. https://www.semanticscholar.org/paper/fbd69ffbc01d6d4bb3d9194914e91a6d3fded86d (accessed on 12th June 2025).

66. Zhang, Z., Zhou, X., Fang, X., Zhou, X., Cheng, Z., & Hu, Y. (2024). Platelet disorders and medication strategies. Thrombosis and Haemostasias. https://www.semanticscholar.org/paper/efa8f43d71feab895dd9309363810ead982abb4f (accessed on 12th June 2025).

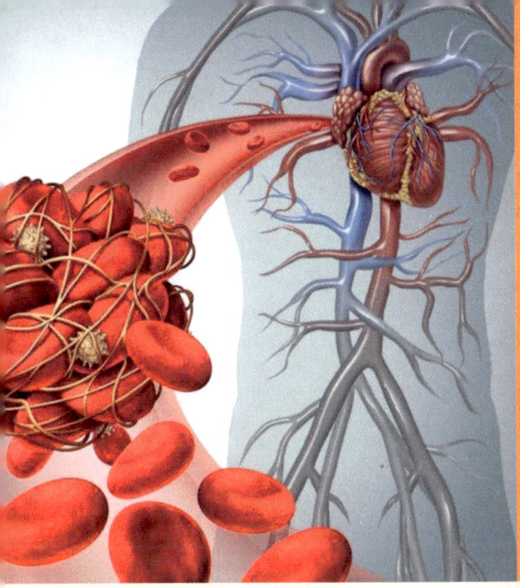

Chapter 9

COAGULATION DISORDERS

Contents

Introduction....207
9.1. Types of Coagulation Disorders....208
9.2. Causes and Risk Factors....213
9.3. Symptoms and Diagnosis....217
9.4. Treatment and Management....221
Summary....228
References....229

Introduction

Coagulation disorders belong to one of the major types of hematological disorders that impair the body's ability to regulate blood clotting. Inappropriate clot formation or excessive bleeding are both hazardous to health. Mutations in genes, environmental factors, or their combination are responsible for coagulation disorders. These disorders are essential to understand because they occur in every age group and population subset, resulting in multiple adverse complications such as hemophilia, von Willebrand's disease, and thrombophilia. A comprehensive review of coagulation disorders reveals that early diagnosis and treatment significantly improve patient recovery. In addition, shifts in paradigms in management plans, advanced therapies, and preventive measures have significantly contributed to transforming the perception and treatment of coagulable disorders. On the whole, a detailed study of coagulation disorders reveals their prevalence and the current advancements in their treatment regimen, making it a significant subject of interest for both medical personnel and patients (Figure 9.1).

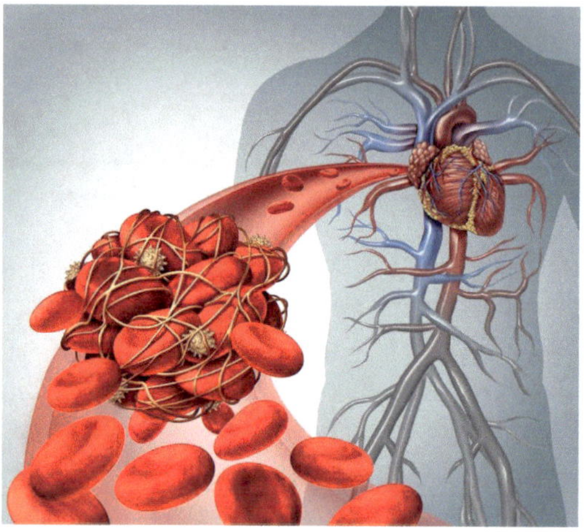

Figure 9.1. Coagulation disorders.

Source: https://www.medicalnote.in/cdn/shop/articles/Blood_Clotting_Factors.jpg?v=1724166944&width=2048.

9.1. Types of Coagulation Disorders

Coagulation disorders consist of many diseases that affect the coagulation of the blood, leading to excessive bleeding or thrombotic events. The disorder can be broadly categorized into two types: inherited and acquired. In the inherited group, RIBDs are rare and cause clinical variability due to deficiencies in factors such as VII, XI, and XIII.

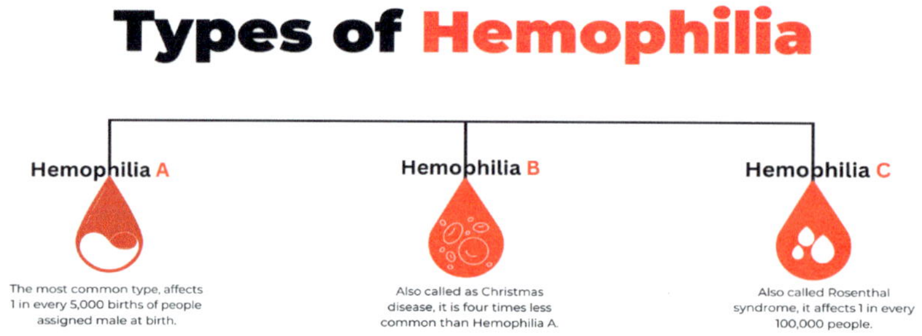

Figure 9.2. Types of hemophilia.

Source: https://media-blog.lalpathlabs.com/apis/ef27dede-b935-4aaa-86a2-8ada561caa2a.png.

For instance, it stated that the most common condition in the study population was factor VII deficiency with, in major bleeding, 23% of the cases (Erthal et al., 2024). The acquired conditions include antiphospholipid syndrome (APS), an autoimmune phenomenon in which the presence of antiphospholipid antibodies interferes with normal coagulation, leading to a predisposition to thrombosis. This further complicates the diagnostic landscape because APS requires a multi-step assay approach due to the variations in sensitivities of available tests (Kumano et al., 2023). Understanding these coagulation disorders can give a way into an efficient management plan for the patient (Figure 9.2).

9.1.1. Hemophilia A

Individuals with hemophilia A, which is caused by a deficiency of clotting factor VIII, face numerous management challenges. The more severe the condition, the lower the levels of the necessary factors, and this can result in unexpected bleeding that may cause significant health problems. There is a significant problem related to treatment, particularly with factor VIII concentrate replacement, which involves the formation of inhibitory alloantibodies. These inhibitors not only complicate hemorrhage management but also increase the associated healthcare costs and disability for patients, highlighting the critical need for vigilant monitoring (Franchini et al., 2017). Additionally, new methods for producing coagulation-factor concentrates have made them safer and less likely to pose infectious disease risks. The shift toward recombinant products, which limit reliance on human plasma, is a pivotal development that addresses these safety concerns while still ensuring effective treatment options for those with Hemophilia A (Bozzette et al., 2006).

9.1.2. Hemophilia B

A lack of clotting factor IX in the blood is what causes Hemophilia B, a genetic bleeding disorder. While Hemophilia A is associated with factor VIII, Hemophilia B accounts for approximately 15% of global hemophilia cases and shares similar challenges in terms of treatment and diagnosis. A significant issue is the underdiagnosis prevalent in many regions, particularly in Asian countries such as Thailand, where the infrastructure and accessibility to specialized care remain limited (Moonla et al., 2023). Treatment strategies for Hemophilia B typically emphasize prophylactic therapies to prevent bleeding episodes, a recommendation endorsed by clinical guidelines (Rezende et al., 2024). Even though factor IX concentrates have greatly improved patient outcomes, many people still encounter difficulties because of financial and geographical barriers. These differences indicate that further efforts are necessary to enhance healthcare systems for hemophilia management worldwide (Figure 9.3).

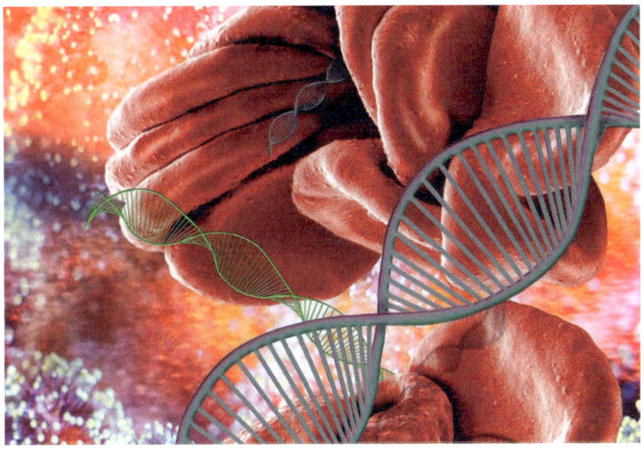

Figure 9.3. Hemophilia B.

Source: https://images.newscientist.com/wp-content/uploads/2022/07/21160938/SEI_115765128.jpg.

9.1.3. Von Willebrand Disease (VWD)

Von Willebrand Disease (vWD) is a hereditary bleeding disorder primarily resulting from a deficiency or dysfunction of von Willebrand factor (vWF), a crucial protein involved in the process of hemostasis. Symptoms of the condition can be as light as minor bleeding from the mucous membranes or as severe as large hemorrhages, mainly during surgery or when someone is injured. Notably, vWD affects platelet adhesion and also helps stabilize factor VIII in the coagulation process, making its regulation necessary to maintain hemostatic balance. In most cases, desmopressin is used to treat vWD, as it helps increase vWF, primarily in individuals with type 1 vWD. It is sometimes challenging to diagnose bleeding disorders since their symptoms are similar to those of other coagulation disorders, and labs are needed to make an accurate distinction. Recent guidelines have emphasized the importance of individualized therapeutic strategies and prompted further research into the molecular mechanisms underlying vWD to enhance patient outcomes (Patrick et al., 2020; Baumgartner et al., 2020).

9.1.4. Factor V Leiden Mutation

Among the various coagulation disorders, the Factor V Leiden mutation is a significant genetic abnormality that heightens the risk of venous thromboembolism (VTE). As a result of this mutation, Factor V becomes altered, making it less susceptible to the effects of activated protein C, which is responsible for regulating blood clotting. Therefore, those with the mutation have a higher chance of getting deep vein thrombosis and pulmonary embolism (PE) than those without it. Such risks are further exacerbated in cases where patients are exposed to additional thrombotic factors such as hormone replacement therapy (HRT); the combination of HRT and APC resistance notably increases VTE risk to approximately thirteenfold in susceptible populations (Daly et al., 2000). Understanding this interplay is crucial for identifying at-risk individuals and guiding clinical management, especially since many women with thrombophilias, including Factor V Leiden, require careful counseling regarding therapeutic interventions (Marquardt et al., 2018) (Figure 9.4).

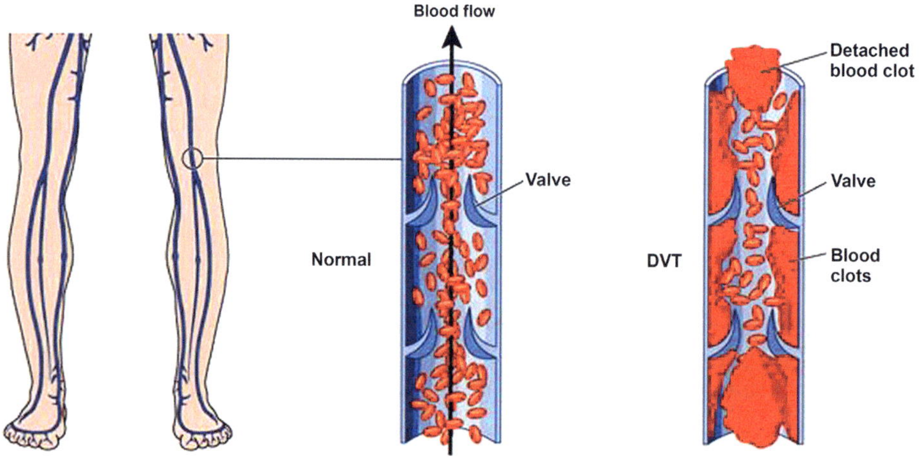

Figure 9.4. Factor V Leiden mutation.

Source: https://medlineplus.gov/images/PX00015W_PRESENTATION.jpeg.

9.1.5. Antiphospholipid Syndrome (APS)

APS stands out as a significant acquired coagulation disorder characterized by the presence of antiphospholipid antibodies (aPL) that predispose patients to both arterial and venous thrombotic events. Since APS can show various symptoms like blood clots and problems in pregnancy, it is hard to diagnose and treat effectively. Recent studies suggest that the clinical implications of aPL extend beyond thrombosis, indicating a potential link to non-thrombotic autoimmune conditions, like multiple sclerosis and immune thrombocytopenic purpura (ITP) (Minagar et al., 2009). Improved diagnostic methods and protocols are essential for accurately identifying APS, especially since inherited thrombophilic disorders can exacerbate its severity (Loh et al., 2011). Understanding how APS works and how its antibodies interact with the body can inform the development of treatments that may reduce the complications associated with this disease. So, using a comprehensive approach to APS is necessary when looking at coagulation disorders in general.

9.1.6. Disseminated Intravascular Coagulation (DIC)

Understanding Disseminated Intravascular Coagulation (DIC) is crucial in the context of coagulation disorders, as this condition exemplifies the complex interplay between thrombosis and hemorrhage. DIC is characterized by the activation of the coagulation system in multiple locations, often due to severe infections, trauma, or malignancies, which causes microthrombi to form in the blood vessels.

These microthrombi consume platelets and coagulation factors, resulting in secondary bleeding due to the depletion of these essential components (Montes et al., 1998). The clinical manifestations of DIC can be deceptively subtle, ranging from oozing at intravenous sites to catastrophic bleeding, which complicates accurate diagnosis (Chalmers et al., 2009). Because of this, laboratory tests such as coagulation screens and complete blood counts help detect DIC and decide on the appropriate treatment for the patient's condition. Therefore, it is essential to notice and treat this syndrome early to avoid serious outcomes (Figure 9.5).

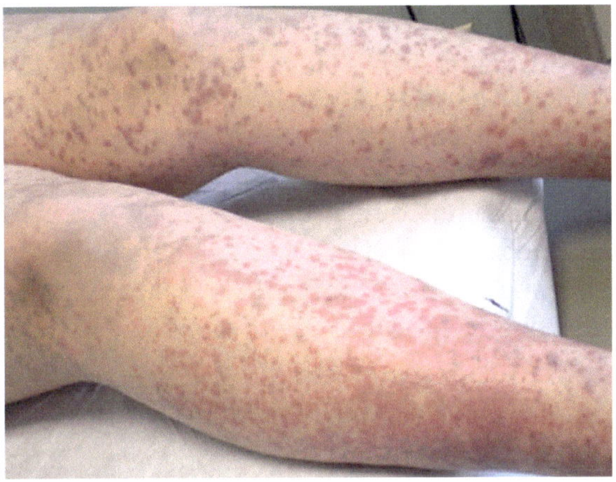

Figure 9.5. Disseminated intravascular coagulation (DIC).

Source: https://ai-care.id/photos/640ebd41a8629.jpg.

9.1.7. Thrombocytopenia

Coagulation disorders become much more difficult when a person has thrombocytopenia and a lower platelet count. Because there are many possible causes, it is essential to know that this condition may result from problems with the immune system, infections, or drugs. Recent findings suggest a potential link between vaccine administration, particularly with mRNA technology, and cases of vaccine-induced thrombosis coupled with thrombocytopenia (VITT) (Sangli et al., 2021). This prompts us to consider the safety of vaccines and the factors that may cause these side effects. Furthermore, thrombocytopenia is often accompanied by a hyperinflammatory response during severe infections, which can exacerbate the condition and complicate management strategies (Copaescu et al., 2020). To manage thrombocytopenia, it is essential to understand its causes and take prompt and appropriate actions to prevent both bleeding and clotting.

9.1.8. Vitamin K Deficiency

A lack of vitamin K is essential in the development

of coagulation disorders, due to the fact that it stops the production of proteins that help blood clot properly. Such a shortage can result in a higher chance of bleeding and hemorrhage, primarily for people with malabsorption syndromes or who have been on anticoagulant drugs for a long time. In addition, recent studies are showing that vitamin K is involved in bone health and vascular function, not only in coagulation. Vitamin K is needed for the process that ensures osteocalcin and matrix Gla-protein function properly in bone mineralization and the prevention of arterial calcification. Thus, addressing vitamin K deficiency not only mitigates the risk of bleeding disorders but may also enhance bone and vascular health outcomes, underlining the coalesce of coagulation and broader physiological health impacts (Petkova et al., 2017; Rajagopal et al., 2023) (Figure 9.6).

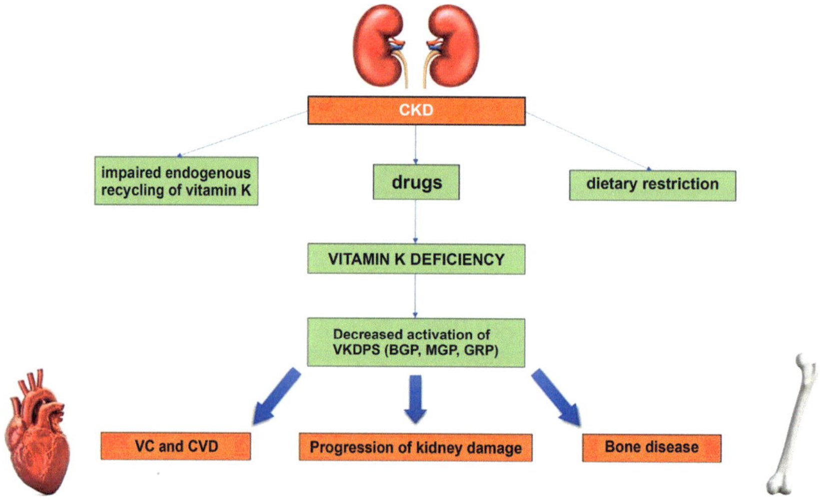

Figure 9.6. Vitamin K deficiency is a critical factor in the development of coagulation disorders, primarily because it impairs the synthesis of vitamin K-dependent proteins essential for effective blood clotting.

Source: https://pub.mdpi-res.com/ijms/ijms-23-05282/article_deploy/html/images/ijms-23-05282-ag.png?1652175010.

9.1.9. Acquired Coagulation Disorders

Because they are complex and related to different health problems, acquired coagulation disorders are challenging to manage. Sometimes, these disorders occur in healthy people and can be viewed as simple deficiencies or as more complex problems with blood clotting. As an example, acquired hemophilia A is an autoimmune disease where autoantibodies against coagulation factor VIII cause the patient to bleed a lot. Likewise, acquired von Willebrand syndrome may happen in patients with heart problems, as the forces on their blood vessels can reduce vWF's ability to aid hemostasis. Moreover, chronic liver diseases bring together factors that help and hinder blood clotting, which makes it challenging to diagnose and treat bleeding problems. Treatments, such as prophylactic emicizumab for hemophilia A, represent advancements in therapy but require careful consideration of each patient's unique circumstances and underlying condition (Lisman et al., 2020; Lisman et al., 2024).

9.2. Causes and Risk Factors

It is essential to know the causes and risk factors of coagulation disorders to prevent and control them. Genetic factors and environmental factors are major contributors to these conditions. Some inherited issues can cause clots to form abnormally, whereas factors such as missing nutrients or other health problems make bleeding more likely. A study highlights specific independent risk factors, including baseline INR levels and nutritional risks, that correlate with increased incidences of coagulation disorders in patients receiving the antibiotic CPZ/SAM (Xu et al., 2025). Furthermore, the role of platelets in coagulation highlights how their dysfunction or reduction can increase bleeding risks, underscoring the importance of monitoring platelet aggregation during diagnosis and therapy (Han et al., 2024). When healthcare providers understand the causes and risks, they can develop more effective interventions to prevent adverse outcomes for patients with coagulation disorders.

9.2.1. Genetic Factors

It is essential to understand the role of genetics in coagulation disorders, since most of these conditions are caused by inherited changes in blood clotting. Many genetic changes can cause problems with important coagulation factors, which may result in either too much bleeding or blood clots. For example, when genetic anomalies are identified in the genes that produce these factors, doctors can make an accurate diagnosis and select suitable treatment plans. Genetic testing is essential, as it gives information about the patient and also about the ways health problems can be inherited in the family. As highlighted, advanced hematological investigations such as coagulation screens can aid in unraveling these complex genetic underpinnings, thereby enhancing our understanding of coagulation disorders (Chalmers et al., 2009). Furthermore, the ramifications of genetic disorders extend to broader physiological processes, influencing systemic conditions such as ectopic mineralization, which can complicate treatment (Vilder et al., 2015) (Figure 9.7).

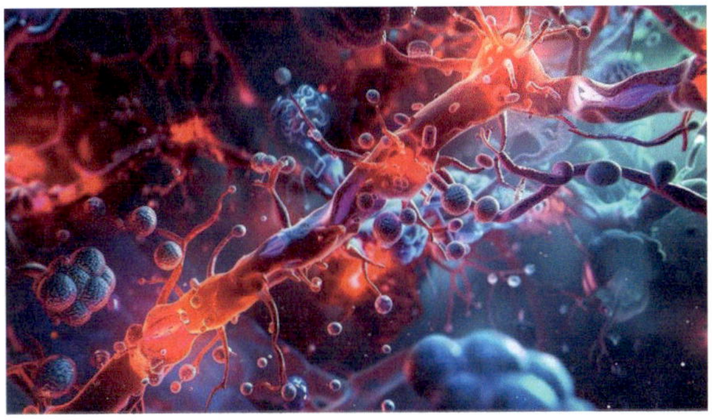

Figure 9.7. Numerous genetic mutations can lead to deficiencies or dysfunctions in key coagulation factors, resulting in either excessive bleeding or thrombosis.

Source: https://t4.ftcdn.net/jpg/07/99/70/51/360_F_799705163_Ecx1LaVPuO7dSUjA2moKwH94fPuaAOl2.jpg.

9.2.2. Environmental Influences

It is essential to understand environmental factors to comprehend how coagulation disorders can be exacerbated by external influences. For example, numerous studies have examined the relationship between hemostasis and inflammation, demonstrating that external factors can stimulate the activity of coagulation factors. Specifically, in the context of multiple sclerosis, the crosstalk between inflammation and the coagulation cascade has been shown to be a significant contributor to disease pathophysiology, with abnormal fibrin deposition and breakdown of the blood-brain barrier (Fornasiero et al., 2019). Furthermore, environmental toxins and lifestyle choices, such as an unhealthy diet and physical inactivity, can disrupt the delicate balance of procoagulants and anticoagulants in the circulatory system, leading to an increased risk of clot formation and associated complications (Pilli et al., 2018). For this reason, a comprehensive study of coagulation disorders should consider environmental factors to enhance prevention and treatment methods.

9.2.3. Medications and Their Effects

Many medications are used to manage coagulation disorders, helping to regulate or enhance blood clotting function. For individuals with hemophilia, who lack the necessary clotting factors, receiving clotting factor replacements is crucial. Also, the mental impact of using medication is important, as shown by the link between joint pain and taking medicine as prescribed in hemophilia patients. Research indicates that a reduction in pain intensity is correlated with an improved physical quality of life, emphasizing the importance of effective pain management alongside factor treatments (Acharya et al., 2014). Furthermore, medications like intracameral bevacizumab demonstrate rapid effects in managing ocular complications associated with bleeding disorders, illustrating a direct link between pharmacological interventions and patient outcomes. However, the treatment effect is often short-lived, necessitating further interventions (Haritoglou et al., 2011). As a result, it is necessary to understand how medications work in many ways to give the best care to those with coagulation disorders (Figure 9.8).

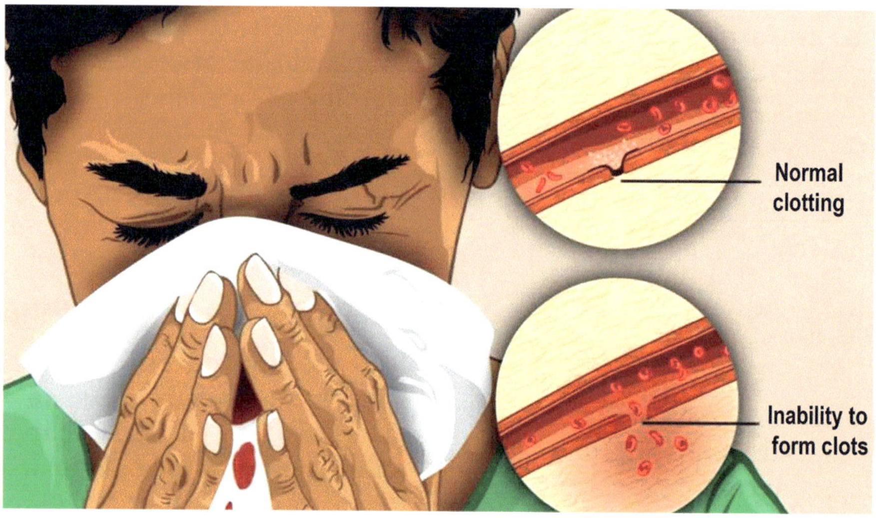

Figure 9.8. The use of clotting factor replacements is crucial for individuals with conditions such as hemophilia, where the body lacks specific factors necessary for proper coagulation.

Source: https://myhematology.com/wp-content/uploads/2024/05/Bleeding.jpg.

9.2.4. Chronic Diseases and Conditions

The connection between chronic diseases and coagulation disorders shows that they have a major impact on patient outcomes. Chronic conditions, such as multiple sclerosis (MS), have been linked to significant alterations in the coagulation pathways. Research indicates that fibrin(ogen) deposition closely correlates with clinical manifestations of MS, suggesting that thrombin and inflammatory responses play pivotal roles in the disease's progression (Adams et al., 2018). Furthermore, chronic multisymptom illnesses (CMI), including conditions like Chronic Fatigue Syndrome and fibromyalgia, may also reflect similar underlying mechanisms involving oxidative stress and mitochondrial dysfunction. The consistent identification of these pathophysiological processes in overlapping conditions suggests shared vulnerabilities that complicate treatment and management strategies for affected individuals (Beatrice, 2012). Studying these relationships helps us identify the different aspects of coagulation disorders and find possible treatments to ease symptoms and improve quality of life.

9.2.5. Lifestyle Factors

Our daily habits and lifestyle choices play a significant role in controlling coagulation disorders and influencing their occurrence and progression. A person's eating habits, physical activity, and substance use can impact both hemostasis and inflammation, potentially altering the clotting process. Including plenty of omega-3 fatty acids and little saturated fat in your diet can help improve your blood clotting. On the other hand, drinking too much alcohol and smoking can worsen clotting problems, which may cause more cases of thrombosis. Besides, not being physically active is connected to obesity, a condition that is more likely to result in VTE.

Recognizing these lifestyle factors enables the selection of the most effective ways to prevent illness and tailor treatments to each patient. By integrating lifestyle modifications alongside traditional treatments, healthcare providers can enhance patient outcomes and mitigate the risk of complications related to coagulation disorders, as highlighted by emerging studies on the interactions between lifestyle and disease dynamics (Bozzette et al., 2006; Vilder et al., 2015) (Figure 9.9).

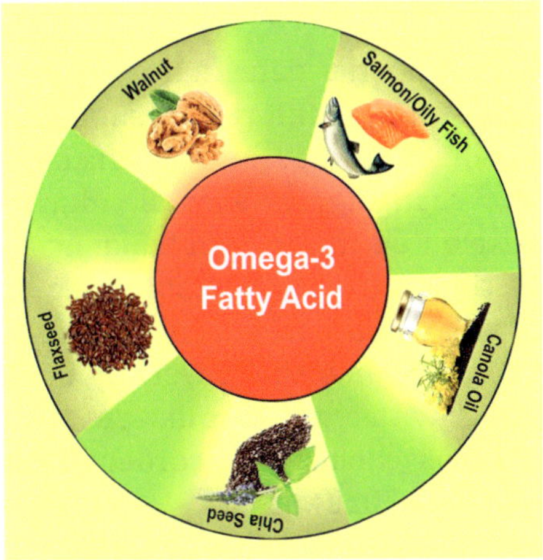

Figure 9.9. A diet high in omega-3 fatty acids and low in saturated fats has been shown to promote healthier blood coagulation profiles.

Source: https://pub.mdpi-res.com/life/life-13-01322/article_deploy/html/images/life-13-01322-g001.png?1686040263.

9.2.6. Age-Related Changes

As people get older, there are significant changes in the body, mainly in the coagulation system. It is essential to note that older individuals are more susceptible to coagulation disorders, primarily due to alterations in both blood clotting and the condition of blood vessels. Age-related changes can lead to an increased risk of hyperfibrinolysis, as observed in surgical settings such as orthotopic liver transplantation, where a drastic increase in tissue-type plasminogen activator activity can disrupt hemostasis (Bontempo et al., 1989). Additionally, elderly patients may develop inhibitory alloantibodies, which can compromise the effective management of bleeding disorders and complicate treatment options (Franchini et al., 2017). They point out the interaction between aging and the coagulation process, which means that older people with coagulation disorders need special treatments. Knowing about these changes in older people is important for better results in healthcare.

9.2.7. Gender Differences in Prevalence

It is clear from the data that gender plays a significant role in the occurrence of coagulation disorders, so these differences should be examined further. It is shown by research that women are more likely to develop certain blood clotting problems, such as VTE, when their hormone levels are changing, for example, during pregnancy and menopause. The increased risk can be partly attributed to the hypothalamic-pituitary-gonadal axis, as hormone imbalances affect both reproductive health and cardiovascular function. Specifically, (Donald et al., 2024) highlights how women with conditions like hypopituitarism face elevated cardiovascular risks, diverging from the trends observed in men. Conversely, studies suggest that men may experience different patterns of comorbidity with conditions like posttraumatic stress disorder, where gender affects the prevalence of specific psychological disorders that exacerbate physical health issues, as demonstrated in (Kristen et al., 2022). It is very important to understand these gender differences when planning screening and treatment for coagulation disorders.

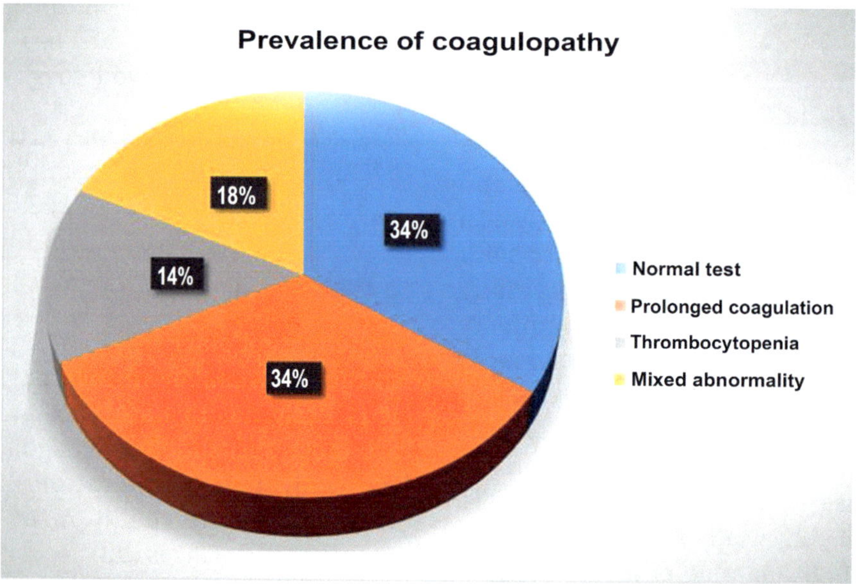

Figure 9.10. The influence of gender on the prevalence of coagulation disorders reveals significant disparities that warrant closer examination.

Source: https://media.springernature.com/lw685/springer-static/image/art%3A10.1186%2Fs12959-021-00287-6/MediaObjects/12959_2021_287_Fig1_HTML.png.

9.2.8. Family History and Inheritance Patterns

Family history is crucial in managing coagulation disorders, as these conditions are often inherited in specific ways that can significantly impact a patient's condition. Because many cases of hemophilia are passed on through families, people with this condition usually need extensive family research to identify those who carry or have the disorder. It is essential for couples who are planning to have children, since prenatal genetic testing can show the chances of passing on a disorder to their kids. As noted, the uptake of prenatal diagnosis and termination of an affected pregnancy is low in carriers of hemophilia, demonstrating the complex interplay of cultural and familial influences on reproductive choices (Abdul-Kadir et al., 2000). Moreover, family history can inform clinicians of potential complications during pregnancy and childbirth, underscoring the necessity of tailored management strategies for affected women (Felice et al., 2002).

9.2.9. Impact of Obesity on Coagulation

Obesity affects the coagulation system, increasing the risk of thrombosis. The main feature of this condition is constant inflammation that results in more procoagulant factors and fewer natural anticoagulants. It has been found that in obese individuals, fibrinogen and factor VIII levels are higher than normal, and these are essential for the blood clotting process. Additionally, being overweight can disrupt the balance between coagulation and fibrinolysis, thereby increasing the risk of blood clots. Because of these factors, the environment is more likely to cause VTE, a condition that is common among obese people. Guidelines emphasize that while genetic predispositions to thrombosis exist, acquired factors like obesity represent significant modifiable risks in managing coagulation disorders (Deepa et al., 2022). Observational studies further highlight the necessity for proactive monitoring and management strategies tailored for obese patients, particularly during surgical interventions or periods of immobility (Wichmann, 2020) (Figure 9.11).

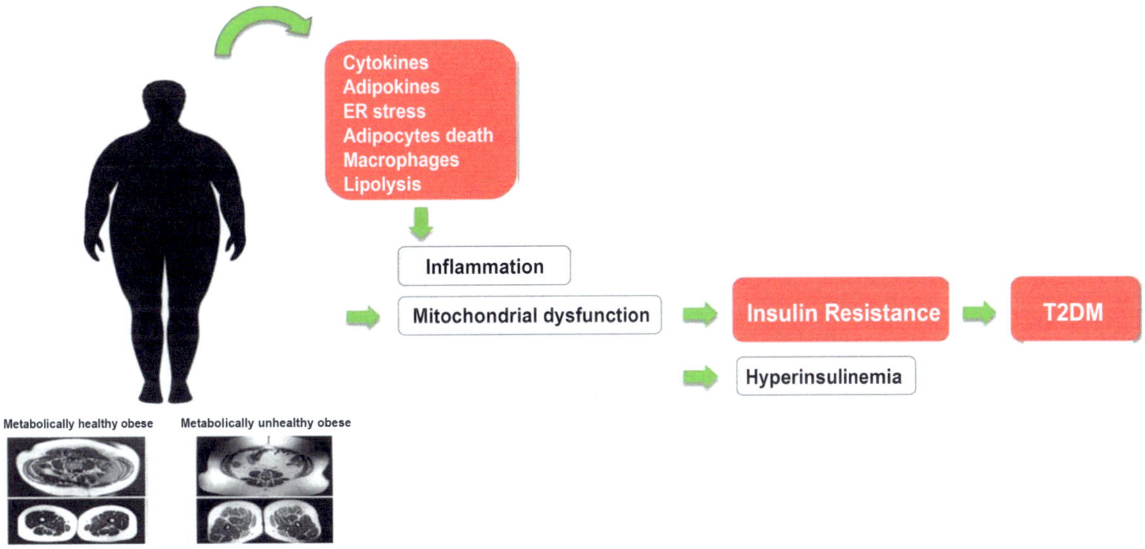

Figure 9.11. Obesity significantly influences the coagulation system, contributing to an increased risk of thrombosis.

Source: https://www.diabetesresearchclinicalpractice.com/cms/10.1016/j.diabres.2023.110773/asset/844a9d64-d173-47c6-83db-153fcf9d097a/main.assets/gr1_lrg.jpg.

9.3. Symptoms and Diagnosis

It is essential to recognize symptoms of coagulation disorders, as these conditions can lead to a wide range of bleeding issues. Clinical symptoms may include recurrent epistaxis, soft tissue bleeding, and joint bleeding, with the latter being particularly prevalent among patients with rare bleeding disorders (RBDs) (Solğun, 2025). For example, a 2-year-old boy exhibiting recurrent epistaxis was diagnosed with hypoprothrombinemia-lupus anticoagulant syndrome after a series of coagulation tests revealed prolonged activated partial thromboplastin time (APTT) and low prothrombin activity (Li et al., 2022).

Proper identification of the deficiency depends on detailed laboratory tests, such as APTT correction and factor level tests, which help doctors determine the appropriate treatment. It is essential to notice these symptoms and follow exact diagnostic steps to help patients and reduce the risks of coagulation disorders..

9.3.1. Common Symptoms of Coagulation Disorders

A variety of common symptoms can develop in coagulation disorders, having a significant impact on a person's health. Excessive bleeding or bruising is common for patients, such as regular nosebleeds, heavy menstrual periods, and spontaneous bruises on the skin. Bleeding inside joints, known as hemarthrosis, is another serious sign that causes significant pain and swelling, and may restrict a person's ability to move freely.

Additionally, thrombosis may occur, resulting in unwanted blood clots that can lead to serious complications such as stroke or PE, especially in conditions like APS where hypercoagulability is a hallmark (Marquardt et al., 2018). The intricacy of these disorders may also contribute to system-wide symptoms, including fatigue and weakness, as observed in overlapping chronic multisymptom illnesses (CMI) like Chronic Fatigue Syndrome (CFS), where oxidative stress and mitochondrial dysfunction play a significant role (Beatrice, 2012). The various symptoms demonstrate the importance of accurately diagnosing and managing coagulation disorders (Figure 9.12).

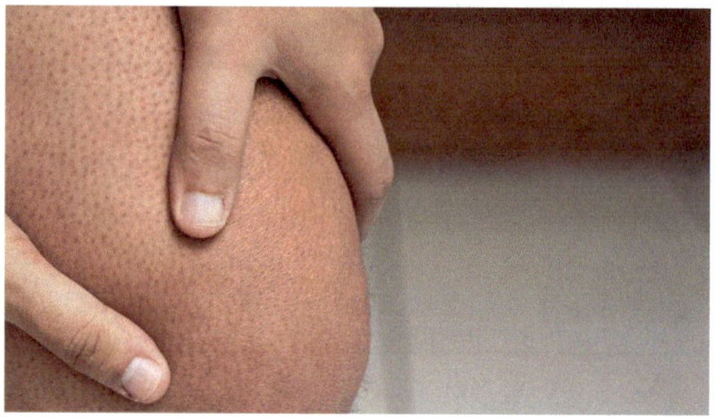

Figure 9.12. Hemarthrosis, or bleeding into joints, is another alarming symptom, leading to severe pain and swelling, which can impede mobility.

Source: https://arthritiskneepain.com/jjwp/wp-content/uploads/2024/06/swollen-knee-on-adult-male.jpg.

9.3.2. Diagnostic Tests for Coagulation Disorders

Several tests are necessary to help diagnose the causes of coagulation disorders. A fundamental tool in this process is the complete blood count (CBC), which provides essential insights into the overall blood profile and can reveal abnormalities in cell counts that may indicate a coagulation issue.

Apart from the CBC, tests are often performed to evaluate specific clotting factors and the entire coagulation process. These tests are vital in differentiating between various hematological abnormalities, as discussed in pediatric clinical practice (Chalmers et al., 2009).

Furthermore, in patients with liver disease, such as cirrhosis, the evaluation of coagulation profiles becomes critical due to the disease's impact on hemostasis and its potential complications, including severe bleeding during surgical interventions (Bacalbașa et al., 2019). For this reason, a planned approach to using these tests is crucial for controlling coagulation disorders.

9.3.3. Role of Blood Tests in Diagnosis

Blood tests help doctors diagnose coagulation disorders and give important details for treating the condition. By conducting various laboratory tests, healthcare professionals can identify any clotting factor issues and assess a person's risk of bleeding. For instance, remote diagnostic programs have been implemented to enhance the accessibility of blood testing for conditions such as VWD, where samples collected from patients are analyzed for von Willebrand factor (vWF) levels and activity (Poletaev et al., 2024).

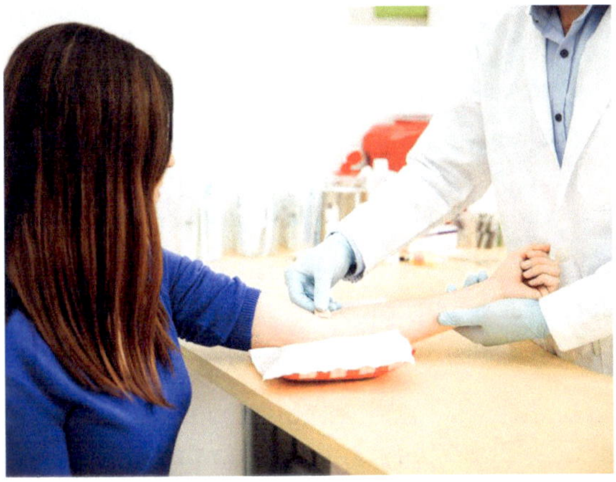

Figure 9.13. Blood tests play a critical role in the diagnosis of coagulation disorders, providing essential information that guides clinical management.

Source: https://media.post.rvohealth.io/wp-content/uploads/2020/08/coagulation-tests_thumb.jpg.

Additionally, advanced genetic testing initiatives, such as those undertaken by the American Thrombosis and Hemostasis Network (ATHN), have shed light on ultra-rare bleeding disorders, uncovering novel genetic variants that may compound existing deficiencies or result in unique bleeding phenotypes (Diane et al., 2024). Using all these diagnostic tools together enables the accurate identification and description of coagulation disorders, as well as the selection of the most suitable treatment plan for each patient (Figure 9.13).

9.3.4. Imaging Studies and Their Relevance

Imaging tests help doctors identify and manage coagulation disorders by detecting any related issues, such as joint damage and bleeding. In situations such as Hemophilia A, X-ray imaging is considered a simple and affordable way to assess joint strength. Research indicates that a majority of patients with Hemophilia A present with significant joint abnormalities, often categorized under the Arnold–Hilgartner classification, demonstrating the correlation between disease progression and radiographic findings, including joint space narrowing and bone degeneration (Faezovich, 2025). In addition, new imaging methods can help identify platelet secretion disorders, which are characterized by varying bleeding tendencies due to issues with platelet granule release. The integration of specialized imaging modalities enhances the diagnostic accuracy and therapeutic strategies employed for managing these complex coagulation disorders (Shahbazi et al., 2024).

9.3.5. Clinical Evaluation and Patient History

It is essential to review the patient's health history and conduct a thorough clinical assessment to diagnose coagulation disorders, since they play a key role in guiding treatment. For instance, in cases where symptoms such as ecchymoses or abnormal bleeding patterns are present, a thorough history is essential to discern whether these manifestations arise from a bleeding disorder or other causes, such as potential child abuse, as exemplified in reports of toddlers exhibiting bruising due to severe type I VWD (Marcos et al., 2015). Additionally, the implications of specific conditions, like Glanzmann's thrombasthenia, underscore the necessity of a detailed patient history, especially in emergency situations involving hemorrhagic cysts; improper assessments could lead to inappropriate surgical interventions (Meena et al., 2016). Combining the patient's history with the results of clinical examinations helps healthcare providers choose the right treatment, which in turn benefits the patient with coagulation disorders (Figure 9.14).

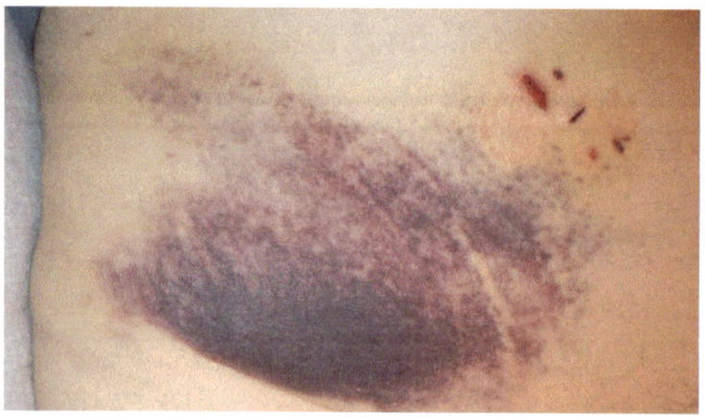

Figure 9.14. Ecchymoses.

Source: https://images-prod.healthline.com/hlcmsresource/images/Image-Galleries/Ecchymosis-gallery/2231-large_ecchymosis_of_the_flank-1296x728-slide3.jpg.

9.3.6. Differential Diagnosis Considerations

It is crucial to consider differential diagnosis in coagulation disorders, as these conditions can exhibit similar symptoms that can confuse the diagnosis. For instance, the distinguishing features between cytokine release syndrome (CRS) and immune effector cell-associated neurotoxicity syndrome (ICANS), as well as infectious complications, are paramount for effective patient care. Recent findings suggest that altered fibrinogen and D-dimer levels can serve as novel diagnostic markers, differentiating CRS/ICANS from infections following CAR-T therapy, potentially improving diagnosis accuracy in patients with hematologic malignancies (Yin et al., 2024). In the case of systemic diseases such as COVID-19, patients can show myocarditis and acute myocardial injury, which may also be similar to coagulation problems. This necessitates a nuanced approach to differential diagnosis, utilizing advanced imaging techniques and biomarkers to accurately identify the underlying pathology (Pleshko et al., 2023). Being detailed is crucial in providing patients with coagulation disorders the best possible treatment outcomes.

9.3.7. Importance of Early Detection

If coagulation disorders are found early, it helps improve the patient's condition and reduces the risk of complications.

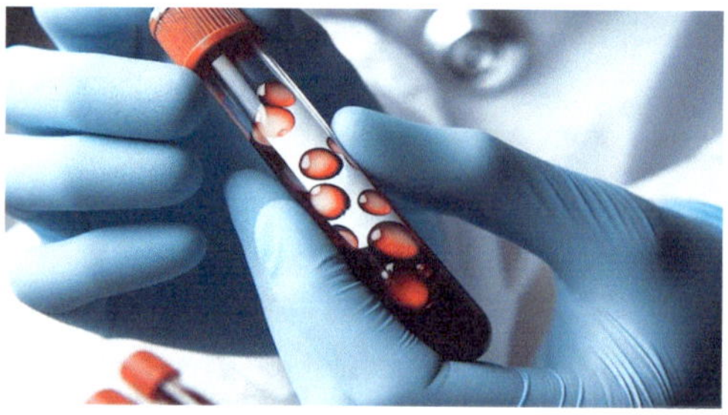

Figure 9.15. Early detection of coagulation disorders is paramount for improving patient outcomes and minimizing complications.

Source: https://medicalbuyer.co.in/wp-content/uploads/2024/04/Coagulation.png.

As seen in various studies, including those highlighting the implications of genetic factors such as ABCC6 gene duplications, timely identification of coagulation abnormalities can significantly enhance therapeutic interventions and risk stratification for patients (Arányi et al., 2010). For instance, a retrospective cohort study on snakebite victims demonstrated that markers like APTT and Prothrombin Time (PT) not only provide crucial insights into the severity of coagulopathy but also effectively predict adverse clinical outcomes such as severe bleeding and organ failure (Patange et al., 2023). Applying these tools enables doctors to initiate treatment for coagulation disorders earlier, thereby improving their management. For this reason, it is essential to incorporate early detection into medical practice to assist patients and alleviate the burden of these diseases (Figure 9.15).

9.3.8. Challenges in Diagnosing Coagulation Disorders

There are several challenges in diagnosing coagulation disorders, which can delay proper treatment. Many regions with little access to healthcare are struggling to identify and treat people with hemophilia. For instance, a study highlighted that in Thailand, discrepancies in diagnostic practices among general practitioners and specialists contribute to a significant underreporting of hemophiliacs within the healthcare system (Moonla et al., 2023). The situation becomes more complicated due to the complex procedures required to determine which coagulation factors are lacking. Moreover, emerging research suggests that diagnostic methodologies initially developed for other conditions, like multidrug-resistant tuberculosis, have revealed links between coagulation pathways and disease mechanisms, indicating potential overlaps that complicate the diagnostic landscape (Chen et al., 2020). Resolving these issues is necessary to help patients with coagulation disorders and provide them with proper care.

9.3.9. Advances in Diagnostic Technology

The use of advanced diagnostic tools has made it easier to identify and treat coagulation disorders, resulting in improved care for each patient. With point-of-care testing and advanced imaging, clinicians can quickly assess a patient's coagulation status and identify any factors that could cause excessive bleeding or the development of a blood clot. Due to these technologies, medical staff can respond quickly to emergencies and potentially alter the outcomes for patients. Additionally, utilizing AI in data analysis enables the detection of complex patterns in coagulation, leading to the identification of new biomarkers crucial for various bleeding disorders. The latest studies indicate that understanding hemostatic processes is crucial for developing more effective treatments for patients. In particular, addressing challenges related to thromboembolic complications, such as those highlighted during the COVID-19 pandemic, underscores the importance of continuous innovation in diagnostic tools (Guarnieri et al., 2024; Azi et al., 2024).

9.4. Treatment and Management

Treatment and management of coagulation disorders should be tailored to the specific type of disorder and its underlying causes. In fulminant myocarditis, it is essential to act fast because the illness can lead to severe blood clotting problems and increase the risk of death. This emphasizes the importance of promptly correcting coagulation dysfunction through targeted therapies (Dong et al., 2025). Also, since schizophrenia is generally treated with antipsychotic drugs for a long time, it brings up another issue because these drugs may increase the risk of blood clots. Understanding the mechanisms linking these medications to coagulation changes is crucial for clinicians, who must closely monitor patients and implement preventive measures to mitigate these risks (Hasni et al., 2024). In general, using both medications and lifestyle changes is crucial for effectively managing coagulation disorders.

9.4.1. Replacement Therapy for Hemophilia

Hemophilia replacement therapy is a cornerstone of the treatment of this bleeding disorder, primarily comprising the infusion of clotting factors VIII or IX to avoid complications of bleeding episodes. However, a critical limitation of this therapy is the induction of inhibitory antibodies against the infused factors, which complicates clinical management by drastically reducing the efficacy of the therapy and increasing the likelihood of adverse complications (Franchini et al., 2017). This response not only increases the difficulty in achieving hemostasis but also contributes to a significant increase in healthcare costs and patient disability. In addition, gene therapy is being investigated to overcome these constraints, which could lead to long-term correction of factor deficiencies through the cure of underlying genetic diseases (Buckley et al., 2011). As such, research into conventional replacement therapy and new gene-editing techniques continues at a rapid pace and is of paramount importance for advancing patient outcomes in hemophilia (Figure 9.16).

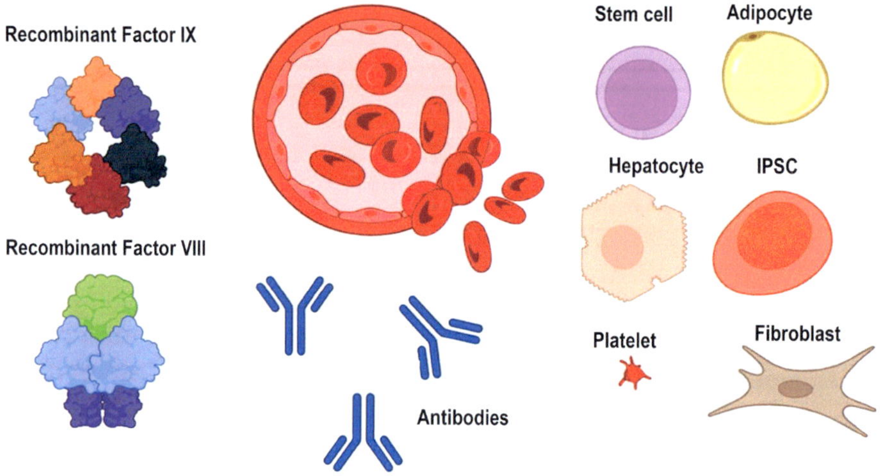

Figure 9.16. Replacement therapy for hemophilia represents a cornerstone in the management of this coagulation disorder, primarily involving the infusion of clotting factors VIII or IX to mitigate the risk of bleeding episodes.

Source: https://www.mdpi.com/biomolecules/biomolecules-14-00854/article_deploy/html/images/biomolecules-14-00854-g002.png.

9.4.2. Anticoagulant Medications

The involvement of anticoagulant drugs in managing coagulation disorders is increasingly identified as imperative, most importantly, preventing thromboembolic complications that may cause dire situations like stroke. Such drugs, including warfarin and non-vitamin K oral anticoagulants, block specific steps of the coagulation cascade to inhibit excessive clot formation. Although effective, patient management on anticoagulants is problematic, particularly in the case of invasive procedures where the risk of bleeding needs to be weighed with great caution. Today's education emphasizes that most patients on anticoagulants are at risk of excessive bleeding, with the interaction between systemic states and oral hemostasis tending to be misrepresented (Barber et al., 2003). In addition, malignancy patients are also vulnerable to such complications because coagulopathy can also present in the form of thrombosis, hence putting them at risk of ischemic events such as stroke (Paris et al., 2015). Therefore, effective management necessitates a fine balancing act between avoiding thrombotic complications and reducing bleeding risk.

9.4.3. Lifestyle Modifications and Self-care

Lifestyle modifications and self-care play a crucial role in managing coagulation disorders, as these conditions often necessitate patients to adopt daily practices that promote their overall health and well-being. For instance, individuals diagnosed with these disorders benefit from maintaining a balanced diet, engaging in regular physical activity, and monitoring their health metrics, which can significantly reduce complications. Research indicates that systematic health education empowers patients to adopt effective self-care management, fostering autonomy in their treatment plans (Nadatien et al., 2024).

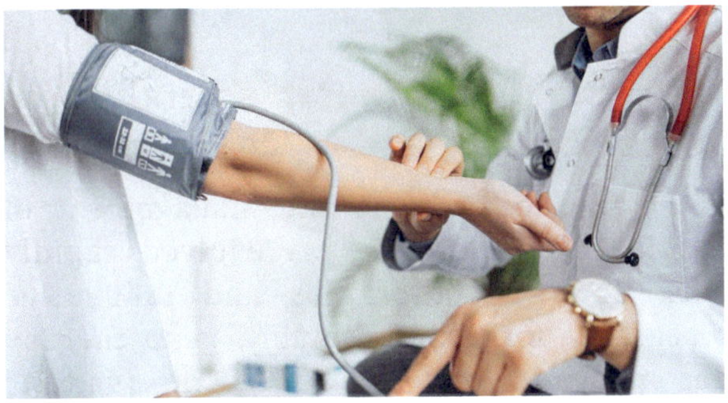

Figure 9.17. Lifestyle modifications and self-care play a pivotal role in managing coagulation disorders, as these conditions often require patients to implement daily practices that enhance their overall health and well-being.

Source: https://www.apexhospitals.com/_next/image?url=https%3A%2F%2Fbed.apexhospitals.com%2Fuploads%2Fhealth_packages2_4949864613.jpg&w=1920&q=75.

Moreover, adherence to established self-care practices is closely linked to educational background and access to healthcare resources, as demonstrated in studies focusing on chronic conditions like diabetes, where individuals with higher education levels exhibit better self-management behaviors (Endale et al., 2025). Thus, inclusion of holistic lifestyle modifications into any patient care enhances the outcomes of all patients additionally reducing the long-term effects of coagulation disorders (Figure 9.17).

9.4.4. Role of Physical Therapy

Physical therapy is a significant component of overall management for disorders of coagulation, particularly in facilitating mobility and correcting the physical complications associated with these conditions. Bleeding disorders such as hemophilia tend to result in pain and impairment of joints as a result of repeated hemorrhages that might eventually cause permanent damage to the musculoskeletal system. Tailored physical therapy interventions can help overcome such challenges by assisting with strength training, flexibility exercises, and gait reeducation to improve joint function, reduce risk, and prevent additional bleeding episodes. Patients and their families can also be educated by physical therapists about safe exercises, ensuring that exercise activities remain both beneficial and low-risk. As validated in recent recommendations, multidisciplinary management, of which physical therapy is a part, is necessary for changing the natural course of bleeding disorders and treating individuals with these conditions holistically (François Mach et al., 2019; Srivastava et al., 2020). Therefore, incorporating physical therapy is imperative for maximizing the outcome in patients with coagulation disorders.

9.4.5. Management of Bleeding Episodes

Effective management of bleeding episodes in individuals with coagulation disorders necessitates a nuanced understanding of the underlying pathology, as well as a comprehensive approach tailored to the specific condition. Clinicians are tasked with balancing the prevention of hemorrhagic events while minimizing the risk of thrombosis, particularly in cases characterized by both coagulation and fibrinolytic system impairments (Crispino, 2023). The complexity of this management is highlighted by the inconsistent correlation between coagulation factor activity levels and bleeding severity observed in rare bleeding disorders, necessitating further investigation and individual assessment (Tavasoli et al., 2024). Treatment strategies may include the administration of clotting factor concentrates, antifibrinolytics, and supportive care, depending on the severity of the disorder and the patient's overall health status. Ultimately, an individualized treatment plan that takes into account patient-specific factors and bleeding history is integral for optimizing outcomes in managing these challenging conditions (Figure 9.18).

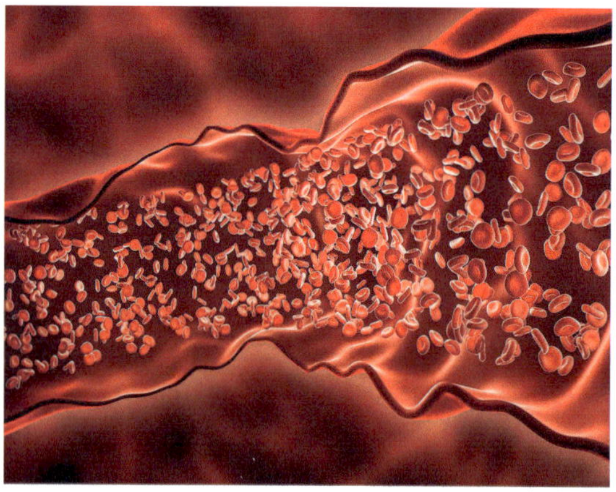

Figure 9.18. Management of bleeding episodes.

Source: https://ameripharmaspecialty.com/wp-content/uploads/2022/11/hemophilia.jpg.

9.4.6. Education and Support for Patients

Effective education and support for patients with coagulation disorders is paramount in enhancing their understanding of their condition and improving health outcomes. Providing patients with comprehensive education about the nature of their disorder, treatment options, and the importance of adherence to prescribed therapies can significantly reduce the risks associated with these conditions. Moreover, support systems such as peer groups and access to health care professionals can create a sense of community, which takes away feelings of isolation. Use of Diagnostic Management Teams, which provide pre-test counseling on what testing is necessary and how it should be interpreted, can ease the process of diagnosis, thereby improving patient care and conserving health care resources (Velazquez et al., 2018). Additionally, understanding biomarkers related to coagulation disorders can empower patients to monitor their health effectively, as evident in the correlations found between migraine types and vascular disease markers (Ferrari et al., 2018). Thus, education and support play a critical role in managing coagulation disorders effectively.

9.4.7. Emerging Therapies and Research

The new landscape of the management of coagulation disorders has evolved rapidly with emergent therapies and innovative research approaches. Notably, gene therapy has proven good at addressing genetic factors, such as in certain disorders like Hemophilia A, caused by factor VIII deficiency, which triggers complications such as severe hemophilic arthropathy and thrombosis (Azhar et al., 2021). At the same time, studies on new hemostatic agents are underway for both organic and inorganic substances capable of efficiently stopping bleeding during trauma. These substances work through exploiting special properties like water adsorption from blood, which tends to improve clot formation through localized concentration of key proteins (Guarnieri et al., 2024). Collectively, these advances represent a paradigm shift in treatment strategies, moving beyond merely alleviating symptoms to ultimately improve the quality of life for individuals with coagulation disorders (Figure 9.19).

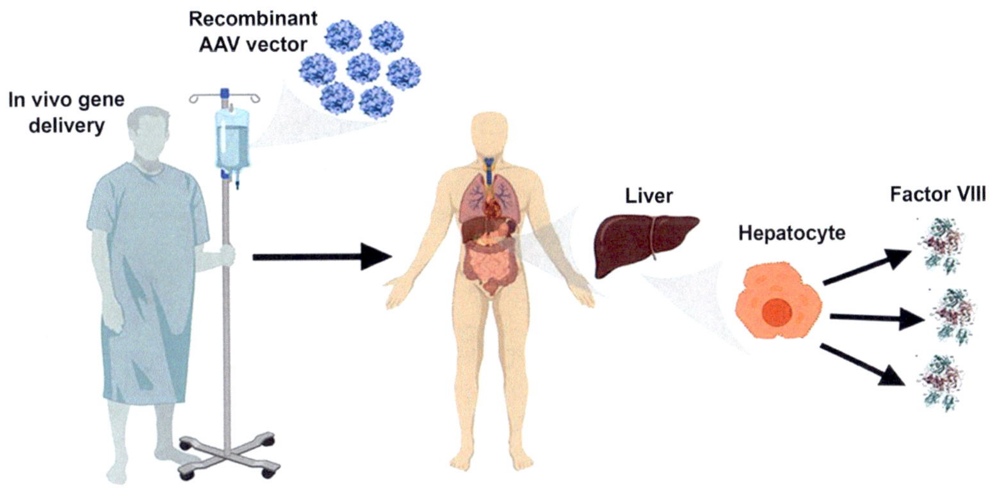

Figure 9.19. The introduction of gene therapy has shown promise in addressing genetic factors underlying conditions like Hemophilia A, which is characterized by factor VIII deficiency and can lead to severe complications such as hemophilic arthropathy and thrombosis.

Source: https://www.frontiersin.org/files/Articles/521124/fimmu-11-00494-HTML/image_m/fimmu-11-00494-g001.jpg.

9.4.8. Psychological Support and Counseling

The intersection of psychological support and counseling with the management of coagulation disorders is a critical area that merits attention. Patients grappling with these disorders often experience unique psychological challenges, including anxiety over bleeding episodes and the implications for daily activities, which can profoundly affect their mental well-being. Effective psychological interventions can mitigate these anxieties, enhancing the patient's quality of life. Preoperative psychological screening and counseling are implemented to prepare patients for the emotional states associated with their treatment, thereby emphasizing control and building resilience (Gupta et al., 2025). Education programs intended to improve patient awareness of the condition can enhance self-acceptance and coping, critical to reducing symptoms of depression (Stanescu et al., 2025). By integrating mental health strategies with conventional medical treatment, healthcare providers can create a comprehensive support system that promotes both physical healing and emotional health.

9.4.9. Importance of Regular Monitoring

Monitoring is crucial in the treatment of coagulation disorders to achieve optimal therapeutic outcomes and minimize associated risks. Anticoagulant-treated patients, such as those receiving warfarin, are most susceptible to variations in coagulation factors, which necessitate repeated monitoring of the international normalized ratio (INR) to ensure continued therapeutic activity and prevent precipitating unwanted events, such as hemorrhage. Research highlights the challenges associated with anticoagulant treatments, particularly Vitamin K antagonists, which necessitate meticulous monitoring due to their interactions with various factors, including diet and other medications (Dockrill et al., 2018). Additionally, comorbid patients highlight the importance of careful monitoring, as underlying conditions can complicate the clinical scenario and impact treatment efficacy and safety profiles. Therefore, structured monitoring protocols significantly enhance patient adherence and satisfaction, which in turn implies better health outcomes in the management of coagulation disorders, as empirical studies report (Cénac et al., 2012) (Figure 9.20).

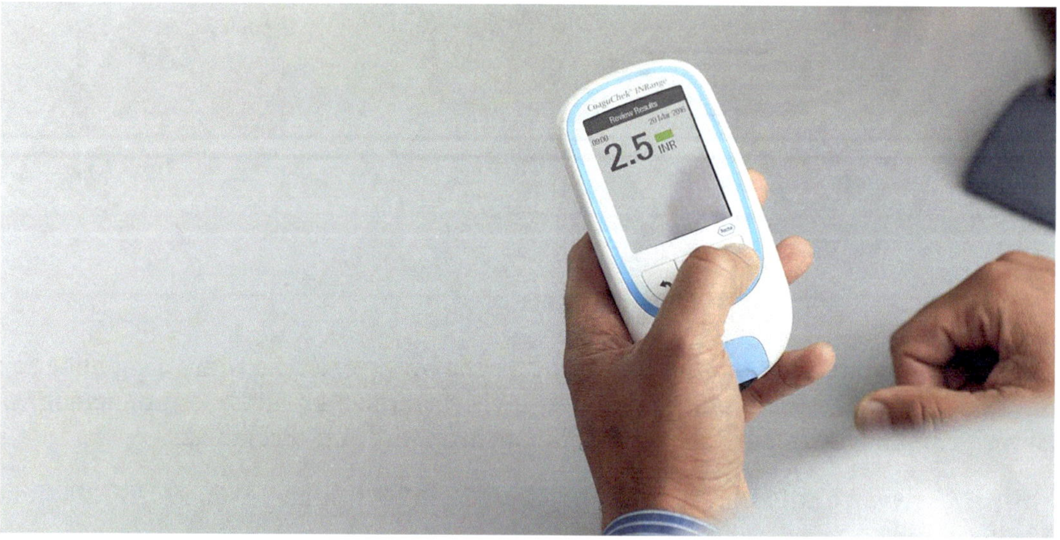

Figure 9.20. Coagulation self-monitoring.

Source: https://roche.scene7.com/is/image/RocheDiaProd/cc-hero-inrange-grey-banner-1?scl=1.

A CLOSER LOOK

VENOUS THROMBOEMBOLISM (VTE)

VTE is an illness characterized by blood clots forming in the veins, typically in the deep veins of the legs or pelvis, referred to as deep vein thrombosis (DVT). When a piece of the clot breaks away and lodges in the lungs, it can result in a possibly fatal pulmonary embolism (PE).

VTE can be precipitated by conditions like prolonged immobility, surgery, certain medical conditions, pregnancy, or inherited blood coagulation disorders. Leg swelling, pain, and redness are symptoms of DVT, whereas PE can cause sudden shortness of breath, chest pain, and palpitations.

Treatment typically involves anticoagulant drugs to prevent clot extension and the formation of new clots, and occasionally, operations to extract or lyse clots in severe cases. Early detection and treatment are crucial to avert potentially life-threatening complications.

SUMMARY

The complexity of coagulation disorders thereby highlights the importance of having an in-depth knowledge and effective management practices. This is well-established through recent research, which has highlighted the alarming interaction between abnormal cerebrovascular mechanisms and cognitive deficits in individuals with these disorders, indicating that various mechanisms, such as neurovascular uncoupling and impaired glymphatic pathways, are involved in these harmful effects (Ackah et al., 2025). Additionally, the heterogeneity of bleeding severity in patients with rare bleeding disorders underscores the challenge of establishing reproducible correlations between coagulation factor activity and clinical features (Tavasoli et al., 2024). Such irreproducibility necessitates further research to elucidate underlying associations, refine screening protocols, and enhance patient-centered care. Ultimately, it will be necessary to have a sophisticated approach that integrates findings from the large-scale studies and more specific case analyses to finally refine treatment modalities and improve quality of life for patients within the spectrum of coagulation disorders.

An examination of coagulation disorders reveals several significant points that advance our understanding of their pathophysiologic basis and potential therapeutic maneuvers. Firstly, certain genetic predispositions, as reflected in recent work, hold important implications between coagulation disorders and other systemic diseases, such as gastrointestinal disease and immune response. For example, the demonstration of pivotal genes associated with these disorders highlights their role in essential biological processes that also converge with immunomodulation (Chen et al., 2025). Aside from genetics, environmental factors such as diet and lifestyle also play a significant role in the development of coagulation disturbances (Wang et al., 2025). In addition, developments in genetic studies form the foundation for personalized medicine strategies, allowing for more precise interventions. Therefore, the convergence of genetic, immunological, and environmental aspects provides an integrative platform for understanding and managing coagulation disorders efficiently.

REFERENCES

1. Economides, D. L., Kadir, R. A., & Lee, C. A. (1999). Inherited bleeding disorders in obstetrics and gynaecology. *BJOG an International Journal of Obstetrics & Gynaecology, 106*(1), 5–13. https://doi.org/10.1111/j.1471-0528.1999.tb08078.xAcharya, A., Barlow, J., Barry, K., Buhrman, B., Buzzard, S., Cour, K., Eckman, E., et al. (2014). A review of evidence about behavioral and psychological aspects of chronic joint pain among people with hemophilia. https://core.ac.uk/download/46171148.pdf (accessed on 12th June 2025).
2. Ackah, J. A., Li, X., Zeng, H., & Chen, X. (2025). Imaging-validated correlates and implications of the pathophysiologic mechanisms of ageing-related cerebral large artery and small vessel diseases: A systematic review and meta-analysis. *Behavioral and Brain Functions: BBF, 21.* https://www.semanticscholar.org/paper/c2e8acd37ad64da0f5e593a4f9768e8c9d9a0662 (accessed on 12th June 2025).
3. Adams, R., Akassoglou, K., Akenami, F. O., Albright, A. V., et al. (2018). A perspective of coagulation dysfunction in multiple sclerosis and in experimental allergic encephalomyelitis. https://core.ac.uk/download/195777098.pdf (accessed on 12th June 2025).
4. Agizew, E., Hundessa, F., Tamru, E., Nigussie, F., & Hailu, M. (2025). Adherence to diabetic self-care management and associated factors among type 2 diabetic patients in North Shewa Zone public hospitals in Amhara Region, Ethiopia. *Frontiers in Clinical Diabetes and Healthcare.* https://www.semanticscholar.org/paper/74934ce4f2d0513bf15bc99e33013f8ea7bc59df (accessed on 12th June 2025).
5. Arachchillage, D. J., Mackillop, L., Chandratheva, A., Motawani, J., MacCallum, P., & Laffan, M. (2022). Thrombophilia testing: A British Society for Hematology guideline. *British Journal of Hematology, 198*, 443–458. https://doi.org/10.1111/bjh.18239 (accessed on 12th June 2025).
6. Arányi, T., Bakos, É., Fülöp, K., Iliás, A., et al. (2010). *Az ABC-fehérjék Tudományos Iskolája: a gének regulációjától a transzport-mechanizmusig = The School of ABC-proteins: From Gene Regulation to Transport Mechanism.* https://core.ac.uk/download/11854978.pdf (accessed on 12th June 2025).
7. Azhar, A. A. M., Banerjee, K. G., Izam, F., Mokhtar, N., et al. (2021). The key complications of hemophilia and recent advancements in their management: An update. https://core.ac.uk/download/539911108.pdf (accessed on 12th June 2025).
8. Azi, C. I., Carsrud, N. D. V., Ezewudo, O., Flores, H., et al. (2024). Hematological conditions associated with COVID-19: Pathophysiology, clinical manifestations, and therapeutic approaches. https://core.ac.uk/download/621451769.pdf (accessed on 12th June 2025).
9. Bacalbașa, N., Banu, P., Bălălău, C., Ghinghină, I., et al. (2019). The risk of bleeding and encephalopathy in surgical patients with liver cirrhosis. https://core.ac.uk/download/216811033.pdf (accessed on 12th June 2025).
10. Barber, A., Lumb, A. B., Kaye, A. D., Turpie, A. G. G., Friedlander, A. H., Schafer, A. I., Ziffer, A. M., et al. (2003). Dental management considerations for the patient with an acquired coagulopathy. Part 1: Coagulopathies from systemic disease. https://core.ac.uk/download/9348885.pdf (accessed on 12th June 2025).
11. Baumgartner, H., De Backer, J., Babu-Narayan, S. V., Budts, W., Chessa, M., Diller, G. P., Lung, B., et al. (2020). 2020 ESC guidelines for the management of adult congenital heart disease.

European Heart Journal, 42, 563–645. https://doi.org/10.1093/eurheartj/ehaa554 (accessed on 12th June 2025).

12. Berumen Velazquez, A., Laposata, M., & Verna, R. (2018). Diagnostic error reduction in the United States and Italy through the intervention of diagnostic management teams. https://core.ac.uk/download/160649042.pdf (accessed on 12th June 2025).
13. Bontempo, F. A., Kang, Y. G., Knot, E. A. R., Lewis, J., et al. (1989). Systemic effects of tissue plasminogen activator-associated fibrinolysis and its relation to thrombin generation in orthotopic liver transplantation. https://core.ac.uk/download/12204422.pdf (accessed on 12th June 2025).
14. Bozzette, S., Diamond, M., Koerper, M. A., Kulkarni, R., et al. (2006). Clinical perspectives of emerging pathogens in bleeding disorders. https://core.ac.uk/download/323066967.pdf (accessed on 12th June 2025).
15. Buckley, S. M., Chan, J. K., Howe, S. J., McKay, T., et al. (2011). Perinatal gene transfer to the liver. https://core.ac.uk/download/18302246.pdf (accessed on 12th June 2025).
16. Carolina Wermelinger Erthal, Gabriela Ayres, Thaís Dourado Reis Nóbrega, Rothschild, C., Stefanello, B., Okazaki, E., Prestes, P., et al. (2024). Rare coagulation disorders: A comprehensive study from the largest hospital in Latin America. *Blood*. https://www.semanticscholar.org/paper/1cbaa4643abe2b0f57df3d5cc0a2cde1c31c23ae (accessed on 12th June 2025).
17. Cénac, A., Gutenberg, A., Lecube, A., Zargar, A. H., Ajith, C., Castle, D., Sidibe, E. H., et al. (2012). Post-partum pituitary insufficiency and livedo reticularis presenting a diagnostic challenge in a resource limited setting in Tanzania: A case report, clinical discussion and brief review of existing literature. https://core.ac.uk/download/pdf/16666922.pdf (accessed on 12th June 2025).
18. Chalmers, E. A., & Halsey, C. (2009). Hematological investigations in children. https://core.ac.uk/download/110273.pdf (accessed on 12th June 2025).
19. Changjing Xu, Junlong Zhu, Kun Tu, Hui Tang, Xinxin Zhou, Qiuyu Li, Kun Chen, et al. (2025). The clinical features and risk factors of coagulopathy associated with cefoperazone/sulbactam: A nomogram prediction model. *Frontiers in Pharmacology, 15*. https://www.semanticscholar.org/paper/68c4fbf81cd69b41df179b28c8dbf3555680186c (accessed on 12th June 2025).
20. Chen, J., Han, Y. S., Yi, W. J., Huang, H., Li, Z., Shi, L., Wei, L., et al. (2020). Serum sCD14, PGLYRP2 and FGA as potential biomarkers for multidrug-resistant tuberculosis based on data-independent acquisition and targeted proteomics. *Journal of Cellular and Molecular Medicine, 24*, 12537–12549. https://doi.org/10.1111/jcmm.15796 (accessed on 12th June 2025).
21. Chen, J., Hou, J., Chen, X., Fan, W., & Sun, P. (2025). Identifying key genes for neurobehavioral disorders caused by long-term sleep deprivation. *Current Analytical Chemistry*. https://www.semanticscholar.org/paper/226aaea61497554fdc3e4ec669387aa3c0f2d43c (accessed on 12th June 2025).
22. Copaescu, A., Smibert, O., Gibson, A., Phillips, E. J., & Trubiano, J. A. (2020). The role of IL-6 and other mediators in the cytokine storm associated with SARS-CoV-2 infection. *Journal of Allergy and Clinical Immunology, 146*, 518–534.e1. https://doi.org/10.1016/j.jaci.2020.07.001
23. Crispino, P. (2023). Hemorrhagic coagulation disorders and ischemic stroke: How to reconcile

both? *Neurology International, 15*, 1443–1458. https://www.semanticscholar.org/paper/8195ad3f7d836922443a1be9d68f94c9e90bb1b0 (accessed on 12th June 2025).

24. Daly, E., Gough, P., Lowe, G., Rumley, A., et al. (2000). Thrombotic variables and risk of idiopathic venous thromboembolism in women aged 45–64 years–Relationships to hormone replacement therapy. https://core.ac.uk/download/9350045.pdf (accessed on 12th June 2025).

25. De Vilder, E., & Vanakker, O. (2015). From variome to phenome: Pathogenesis, diagnosis and management of ectopic mineralization disorders. https://core.ac.uk/download/55848035.pdf (accessed on 12th June 2025).

26. Dockrill, S. J., Gorog, D., & Vimalesvaran, K. (2018). Role of rivaroxaban in the management of atrial fibrillation: Insights from clinical practice. https://core.ac.uk/download/287581671.pdf (accessed on 12th June 2025).

27. Dong, S., Peng, Q., Lu, K., Wei, Q., & Yang, J. (2025). Successful management of coagulation dysfunction in a patient with fulminant myocarditis: A case report. *Frontiers in Cardiovascular Medicine, 11*. https://www.semanticscholar.org/paper/0f4a1294505803f05361e36b1871ad05abf83360 (accessed on 12th June 2025).

28. Elendu, C., Amaechi, D. C., Alakwe-Ojimba, C. E., Elendu, T. C., Elendu, R. C., Ayabazu, C. P., Aina, T. O., Aborisade, O., & Adenikinju, J. S. (2023). Understanding sickle cell disease: Causes, symptoms, and treatment options. *Medicine (Baltimore), 102*(38), e35237. https://doi.org/10.1097/MD.0000000000035237 (accessed on 12th June 2025).

29. Faezovich, V. F. (2025). X-ray diagnostics of femoral head destruction in patients with hemophilia A. *International Journal for Research in Applied Science and Engineering Technology*. https://www.semanticscholar.org/paper/48694b63d7421b2ca8aef44b9bad9462c43e873b (accessed on 12th June 2025).

30. Felice, A. (2002). Molecular biology at the bedside: The impact of genomics on the practice of medicine. https://core.ac.uk/download/46601830.pdf (accessed on 12th June 2025).

31. Ferrari, M. D., Herial, N., Khubchandani, J., Koppen, H., et al. (2018). Migraine and vascular disease biomarkers: A population-based case-control study. https://core.ac.uk/download/213449740.pdf (accessed on 12th June 2025).

32. Fornasiero, A., Ristori, G., Salvetti, M., Buscarinu, M. C., Ferraldeschi, M., Umeton, R., et al. (2019). Genome-wide multiple sclerosis association data and coagulation. https://core.ac.uk/download/195777097.pdf (accessed on 12th June 2025).

33. Franchini, M., Liumbruno, G. M., Marano, G., Mengoli, C., et al. (2017). Inhibitors in patients with congenital bleeding disorders other than hemophilia. https://core.ac.uk/download/153367572.pdf (accessed on 12th June 2025).

34. Golomb, B. A. (2012). Oxidative stress and mitochondrial injury in chronic multisymptom conditions: From Gulf War illness to autism spectrum disorder. https://core.ac.uk/download/pdf/290596.pdf (accessed on 12th June 2025).

35. Goswami, Y., & Gaurkar, S. (2023). Ramsay Hunt syndrome: An introduction, signs and symptoms, and treatment. *Cureus, 15*. https://www.semanticscholar.org/paper/d1156ab20a108fe569a25ebe45da0fbcb5caf864 (accessed on 12th June 2025).

36. Guarnieri, G. de P., & Nery, J. G. (2024). Reflections on the potential of applying artificial intelligence (AI) and machine learning (ML) for screening topical hemostatic agents based

on inorganic solids for hemorrhage control. https://core.ac.uk/download/636476028.pdf (accessed on 12th June 2025).

37. Gupta, R., Bansal, P., Chaudhury, G., Gupta, R., Keshari, A., & Sharma, P. (2025). Psychological determinants of patient satisfaction in aesthetic surgery: The impact of preoperative screening and counselling. *International Journal of Aesthetic Plastic Surgery, 1*, 57–62. https://www.semanticscholar.org/paper/368beecd27f53807c154bcc18400cd42091de1e1 (accessed on 12th June 2025).

38. Han, J., Yoon, I., & Jeon, H. J. (2024). Microfluidic system-based quantitative analysis of platelet function through speckle size measurement. *Biomolecules, 14*. https://www.semanticscholar.org/paper/a26c86b0fea0fde3dcd2887ff05c30b2b337bd9f (accessed on 12th June 2025).

39. Haritoglou, C., Jagow, B. von, Ulbig, M., Wolf, A., et al. (2011). Intracameral injection of bevacizumab for the treatment of neovascular glaucoma. https://core.ac.uk/download/16432295.pdf (accessed on 12th June 2025).

40. Hasni, D., Anggraini, D., Anissa, M., & Khan, M. S. S. (2024). A review of antipsychotic medications on hypercoagulability in schizophrenia: Pathophysiology, risks, and management strategies. *Journal of Angiotherapy*. https://www.semanticscholar.org/paper/a2fe1d2b9c6f111f045c80b8ba89b95b1612d813 (accessed on 12th June 2025).

41. Kumano, O., Peyrafitte, M., & Amiral, J. (2023). Update on laboratory practice for the diagnosis of lupus anticoagulant and the antiphospholipid syndrome. *Exploration of Immunology*. https://www.semanticscholar.org/paper/30079556463953a4d2cc15021e9483cc45bf39ab (accessed on 12th June 2025).

42. Li, J. Z., Tian, X., Liao, C. S., He, X., & Zhu, C. (2022). [Recurrent epistaxis with coagulation disorders in a boy aged 2 years]. *Zhonghua Dang Dai Er Ke Za Zhi = Chinese Journal of Contemporary Pediatrics, 24*(7), 817–820. https://www.semanticscholar.org/paper/70960c5ff05666dadb30991ee5ef0fc77c50d46a (accessed on 12th June 2025).

43. Lisman, T., Susen, S., & Tiede, A. (2024). Acquired bleeding disorders. https://core.ac.uk/download/620146008.pdf (accessed on 12th June 2025).

44. Loh, P. K., Ng, K. W. P., & Sharma, V. K. (2011). Role of investigating thrombophilia disorders in young stroke. https://core.ac.uk/download/pdf/8526643.pdf (accessed on 12th June 2025).

45. Mach, F., Baigent, C., Catapano, A. L., Koskinas, K. C., Casula, M., Badimón, L., Chapman, M. J., et al. (2019). 2019 ESC/EAS guidelines for the management of dyslipidemias: Lipid modification to reduce cardiovascular risk. *European Heart Journal, 41*, 111–188. https://doi.org/10.1093/eurheartj/ehz455 (accessed on 12th June 2025).

46. Marquardt, C. W., Pickens, P. V., & Varner, C. K. (2018). Antiphosphatidylserine antibody as a cause of multiple dural venous sinus thromboses and ST-elevation myocardial infarction. https://core.ac.uk/download/213444063.pdf (accessed on 12th June 2025).

47. McDonald, D., McDonnell, T., O'Reilly, M. W., & Sherlock, M. (2024). Replacement with sex steroids in hypopituitary men and women: Implications for gender differences in morbidities and mortality. *Reviews in Endocrine & Metabolic Disorders, 25*, 839–854. https://www.semanticscholar.org/paper/3abbba7f2e2957820dd5524dba0e262a17297e93 (accessed on 12th June 2025).

48. Minagar, A., Maghzi, A. H., Bidot, C. J., Horstman, L. L., Etemadifar, M., Zivadinov, R., Kelley,

R. E., et al. (2009). Antiphospholipid antibodies: Paradigm in transition. https://core.ac.uk/download/pdf/81636382.pdf (accessed on 12th June 2025).

49. Montes, R., Panizo, C., Paramo, J. A., Rocha, E., et al. (1998). Acute generalized, widespread bleeding. Diagnosis and management. https://core.ac.uk/download/83572896.pdf (accessed on 12th June 2025).

50. Moonla, C., Sosothikul, D., Pongtanakul, B., Suwanawiboon, B., Traivaree, C., Natesirinilkul, R., Sirachainan, N., & Angchaisuksiri, P. (2023). Practices and challenges for hemophilia management under resource constraints in Thailand. *Orphanet Journal of Rare Diseases, 18,* 110. https://doi.org/10.1186/s13023-023-02718-1 (accessed on 12th June 2025).

51. Nadatien, I., Puspita, U. N., Kartini, Y., Setiyowati, E., & Hidayah, N. (2024). Does education influence self-care management in diabetes mellitus patients? Systematic review. *Journal of Applied Nursing and Health*. https://www.semanticscholar.org/paper/8259bc16098e13ae1adf8cc86b83e0b6d149786c (accessed on 12th June 2025).

52. Northup, P. G., García-Pagán, J. C., García-Tsao, G., Intagliata, N. M., Superina, R., Roberts, L. N., Lisman, T., et al. (2020). Vascular liver disorders, portal vein thrombosis, and procedural bleeding in patients with liver disease: 2020 practice guidance by the American Association for the Study of Liver Diseases. *Hepatology, 73,* 366–413. https://doi.org/10.1002/hep.31646 (accessed on 12th June 2025).

53. Nugent, D. J., Williams, S., Acharya, S., Ashburner, C., Balasa, V. V., Bhatt, N., Chandler, M., et al. (2024). ATHN 10–Novel variants in persons with rare coagulation disorders across hemophilia treatment centers in the United States. *Blood*. https://www.semanticscholar.org/paper/07091fd83f83995aa09faeb8869def3bcfe95451 (accessed on 12th June 2025).

54. Paris, E. M. (2015). Multiple cerebral infarctions in the context of malignancy. https://core.ac.uk/download/46603036.pdf (accessed on 12th June 2025).

55. Patange, A., Patange, A., & Gauri, T. (2023). The role of activated partial thromboplastin time (APTT) and prothrombin time (PT) in evaluating outcome among hospitalized patients with snake bite. https://core.ac.uk/download/588567297.pdf (accessed on 12th June 2025).

56. Petkova, N., Petrova, K., Bliznakova, M., Paskalev, D., & Galunska, B. (2017). The new face of vitamin K–More than blood clotting factor. *22,* 29–37. https://www.semanticscholar.org/paper/31ec456e1b9c007a3524236f27dcf2ea53174b47 (accessed on 12th June 2025).

57. Pilli, V. S. (2018). Understanding the clotting cascade, regulators, and clinical modulators of coagulation. https://core.ac.uk/download/322436111.pdf (accessed on 12th June 2025).

58. Pimentel Marcos, S., Valério, M., & Vilhena, M. M. (2015). Criança com múltiplas equimoses... Serão maus tratos? *Nascer e Crescer, 24,* 37–40. https://www.semanticscholar.org/paper/2216d077edc240a840b53af78ee1323d5a20b71d (accessed on 12th June 2025).

59. Pleshko, A. A., Petrova, E. B., Grigorenko, E. A., Gorbat, T. V., Gunich, S. V., et al. (2023). Acute myocardial injury in COVID-19 patients: Pathogenetic aspects and differential diagnosis considerations. *Emergency Cardiology and Cardiovascular Risks*. https://www.semanticscholar.org/paper/4263650d7acae4084e7b03299a41ee382857dd75 (accessed on 12th June 2025).

60. Poletaev, A., Zharkov, P. V., Seregina, E., & Dubinina, M. V. (2024). Five-year experience in remote diagnosis of von Willebrand disease in Russia. *Pediatric Hematology/Oncology and Immunopathology.* https://www.semanticscholar.org/paper/752765309f68e9593bb2b7ffbe5ac2c0fbd45067 (accessed on 12th June 2025).

61. Rajagopal, S., Nair, A., Digraskar, R., Allu, A., Naravula, J., Menon, S., Nallapeta, S., et al. (2023). Docking complexes of active phytochemicals with VK-deficient genes. *Current Biotechnology*. https://www.semanticscholar.org/paper/69b2621db319ba8023375f05c2d9083503888086 (accessed on 12th June 2025).
62. Rezende, S. M., Neumann, I., Angchaisuksiri, P., Awodu, O. A., Boban, A., Cuker, A., Curtin, J., et al. (2024). International Society on Thrombosis and Haemostasias clinical practice guideline for treatment of congenital hemophilia A and B based on the Grading of Recommendations Assessment, Development, and Evaluation methodology. *Journal of Thrombosis and Haemostasias, 22*, 2629–2652. https://doi.org/10.1016/j.jtha.2024.05.026 (accessed on 12th June 2025).
63. Sangli, S., Virani, A., Cheronis, N., Vannatter, B., Minich, C., Noronha, S., Bhagavatula, R., et al. (2021). Thrombosis with thrombocytopenia after the messenger RNA-1273 vaccine. *Annals of Internal Medicine, 174*, 1480–1482. https://doi.org/10.7326/l21-0244 (accessed on 12th June 2025).
64. Satia, M. N., Jandhyala, M., More, V., & Shanmukhaiah, C. (2016). Conservative management of a complex ovarian cyst in a case of Glanzmann's thrombasthenia. *International Journal of Reproduction, Contraception, Obstetrics and Gynecology, 5*, 2052–2054. https://www.semanticscholar.org/paper/86e3e35abf798f2ee65a0c8e37e1ed6b4a4180e0 (accessed on 12th June 2025).
65. Shahbazi, M., Ahmadinejad, M., Mahabadi, V., Teimourpour, A., & Golzadeh, K. (2024). Frequency, clinical, and laboratory findings of platelet secretion disorders in patients referred to the specialized coagulation laboratory of the Iranian Blood Transfusion Organization. *Blood Coagulation & Fibrinolysis, 35*, 115–123. https://www.semanticscholar.org/paper/e32498992f480d5dd70c5c431f8bde6651a56a2c (accessed on 12th June 2025).
66. Solğun, H. (2025). Diagnosis, treatment, surgical practices and review of the literature in rare coagulation factor deficiencies. *Italian Journal of Pediatrics, 51*. https://www.semanticscholar.org/paper/452c158f9e3e0ea1c00837c7db870587b3dd35da (accessed on 12th June 2025).
67. Srivastava, A., Santagostino, E., Dougall, A., Kitchen, S., Sutherland, M. L., Pipe, S. W., Carção, M., et al. (2020). WFH guidelines for the management of hemophilia, 3rd edition. *Hemophilia, 26*, 1–158. https://doi.org/10.1111/hae.14046
68. Stanescu, C., Anghel, L., & Tamas, C., & Ciubară, A. (2025). Education of patients and their families to manage emotional impact of skin scars. *BRAIN. Broad Research in Artificial Intelligence and Neuroscience*. https://www.semanticscholar.org/paper/fd568b1552dc35e1a4f6653e18eaea341ba27bf3 (accessed on 12th June 2025).
69. Tavasoli, B., Zangooie, A., Safdari, S. M., Hoseinnezhad, T., Shabannezhad, A., Alikhani, A., Salehi, Z., et al. (2024). Correlation between phenotype and coagulation factor activity level in rare bleeding disorders: A systematic review. *Seminars in Thrombosis and Hemostasis*. https://www.semanticscholar.org/paper/d804edd0e177ec42ae7e45cb6a203c5149fbad58 (accessed on 12th June 2025).
70. Walter, K. H., Levine, J., Madra, N. J., Beltran, J. L., Glassman, L. H., & Thomsen, C. (2022). Gender differences in disorders comorbid with posttraumatic stress disorder among U.S. Sailors and Marines. *Journal of Traumatic Stress, 35*, 988–998. https://www.semanticscholar.org/paper/a334cad57c9c6f07bd983ffa7192232ee318f35f (accessed on 12th June 2025).

71. Wang, Y., Zhao, Z., Wang, R., & Hu, X. (2025). Genetic links between gastrointestinal disorders and kidney stone disease. *Kidney360, 6*, 616–626. https://www.semanticscholar.org/paper/2f9a55cf5ba639b482fd7332b3cc477b20adc646 (accessed on 12th June 2025).

72. Wichmann, D. (2020). Autopsy findings and venous thromboembolism in patients with COVID-19. *Annals of Internal Medicine, 173*, 1030–1030. https://doi.org/10.7326/l20-1206 (accessed on 12th June 2025).

73. Yin, X., Zhang, A.-R., Bao, Y.-T., Wang, Y., Xu, L., Zhang, X., Zhao, X., et al. (2024). Coagulation biomarker signature as a novel differential diagnostic tool for CRS/ICANS and infection post-CAR-T therapy. *Blood*. https://www.semanticscholar.org/paper/22298fea80478a34764f5bbc111322e4ca434bdf (accessed on 12th June 2025).

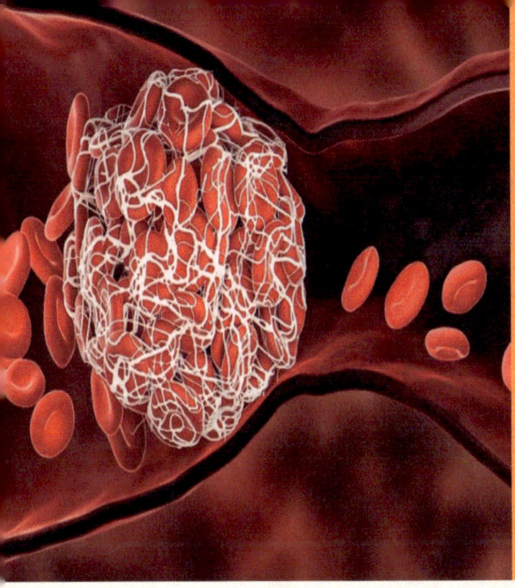

Chapter 10

THROMBOTIC DISORDERS

Contents

Introduction 237
10.1. Types of Thrombotic Disorders 238
10.2. Pathophysiology of Thrombotic Disorders 242
10.3. Diagnosis of Thrombotic Disorders 248
10.4. Treatment and Management of Thrombotic Disorders 252
Summary 259
References 260

Introduction

Thrombotic disorders are a significant focus of attention in the field of hematology, as they encompass a group of conditions characterized by the inappropriate formation of blood clots in the bloodstream. They are likely to cause catastrophic conditions like deep vein thrombosis, pulmonary embolism (PE), and stroke, making thorough knowledge and treatment approaches imperative. With advancing research, numerous treatment modalities, such as pharmacological treatments like Janus kinase (JAK) inhibitors, have been developed with new therapeutic options for the management of these conditions. Nevertheless, the safety profile of these therapies is still essential to assess because they are also associated with risks of bleeding and thrombosis, which can complicate patient treatment (Shahzad et al., 2024). Moreover, innovative therapeutic approaches, such as Kinesio taping, have been suggested as adjunctive measures in managing musculoskeletal disorders that may contribute to thrombotic risk (Mo et al., 2024). These factors underscore the complexity and multifaceted nature of thrombotic disorders, as well as the importance of ongoing research in this vital area of healthcare (Figure 10.1).

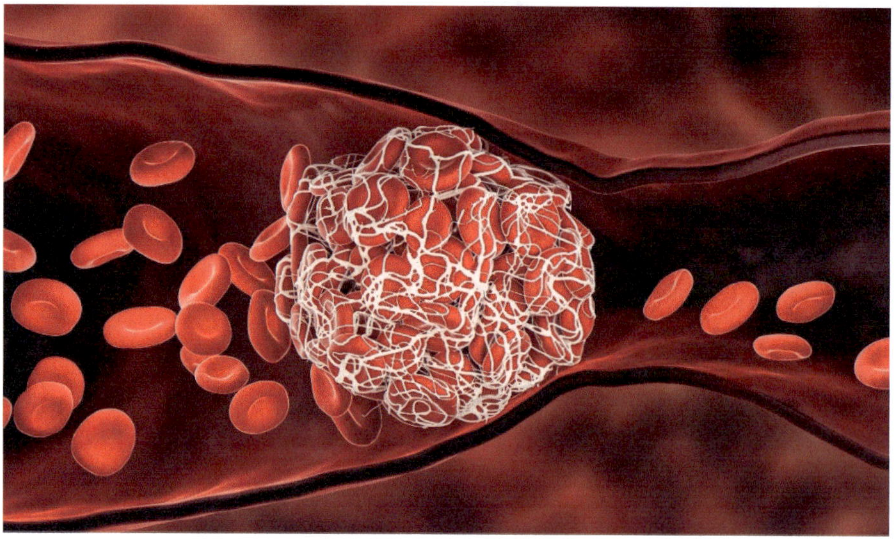

Figure 10.1. Thrombotic disorders.

Source: https://d2jx2rerrg6sh3.cloudfront.net/images/news/ImageForNews_725906_16637949337932688.jpg.

10.1. Types of Thrombotic Disorders

Thrombotic disorders refer to the abnormal development of blood clots, which can lead to a range of complications, including both venous and arterial thrombosis. Among the various thrombotic disorders, Heparin-induced thrombocytopenia (HIT) is a significant condition that develops as a result of antibody-activated platelets, typically induced following heparin administration. This condition can cause both venous and arterial thrombosis as a result of the severe prothrombotic condition that it establishes (Greinacher et al., 2023). Aside from HIT, other thrombotic conditions are inherited disorders such as Factor V Leiden and antiphospholipid syndrome (APS), which make people inappropriately prone to clots. The sub-classification of anti-PF4 antibodies into different types better explains the pathophysiology behind some thrombotic disorders and also clears the fact that these are complex in nature and need therapeutic strategies to be personalized (Greinacher et al., 2023). It becomes easier to plan an effective treatment strategy for the affected individuals by understanding these different types.

10.1.1. Deep Vein Thrombosis (DVT)

A thrombotic disease, deep vein thrombosis, entails the formation of clots in the deep veins, mainly within the legs. This is one of the dangerous health risks because the complications can be potentially severe and may prove fatal, such as PE. Some of the factors contributing to this disease include immobility for long periods and various medical conditions, as well as lifestyle choices such as smoking. Understanding the pathogenic mechanism of DVT is crucial for prevention and management; venous stasis, endothelial injury, and hypercoagulability are integral elements of the Virchow's triad explaining the pathophysiology of this disease. Prevention and early detection in the form of anticoagulation therapy and lifestyle modification are vital in avoiding the development of thrombotic complications of DVT. Therefore, management approaches should be individualized based on the experience of actual risk profiles to combat this very common disease (Nuha et al., 2022; Alexander et al., 2022) (Figure 10.2).

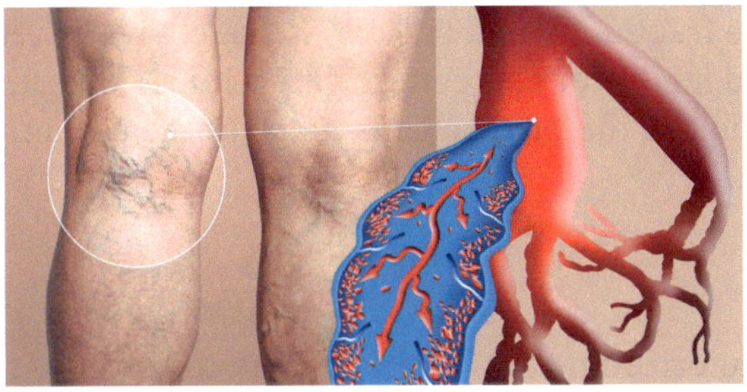

Figure 10.2. Deep vein thrombosis (DVT).

Source: https://s43932.pcdn.co/wp-content/uploads/sites/147/2024/01/Deep-Vein-Thrombosis-min-scaled.jpeg.optimal.jpeg.

10.1.2. Pulmonary Embolism (PE)

Pulmonary embolism (PE) represents a critical manifestation of thrombotic disorders, characterized by the obstruction of pulmonary arteries by blood clots that typically originate from deep vein thrombosis (DVT). This life-threatening condition demands urgent clinical attention, as its symptoms—ranging from sudden shortness of breath and chest pain to hemoptysis—can develop rapidly and unpredictably. The complexity of managing PE is underscored by its multifactorial risk factors, including prolonged immobility, certain genetic conditions, and the presence of arrhythmias like atrial fibrillation, which is detailed in the 2023 ACC/AHA/ACCP/HRS Guideline for the Diagnosis and Management of Atrial Fibrillation (José et al., 2023). Additionally, demographic factors such as age and sex significantly influence the incidence and outcomes of PE, highlighting the need for individualized assessments in clinical practice (Alexander et al., 2022). Recognizing this interplay is essential for effective prevention and management strategies.

10.1.3. Arterial Thrombosis

Arterial thrombosis is a pathophysiologic process of utmost importance where a clot of blood within an artery impedes blood supply to a vital organ, leading to ischemia and possible tissue destruction. The condition is particularly associated with atherosclerosis, where plaque deposition constricts the arterial lumens, triggering the development of thrombi. Hypertension, hyperlipidemia, and diabetes mellitus further increase this risk, requiring thorough management strategies to ward off complications. Current research has highlighted the anticoagulants and antiplatelet therapies in averting arterial thrombosis, with a focus on their value in high-risk groups and those with a cardiovascular disease history (Alexander et al., 2022). Additionally, advances in imaging diagnostics have improved the detection of arterial obstructions, facilitating timely interventions (Patrick et al., 2020). Sustained investigation of the mechanisms of arterial thrombosis is imperative to devise novel therapeutic strategies, thereby improving patient outcomes in thrombosis." (Figure 10.3)

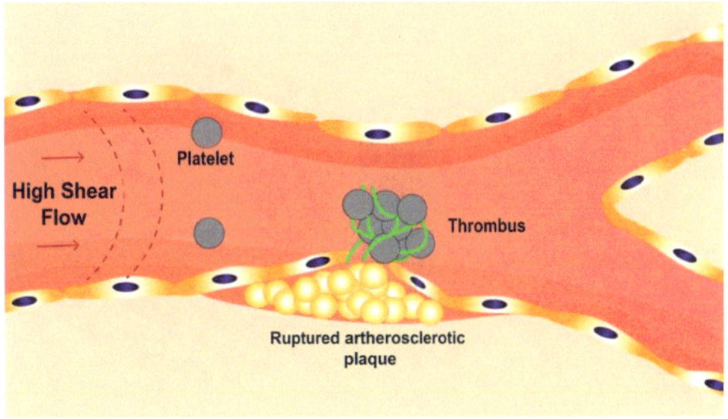

Figure 10.3: Arterial thrombosis.

Source: https://myhematology.com/wp-content/uploads/2023/12/Arterial-thrombosis.jpg.

10.1.4. Thrombophilia

Thrombophilia refers to an increased tendency for abnormal blood clotting. It is a significant contributor to thrombotic disorders, which more often occur in the younger population. It includes inherited and acquired disorders that interfere with normal hemostatic mechanisms. The inherited forms include deficiencies of natural anticoagulants, such as protein C, protein S, and antithrombin III, and mutations like Factor V Leiden. These anomalies predispose individuals to venous thrombosis but less clearly involve arterial events, such as ischemic stroke, which are estimated in only 1-4% of cases that can be definitely and directly attributed to thrombophilia (Abrishamizadeh, 2017). In contrast, acquired thrombophilic conditions, including APS, occur far more frequently and may complicate any strategy to manage them. Diagnosis will need to involve detailed laboratory screening exceptionally because the successful treatment interventions will be dependent on the proper knowledge of the causative thrombotic predisposition (García-García et al., 2020).

10.1.5. Antiphospholipid Syndrome (APS)

APS is a multifaceted autoimmune disease that is characterized by the predisposition to thrombosis, with potential for causing severe complications like stroke and myocardial infarction. The syndrome is in the formation of abnormal thrombi characterized by the presence of antiphospholipid antibodies. It has been demonstrated that this condition is likely linked to complement system mechanisms, particularly in the obstetric presentation of APS, suggesting that complement activation plays a crucial role in the pathogenesis of thrombotic manifestations of the syndrome (Cohen et al., 2024). In addition, studies have demonstrated an elegant interaction between coagulation pathways and inflammation, indicating that the disruption of thrombin and platelet activities plays a significant role in the thrombotic milieu seen in APS (Adams et al., 2018). Thus, understanding such mechanisms is of paramount importance for constructing patient-specific therapeutic strategies to modulate thrombotic risk in the affected individuals (Figure 10.4).

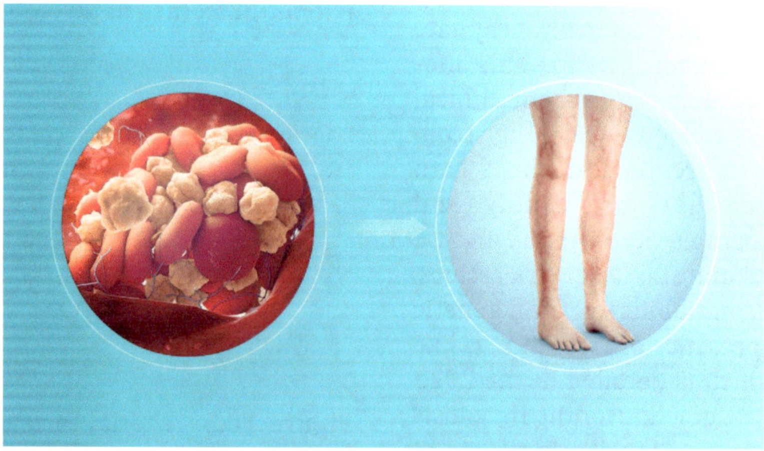

Figure 10.4. Antiphospholipid syndrome (APS).

Source: https://cdn.storymd.com/optimized/ZoBEpMTvAM/original.jpg.

10.1.6. Cerebral Venous Sinus Thrombosis (CVST)

Cerebral venous sinus thrombosis (CVST) is a severe condition resulting from the obstruction of blood flow within the brain's venous sinuses, leading to elevated intracranial pressure and potential neurological impairment. This disease usually presents in connection with several risk factors such as pregnancy, some coagulopathies, and other thrombogenic conditions. Based on Virchow's triad, changes in the dynamics of blood flow, endothelial damage, and hypercoagulability are critical factors in the formation of venous thrombosis, including CVST. In addition, malignancy patients are at increased risk of thrombotic complications, requiring vigilant assessment of anticoagulation therapy to prevent adverse consequences (Taanila et al., 2017). Thereby, this intricacy of all the risk factors poses a high urgency for early diagnosis and suitable management strategies for CVST, as early intervention may significantly improve the outcomes of patients and decrease the possibilities of complications in the long term.

10.1.7. Myocardial Infarction

Myocardial infarction, more popularly referred to as a heart attack, represents a severe outcome of acute cardiovascular events that are dominated by arterial thrombosis. The pathophysiological mechanism responsible for myocardial infarction typically begins with the rupture or erosion of an atherosclerotic plaque, which activates platelets and causes them to aggregate, ultimately leading to the formation of a thrombus. This thrombotic process may occlude coronary arteries, causing impairment of blood supply to cardiac tissue and resulting in tissue ischemia and necrosis. Research indicates that factors influencing platelet reactivity and endogenous fibrinolysis play crucial roles in the severity and outcomes of myocardial infarction. For instance, administration of morphine, often used to manage pain in patients undergoing primary percutaneous coronary intervention, has been associated with impaired spontaneous myocardial reperfusion and larger infarct sizes (Farag et al., 2017). Additionally, the interactions between fibrinolysis and thrombosis are also important, as their imbalance may lead to persistent vessel occlusion, thereby exacerbating myocardial damage (Gorog et al., 2015) (Figure 10.5).

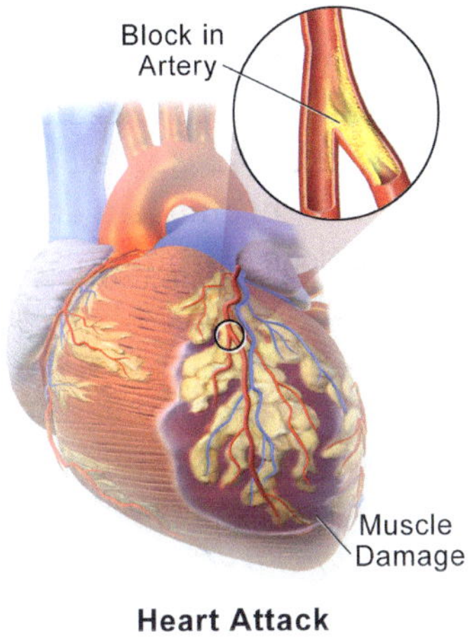

Figure 10.5. Myocardial infarction.

Source: https://upload.wikimedia.org/wikipedia/commons/f/fb/Blausen_0463_HeartAttack.png.

10.1.8. Stroke

Comprehending stroke as a critical aspect of thrombotic diseases involves an understanding of the pathophysiology of arterial thrombosis. Stroke, and especially ischemic stroke, results when a clot in the blood interrupts the delivery of blood to a part of the brain, causing neuronal injury and possible loss of intellect and motor functions. The balance between proaggregatory substances that enhance clotting and fibrinolytic mechanisms that dissolve clots is crucial in determining the outcome of strokes. When the scale shifts toward inordinate platelet activation and the propagation of the thrombus, the risk of an occluding event significantly escalates; however, an optimally regulated fibrinolytic activity would counteract this (Gorog et al., 2015). The latest studies have also highlighted the role of systemic factors, such as hormone therapy, in influencing cardiovascular risks and necessitating further exploration of these connections (Arcelus et al., 2018). Thus, stroke prevention and management strategies must target both thrombotic and fibrinolytic systems to achieve optimal clinical benefits.

10.1.9. Disseminated Intravascular Coagulation (DIC)

Disseminated intravascular coagulation (DIC) represents a complex and critical pathological process characterized by the widespread activation of the coagulation cascade, leading to the paradoxical occurrence of both thrombosis and bleeding. This condition is not a standalone disorder; rather, it often manifests as a complication arising from severe underlying illnesses such as sepsis, trauma, or obstetric emergencies. Therefore, patients usually come to the attention of clinicians with some degree of organ dysfunction resulting from microvascular occlusions due to thrombi formation throughout the circulatory system. Notably, the link between DIC and sepsis emphasizes an essential aspect of its pathophysiology; whilst sepsis can trigger an immune response leading to coagulopathy, the clinical presentation can be far removed from that seen in bacterial sepsis-induced coagulopathy (SIC) (Jarczak et al., 2021). Moreover, distinguishing DIC from other coagulopathies, such as the unique profile seen in COVID-19-associated coagulopathy (CAC), is vital for effective management (Iba et al., 2020) (Figure 10.6).

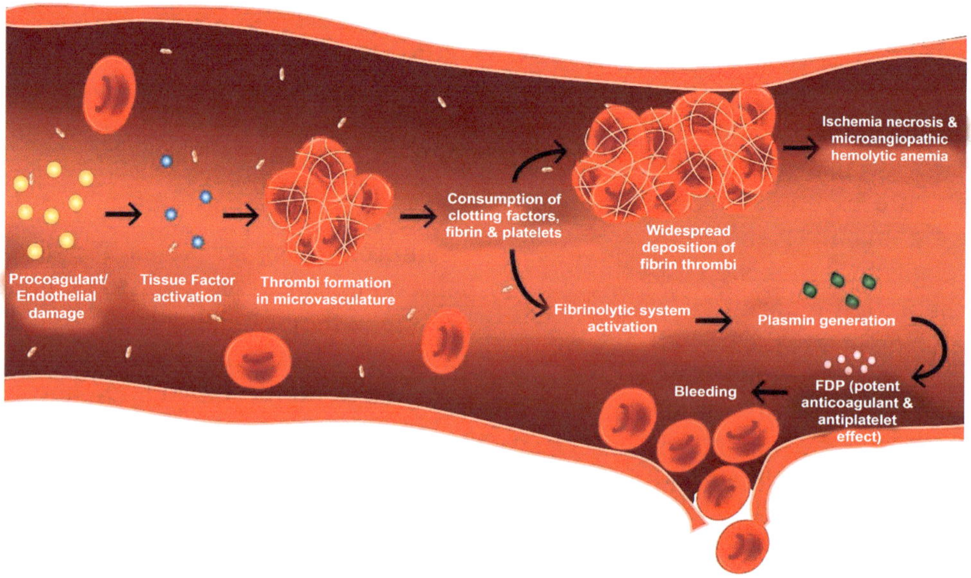

Figure 10.6. Disseminated intravascular coagulation (DIC).

Source: https://myhematology.com/wp-content/uploads/2023/10/DIC-pathophysiology.jpeg.

10.2. Pathophysiology of Thrombotic Disorders

Thrombotic disease, characterized by the hyperproduction of blood clots, is caused by the multifactorial interaction of genetic, environmental, and pathological processes that disrupt normal hemostasis. Underlying this dysregulation are disturbances in the coagulation cascade, platelet function, and the endothelial lining of blood vessels, which cause venous and arterial thrombosis.

For instance, the influence of certain adipokines, such as retinol-binding protein 4 (RBP4), is notable in the context of thrombotic risk, as elevated levels are associated with obesity and cardiovascular diseases, thereby implicating metabolic disturbances in the formation of clots (Zhang et al., 2025). Furthermore, complications arising from COVID-19 highlight the multifactorial nature of thrombosis, where viral-induced immune responses and direct vascular injury contribute to an increased incidence of thrombotic events (Chavhan et al., 2024). Understanding these mechanisms is crucial for developing effective prevention and treatment strategies for thrombotic disorders.

10.2.1. Coagulation Cascade Overview

The coagulation cascade is a crucial component of hemostasis, regulating the complex process of blood clotting that occurs upon injury within the vasculature. The process is separated into two key phases: primary and secondary hemostasis. In primary hemostasis, platelets bind to the injured vessel wall, creating a temporary plug. Secondary hemostasis, on the other hand, constitutes a cascade of enzymatic processes that activate several coagulation factors, culminating in the conversion of fibrinogen into fibrin, which stabilizes the platelet plug. The subtle balance between anticoagulant and procoagulant pathways is vital for normal hemostatic function; derangement may result in thrombotic disorders, including venous thromboembolism (VTE) and myocardial infarction (Lippi et al., 2018). The involvement of thrombin-activatable fibrinolysis inhibitor (TAFI) has come to play a vital role because it regulates fibrinolysis and may delineate an individual's risk for thrombotic events (Boffa et al., 2001). With knowledge of this cascade, effective diagnosis and management of hemostatic disorders can be made possible (Figure 10.7).

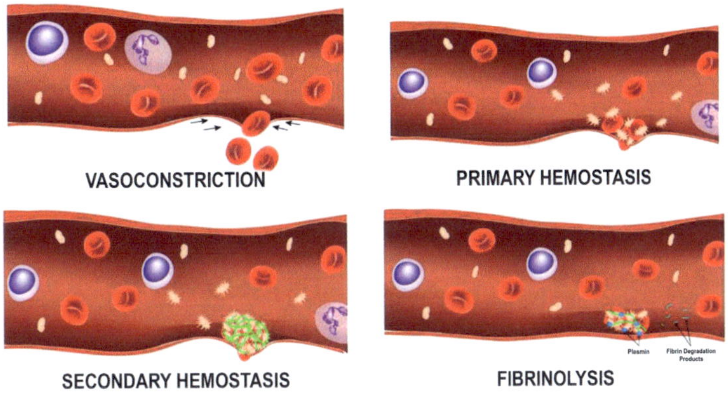

Figure 10.7. The coagulation cascade is a fundamental aspect of hemostasis, orchestrating the complex process of blood clot formation in response to vascular injury.

Source: https://myhematology.com/wp-content/uploads/2023/12/Hemostasis.jpg.

10.2.2. Role of Platelets in Thrombosis

The function of platelets in thrombosis is the key element in the causation of thrombotic disorders. Platelets, long known for their role in hemostasis, play an essential role in the formation of thrombus as they undergo activation and aggregation following vascular injury. In diseases such as chronic myeloproliferative neoplasms (MPN), the prothrombotic state is exacerbated by elevated platelet counts and functional defects, leading to increased thrombus formation. These platelets engage with leukocytes and activated endothelium, forming a self-perpetuating thromboinflammatory cycle that promotes additional thrombosis (Heller et al., 2019). Several studies also exist that investigate the effects of hormonal changes in the climacteric on the level of platelet microparticles, which may impact the risk of thrombosis, particularly among postmenopausal women (Rank et al., 2012). Hence, an in-depth understanding of platelet dynamics is crucial for designing effective intervention strategies that can counteract thrombosis in affected individuals and thereby contribute to improved patient outcomes.

10.2.3. Endothelial Dysfunction

The most critical ingredient in this process is endothelial dysfunction, which upsets the delicate balance of prothrombotic and antithrombotic mechanisms that exist in the vascular tree. It is characterized by a decreased availability of nitric oxide and an increase in pro-inflammatory cytokines, which exacerbate the hypercoagulable state. In MPNs, for instance, heightened cytokine levels perpetuate a proinflammatory condition, which significantly increases the risk of thrombosis, as discussed in Liu et al. (2024). Likewise, in sickle cell disease, multiple mechanisms such as hemolytic anemia-associated chronic organ damage and reduced nitric oxide availability result in endothelial dysfunction, further aggravating the patient's condition and increasing thrombotic risk, as noted in (Hazenberg et al., 2024). Such findings underscore the multifactorial basis of thrombotic disorders, with endothelial dysfunction being a central pathogenic factor that must be targeted in interventions for the prevention of thrombotic events (Figure 10.8).

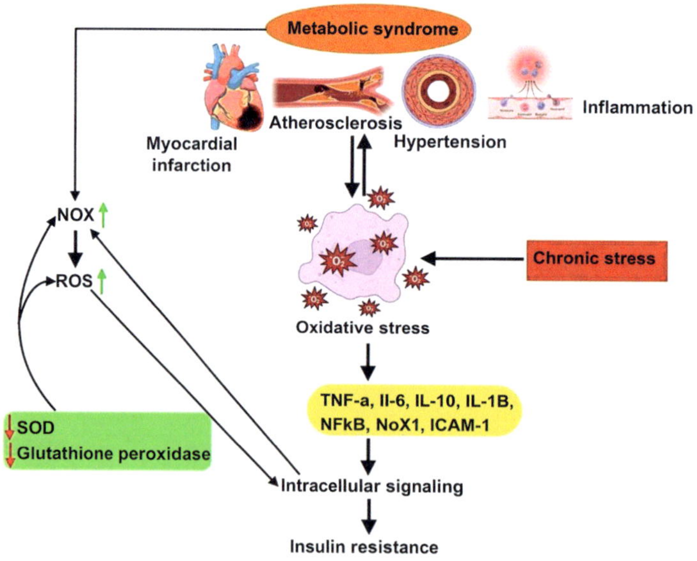

Figure 10.8. Endothelial dysfunction is a crucial factor contributing to thrombotic disorders, as it disrupts the delicate balance between prothrombotic and anticoagulant mechanisms within the vascular system.

Source: https://www.frontiersin.org/files/Articles/1221438/fnut-10-1221438-HTML/image_m/fnut-10-1221438-g001.jpg.

10.2.4. Genetic Factors Contributing to Thrombosis

The contribution of genetic factors to thrombosis is especially significant in MPNs, in which specific mutations have been associated with thrombotic risk. Primarily, the JAK2 V617F mutation largely determines the thrombotic risk in MPN patients, as it favors hypercoagulability through mechanisms that encompass the chronic activation of leukocytes, platelets, and endothelial cells.

Apart from the JAK2 mutation, alterations of other genes like CALR and MPL are also involved in the pathophysiology of thrombosis but to a lesser extent in splanchnic vein thrombosis (SVT) (Heller et al., 2019). These gene mutations, when interacting, promote a pro-inflammatory condition that enhances the potential for thrombosis through elevated blood viscosity and abnormal platelet function, thereby advancing the argument that the complexity of thrombosis is linked to multifactorial disease processes influenced by genetic predispositions (Heller et al., 2019).

10.2.5. Acquired Risk Factors

In the context of thrombotic disorders, acquired risk factors significantly contribute to the increased likelihood of thrombosis. One noteworthy acquired condition is APS, characterized by the presence of antiphospholipid antibodies, which can promote thrombus formation through pathogenic mechanisms leading to both arterial and venous thromboses (Deepa et al., 2022). MPNs, which are clonal expansions of abnormal stem cells that contribute to hemopoiesis, contribute to a cumulative thrombotic risk, often due to mutations such as JAK2 (Patrick et al., 2020). Lifestyle contributory factors include obesity and smoking, which significantly contribute to the occurrence of thrombotic events. These acquired factors not only contribute independently but also interact with inherited thrombophilic states, demonstrating that thrombus formation in affected persons is multifactorial. Knowledge of these acquired risks is crucial for the appropriate management and prevention of thrombotic disease (Figure 10.9).

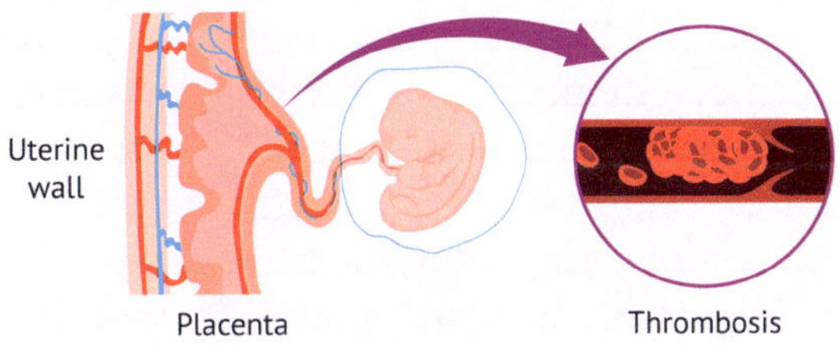

Figure 10.9. Antiphospholipid syndrome (APS).

Source: https://babygest.com/en/wp-content/uploads/2021/01/side-effects-of-antiphospholipid-syndrom.png.

10.2.6. Inflammatory Processes in Thrombosis

This interaction between inflammatory mechanisms and thrombosis is now widely appreciated as an essential determinant of the pathogenesis of thrombotic disorders. Chronic inflammation markedly amplifies the risk of thrombosis; these mechanisms involve enhancing platelet activation and leukocyte recruitment. For example, increased cytokine levels associated with disorders like MPN cause a proinflammatory environment, leading to a hypercoagulable state and thrombotic complications (Heller et al., 2019). In addition, the involvement of thrombin in the inflammatory process highlights how coagulation factors interact with immune responses. Thrombin, which not only causes a clot, also activates microglia, leading to the further release of mediators that exacerbate tissue damage (Adams et al., 2018). Such processes of inflammation need to be understood to develop targeted interventions aimed at reducing thrombotic risks associated with chronic inflammatory diseases.

10.2.7. Hemodynamic Changes Leading to Thrombus Formation

Hemodynamic alterations are a key factor in the pathophysiology of thrombus formation, primarily through changes in blood flow dynamics. When blood flow becomes interrupted due to diseases like atherosclerosis, turbulence can trigger endothelial damage, thereby enhancing platelet activation and aggregation. This phenomenon is potentiated in low shear stress states, where stasis blood can cause the deposition of clotting factors and cellular detritus. Consequently, these hemodynamic changes create a favorable environment for thrombus formation. A notable case illustrates this connection; a 29-year-old woman developed an acute left occipital lobe infarction attributed to iron deficiency anemia, underscoring how physiological blood alterations can precipitate thrombosis despite the absence of traditional vascular risk factors (Nace et al., 2020). In addition, emerging therapies employing laser technology have demonstrated that regulating certain hemodynamic factors, such as photodynamic therapy, is capable of lowering thrombotic complications and favorably influencing outcomes (Bragina et al., 2017) (Figure 10.10).

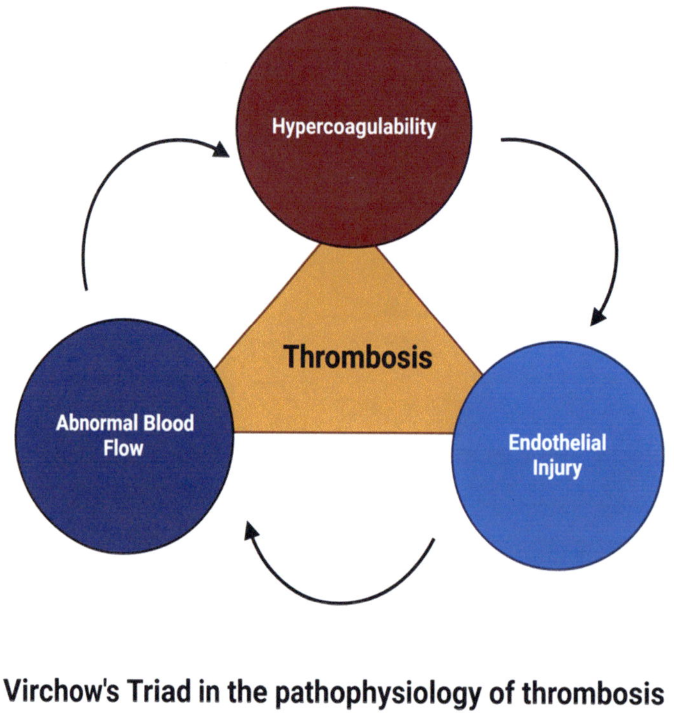

Figure 10.10. The formation of DVT is a complex process that is influenced by three key factors: endothelial damage/vascular injury, blood flow turbulence, and hypercoagulability of the blood.

Source: https://assets.cureus.com/uploads/figure/file/1204773/article_river_f95702707fb211efb21ea7c5841cc0c6-49497f89-aa76-4b48-95f6-acd0fbbadb44.png.

10.2.8. Interaction between Coagulation and Fibrinolysis

Maintaining balance in blood clotting and dissolving is very important in the context of thrombotic disorders. Coagulation quickly forms fibrin clots after a wound to a blood vessel, and fibrinolysis breaks them down once they are no longer required, allowing normal circulation to resume. If the balance in the body is disturbed, it can increase someone's risk of thrombosis. For instance, certain autoimmune skin diseases, such as chronic spontaneous urticaria and angioedema, have been shown to exhibit an increased presence of thrombin generation and inflammatory markers during flare-ups, indicating active coagulation processes that may increase the risk of thrombosis (Borghi et al., 2019). Similarly, patients with cirrhosis experience a complex dysregulation of hemostasis, resulting in a paradoxical tendency toward both bleeding and thrombosis due to altered coagulant and anticoagulant factors (Stefano et al., 2009). It is essential to understand these interactions to design good treatment methods for thrombotic disorders..

10.2.9. Impact of Lifestyle Factors on Thrombotic Risk

Lifestyle determinants are closely entangled with thrombotic conditions, which significantly influence a person's risk profile. Physical inactivity, obesity, and poor diet have been found to play a crucial role in the pathogenesis of thrombotic events.

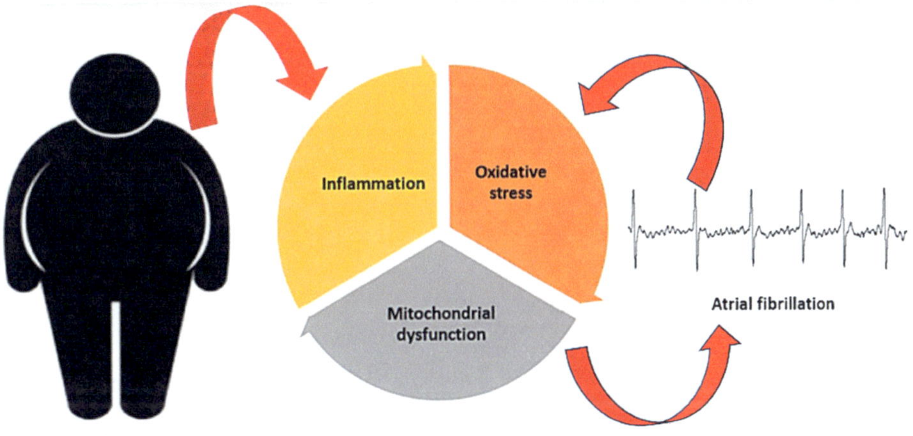

Figure 10.11. A high body mass index (BMI) is associated with increased levels of inflammatory markers and endothelial dysfunction, which are known precursors to thrombosis.

Source: https://www.mdpi.com/antioxidants/antioxidants-13-00117/article_deploy/html/images/antioxidants-13-00117-g001.png.

For instance, a high body mass index was strongly linked with elevated levels of inflammatory markers and endothelial dysfunction, which are established predictors of thrombosis. Moreover, smoking elevates the likelihood of VTE by promoting vascular inflammation and hypercoagulability. Conversely, regular physical activity and a balanced diet rich in omega-3 fatty acids and antioxidants can mitigate these risks. The systemic implications of lifestyle on thrombotic disorders are also evident in more severe contexts, such as pregnancy-related complications like pre-eclampsia, where lifestyle factors can exacerbate risks, linking increased thrombotic tendencies to cardiovascular consequences both during and after pregnancy (Palmiero et al., 2025). Additionally, in patients with COVID-19, lifestyle-related health status has been shown to influence thrombotic outcomes significantly (Yachi et al., 2023) (Figure 10.11).

10.3. Diagnosis of Thrombotic Disorders

Diagnosis of thrombotic disorders is a multifaceted process that generally involves a rigorous evaluation of clinical presentation and laboratory findings. Risk factor screening, including genetic predisposition, lifestyle, and underlying medical conditions that may contribute to thrombus development, is typically the initial step. Clinicians often use a combination of imaging and coagulation studies to establish the presence of thrombosis and evaluate the risk of complications. For instance, although vitamin K antagonists, such as warfarin, are vital to the treatment of these disorders, their complex pharmacokinetics require strict monitoring and dose adjustments according to the patient's international normalized ratio (INR) value (Galliazzo et al., 2023). In addition, some transplant-related syndromes, such as transplant-related thrombotic microangiopathy, emphasize the need for sharp diagnosis and personalized therapeutic regimens, demonstrating the multifaceted character of management of thrombotic disorders (McEwan et al., 2023).

10.3.1. Clinical Assessment and History Taking

Effective clinical assessment and thorough history-taking are crucial components in managing thrombotic disorders, as they enable healthcare professionals to identify patients at an elevated risk for thromboembolic events.

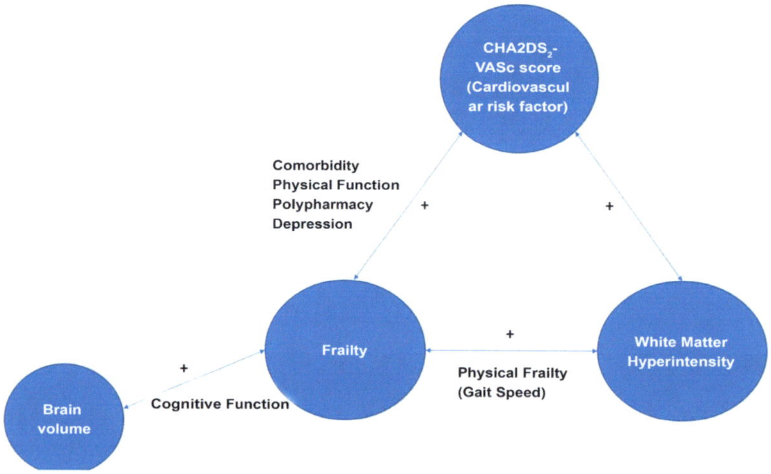

Figure 10.12. Tools like the CHA2DS2-VASc and HAS-BLED scores can be utilized during this assessment to systematically classify the thrombotic and bleeding risks associated with individual patients.

Source: https://media.springernature.com/full/springer-static/image/art%3A10.1038%2Fs41598-020-75256-6/MediaObjects/41598_2020_75256_Fig1_HTML.png.

A comprehensive history includes not only the patient's medical background and previous incidents of VTE but also the evaluation of potential risk factors such as genetic predispositions, obesity, and age, which can significantly influence thrombotic risk. Tools like the CHA2DS2-VASc and HAS-BLED scores can be utilized during this assessment to systematically classify the thrombotic and bleeding risks associated with individual patients. Additionally, the integration of evidence-based guidelines, as described by the American Physical Therapy Association, enhances the clinical decision-making process, allowing for targeted interventions to prevent complications from conditions such as lower extremity deep vein thrombosis (Auten et al., 2016). Furthermore, protocols such as CoRaMaPicc have been developed to mitigate procedural risks and ensure optimal patient outcomes in individuals with high cardiovascular risk profiles (Giacopelli et al., 2018) (Figure 10.12).

10.3.2. Imaging Techniques (e.g., Ultrasound, CT)

Advanced imaging modalities, including ultrasound and computed tomography (CT), are crucial in the diagnosis and treatment of thrombotic disorders. They enable clinicians to visualize vascular structures and detect obstructions caused by thrombi, facilitating timely intervention. For example, ultrasound is particularly useful because it offers real-time imaging, making it possible to evaluate venous thrombosis in the extremities. Conversely, CT scans can provide cross-sectional images of the internal body structures; therefore, they are critical in diagnosing PE or deep vein thrombosis. The integration of both methods ensures the precise diagnosis of the disease and enables physicians to prescribe appropriate measures to address it. In addition, the development of new imaging technology continues to evolve with the demand for research and development in this field in an effort to improve patient outcomes for thrombotic disorders (Kitsiou et al., 2013).

10.3.3. Laboratory Tests (e.g., D-dimer, Coagulation Profile)

Laboratory tests play a significant role in the diagnosis and management of thrombotic disorders, particularly in assessing D-dimer levels and coagulation profiles.

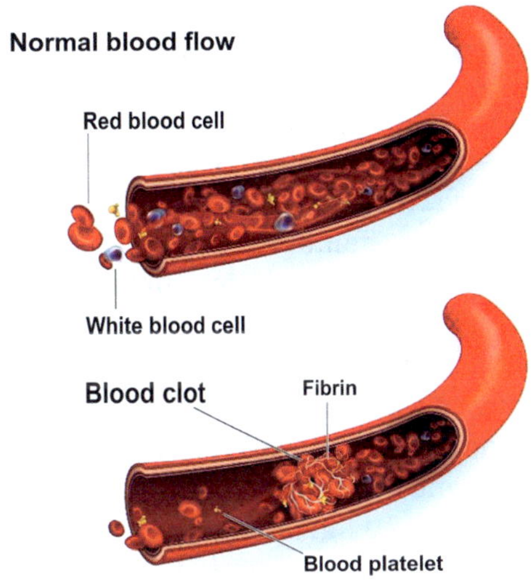

Figure 10.13. D-dimer test.

Source: https://my.clevelandclinic.org/-/scassets/images/org/health/articles/22045-d-dimer-test-blood-clot-final.

D-dimer, a fibrin degradation product, is a sensitive marker of thrombosis, and an increased level can indicate active clot formation and dissolution within the body, warranting further investigation in the instance of suspected embolism or thrombosis. In addition, a standardized coagulation profile with coagulation parameters (prothrombin time, activated partial thromboplastin time (APTT), and certain antibody assays) is needed to determine underlying hemostatic derangements that may be predisposing the patient to thrombotic events. For example, abnormal coagulation tests in association with high antiphosphatidylserine IgM antibodies can be found in patients who present with recurrent thrombosis, even when standard assays are normal (Marquardt et al., 2018). Further understanding of the balance between coagulation and fibrinolysis through global hemostatic assays would contribute to risk stratification of ischemic stroke patients (Rooth et al., 2012) (Figure 10.13).

10.3.4. Risk Assessment Models

Among the diverse strategies employed to improve patient outcomes in thrombotic disorders, risk assessment models play a crucial role in stratifying patients based on their risk of exacerbating complications. The models typically use demographic factors, genetic predispositions, and clinical history to assess individual risk levels. For instance, research indicates that non-O blood types show a significant correlation with increased thrombotic risk, suggesting that ABO blood group antigens may influence factors such as von Willebrand factor (vWF) and inflammatory cytokines, which are critical in clot formation (Catalano et al., 2017). Moreover, gender, ethnicity, and lifestyle variables, including smoking and immobility, have been identified as key predictors of venous events such as deep vein thrombosis and PE, thus highlighting the importance of complete models that include these factors (Chan et al., 2014). With this customized approach to prevention strategies, healthcare professionals can manage and prevent thrombotic episodes more effectively, ultimately enhancing patient care.

10.3.5. Differential Diagnosis Considerations

In the context of thrombotic disorders, differential diagnosis considerations are paramount for ensuring accurate identification and management of conditions with overlapping clinical features. For instance, atypical hemolytic uremic syndrome (aHUS) often presents similarly to thrombotic thrombocytopenic purpura (TTP) and other thrombotic microangiopathies, which can complicate the diagnostic process in acute settings, particularly in intensive care units, where time is critical (Abroug et al., 2017). Moreover, knowledge of the patient's clinical history and presenting symptoms is necessary to avoid missing a diagnosis; as in the case of a 54-year-old man with hemoglobin SC disease, whose manifestations had to be carefully evaluated to exclude infections or other co-morbid conditions (Devnani et al., 2016). Therefore, a thorough understanding of the clinical discriminators between these diseases enables clinicians to institute appropriate interventions and improve patient outcomes (Figure 10.14).

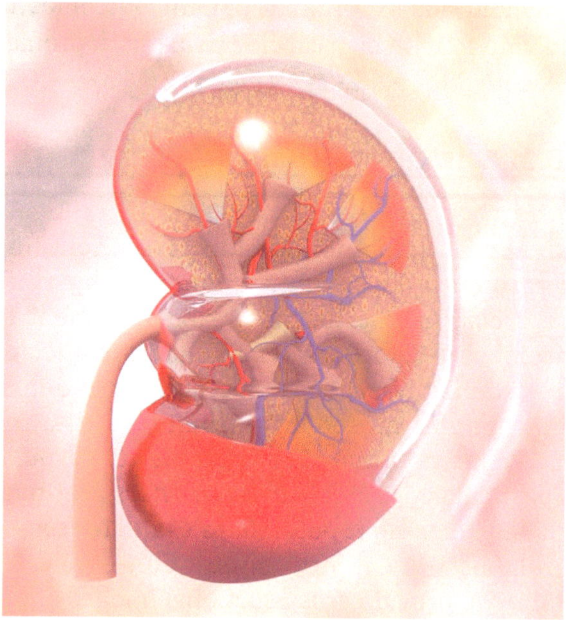

Figure 10.14. Atypical hemolytic uremic syndrome (aHUS).

Source: https://www.sskidneyhospital.com/img/atypical-hemolytic-uremic-syndrome-hospital-in-rewari.jpg.

10.3.6. Importance of Early Detection

Early diagnosis of thrombotic disorders is crucial for effective management and improved patient outcomes. Detection of these disorders at an early stage can prevent serious complications, like stroke or myocardial infarction, arising from occult thrombosis. Additionally, early treatment enables clinicians to implement appropriate therapeutic measures, such as anticoagulation therapy, which can prevent further clotting and related morbidity. The subtlety of thrombotic disorders has its own 'complexity' in etiology and clinical presentation, which calls for the personalization of screening approaches. For instance, new advancements in machine learning models are providing new avenues for earlier detection, aligning with other discoveries that claim early identification is key to everything. As with other illnesses, e.g., as in (Hasan et al., 2024), early detection is essential; similarly, in the case of thrombotic disorders, it can transform patient care trajectory and enhance quality of life.

10.3.7. Role of Biomarkers in Diagnosis

Increasingly, there is recognition of the pivotal role of biomarkers in the diagnosis of thrombotic disorders, which enhances patient outcomes.

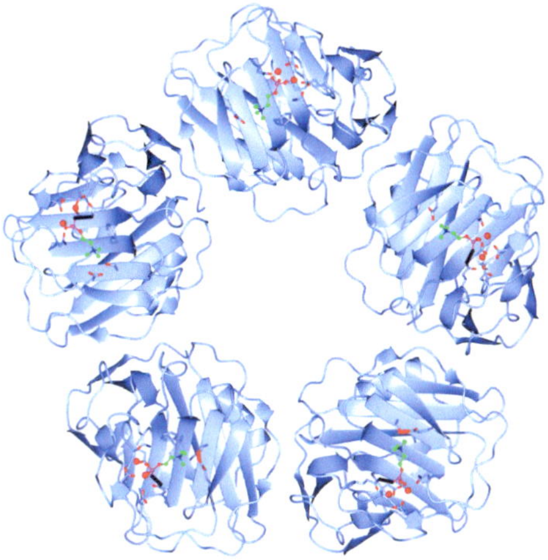

Figure 10.15. C-reactive protein (CRP).

Source: https://pub.mdpi-res.com/diseases/diseases-11-00132/article_deploy/html/images/diseases-11-00132-g001.png?1696850239.

Biomarkers, including inflammatory markers, offer a non-invasive approach for identifying patients with a higher potential for developing such conditions, which are often asymptomatic until a serious event occurs. For instance, elevated levels of leukocytes and C-reactive protein (CRP) have been correlated with the subsequent development of various thrombotic events, underscoring the potential of these indicators in early detection (Zeng et al., 2024). Moreover, the identification of specific biomarkers can facilitate personalized treatment approaches, enabling tailored therapies that target the underlying pathophysiological mechanisms of thrombotic disorders. With further research to refine the roles of biomarkers, improvements are likely to enhance the diagnostic capabilities of the medical community, potentially reducing the morbidity associated with these prevalent conditions (Celeski et al., 2024). In this regard, the integration of biomarkers into routine diagnostics is a vital breakthrough in managing thrombotic disorders (Figure 10.15).

10.3.8. Challenges in Diagnosing Thrombotic Disorders

Thrombotic disorder diagnosis is plagued by multidimensional challenges that will take a long time to treat properly. Among the significant issues here is one that starts in the rarity and complexity of certain conditions, e.g., complement-mediated thrombotic microangiopathies (CM-TMA), because they are often misdiagnosed owing to symptoms that overlap with other disorders like TTP. Medical practitioners frequently lack experience and knowledge of such uncommon disorders, and hence are afflicted by severe gaps in care, like delay in diagnosis, inadequate response to therapy (Kuter et al., 2024). Lastly, advances in genetics and immunology, which enhance the understanding of this type of disorder, also continue to necessitate revisions to professional education on how to utilize new therapies and diagnostic techniques optimally (Musalem, 2025). Therefore, incorporating current information on optimally proven practices is essential for improving diagnostic precision and optimizing patient management in the field of thrombotic disorders.

10.3.9. Guidelines for Diagnostic Protocols

The establishment of comprehensive guidelines for diagnostic protocols in thrombotic disorders is essential to ensure the accurate identification and management of complex conditions. This process begins with the evaluation of a patient's medical history, which includes any risk factors such as family history, previous episodes of thrombosis, and underlying medical conditions. Diagnostic tests should not be standardized across the board; instead, they must be tailored to individual patient circumstances. For example, the requirement of including better imaging techniques, such as ultrasound and computed tomography, along with laboratory investigations like D-dimer assays, is most important for the proper establishment of the existence of thrombi. According to recent research published in scientific journals, the use of specific diagnostic protocols will further improve outcomes by ensuring timely interventions, as it is essential for hierarchical success involving both anatomical and systemic factors (Gitto et al., 2025). Therefore, strengthening multidisciplinary work is crucial in developing these guidelines and enhancing the outcomes of patient care in thrombotic disorders (Figure 10.16).

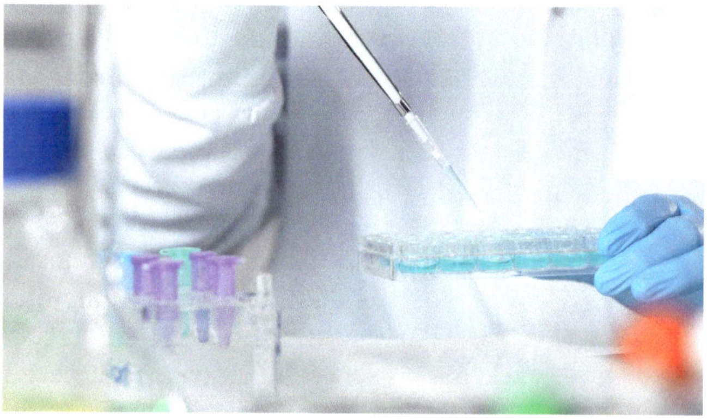

Figure 10.16. Diagnostic tests should not be standardized across the board; rather, they must be tailored to individual patient circumstances.

Source: https://www.pewtrusts.org/-/media/post-launch-images/2019/05/gettyimages-556421529/16x9_m.jpg.

10.4. Treatment and Management of Thrombotic Disorders

Effective treatment and management of thrombotic disorders require a nuanced understanding of both the underlying pathophysiology and patient-specific factors. The emergence of immune-mediated mechanisms, such as anti-platelet factor 4 (PF4) immunothrombotic, for instance, highlights the complexity of these conditions, especially in patients with comorbidities like antineutrophil cytoplasmic antibody (ANCA)-associated vasculitis (AAV) (Remez-Gabay et al., 2025). Therapeutic approaches need to evolve in response to these challenges, particularly through the use of intravenous immunoglobulin (IVIG) for the control of hypercoagulability and NETosis. Additional considerations in treatment involve confronting the multifaceted nature of hypercoagulability, which is influenced by both genetic and environmental factors that disrupt the delicate balance between pro-coagulant and anticoagulant pathways (Jaafari et al., 2024). This comprehensive strategy underscores the importance of early diagnosis, risk assessment, and individualized anticoagulant therapy in preventing morbidity and enhancing outcomes in patients with thrombotic disorders.

10.4.1. Anticoagulant Therapy

Anticoagulant therapy is, therefore, central to the control of thrombotic disease, particularly in patients with a high risk of thromboembolism. Internal and external patient factors in liver disease increase the thrombotic complications. Thus, selection and monitoring of anticoagulant therapy should be done cautiously in such patient groups. The American Gastroenterological Association guidelines emphasize the importance of individualized management plans for these patients, which may also involve the use of low-molecular-weight heparin to prevent VTE while balancing the risk of hemorrhage (Arykan et al., 2022). Likewise, the COVID-19 pandemic has revealed a critical hypercoagulable condition in affected individuals, and for this reason, the heightened utilization of heparin has not only been due to its anticoagulant function but also because of its anti-viral and anti-inflammatory activities (Lucatelli et al., 2021). Generally, the intricacies of anticoagulant therapy underscore the importance of careful assessment and personalized treatment in thrombotic disorders (Figure 10.17).

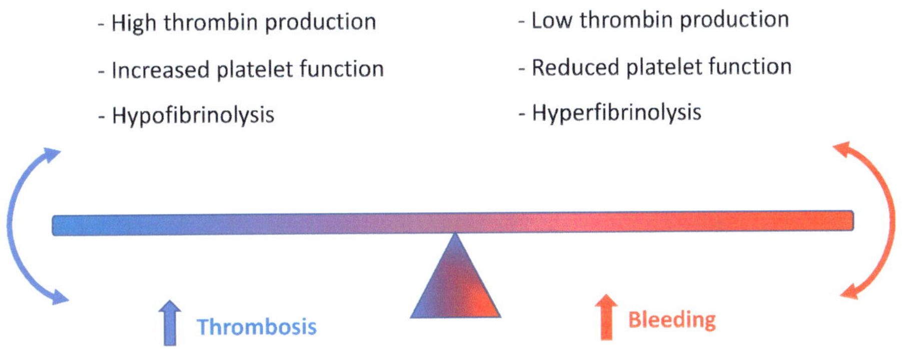

Figure 10.17. Anticoagulant therapy plays a crucial role in managing thrombotic disorders, particularly in patient populations who are at heightened risk of thromboembolic events.

Source: https://pub.mdpi-res.com/jcm/jcm-12-05955/article_deploy/html/images/jcm-12-05955-g001.png?1694659676.

10.4.2. Thrombolytic Therapy

Thrombolytic therapy is a significant intervention in the treatment of thrombotic illness, particularly in acute conditions such as ischemic stroke and myocardial infarction. As a result of their mechanism for dissolving blood clots that cause disruptions in blood flow, these treatments play a critical role in reducing the morbidity and mortality rates of thrombotic diseases. Traditional agents, such as tissue plasminogen activators and streptokinase, have demonstrated impressive efficacy in clinical settings; however, they are associated with risks of serious complications, including hemorrhage and allergic reactions. Recent research highlights the potential of alternative therapies, such as the ethanolic extract from Nelumbo nucifera leaves, which has demonstrated promising thrombolytic and antioxidant properties, achieving a clot lysis rate of 94.34% in vitro (Aditi et al., 2025). This suggests an increasing interest in complementary and less toxic thrombolytic alternatives, necessitating novel approaches to enhance efficacy and safety in the treatment of thrombotic disorders (Benemei et al., 2024).

10.4.3. Surgical Interventions (e.g., Thrombectomy)

Surgical interventions, particularly thrombectomy, play a crucial role in the management of thrombotic disorders, especially in cases involving acute ischemic stroke. This procedure aims to swiftly remove the thrombus obstructing cerebral blood flow, thereby minimizing potential neurological damage. A recent study conducted in 2023-2024 highlights the multifaceted effects of thrombectomy, indicating that while it is a critical life-saving intervention, patients often experience significant changes in their affective state during the early postoperative period. Evaluations conducted seven days post-surgery revealed a notable dissociation between patients' self-perceptions of anxiety and depression and objective assessments thereof, employing scales such as the Hamilton Anxiety Rating Scale (HARS) and Hamilton Depression Rating Scale (HDRS) (Rehush, 2024). Ultimately, understanding these psychological effects is essential for devising comprehensive rehabilitation strategies tailored to address both the physiological and psychological aftermath of thrombectomy procedures (Regusch, 2024) (Figure 10.18).

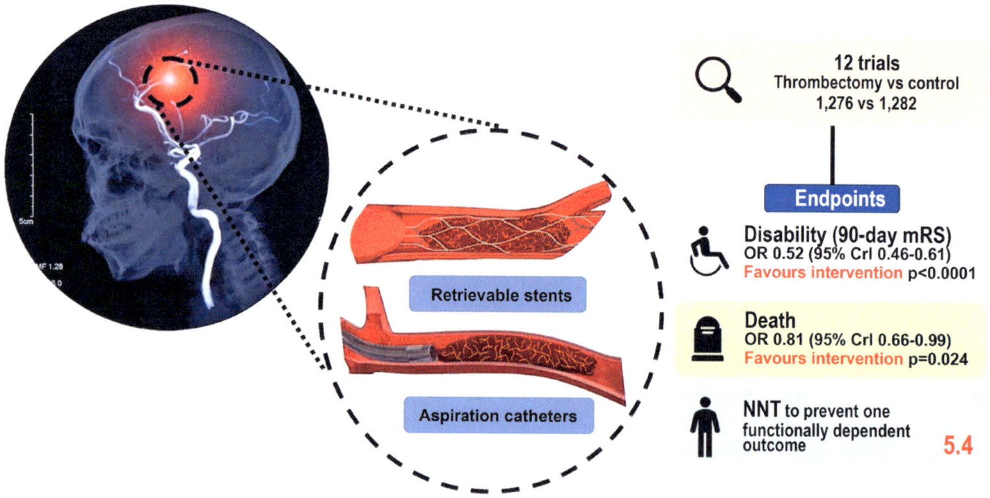

Figure 10.18. Surgical interventions, particularly thrombectomy, play a crucial role in the management of thrombotic disorders, especially in cases involving acute ischemic stroke.

Source: https://eurointervention.pcronline.com/storage/issues/EIJ204e/223_EIJ-D-21-00343_Rajkumar_204e/medias/227234/00_Rajkumar_204.jpg.

10.4.4. Long-Term Management Strategies

Long-term management strategies for thrombotic disorders necessitate a comprehensive and individualized approach, as the underlying pathology can vary widely among patients. Effective management is marked by the careful monitoring of patients who have experienced events such as TTP or hemolytic uremic syndrome (HUS), which often necessitates understanding the unique precipitating factors behind these conditions, such as infections or immunosuppression, as highlighted in (Young et al., 2007). Furthermore, patients presenting with concomitant cardiac and hematologic disorders require meticulous attention, as their treatment may involve balancing anticoagulation management with the risks associated with potential surgery. This necessitates a thorough understanding of their overall health status and treatment history, as noted in Goldhammer et al. (2016). By integrating these strategies, healthcare providers can enhance patient outcomes while reducing the risk of recurrent thrombotic events.

10.4.5. Patient Education and Lifestyle Modifications

Effective patient education and lifestyle modifications are crucial components in managing thrombotic disorders, as they empower individuals to take control of their health. Engaging patients in understanding their condition enhances adherence to prescribed health regimens and fosters proactive behavior, such as managing weight and increasing physical activity. Lifestyle changes, including dietary adjustments and smoking cessation, significantly reduce the risk of thrombus formation by improving cardiovascular health. However, the resource materials available for patient education often fall short in meeting the health literacy levels of the general population; for instance, many online resources exceed the readability suitable for average adults and inadequately outline actionable steps for managing their health (Bhatt et al., 2024). Therefore, developing accessible and comprehensible educational tools is essential to bridge this gap, ensuring that patients can effectively implement lifestyle modifications necessary for reducing the risk of complications associated with thrombotic disorders (Bucan et al., 2025) (Figure 10.19).

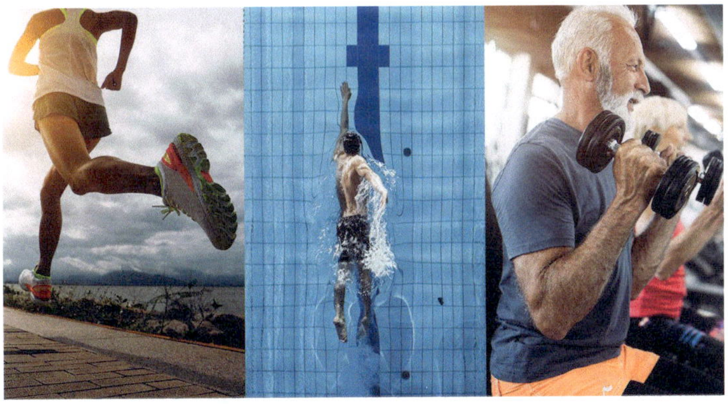

Figure 10.19. Engaging patients in understanding their condition enhances adherence to prescribed health regimens and fosters proactive behavior, such as managing weight and increasing physical activity.

Source: https://gwdocs.com/sites/g/files/zaskib551/files/styles/1140x600/public/2024-04/physical-activity-main-1140x600.jpg?itok=Ukm120r1.

10.4.6. Monitoring and Follow-Up Care

Effective monitoring and follow-up care are crucial for managing thrombotic disorders, particularly in preventing complications associated with VTE. After the initial diagnosis and treatment of conditions such as lower extremity deep vein thrombosis (LE DVT), patients require continuous assessment to evaluate their response to therapy and adjust treatment as needed. This ongoing care can significantly reduce the risk of recurrence and improve long-term outcomes. In this context, physical therapists play an essential role by adhering to clinical practice guidelines that focus on the prevention, screening, and treatment of VTE. These guidelines help in structuring a patient-centric follow-up plan that incorporates key action statements designed to enhance clinical decision-making and patient engagement. By implementing these evidence-based protocols, healthcare professionals can ensure a comprehensive approach to monitoring that supports both immediate recovery and long-term health (Kitsiou et al., 2013; Auten et al., 2016).

10.4.7. Management of Complications

The management of complications arising from thrombotic disorders necessitates a multifaceted approach, particularly in high-risk populations such as women with MPNs and those experiencing membranous nephropathy (MN). In the context of MPNs, effective management strategies must address the heightened risk of thrombosis and bleeding while also considering reproductive health, as these patients often navigate unique challenges during pregnancy. With rates of complications including increased preterm births and cesarean sections, tailored interventions such as low-dose aspirin and low-molecular-weight heparin are critical to optimizing maternal and fetal outcomes (Chiasakul et al., 2025). Similarly, complications like renal vein thrombosis (RVT) in MN patients require prompt recognition and management, often involving anticoagulation and immunosuppressive therapy to mitigate acute kidney injury (Kashiv et al., 2024). Ultimately, an individualized approach grounded in evidence-based guidelines is essential for enhancing patient outcomes and navigating the complex landscape of thrombotic disorders (Figure 10.20).

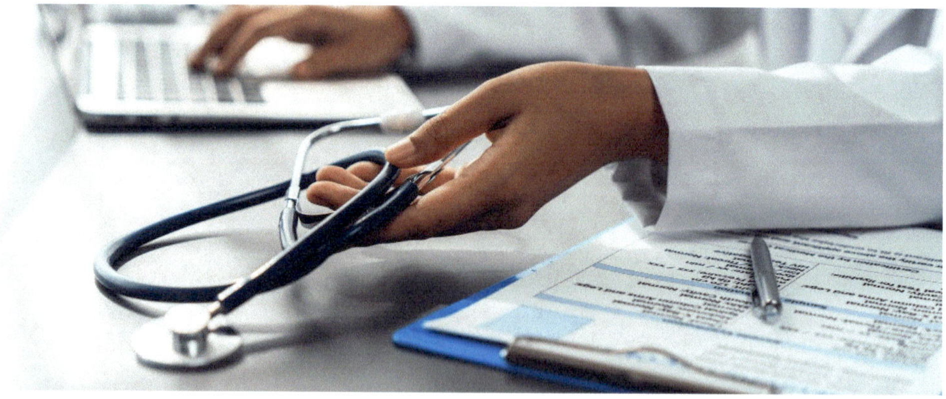

Figure 10.20. Complications like renal vein thrombosis (RVT) in MN patients require prompt recognition and management, often involving anticoagulation and immunosuppressive therapy to mitigate acute kidney injury

Source: https://sp-ao.shortpixel.ai/client/to_webp,q_glossy,ret_img/https://kch.sa/wp-content/uploads/2024/06/Overview.jpg.

10.4.8. Emerging Therapies and Research

In the realm of thrombotic disorders, emerging therapies and research are reshaping the landscape of treatment options. Advances in molecular docking techniques have opened new avenues for understanding the underlying mechanisms of thrombus formation, allowing for the identification of specific molecular targets that can be exploited for therapeutic intervention. For instance, the 2023 ACC/AHA/ACCP/HRS Guideline for the Diagnosis and Management of Atrial Fibrillation emphasizes the integration of innovative treatment approaches tailored to patient-specific needs, which could significantly enhance management strategies for those at risk of thrombotic events (José et al., 2023). Moreover, ongoing studies into nutraceuticals show promise in modulating biochemical pathways associated with thrombotic disorders. The application of molecular docking not only aids in assessing the efficacy of these bioactive substances but also accelerates the development of new therapies aimed at attenuating thrombus-related complications, thereby improving patient outcomes (Agu et al., 2023).

10.4.9. Role of Multidisciplinary Teams in Management

The management of thrombotic disorders necessitates a robust multidisciplinary team (MDT) approach, which is essential for effectively addressing the complexities associated with these conditions. Thrombotic disorders often involve a variety of etiologies and risk factors, necessitating collaboration among specialists in hematology, cardiology, vascular medicine, and other relevant fields. Such teamwork facilitates comprehensive assessments and tailored treatment plans that consider patients' unique health statuses and potential comorbidities. Previous research has highlighted that integrated care models led by MDTs enhance medical decision-making, particularly in complex cases where standard protocols may fall short (Chen et al., 2024). Additionally, effective communication among team members and with patients significantly improves adherence to recommended treatment regimens, ultimately optimizing patient outcomes (Daniela, 2025). Therefore, harnessing the collective expertise of an MDT not only enriches clinical practice but also elevates the standard of care for individuals grappling with thrombotic disorders.

A CLOSER LOOK

JANUS KINASE (JAK) INHIBITORS

Janus kinase (JAK) inhibitors belong to a class of drugs that inhibit the action of Janus kinases. These are enzymes involved in the signaling pathways of various cytokines and growth factors, which are crucial for immune function and blood cell production. These drugs help reduce inflammation and abnormal immune responses by inhibiting JAK enzymes.

Most common JAK inhibitors are currently used for the treatment of autoimmune diseases, including rheumatoid arthritis and psoriatic arthritis, and certain blood disorders, such as myelofibrosis and polycythemia vera. Examples of JAK inhibitors include tofacitinib, ruxolitinib, and baricitinib.

As they work on the immune system, JAK inhibitors can make patients susceptible to infection and should be closely monitored during their use.

SUMMARY

The complex landscape of thrombotic disorders necessitates ongoing research and clinical vigilance to improve diagnostic accuracy and therapeutic outcomes. As evidenced by recent studies, including those evaluating the safety of JAK inhibitors, the incidence of thrombotic events remains a significant concern, with a reported rate of 5.7%, primarily due to VTE (Shahzad et al., 2024). Moreover, advancements in imaging technology, as well as insights into diseases in the pelvic venous area, have revealed improved diagnostic criteria and methodologies that can lead to better identification and treatment management of these conditions (Sergey et al., 2025). Tailored interventions and monitoring strategies, hence, become critical observations that would less likely expose patients to risks related to both thrombotic events and their treatment. Ultimately, an integrated strategy that includes comprehensive diagnostics and individualized treatment is crucial for enhancing the outcomes of thrombotic diseases.

In examining thrombotic disorders, it is crucial to highlight several key points that underscore their complexity and impact on patient health. Thrombotic conditions often manifest as a direct result of an interplay between genetic and environmental factors, necessitating a comprehensive understanding of their pathophysiology. For instance, the prevalence of thrombosis increases notably with age, particularly in individuals aged 65-74 years, where the incidence is further amplified by comorbidities such as chronic myeloid leukemia and the presence of cardiac implantable electronic devices, which can complicate therapeutic approaches (Alexander et al., 2022). Furthermore, the development of diagnostic techniques like cardiac magnetic resonance imaging helps detect thrombotic events as early as possible, consequently improving management and outcomes. Collaborating with experts in the field opens a way to learn more about the necessity for a collaborative approach towards care, as well as about the adaptation of preventive and treatment strategies for such conditions (Halvorsen et al., 2022).

REFERENCES

1. Abrishamizadeh, A. (2017). Thrombophilia and arterial ischemic stroke. *Advances in Bioscience and Clinical Medicine*, 45. https://doi.org/10.7575/aiac.abcmed.ca1.45Abroug, F., Azoulay, E., Benoit, D., Eggimann, P., et al. (2017). Expert statements on the standard of care in critically ill adult patients with atypical hemolytic uremic syndrome. https://core.ac.uk/download/141525591.pdf (accessed on 12th June 2025).
2. Adams, R., Akassoglou, K., Akenami, F. O., Albright, A. V., et al. (2018). A perspective of coagulation dysfunction in multiple sclerosis and in experimental allergic encephalomyelitis. https://core.ac.uk/download/195777098.pdf (accessed on 12th June 2025).
3. Agu, P. C., Afiukwa, C. A., Orji, O. U., Ezeh, E. M., Ofoke, I. H., Ogbu, C. O., Ugwuja, E. I., et al. (2023). Molecular docking as a tool for the discovery of molecular targets of nutraceuticals in diseases management. *Scientific Reports, 13*. https://doi.org/10.1038/s41598-023-40160-2 (accessed on 12th June 2025).
4. Arachchillage, D. J., Mackillop, L., Chandratheva, A., Motawani, J., MacCallum, P., & Laffan, M. (2022). Thrombophilia testing: A British Society for Hematology guideline. *British Journal of Hematology, 198*, 443–458. https://doi.org/10.1111/bjh.18239 (accessed on 12th June 2025).
5. Arcelus, J., Gooren, L., Klink, D., T'Sjoen, G., et al. (2018). Endocrinology of transgender medicine. https://core.ac.uk/download/162667742.pdf (accessed on 12th June 2025).
6. Arykan, N., Shestopalov, A., Khvorostinina, E. E., Alekseeva, A. O., & Asaturyan, K. S. (2022). Selecting anticoagulant therapy in patients with cirrhosis. *Russian Medical Inquiry*. https://www.semanticscholar.org/paper/b408d1cd990af7df967b93051dbb6d1035ff54b1 (accessed on 12th June 2025).
7. Auten, B., Frese, E. M., Hillegass, E., Puthoff, M., et al. (2016). Role of physical therapists in the management of individuals at risk for or diagnosed with venous thromboembolism: Evidence-based clinical practice guideline. https://core.ac.uk/download/213061294.pdf (accessed on 12th June 2025).
8. Benemei, S., Gatto, F., Marcucci, R., & Gresele, P. (2024). Emerging thrombotic disorders associated with virus-based innovative therapies: From VITT to AAV gene therapy–related thrombotic microangiopathy. *Thrombosis and Haemostasias*. https://www.semanticscholar.org/paper/af6555798fc722145b9e9f220bc612fd7901c66b (accessed on 12th June 2025).
9. Bhatt, C., Lin, E., Ferreira-Legere, L., Jackevicius, C. A., Ko, D. T., Lee, D. S., Schade, K., et al. (2024). Evaluating readability, understandability, and actionability of online printable patient education materials for cholesterol management: A systematic review. *Journal of the American Heart Association: Cardiovascular and Cerebrovascular Disease, 13*. https://www.semanticscholar.org/paper/e68e06016cc68a31b2b162f9385748bdde38d845 (accessed on 12th June 2025).
10. Boffa, M., Nesheim, M., & Koschinsky, M. (2001). Thrombin activable fibrinolysis inhibitor (TAFI): Molecular genetics of an emerging potential risk factor for thrombotic disorders. *Current Drug Targets. Cardiovascular & Hematological Disorders, 1*(2), 59–74. https://www.semanticscholar.org/paper/18b171737a3e9e24279f9966345b20b9ddfd11c6 (accessed on 12th June 2025).

11. Borghi, A., Marzano, A. V., Cugno, M., & Garcovich, S. (2019). Coagulation and skin autoimmunity. https://core.ac.uk/download/225134758.pdf (accessed on 12th June 2025).
12. Bragina, O. A., Gekaluyk, A. S., Goltsov, A., Rafailov, E., et al. (2017). Laser-induced generation of singlet oxygen and its role in the cerebrovascular physiology. https://core.ac.uk/download/228178032.pdf (accessed on 12th June 2025).
13. Bucan, J. I., Braut, T., Kršek, A., Sotošek, V., & Batičić, L. (2025). Updates in gastroesophageal reflux disease management: From proton pump inhibitors to dietary and lifestyle modifications. *Gastrointestinal Disorders*. https://www.semanticscholar.org/paper/a5ad244b16a71a2aecc0725d60b8efabb4a823a2 (accessed on 12th June 2025).
14. Catalano, L., Franchini, M., Liumbruno, G. M., Marano, G., et al. (2017). The role of ABO blood type in thrombosis scoring systems. https://core.ac.uk/download/98343593.pdf (accessed on 12th June 2025).
15. Celeski, M., Segreti, A., Crisci, F., Cricco, R., Piscione, M., Di Gioia, G., Nusca, A., et al. (2024). The role of cardiac troponin and other emerging biomarkers among athletes and beyond: Underlying mechanisms, differential diagnosis, and guide for interpretation. *Biomolecules, 14*. https://www.semanticscholar.org/paper/8f704ca46c6a1913fc70b000c8f9ebb1800ee419 (accessed on 12th June 2025).
16. Chan, V. T., Criqui, M. H., Denenberg, J. O., Golomb, B. A., et al. (2014). Risk marker associations with venous thrombotic events: A cross-sectional analysis. https://core.ac.uk/download/323065917.pdf (accessed on 12th June 2025).
17. Chavhan, R., Wanjari, A., Kumar, S., Acharya, S., Rathod, N., Reddy, H., & Gemnani, R. R. (2024). A comprehensive review on navigating the neurological landscape of COVID-19: Insights into etiopathogenesis and clinical management. *Cureus, 16*. https://www.semanticscholar.org/paper/5a3e644519efc6399a064575e5cec7b537e56c40 (accessed on 12th June 2025).
18. Chen, J., Yao, Q., Wang, X., Jiang, J., Zhu, H., & Yu, D. (2024). Significance of multidisciplinary teams for patients with oral and maxillofacial surgical diseases: An observational retrospective study in a general hospital in China. *Journal of Multidisciplinary Healthcare, 17*, 6187–6198. https://www.semanticscholar.org/paper/344d73a2669ac8d7fda087b68588b6d6be522abe (accessed on 12th June 2025).
19. Chiasakul, T., & Baker, R. (2025). Management of bleeding, thrombotic and pregnancy-related complications in women with myeloproliferative neoplasms: A case-based review focusing on sex-specific challenges. *Journal of Clinical Medicine, 14*. https://www.semanticscholar.org/paper/0fa867801a9a8e62497a50f6f1cdeaa10865ccad (accessed on 12th June 2025).
20. Chubchenko, S. V., Alenichev, A. V., & Gavrilov, S. G. (2025). Current diagnosis of pelvic venous diseases (literature review). *University Proceedings. Volga Region. Medical Sciences*. https://www.semanticscholar.org/paper/03bf8dd2f63e578b8afa676e893b85cd570d5b10 (accessed on 12th June 2025).
21. Cohen, H., Efthymiou, M., Isenberg, D. A., Maranini, S., et al. (2024). Can complement activation be the missing link in antiphospholipid syndrome? https://core.ac.uk/download/603250286.pdf (accessed on 12th June 2025).
22. Darade, A. S., Pandey, A. M., & Agrawal, S. A. (2025). Thrombolytic potential and antioxidant efficacy of *Nelumbo nucifera* leaf extract. *Indian Drugs*. https://www.semanticscholar.org/paper/ea5e8764ca40a8a99fe90673d80d61f774d0e0ed (accessed on 12th June 2025).

23. De Stefano, V., Gasbarrini, A., & Ponziani, F. R. (2009). Viral cirrhosis: An overview of hemostatic alterations and clinical consequences. https://core.ac.uk/download/pdf/8522693.pdf (accessed on 12th June 2025).

24. Devnani, R., Kammeyer, R., & Mehta, R. (2016). Cerebral fat embolism syndrome mimicking thrombotic thrombocytopenic purpura in a patient with Hemoglobin SC disease. https://core.ac.uk/download/84831018.pdf (accessed on 12th June 2025).

25. ElSayed, N. A., Aleppo, G., Aroda, V. R., Bannuru, R. R., Brown, F. M., Bruemmer, D., Collins, B. S., et al. (2022). 15. Management of diabetes in pregnancy: *Standards of Care in Diabetes—2023. Diabetes Care, 46,* S254–S266. https://doi.org/10.2337/dc23-s015 (accessed on 12th June 2025).

26. Farag, M., Gorog, D. A., Spinthakis, N., Srinivasan, M., et al. (2017). Morphine analgesia pre-PPCI is associated with prothrombotic state, reduced spontaneous reperfusion and greater infarct size. https://core.ac.uk/download/287581512.pdf (accessed on 12th June 2025).

27. Feijão, D. de M. (2025). Home-based palliative care for the elderly: Challenges, strategies, and the role of family and healthcare teams. *International Seven Journal of Multidisciplinary.* https://www.semanticscholar.org/paper/bbd69936c56abc085dd576bf2d55fab51e0863e0 (accessed on 12th June 2025).

28. Galliazzo, S., Bucciarelli, P., Barcellona, D., Ciampa, A., Grandone, E., Malcangi, G., Rescigno, G., et al. (2023). Practical suggestions for an optimal management of vitamin K antagonists: Italian Federation of Centers for the Diagnosis of Thrombotic Disorders and the Surveillance of the Antithrombotic Therapies (FCSA) position paper. *Thrombosis and Haemostasias, 124,* 803–809. https://www.semanticscholar.org/paper/8a82ec7593cf9bf618e8abd63241efd33ca3b5c5 (accessed on 12th June 2025).

29. García-García, I., Jiménez, M., Valcárcel, D., Mingot-Castellano, M., Pascual Izquierdo, M. C., Viejo, A., Lozano, M., et al. (2020). Caplacizumab as new paradigm-changing therapy for patients with autoimmune thrombotic thrombocytopenic purpura (aTTP): Real-world data from TTP Spanish Registry. *Blood, 136,* 20–21. https://www.semanticscholar.org/paper/b05bb94d65ced53e22ca0b6de1521e1f5d17822e (accessed on 12th June 2025).

30. Giacopelli, P., Marchitto, N., Panfilio, S., Piovanello, M., et al. (2018). Stratification of thrombotic risk in patients that are undergoing to PICC implantation: The "CoRa-MaPiCC STUDY." https://core.ac.uk/download/158328407.pdf (accessed on 12th June 2025).

31. Gitto, M., Motta, N., Aldè, M., Zanetti, D., & Di Berardino, F. (2025). Auditory processing disorders: Navigating the diagnostic maze of central hearing losses. *Journal of Clinical Medicine, 14.* https://www.semanticscholar.org/paper/5e5d2bf4b4ab20ce98451f4dae26ef6cb3787179 (accessed on 12th June 2025).

32. Goldhammer, J. E., & Kohl, B. A. (2016). Coexisting cardiac and hematologic disorders. https://core.ac.uk/download/83049377.pdf (accessed on 12th June 2025).

33. Gorog, D. A., & Okafor, O. N. (2015). Endogenous fibrinolysis: An important mediator of thrombus formation and cardiovascular risk. https://core.ac.uk/download/287581705.pdf (accessed on 12th June 2025).

34. Greinacher, A., & Warkentin, T. E. (2023). Thrombotic anti-PF4 immune disorders: HIT, VITT, and beyond. *Hematology. American Society of Hematology. Education Program, 2023*(1), 1–10.

https://www.semanticscholar.org/paper/7d35087552e0d3c8c860add67e1cc40e90d26753 (accessed on 12th June 2025).

35. Halvorsen, S., Mehilli, J., Cassese, S., Hall, T. S., Abdelhamid, M., Barbato, E., De Hert, S., et al. (2022). 2022 ESC guidelines on cardiovascular assessment and management of patients undergoing non-cardiac surgery. *European Heart Journal, 43*, 3826–3924. https://doi.org/10.1093/eurheartj/ehac270 (accessed on 12th June 2025).

36. Hasan, S. M. M., Uddin, M. P., Al Mamun, M., Sharif, M. I., Ulhaq, A., & Krishnamoorthy, G. (2024). A machine learning framework for early-stage detection of autism spectrum disorders. *IEEE Access, 11*, 15038–15057. https://www.semanticscholar.org/paper/4d864a38c32229b18222882d13317e54e021f347 (accessed on 12th June 2025).

37. Hazenberg, E., Herrera, D., Aston, H., Price, E., Raval, G., Gollan, S., Xu, H., et al. (2024). Pulmonary hypertension and hemoglobin F values in patients with sickle cell disease. *Blood*. https://www.semanticscholar.org/paper/726afaf601ab71bd92132f646db37a1dcd5ad782 (accessed on 12th June 2025).

38. Heller, P. G., & Marin Oyarzún, C. P. (2019). Platelets as mediators of thromboinflammation in chronic myeloproliferative neoplasms. https://core.ac.uk/download/323211431.pdf (accessed on 12th June 2025).

39. How, J., Oh, S. T., & Zhou, A. (2016). Splanchnic vein thrombosis in myeloproliferative neoplasms: Pathophysiology and molecular mechanisms of disease. https://core.ac.uk/download/80495017.pdf (accessed on 12th June 2025).

40. Iba, T., Levy, J. H., Connors, J. M., Warkentin, T. E., Thachil, J., & Levi, M. (2020). The unique characteristics of COVID-19 coagulopathy. *Critical Care, 24*. https://doi.org/10.1186/s13054-020-03077-0 (accessed on 12th June 2025).

41. Jaafari, A. S. A., Alajmi, K. H. A., Althabaity, A. M., Salem, K. S. A., Alhargan, M. S., Alotaibi, H. F. A., Almutairi, N. A., et al. (2024). Hypercoagulability: An updated overview for healthcare providers. *Journal of Eco Humanism*. https://www.semanticscholar.org/paper/2be4318be42f4d35e1d62ab85013d810e8516413 (accessed on 12th June 2025).

42. Jarczak, D., Kluge, S., & Nierhaus, A. (2021). Sepsis—Pathophysiology and therapeutic concepts. *Frontiers in Medicine, 8*. https://doi.org/10.3389/fmed.2021.628302 (accessed on 12th June 2025).

43. Joglar, J. A., Chung, M. K., Armbruster, A. L., Benjamin, E. J., Chyou, J. Y., Cronin, E. M., Deswal, A., et al. (2023). 2023 ACC/AHA/ACCP/HRS guideline for the diagnosis and management of atrial fibrillation: A report of the American College of Cardiology/American Heart Association Joint Committee on Clinical Practice Guidelines. *Circulation, 149*. https://doi.org/10.1161/cir.0000000000001193 (accessed on 12th June 2025).

44. Kashiv, P., Malde, S., Gupta, S., Dubey, S., Sejpal, K., Pawar, T., Mahajan, V., et al. (2024). A case of NELL-1-positive membranous nephropathy with acute kidney injury due to bilateral renal vein thrombosis. *Cureus, 16*. https://www.semanticscholar.org/paper/8d0433bbd918a8042ea9e7f1f879593583e297c3 (accessed on 12th June 2025).

45. Kitsiou, A., Caforio, A. L. P., Porta-Sanchez, A., Vahanian, A., Iung, B., Carrera, C., Szymanski, C., et al. (2013). ESC core curriculum for the general cardiologist (2013). https://core.ac.uk/download/55756305.pdf (accessed on 12th June 2025).

46. Kuter, D., Cataland, S., Broome, C. M., & Neunert, C. E. (2024). The latest insights into rare blood disorders: Diagnosis and treatment strategies. *American Journal of Hematology*. https://www.semanticscholar.org/paper/473714453ac2a6fbfe1d16e3f739da8b351c8583 (accessed on 12th June 2025).

47. Lippi, G., & Favaloro, E. (2018). Laboratory hemostasis: From biology to the bench. *Clinical Chemistry and Laboratory Medicine (CCLM), 56*, 1035–1045. https://www.semanticscholar.org/paper/af79152abb8c105d62cc11e88b135594a2aeb44f (accessed on 12th June 2025).

48. Liu, Y., Wang, Y., Huang, G., Wu, S., Liu, X., Chen, S., Luo, P., et al. (2024). The role of leukocytes in myeloproliferative neoplasms thromboinflammation. *Journal of Leukocyte Biology*. https://www.semanticscholar.org/paper/82a26373f53ffb42148665aaeaa656dc61d20e14 (accessed on 12th June 2025).

49. Lucatelli, P., Rocco, B., Nardis, P., Cannavale, A., Bezzi, M., Catalano, C., & Corona, M. (2021). Bleeding in COVID patients: What we have understood so far. *Cardiovascular and Interventional Radiology, 44*, 666–668. https://www.semanticscholar.org/paper/4c9defc2dfc15ccf8558ae606ab8ec2ed2e57a43 (accessed on 12th June 2025).

50. Lyon, A. R., López-Fernández, T., Couch, L. S., Asteggiano, R., Aznar, M. C., Bergler-Klein, J., Boriani, G., et al. (2022). 2022 ESC guidelines on cardio-oncology developed in collaboration with the European Hematology Association (EHA), the European Society for Therapeutic Radiology and Oncology (ESTRO) and the International Cardio-Oncology Society (IC-OS). *European Heart Journal, 43*, 4229–4361. https://doi.org/10.1093/eurheartj/ehac244 (accessed on 12th June 2025).

51. Marquardt, C. W., Pickens, P. V., & Varner, C. K. (2018). Antiphosphatidylserine antibody as a cause of multiple dural venous sinus thromboses and ST-elevation myocardial infarction. https://core.ac.uk/download/213444063.pdf (accessed on 12th June 2025).

52. McEwan, A., Greenwood, M., Ward, C., Ritchie, D., Szer, J., Gardiner, E., Colic, A., et al. (2023). Diagnosis and management of endothelial disorders following hematopoietic stem cell transplantation. *Internal Medicine Journal, 53*. https://www.semanticscholar.org/paper/6468e682fdcc66a48a57a49f4991f39b7bb98be6 (accessed on 12th June 2025).

53. Mo, Q., Xu, S., Hu, F., & Zheng, X. (2024). Effectiveness and clinical relevance of kinesio taping in musculoskeletal disorders: A protocol for an overview of systematic reviews and evidence mapping. *BMJ Open, 14*. https://www.semanticscholar.org/paper/6f79dd17daec88cfaa4bfd58064e1564b4b2c037 (accessed on 12th June 2025).

54. Musalem, P. (2025). Ten tips for managing complement-mediated thrombotic microangiopathies (formerly atypical hemolytic uremic syndrome): Narrative review. *BMC Nephrology, 26*. https://www.semanticscholar.org/paper/85d72f4c33a9384bf23ed454422d4beba337ff3d (accessed on 12th June 2025).

55. Nace, T. C., O'Sullivan, C., Shan, K. S., Zhang, L., et al. (2020). Iron deficiency anemia: An unexpected cause of an acute occipital lobe stroke in an otherwise healthy young woman. https://core.ac.uk/download/322850195.pdf (accessed on 12th June 2025).

56. Northup, P. G., García-Pagán, J. C., García-Tsao, G., Intagliata, N. M., Superina, R., Roberts, L. N., Lisman, T., et al. (2020). Vascular liver disorders, portal vein thrombosis, and procedural bleeding in patients with liver disease: 2020 practice guidance by the American Association

for the Study of Liver Diseases. *Hepatology, 73*, 366–413. https://doi.org/10.1002/hep.31646 (accessed on 12th June 2025).

57. Ohkouchi, S., Morimoto, Y., Suganuma, N., Kurosawa, H., Azuma, K., Omori, H., Tamura, T., et al. (2025). Importance of early detection and treatment of occupational hypersensitivity pneumonia. *Journal of Occupational Health*. https://www.semanticscholar.org/paper/bd425a568deed2fa29e8207e74487a1cd5d8ede0 (accessed on 12th June 2025).

58. Palmiero, P., Caretto, P., Ciccone, M. M., Maiello, M., et al. (2025). Long-term cardiovascular risk and maternal history of pre-eclampsia. *Journal of Clinical Medicine, 14*. https://www.semanticscholar.org/paper/455fd296ab369889d55444260e65e6db6e08ec3d (accessed on 12th June 2025).

59. Rank, A., Bal, L., Berckmans, R. J., Toth, B., Biro, E., Corada, M., et al. (2012). Climacteric lowers plasma levels of platelet-derived microparticles: A pilot study in pre-versus postmenopausal women. https://core.ac.uk/download/16432947.pdf (accessed on 12th June 2025).

60. Regusch, A. V. (2024). Early affective disorders in patients who underwent thrombectomy for thrombotic occlusion: Comparison of objective and subjective assessments. *Psychiatry Neurology and Medical Psychology*. https://www.semanticscholar.org/paper/9d863e5d9c84d955109a42a1fada258a0cb224b3 (accessed on 12th June 2025).

61. Rehush, A. (2024). Early affective disorders after thrombectomy for thrombotic occlusion: An objective assessment. *Ukrains'kyi Visnyk Psykhonevrolohii*. https://www.semanticscholar.org/paper/f2886819ce78a8c8a3e9a6bc010dfe4a1bd24fbe (accessed on 12th June 2025).

62. Remez-Gabay, L., Vdovich, O., Akria, L., & Kruzel-Davila, E. (2025). Case report: Anti-platelet factor 4–mediated immunothrombosis in a patient with ANCA vasculitis–A shared mechanism of NETosis. *Frontiers in Immunology, 16*. https://www.semanticscholar.org/paper/5b4039f26756a7ebd83bcec4532a4664de8b83e0 (accessed on 12th June 2025).

63. Rooth, E. (2012). Hemostatic disturbances in acute ischemic stroke. https://core.ac.uk/download/70340028.pdf (accessed on 12th June 2025).

64. Shahzad, M., Amin, M. K., Basharat, A., Noor, J., Khalid, M. F., Zaidi, M., Park, R., et al. (2024). Uncovering the risks: Bleeding and thrombotic complications of JAK inhibitors in hematological conditions: A comprehensive systematic review and meta-analysis. *Blood*. https://www.semanticscholar.org/paper/3f1f2cde11e1d3d0ea397cb6f0081ac6e1ec5f1d (accessed on 12th June 2025).

65. Taanila, A. (2017). The role of a malignancy in the treatment of a venous thromboembolism and superficial thrombophlebitis. https://core.ac.uk/download/84364043.pdf (accessed on 12th June 2025).

66. Thawabteh, A., Jibreen, A., Karaman, D., Thawabteh, A., & Karaman, R. (2023). Skin pigmentation types, causes and treatment—A review. *Molecules, 28*. https://www.semanticscholar.org/paper/bb0cbb024086d33c5d970198aeb906c00c881170 (accessed on 12th June 2025).

67. Yachi, S., Takeyama, M., Nishimoto, Y., Tsujino, I., Nakamura, J., Yamamoto, N., Nakata, H., et al. (2023). Risk factors and impact on outcomes of thrombosis in patients with COVID-19 in Japan: From the CLOT-COVID Study. *Annals of Vascular Diseases, 16*, 31–37. https://www.semanticscholar.org/paper/6a7bb3d91457839533a8470d51f03a990dbd4eda (accessed on 12th June 2025).

68. Young, D., Hosler, K. G. J., Pollock, T. J., Marques, I., Sadler, M., Beattie, T. J., Tarr, P. I., et al. (2007). Clinical surveillance of thrombotic microangiopathies in Scotland, 2003–2005. https://core.ac.uk/download/9023772.pdf (accessed on 12th June 2025).

69. Zeng, Y., Chourpiliadis, C., Hammar, N., Seitz, C., Valdimarsdóttir, U., Fang, F., Song, H., et al. (2024). Inflammatory biomarkers and risk of psychiatric disorders. *JAMA Psychiatry*. https://www.semanticscholar.org/paper/525e6dc4203824c4f3c433c788bb0f0bf2e1e678 (accessed on 12th June 2025).

70. Zhang, K., Wang, L., Gao, W., & Guo, R. (2025). Retinol-binding protein 4 in skeletal and cardiac muscle: Molecular mechanisms, clinical implications, and future perspectives. *Frontiers in Cell and Developmental Biology, 13*. https://www.semanticscholar.org/paper/a2a49eae85306b3bc9506b9a258f05e856d20e2b (accessed on 12th June 2025).

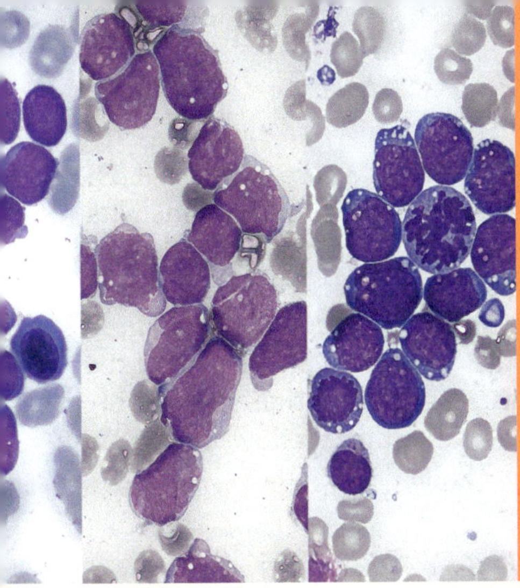

Chapter 11

ACUTE LEUKEMIAS

Contents

Introduction 267
11.1. Types of Acute Leukemias 268
11.2. Symptoms and Diagnosis 272
11.3. Treatment Options 277
11.4. Prognosis and Outcomes 281
Summary 288
References 289

Introduction

It is essential to comprehend the nature of acute leukemias to understand the characteristics of hematological malignancies, a heterogeneous family of disorders characterized by the rapid proliferation of immature blood cells. The acute leukemias comprise two broad groups: acute lymphoblastic leukemia (ALL) and acute myeloid leukemia (AML), each of which is associated with specific pathophysiologic features and clinical presentations. The pathogenesis of such leukemias is typically associated with specific genetic mutations and chromosomal lesions that lead to the uncontrolled proliferation of leukemic cells. Moreover, secondary leukemias are additionally caused by former irradiation therapy, which also poses additional challenges in management and treatment (Davoren et al., 2014). Considering their complexity and multi-factorial nature of potential inducers, the elucidation of acute leukemia pathogenesis is important, essential to optimize treatments and diagnostic methods that eventually lead to optimizing patient outcomes in such a high-priority research area (Brys et al., 2015).

11.1. Types of Acute Leukemias

Being aware of the different subtypes of acute leukemias helps one in proper diagnosis and treatment. These malignancies are further classified under two major groups, which are ALL and AML, originating from different lineages of hematopoietic cells. ALL essentially targets lymphoid precursors and may be prevalent predominantly among child populations, thereby necessitating intricate diagnosis protocols due to its nonspecific symptomatology, which can be misleading at times (Devi et al., 2024). AML, on the other hand, emerges from myeloid precursors and affects more adults than children, with variants that may differ depending on cytogenetic abnormalities. The fifth edition of the classification of diseases from the World Health Organization delivers the latest information regarding these leukemias, placing significant emphasis on accurate diagnosis in the determination of prognosis and individually adjusted treatment plans (Valiev et al., 2025). Each type's distinctive characteristics and dangers provide a gateway to the more specific therapeutic approaches, highlighting the need to actualize and understand their differentiation.

11.1.1. Acute Lymphoblastic Leukemia (ALL)

ALL is a heterogeneous collection of hematological cancers distinguished by the aggressive growth of immature lymphoid cells. It mainly affects children, but the condition does occur in adults, with a difference in genetic and clinical consequences. Among the distinct subtypes of ALL, T cell acute lymphoblastic leukemia (T-ALL) occurs due to the oncogenic transformation of T cell progenitors following a multistep oncogenic process involving genetic changes and sustained activation of NOTCH signaling (Ferrando et al., 2012). Current literature emphasizes the demographical and clinical features of T-ALL, where about 17.22% of ALL in the Pakistani population presents with this subtype, mainly in young males (Adil et al., 2005). Such finer points must be considered in the development of successful treatment protocols and the improvement of prognostic outcomes in these affected patients, reflecting the ongoing need for routine follow-up care in acute leukemias (Figure 11.1).

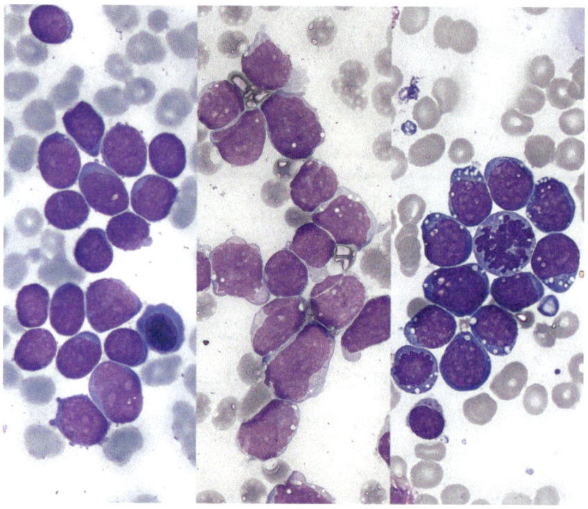

Figure 11.1. Acute Lymphoblastic Leukemia (ALL) represents a heterogeneous group of hematological malignancies characterized by the rapid proliferation of immature lymphoid cells.

Source: https://upload.wikimedia.org/wikipedia/commons/f/f9/Morphological_types_of_acute_lymphoblastic_leukemia.jpg.

11.1.2. Acute Myeloid Leukemia (AML)

AML is an aggressive and heterogeneous type of blood cancer that involves accelerated growth of aberrant myeloid cells. Even with significant developments in therapeutic approaches, the outlook for AML patients remains poor, especially for those with certain genetic aberrations, such as KMT2A rearrangements and NPM1 mutations. These genetic determinants are responsible not only for the leukemogenic process but also for the difficulties in obtaining satisfactory treatment responses, as reported in research, which has yielded unfavorable outcomes for the afflicted patients (Li et al., 2025). New therapeutic approaches, including the activation of thermogenic adipose tissues, have shown promise in preclinical models, significantly inhibiting leukemic cell growth and enhancing survival in mice (Chen et al., 2024). Such findings underscore the need to continue researching the development of targeted therapies for addressing the complex molecular pathways involved in AML, as this could yield better treatment options for combating this formidable disease (Figure 11.2).

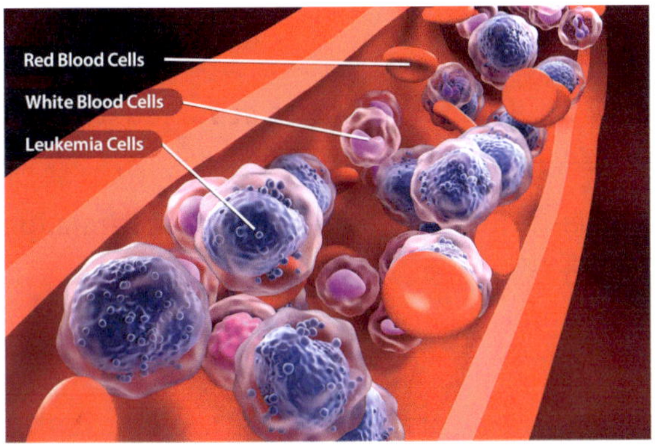

Figure 11.2. Acute myeloid leukemia (AML).

Source: https://img.lb.wbmdstatic.com/vim/live/webmd/consumer_assets/site_images/article_thumbnails/BigBead/acute-myeloid-leukemia-aml-bigbead/1800x1200-acute-myeloid-leukemia-aml-bigbead.jpg.

11.1.3. Differences between ALL and AML

ALL and AML are two distinct types of acute leukemias, characterized by unique cellular origins, clinical presentations, and genetic profiles. ALL primarily originates from B or T lymphocyte precursors, typically presenting in children, thereby emphasizing its higher prevalence among pediatric populations compared to adults. In contrast, AML arises from the progenitor cells of the myeloid lineage and is diagnosed more frequently in elderly individuals, indicating an age bias in occurrence rates. The biological processes of the diseases also serve to distinguish them; for example, dysregulation of the mammalian target of rapamycin (mTOR) signaling has been reported in both AML and ALL, and investigators are currently developing research aimed at exploiting mTOR inhibitors for therapeutic use (Bianchi et al., 2018). Moreover, radiation exposure has been linked to secondary leukemias such as AML, necessitating robust animal models for effective research (Davoren et al., 2014). Understanding these differences is crucial for tailoring treatment strategies and improving patient outcomes.

11.1.4. Risk Factors Associated with Each Type

The key to an appropriate management and treatment strategy is to know the risk factors for different types of acute leukemia. AML and ALL have distinct risk profiles that are significantly influenced by genetic, environmental, and treatment-related factors. In AML, older age and previous exposure to cytotoxic chemotherapy or radiation are significant contributors, whereas ALL is often associated with genetic predispositions and environmental exposures, particularly in children. Furthermore, the development of venous thromboembolism (VTE) is a notable complication in hematological cancers, with unique risk factors varying by leukemia type that necessitate tailored thromboprophylaxis protocols; for instance, ALL patients might have heightened risks due to treatment-related factors (Chan et al., 2020). Additionally, the role of allogeneic hematopoietic stem cell transplantation (allo-HSCT) adds complexity and necessitates careful consideration of treatment efficacy and patient outcomes in this context (Couturier et al., 2024) (Figure 11.3).

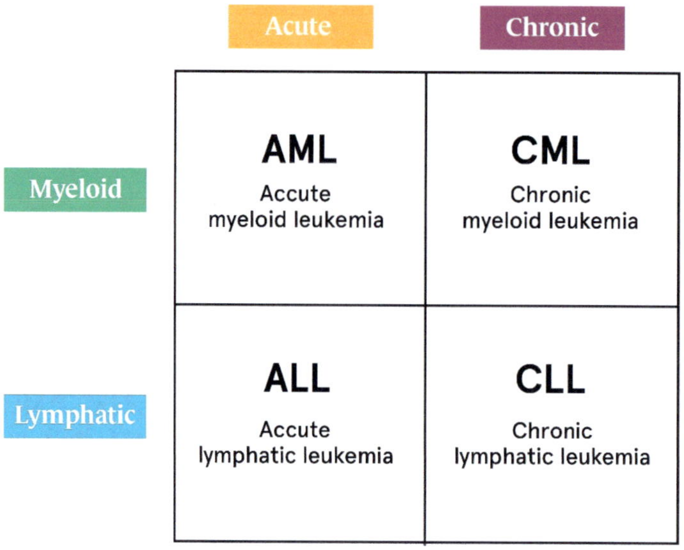

Figure 11.3. Understanding the risk factors associated with different types of acute leukemias is essential for effective management and treatment strategies.

Source: https://www.rockymountaincancercenters.com/hs-fs/hubfs/RMCC-TypesOfLeukemia.jpg?width=2485&height=1924&name=RMCC-TypesOfLeukemia.jpg.

11.1.5. Age Demographics Affected by Each Type

Acute leukemias are known for being aggressive and progressing rapidly, and their age distribution varies by subtype. For instance, AML shows a pronounced incidence in older adults, with median ages often surpassing 70 years, especially among those with genetic alterations such as NPM1 and KMT2A, which predominantly affect this age group (Borate et al., 2024). In contrast, ALL is more prevalent in younger populations, particularly children and young adults, illustrating a stark age dichotomy within acute leukemias. Additionally, myeloid sarcoma (MS) and extramedullary acute myeloid leukemia (eAML) also present significant age variations, with a median patient age of approximately 40 years, indicating that while some forms of leukemia are age-related, others can affect a broader demographic spectrum (Shatilova et al., 2024). It is necessary to understand these demographic trends to create the proper prevention and therapy for people at any age.

11.1.6. Genetic Mutations Linked to Acute Leukemias

The function of genetic mutations in the development of acute leukemia is a multifaceted interaction of numerous molecular processes that play a crucial role in disease etiology. Specifically, BRCA1 and BRCA2 gene mutations have been shown to increase the risk of myeloid leukemia, particularly in individuals inheriting defects in both alleles of the genes, such as in children, where the rate of AML increases significantly (Friedenson, 2011). Additionally, chromosomal translocations involving the RUNX1 gene have been implicated in the initiation of leukemia, specifically through the production of fusion proteins such as TEL-RUNX1 and RUNX1-ETO, which disrupt normal cellular growth control mechanisms and evade senescence (Anderson et al., 2018). These collectively emphasize the need for early diagnosis to mutations that impart risk for acute leukemia, thus opening new targeted therapies that can potentially overcome disease progression and be of advantage to the patient (Figure 11.4).

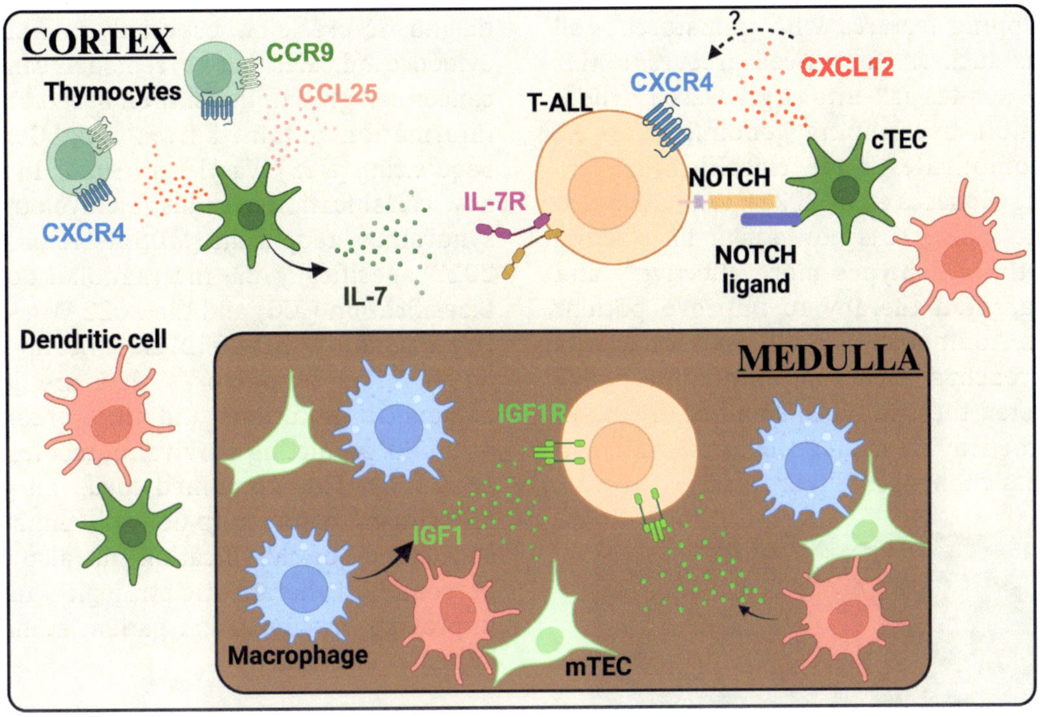

Figure 11.4. The thymic TME promotes survival and proliferation of T-ALL cells by providing pro-leukemic signals such as IL-7, NOTCH ligands, and IGF1.

Source: https://www.nature.com/articles/s12276-024-01335-7.

11.1.7. Subtypes of Acute Lymphoblastic Leukemia

ALL is a variety of different subtypes, mainly classified based on the type of malignant lymphoid cells, for example, B-cell and T-cell ALL, with their unique responses to therapy and biology. T-cell ALL (T-ALL), for instance, arises from the malignant transformation of hematopoietic progenitors and is characterized by complex genetic alterations that activate critical oncogenic pathways, such as NOTCH signaling, thus defining unique molecular groups with specific clinicobiological features (Ferrando et al., 2012). Another mechanism that uses this classification is the B-cell precursor ALL (B-ALL), which further has genetic mutations for other classifications. Examples include the Philadelphia chromosome, linked to a bad prognosis, where aberrant signaling pathways, including PI3K/AKT/mTOR, contribute to therapy resistance (Badura et al., 2013). It is essential to classify these subtypes so that a treatment can be developed that specifically addresses the unique nature of each type and supports patients with acute leukemia.

11.1.8. Subtypes of Acute Myeloid Leukemia

The AML subtypes encompass a diverse range of hematological malignancies characterized by unique morphological, phenotypic, and genetic features. A challenging subset is acute leukemias that are minimally differentiated and tend to cross over the distinction between AML and ALL, which pose diagnostic challenges because of overlapping features with immature T-cell leukemias such as early T-cell precursor ALL. These leukemias fall into a gray area, where they exhibit overlapping genomic changes, which complicates their classification and treatment (Genescà et al., 2022). With advances in genetic typing, it is now easier for doctors to treat these subtypes more effectively and utilize targeted therapy to improve patient outcomes. Additionally, identifying novel agents and approaches, including immunotherapies and targeted therapies, can significantly aid in shifting the way we manage high-risk AML and address its challenges (Figure 11.5).

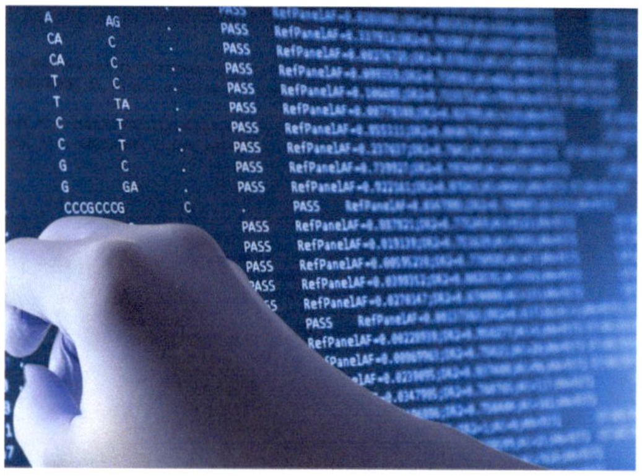

Figure 11.5. Advancements in genetic profiling provide a promising avenue for better management of these subtypes, facilitating more personalized therapeutic approaches and improving patient outcomes.

Source: https://cdn.prod.website-files.com/65b10cf2a9c7f9d23b4bb47d/65b10cf2a9c7f9d23b4bb4dc_comprehensive-guide-to-cancer-types-analyzed-by-ngs-testing.jpg.

11.1.9. Emerging classifications in Acute Leukemias

The landscape of acute leukemias is rapidly evolving, with the emergence of new classifications that enable us to define these complex diseases with greater precision. New developments in genomic profiling and machine learning methodologies have, in turn, improved diagnostic precision, especially in ALL, where evidence indicates that novel models can forecast cancer cell growth in children based on clinical information obtained from Next Generation Sequencing (NGS) (Vasyl et al., 2024). In addition, new classification systems for myelodysplastic syndromes/neoplasms (MDS) were provided in 2022, specifically the International Consensus Classification (ICC) and the 2022 World Health Organization (WHO-2022) classification system, which offer frameworks that are inclusive of genetic mutations and the percentage of blasts in predicting survival outcomes (Lee et al., 2024). This combined focus on genomic and clinical parameters not only enhances the consistency of classification but also leads to personalized therapeutic strategies, ultimately improving prognosis and patient management in acute leukemias.

11.2. Symptoms and Diagnosis

The symptoms and diagnosis of acute leukemias present a complex interplay of clinical manifestations and diagnostic challenges. Patients commonly exhibit generalized fatigue, fever, and frequent infections, which stem from hematological abnormalities such as leukocytosis or leukopenia. Physical examinations may reveal splenomegaly, hepatomegaly, and lymphadenopathy, indicating systemic involvement. Early and accurate diagnosis is critical, as it can significantly affect treatment outcomes. Diagnostic methods, such as bone marrow biopsies and whole blood counts, are often performed to distinguish between various leukemic phenotypes. Notably, new in vivo models of leukemia have provided insightful findings, demonstrating that it is possible to examine a number of populations of leukemic initiating cells (LIC) in cases of childhood ALL, thereby raising our knowledge of the disease's pathophysiology (Blair et al., 2013). Additionally, the identification of suitable animal models remains central to the development of therapeutic management, particularly given the multifactorial nature of leukemic emergence (Davoren et al., 2014).

11.2.1. Common Symptoms of Acute Leukemias

Usual signs of acute leukemia can have a dramatic impact on a patient's life and result in rapid diagnosis. Because the bone marrow is less capable of producing blood cells, patients often become tired, develop a fever, and frequently experience infections. Sometimes, unexpected bruising or bleeding might occur due to the low platelet count associated with these malignancies. Other signs that can be mistaken for something else are losing weight, having night sweats, and feeling pain in the bones or joints. As scientists learn more about acute leukemias, it is evident that noticing these symptoms early is very important for successful treatment. Clinical studies underscore this need, demonstrating that awareness and appropriate management can mitigate adverse outcomes associated with delayed treatment initiation (Matar et al., 2025; Han et al., 2024) (Figure 11.6).

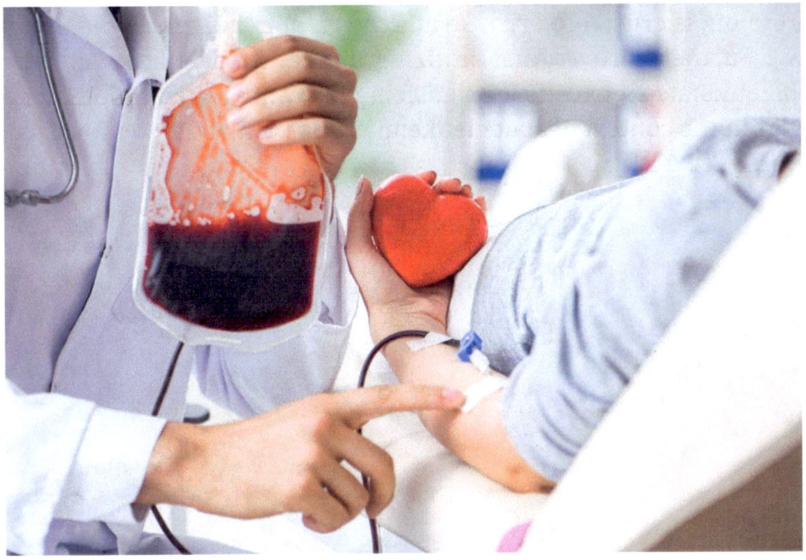

Figure 11.6. Patients may experience fatigue, fever, and recurrent infections due to the compromised bone marrow function that hampers blood cell production.

Source: https://www.homage.com.my/wp-content/uploads/sites/2/2021/07/Article-Images-21-scaled.jpg.

11.2.2. Diagnostic Tests Used for Identification

The identification and classification of acute leukemias hinge significantly on the application of various diagnostic tests, which help delineate the specific subtype and inform treatment strategies. Cytogenetic analyses, such as fluorescence in situ hybridization (FISH), are crucial for detecting chromosomal abnormalities like the t(7;12; q36;p13) translocation, commonly associated with poor outcomes in infant AML cases (Naiel et al., 2013). Additionally, the Philadelphia chromosome, which identifies a specific subtype of ALL, is evaluated through genetic analysis that reveals rearrangements, determining therapeutic responses. For instance, overexpression of cytokine receptor-like factor 2 (CRLF2) has been identified as responsible for cases of Ph-like ALL, indicating the necessity of tailored treatment due to glucocorticoid resistance, which contributes to further poor prognoses in these patients (Delgado-Martin et al., 2019). This means that these advanced diagnostic techniques become crucial for introducing appropriate treatment strategies among the patients admitted with acute leukemias.

11.2.3. Role of Blood Tests in Diagnosis

Blood tests play a crucial role in determining whether someone has acute leukemia, as they reveal the characteristic blood changes associated with these cancers. Initially, a complete blood count (CBC) can reveal essential variations, including increased white blood cell (WBC) counts, reduced RBCs, and abnormal platelets, indicating hematological disturbance. Additionally, certain biomarkers identified through advanced blood tests enable doctors to distinguish between the different types of acute leukemia, which is crucial for selecting the most effective treatment. For instance, the identification of the Philadelphia chromosome or genetically distinct markers, such as CRLF2 overexpression, is crucial for risk stratification and treatment planning in ALL (Delgado-Martin et al., 2019). Furthermore, studies utilizing animal models have shown the efficacy of in vivo assessments of leukemic stem cells, emphasizing how integrated blood test results can inform therapeutic strategies in the context of acute leukemias and contribute to improved clinical outcomes (Blair et al., 2013) (Figure 11.7).

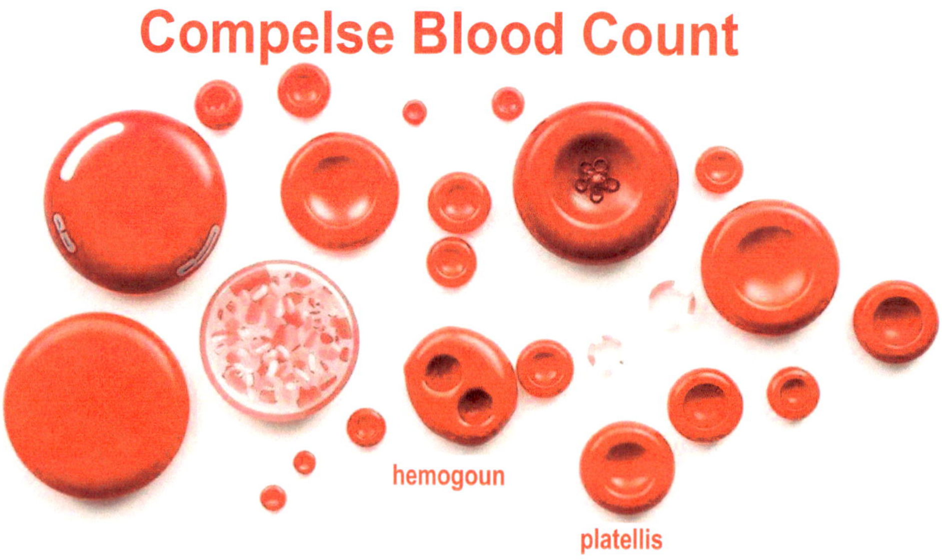

Figure 11.7. Initially, a complete blood count (CBC) can reveal essential variations, including increased white blood cell counts, reduced red blood cells, and abnormal platelets, indicating hematological disturbance.

Source: https://referrallabs.in/wp-content/uploads/2024/12/image-1-1024x585.jpeg.

11.2.4. Bone Marrow Biopsy Procedures

Bone marrow biopsy tests are a critical component of the diagnostic evaluation of acute leukemias, providing important information about cellular constituency and bone marrow architecture. Bone marrow aspiration (BMA) and bone marrow trephine biopsy (BMB) are typically performed in conjunction with each other. The BMA insight is in its cytological features and cell counts. At the same time, BMB is a treasure trove of spatial cell relationships and the general structure of bone marrow, which proves to be particularly significant in leukemic states (Mishra et al., 2024). The combination of these testing methods significantly enhances the assessment of measurable residual disease (MRD), a valuable factor to consider when analyzing treatment response and the risk of relapse in AML patients (John et al., 2025). Together, the utilization of BMA and BMB enhances not just diagnostic accuracy, but also therapeutic decision-making in treating acute leukemias appropriately..

11.2.5. Imaging Studies and Their Significance

The inclusion of imaging in the management of acute leukemias facilitates early detection and aids in evaluating disease progression, thereby greatly favoring the patient. Techniques like magnetic resonance imaging and computed tomographic scans provide critical information regarding the central nervous system, where CNSL complications tend to occur. Studies show that flow cytometry (FCM) offers higher sensitivity in detecting CNSL compared to conventional cytomorphology (CM), highlighting the need for advanced imaging for accurate diagnosis and strategic treatment planning (Tang et al., 2024). Furthermore, detailed imaging investigations assist physicians in monitoring how the patient responds to therapy, evaluating how effective the therapies are, and modifying the treatment plan as needed. As the landscape in leukemia management evolves, so will the need for advanced imaging modalities, not only in making the diagnosis but also in individualizing patient-specific care strategies for optimal survival benefits and improvement in quality of life (Fernández Alfonso et al., 2024) (Figure 11.8).

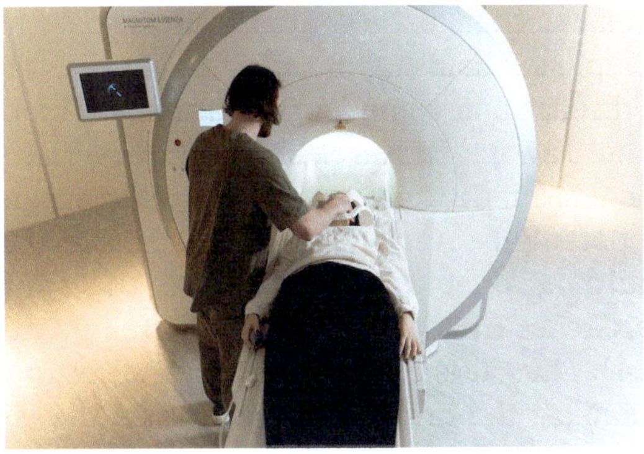

Figure 11.8. Techniques such as magnetic resonance imaging (MRI) and computed tomography (CT) scans provide critical insights into the central nervous system.

Source: https://cdn.flabs.in/webassets/51df92626a2314268279.jpg.

11.2.6. Differential Diagnosis Considerations

The differential diagnosis of acute leukemias necessitates a comprehensive understanding of various hematological disorders that may present with similar clinical features. Conditions such as hypereosinophilic syndrome (HES) can complicate the diagnostic process, as HES encompasses a range of disorders characterized by elevated eosinophil levels without a clear underlying cause, potentially mimicking leukemia symptoms. A thorough examination of peripheral blood smears and bone marrow aspiration is crucial in distinguishing acute leukemia from other conditions, as both may present with abnormal cell proliferation. Furthermore, the cancer stem cell hypothesis highlights the need to examine self-renewal characteristics of these cells, especially in acute leukemias, since this can have implications on treatment outcomes and disease evolution. Hence, differential diagnosis requires an appropriate clinical assessment, in addition to understanding the intricate biological mechanisms underlying leukemogenesis and related syndromes, such as HES, which poses a significant challenge to clinicians (Brys et al., 2015; Busse et al., 2016).

11.2.7. Importance of Early Symptom Recognition

Noticing the first symptoms in acute leukemias as soon as possible is very important, since quick action can change the course of the disease for the better. Typically, people first notice fatigue, fever, and unusual bruising, which may indicate that something is amiss. A late diagnosis can exacerbate the disease and complicate treatment, which is why both healthcare providers and patients should be more aware. Research shows that barriers to symptom recognition can impede timely responses, which may ultimately result in a poorer prognosis (Oppong et al., 2024). Furthermore, understanding the potential severity of symptoms associated with acute leukemias, as well as other concurrent conditions, enables quick referrals and appropriate management strategies, similar to the urgent approaches in acute cholecystitis treatment, which prioritize early intervention (Mencarini et al., 2024). Thus, it is essential to create a setting where early recognition of symptoms is given priority to manage the disease well and raise the chance of survival (Figure 11.9).

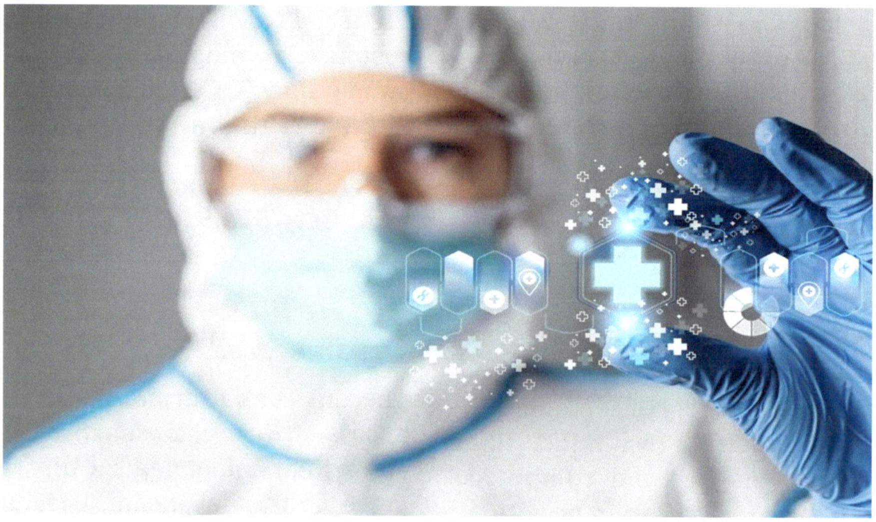

Figure 11.9. Delayed diagnosis can lead to disease progression and exacerbate treatment challenges, emphasizing the crucial role of heightened awareness among both healthcare providers and patients.

Source: https://www.financialexpress.com/wp-content/uploads/2024/02/medical-banner-with-doctor-wearing-equipment.jpg.

11.2.8. Challenges in Diagnosing Acute Leukemias

It is quite to identify acute leukemias because of several issues that hinder the process. The most significant among them is the reliance on traditional diagnostic techniques, such as immunophenotyping by multiparameter flow cytometry (FCM), which, although successful, is typically time-consuming and, to some degree, subjective, thereby increasing the likelihood of misdiagnosis or treatment delay (Dworzak et al., 2024). Also, since acute leukemia patients have weak immune systems, they are more likely to get infections, so it is necessary to watch for complications during diagnosis. As reported, bloodstream infections can adversely affect patient outcomes and delay necessary intervention (Kjellander et al., 2016). Even though automated FCM diagnostics can help address these problems, widespread adoption requires creating standard guidelines and training more personnel. All in all, these points demonstrate the necessity of updating diagnostic methods for patients with acute leukemia.

11.3. Treatment Options

The treatment landscape for acute leukemias is constantly changing, especially with the integration of targeted therapies that improve patient outcomes and overcome challenges developed by traditional regimens. For adults with ALL, innovative strategies have significantly improved survival rates. For example, modern pediatric-type regimens achieve roughly a 60% survival rate in young adults, far exceeding the previous standard (Bassan et al.). Despite this, approximately 60% of adult patients remain at a dismal prognosis, highlighting the necessity for personalized treatment regimens taking into account unique disease parameters (Capitani et al., 2018). The investigation of new drugs, such as monoclonal antibodies and immunomodulators, and the judicious application of tyrosine kinase inhibitors (TKI) for Philadelphia chromosome-positive individuals is a promising area to explore. These developments aim to improve the efficacy of treatments but also try to reduce long-term side effects, which will offer a more patient-friendly approach in the treatment of acute leukemias.

11.3.1. Overview of Treatment Modalities

Treating acute leukemia calls for a variety of approaches, usually using chemotherapy, targeted drugs, and supportive care that are chosen based on the patient's type and genetic makeup of the leukemia. Traditional chemotherapy is still the primary treatment, using chemicals to help patients go into remission; yet, targeted therapies have significantly improved results for some subtypes, mainly those with unique genetic changes. Notably, patients with therapy-related myeloid neoplasms (t-MN), which can arise from previous treatments, face additional challenges due to their complex genetic abnormalities and resistance to standard therapies, resulting in poorer prognoses compared to de novo cases of AML (Larson et al., 2011). Furthermore, immunophenotyping plays a pivotal role in diagnosing and stratifying acute leukemias, enabling clinicians to classify patients accurately and determine the most effective treatment regimen (Kabera et al., 2014). All in all, being well-informed about treatment options is important for better results in patients with acute leukemias (Figure 11.10).

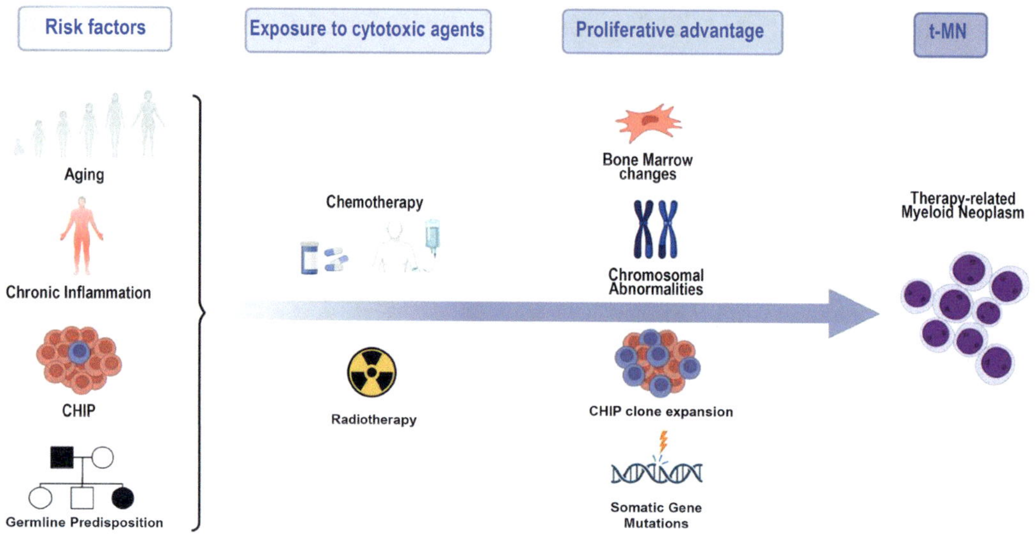

Figure 11.10. Therapy-related myeloid neoplasms (t-MN).

Source: https://www.mdpi.com/biomedicines/biomedicines-12-01054/article_deploy/html/images/biomedicines-12-01054-g001.png.

11.3.2. Chemotherapy Regimens for Acute Leukemias

The efficacy of chemotherapy regimens for acute leukemias, particularly AML and ALL, is a critical area of ongoing research and clinical innovation. Usually, the standard approach includes strong chemotherapy that works to clear the cancer while limiting side effects to help people enjoy a better life. Recent studies emphasize the necessity for personalized approaches, tailoring chemotherapy based on individual genetic profiles and disease characteristics to achieve optimal outcomes (Czajka et al., 2024). Furthermore, special considerations arise in unique patient populations, such as pregnant women, where the administration of cytotoxic agents during different trimesters can lead to varying risks of teratogenicity and maternal complications (Al-Anazi et al., 2015). As researchers discover more about leukemia's biology, using personalized medicine in chemotherapy becomes more important, which leads to better and safer ways to treat acute leukemia.

11.3.3. Role of Targeted Therapy

Targeted therapy has dramatically improved the way acute leukemias are treated, mainly through precision medicine. Targeted therapies are designed to stop the growth of cancer cells by targeting specific changes in their molecules, while sparing healthy tissues. For example, the BCR-ABL fusion protein observed in Chronic Myeloid Leukemia (CML) has now become a target of choice for therapies like imatinib, which acts by binding to the protein's tyrosine kinase domain, thereby inhibiting its function and resulting in better patient outcomes (Aljabali et al., 2024). Furthermore, individualized chemotherapy regimens tailored to a person's genetic profile optimize efficacy while reducing toxicity, thereby enhancing compliance and quality of life (Czajka et al., 2024). The trend in personalized therapy for leukemia suggests that targeted therapies are indeed working miracles, and that there is still room for improvement in cancer treatment (Figure 11.11).

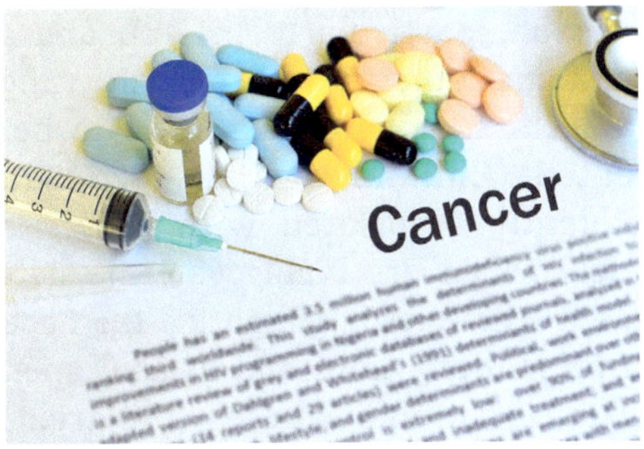

Figure 11.11. By focusing on specific molecular abnormalities within cancer cells, targeted therapies aim to inhibit the growth of malignant cells more effectively while sparing healthy tissues.

Source: https://www.regionalcancercare.org/wp-content/uploads/2021/08/rcca-targeted-therapy.jpg.

11.3.4. Stem Cell Transplantation Procedures

The methods of stem cell transplantation (HSCT) form the cornerstone of the treatment of acute leukemias, offering potential curative strategies for patients with these acute hematological malignancies. HSCT can be performed using stem cells derived from three primary sources: bone marrow, peripheral blood, and umbilical cord blood, each with unique advantages and limitations. Evidence suggests that although peripheral blood stem cell transplants may result in better disease-free survival and reduced relapse risk, they also present a higher rate of severe graft-versus-host disease (GVHD) compared to bone marrow transplants (Cheuk et al., 2013). Additionally, psychological effects on patients receiving HSCT are considerable; survivors frequently report poorer quality of life and different levels of distress many years following their treatment (Basso et al., 2017). Thus, successful patient counseling regarding the choice of stem cell sources and management of potential complications is crucial in the multidisciplinary management of acute leukemias.

11.3.5. Radiation Therapy Applications

The use of radiation therapy in the treatment of acute leukemias is both a chance and a challenge in the medical management of these complex conditions. Radiation is mainly used as part of the preparative regimen for HSCT, efficiently destroying malignant cells and allowing for engraftment of healthy HSCs.

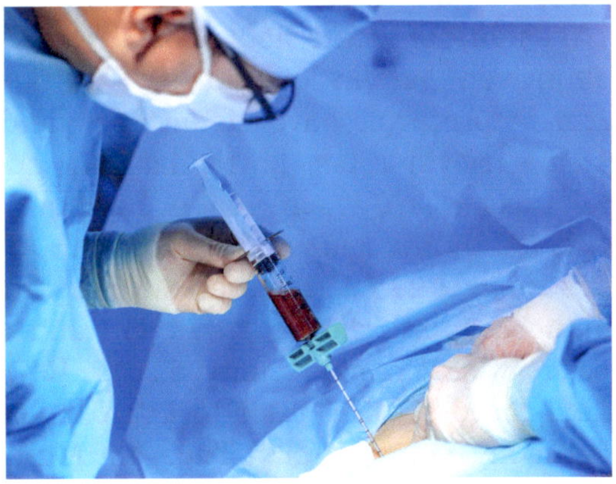

Figure 11.12. Radiation is primarily utilized as a part of the preparative regimen for hematopoietic stem cell transplantation, effectively eradicating malignant cells and enabling the engraftment of healthy hematopoietic stem cells.

Source: https://news.cancerconnect.com/.image/ar_4:3%2Cc_fill%2Ccs_srgb%2Cfl_progressive%2Cq_auto:good%2Cw_1200/MTk3NDI3OTExMTM1ODY0NzMx/sct.jpg.

This is especially vital in high-risk scenarios where systemic therapies will likely be inadequate. Advances in the radiation techniques have also come with sharp precision in targeting cancerous tissues with less damage to the healthy organs that may complicate the treatment. Apart from such trends, others suggest that integrating radiation therapy with advancements in cytogenetics will be necessary, underlining the need for modern methodologies to improve both the accuracy of diagnostics and the efficacy of treatment for acute leukemias. As a consequence, ongoing research into optimizing radiation treatment regimens is vital to improving survival outcomes and minimizing toxicity in this vulnerable patient population (Askin et al., 2017) (Figure 11.12).

11.3.6. Clinical Trials and Experimental Treatments

Innovations in clinical trials and experimental treatments are crucial for advancing the management of acute leukemias, resulting in improved patient outcomes. Traditional treatment protocols have historically yielded limited survival rates, particularly in adult populations, where a mere 40% overall survival is observed for ALL compared to the 80-90% cure rates seen in children. However, the integration of modern approaches, such as TKI and the assessment of minimal residual disease (MRD), has enhanced survival rates to approximately 60% among young adults. Thus, in addition to the above, the development of targeted therapies focused on the phosphatidylinositol 3-phosphate kinase (PI3K)/Akt/mTOR signaling pathway shows promising preclinical efficacy and is currently undergoing rigorous evaluation in clinical trials aimed at reducing treatment-related toxicities and optimizing event-free survival (Capitani et al., 2018). With continued research and the advent of new agents, such as monoclonal antibodies and chimeric antigen receptor T cells, a revolutionary period in precision medicine for acute leukemias is underway (Bassan et al.).

11.3.7. Supportive Care and Symptom Management

Symptom management and supportive care are at the forefront of acute leukemias treated by care teams to enhance the patient's quality of life and outcomes. The new agents on the horizon, particularly in ALL and AML, herald a monumental rise in the range of toxic effects, a significant burden to be well delineated. Childhood ALL, for example, is frequently associated with severe acute toxicities, which are highly variable between treatment strategies, highlighting the necessity for universal definitions and measurements to enable international studies and treatment modifications (Attarbaschi et al., 2016). Moreover, the integration of early palliative care (EPC) has shown promise in alleviating the physical and psychological burdens faced by AML patients, improving quality of life while promoting adaptive coping strategies (Bandieri et al., 2022). Consequently, prioritizing supportive care not only addresses immediate symptoms but also fosters a holistic approach to leukemia treatment, ultimately improving patient experiences throughout their journey (Figure 11.13).

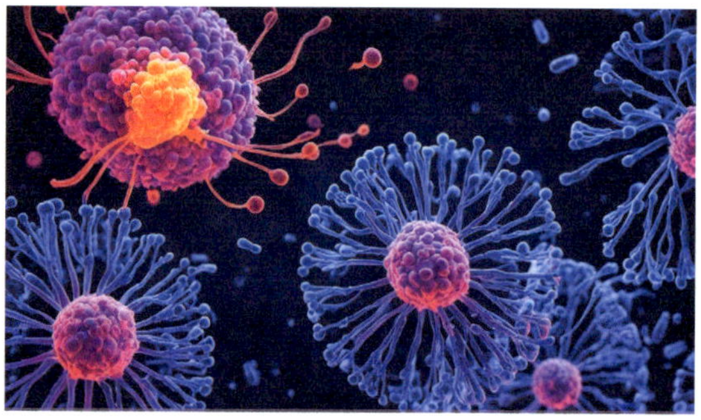

Figure 11.13. As new therapies emerge, particularly in acute lymphoblastic leukemia (ALL) and acute myeloid leukemia (AML), the spectrum of toxic effects becomes increasingly complex, necessitating a robust framework for addressing these challenges.

Source: https://oasismedicalinstitute.com/wp-content/uploads/Ozone-Treatment-Leukemia.jpg.

11.3.8. Long-Term Management Strategies

Management strategies in the long term for acute leukemias are best addressed by an interdisciplinary team, considering both the biology of the disease and the individual patient's needs. An enhanced understanding of the molecular pathways that underlie diseases, particularly in Philadelphia chromosome-positive disease, emphasizes the possibility of targeted therapy, such as TKIs, with consequent noteworthy improvements in patient outcomes. The use of dual PI3K/mTOR inhibitors has emerged as a promising new therapeutic direction, exhibiting marked antileukemic effects across all genetic subtypes, thereby establishing the need for tailoring treatment regimens (Badura et al., 2013). In addition, conventional management regimens have shown a mean survival rate of approximately 40% in the adult form of ALL; however, updated versions of pediatric regimens have increased this rate to around 60% in young adults (Bassan et al.). These approaches reflect a growing tendency towards precision medicine, prompting tailor-made interventions according to individuals' genetic makeup, thereby enhancing efficacy in long-term treatment of acute leukemias.

11.3.9. Challenges in Treatment Adherence

Treatment of acute leukemias is not without problems, particularly with regard to patient compliance. It is difficult for patients to adhere to the planned regimen due to the severity of side effects, psychological issues such as depression and anxiety, and a general lack of knowledge regarding their value in treatment regimens. The review suggests that customized chemotherapy regimens incorporating the individual's genotypic features are essential for reducing these burdens, thereby enhancing treatment effectiveness and minimizing toxicities (Czajka et al., 2024). More importantly, there is a need for multi-level support interventions, comprising education, symptom management, and the removal of barriers to care, to encourage adherence (Czajka et al., 2024). Furthermore, experiences from multinational studies indicate that understanding local contexts and patient perspectives can significantly inform adherence strategies, providing insights that might also aid other research efforts in similar fields. Addressing these adherence challenges is crucial for enhancing treatment outcomes in patients with acute leukemia (Figure 11.14).

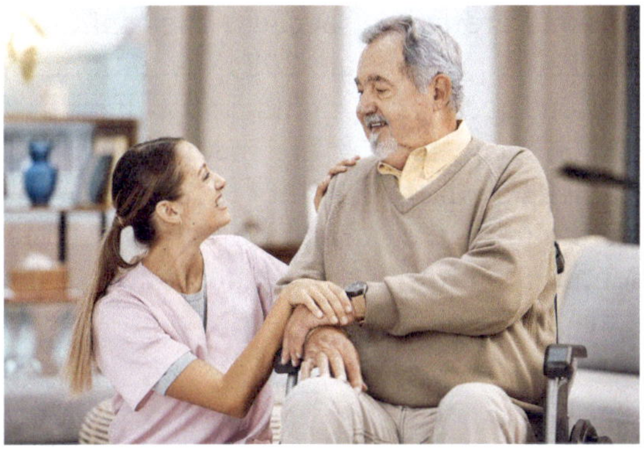

Figure 11.14. The necessity for multifaceted support strategies—encompassing education, symptom management, and addressing barriers to care—is crucial for fostering adherence

Source: https://www.amba.co/wp-content/uploads/2024/03/meds.jpg.

11.4. Prognosis and Outcomes

The prognosis and outcomes for patients diagnosed with acute leukemias, particularly ALL and AML, significantly hinge upon genetic and molecular characteristics identified at diagnosis. In ALL, the presence of the Philadelphia chromosome-like subtype underscores a troubling prognosis, with research indicating that the overexpression of cytokine receptor-like factor 2 (CRLF2) is correlated with inferior clinical outcomes and glucocorticoid resistance, thereby complicating treatment strategies (Delgado-Martin et al., 2019). As in AML, particular clonal gene rearrangements identified at presentation are significant prognosticators; for example, improved survival is often seen in those patients with rearrangements in the T cell receptor (TcR)-beta gene, and generally more severe are those cases which do involve rearrangement of IL-3 or GM-CSF, as noted by Braun et al. (2000). Collectively, these point towards the necessity of intensive genetic evaluation to allow proper therapeutic options and thus improved patient outcomes in acute leukemias.

11.4.1. Factors Influencing Prognosis

The prognosis for acute leukemias is multifactorial, involving both genetic, molecular, and environmental factors. Certain genetic mutations, such as in AML, are also crucial in influencing the response to the therapy and will be reflected in the final outcomes. For instance, FLT3 and NPM1 mutations are crucial because they influence other kinds of future prognoses and direct therapy measures (Agurto et al., 2024). Additionally, the socioeconomic and healthcare contexts in which treatment occurs can significantly affect decision-making and patient outcomes. A comprehensive analysis suggests that the medical decision-making process regarding innovative treatments is influenced by the availability of resources and the broader healthcare environment (Kenneth). Thus, understanding the intricate interplay between genetic markers and the socioeconomic landscape is essential for improving prognosis and tailoring effective interventions in cases of acute leukemia (Figure 11.15).

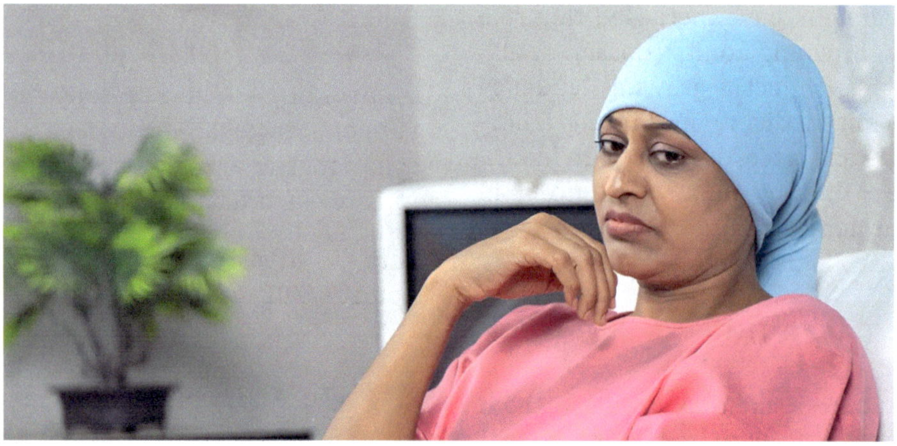

Figure 11.15. Specific genetic mutations, such as those identified in acute myeloid leukemia (AML), play a pivotal role in determining treatment responsiveness and overall outcomes.

Source: https://bmchrc.org/speciality/667e459d5b83bAcute%20Myeloid%20Leukemia%20(AML)%20at%20BMCHRC.webp.

11.4.2. Survival Rates for Different Types

Survival rates for different types of acute leukemias exhibit notable variability, influenced by factors such as genetic predisposition, environmental exposures, and advancements in treatment. ALL, predominantly affecting children, generally boasts a higher survival rate compared to AML, which tends to be more prevalent in adults. Studies have shown that the use of targeted therapies, including mTOR inhibitors, has promise in altering outcomes among patients with leukemia, most notably by modulating key pathways participating in leukemogenesis (Bianchi et al., 2018). Environmental hazards, including exposure to benzene, have also been linked to chromosome aberrations that increase the risk of leukemia, underscoring the importance of understanding these risk factors to enhance survival chances (Smith et al., 1998). Generally, further developments in the understanding of acute leukemias will be essential in helping to improve treatment and, consequently, survival rates among various leukemia types.

11.4.3. Impact of Age on Outcomes

Age has a profound impact on the prognosis of acute leukemias, especially regarding the efficacy of treatment and survival rates. Research has shown that ALL yields higher cure rates among children as opposed to adults. This is partly due to the differences in leukemia molecular subtypes and the age-related response to chemotherapy agents, as evident in findings that show varying sensitivities to drugs between groups (Yoshimura et al., 2024). Moreover, AML is more problematic in the elderly, as the incidence rates are found to increase gradually with age based on the epidemiological data, along with a marginally low survival rate for those over 65 years by Han et al., 2024. This highlights the need for age-specific treatment protocols and further research on the molecular basis of age-related differences in therapeutic responses. Ultimately, it is imperative to understand these subtleties to optimize treatment strategies across age demographics in acute leukemias (Figure 11.16).

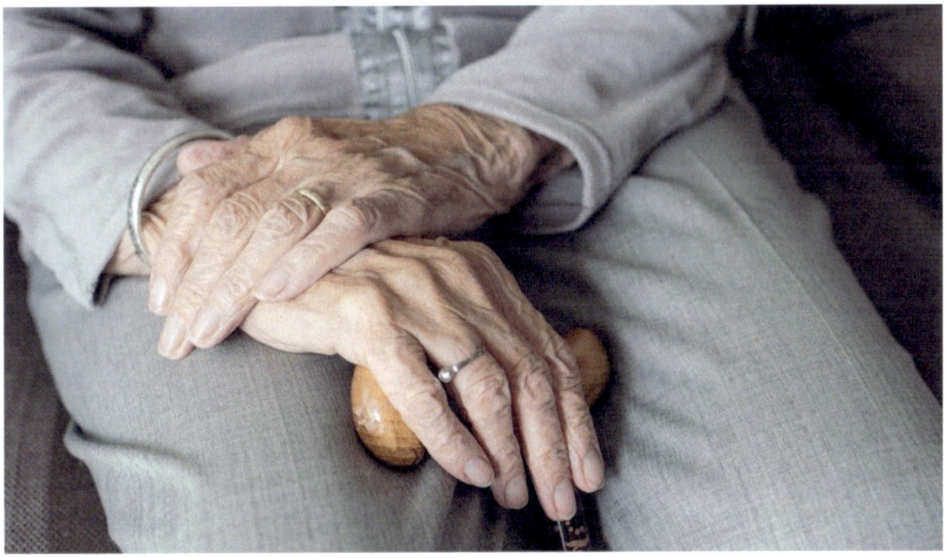

Figure 11.16. Age significantly influences the outcomes of acute leukemias, particularly in the context of treatment effectiveness and overall survival rates.

Source: https://assets.technologynetworks.com/production/dynamic/images/content/386675/older-adults-show-improved-survival-with-standard-treatment-for-aggressive-blood-cancer-386675-960x540.jpg?cb=12815109.

11.4.4. Role of Genetic Factors in Prognosis

The prognosis of acute leukemias, especially AML, is highly dependent on the underlying genetic factors that determine the heterogeneity of the disease and responsiveness to treatment. The research highlights the significance of specific genetic markers, such as the FHL1 gene, which has been shown to be a strong prognostic biomarker. The elevated expression of FHL1 correlates with poor patient outcomes, and enhancing conventional chemotherapeutic drugs, such as cytarabine and daunorubicin, has been identified as a promising target for therapeutic approaches (Luo et al., 2025). Moreover, recent advancements utilizing computational tools like OncoSplice have enabled the identification of molecular subtypes within AML based on splicing profiles, revealing a dominant splicing subtype that predicts adverse prognoses even in the absence of traditional mutations (Venkatasubramanian et al., 2025). Collectively, these genetic insights not only elucidate the complexities of leukemia pathology but also pave the way for targeted interventions that aim to improve patient survival outcomes.

11.4.5. Quality of Life Considerations Post-Treatment

The aftermath of acute leukemia treatment necessitates a comprehensive evaluation of quality of life, particularly as survivors grapple with various physical and psychological challenges. Survivors often contend with long-term side effects, including oral health complications like mucositis, xerostomia, and gingival bleeding, which significantly impact their overall well-being and life satisfaction (Aroso et al., 2017). Additionally, the emergence of therapy-related myeloid neoplasms in patients exposed to cytotoxic therapies underscores the necessity for tailored follow-up care and fitness assessments, taking into account individual patient histories and comorbidities (Buccisano et al., 2023). Such personalized approaches not only optimize treatment outcomes but also enhance the quality of life by addressing the unique needs of survivors. Thus, integrating dental care and psychosocial support in post-treatment plans is essential to improving health-related quality of life in individuals recovering from acute leukemias (Figure 11.17).

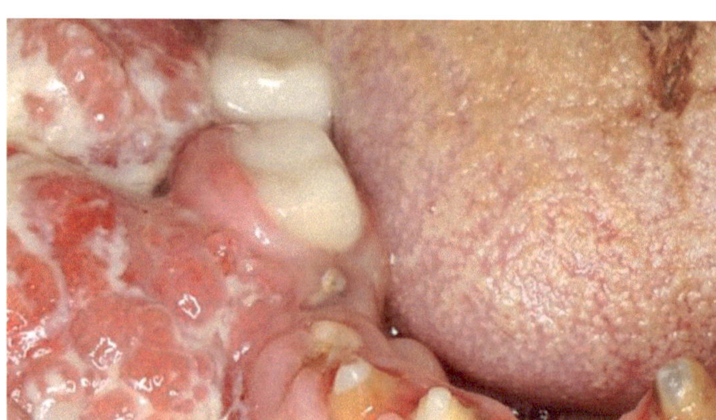

Figure 11.17. Survivors often contend with long-term side effects, including oral health complications like mucositis, xerostomia, and gingival bleeding, which significantly impact their overall well-being and life satisfaction

Source: https://decisionsindentistry.com/wp-content/uploads/2023/11/28-Figure-1-oral-cancer.jpg.

11.4.6. Recurrence Rates and Monitoring

Successful surveillance of relapse rates in acute leukemias is essential to enhance outcomes of patients and direct treatment practices. The availability of MRD quantitation has significantly altered the way clinicians assess relapse risk, particularly after HSCT. By identifying residual leukemic cells, physicians can make informed decisions regarding the necessity and timing of interventions to prevent recurrence, as highlighted by recent reviews of post-transplantation strategies (de Lima et al., 2014). Advancements in therapies, including the development of targeted therapies such as TKIs, have also produced improved survival results through treatment specifically based on risk assessment, which is indeed different between patients, as the case may be, particularly in Philadelphia chromosome-positive ALL (Bassan et al.). Therefore, a robust monitoring framework, leveraging MRD insights, is vital for the successful management of recurrence in acute leukemia patients, ultimately aiming to mitigate relapse and enhance long-term survival.

11.4.7. Psychological Impact on Patients and Families

The psychological impact of acute leukemias on patients and their families can be profound and multifaceted, shaping their daily lives and emotional well-being. Patients often grapple with anxiety, fear of mortality, and uncertainty regarding treatment outcomes, which can severely affect their quality of life. As highlighted in research, family caregivers experience significant psychological distress themselves, often struggling with feelings of helplessness and the burden of caregiving responsibilities. These are emotional challenges, however, which can result in heightened stress and anxiety levels among caregivers, requiring specific support programs tailored to their specific needs and fostering resilience. Open communication with healthcare providers and involvement in support groups have been demonstrated to reduce some of these problems and create a support environment that allows for coping mechanisms. In general, addressing the psychological effects, as studied in IMPACT-AML and other studies, is crucial for enhancing the health and well-being of leukemia patients and caregivers (Maturo et al., 2024; Charalambous et al., 2024) (Figure 11.18).

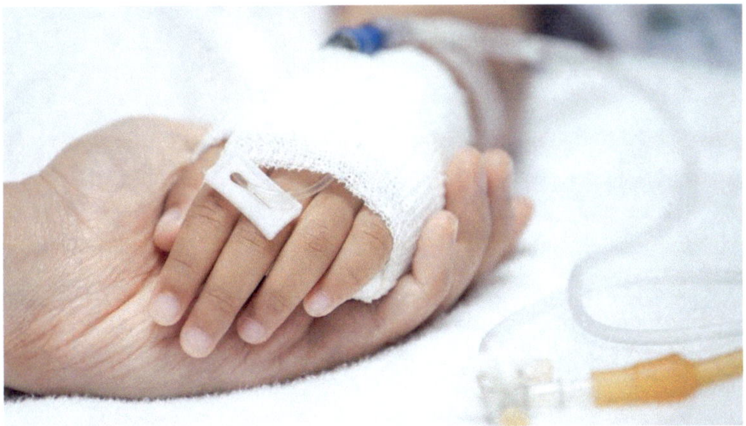

Figure 11.18. The psychological impact of acute leukemias on patients and their families can be profound and multifaceted, shaping their daily lives and emotional well-being.

Source: https://www.britishjournalofnursing.com/media/e5dh3brf/sick_child_1000x667.jpg?width=1002&height=564&v=1d90a21c728aaf0.

11.4.8. Advances in Research Affecting Outcomes

The evolution of classification systems for acute leukemias has been fundamentally shaped by advances in research that significantly impact patient outcomes. The integration of genetic and molecular insights has led to more precise diagnostic criteria, enabling tailored therapeutic approaches that enhance survival rates. As highlighted by Rebecca et al. (2024), improvements in understanding the biological underpinnings of acute leukemias have transformed treatment paradigms, enabling earlier detection and more effective therapies. Furthermore, the WHO's ongoing efforts to unify classification criteria promote international collaboration, as evidenced by initiatives such as the International Consensus Classification (ICC) for hematologic malignancies, which aims to standardize diagnostic practices across global healthcare systems. Not only will such advancements expedite treatment decisions, but they will also address the inequities in access and promote health equity for diverse populations facing acute leukemias (Daniel et al., 2022). The progression of integrating research into clinical practice rewrites a lot of new pages on the management of acute leukemia and into the future.

11.4.9. Future Directions in Improving Prognosis

Advancements in understanding the molecular etiology of acute leukemias are paving the way for targeted therapeutic strategies that aim to improve patient prognosis. The challenge remains in treating relapsed cases, particularly in B-lineage acute lymphoblastic leukemia (B-ALL) and T-cell acute lymphoblastic leukemia (T-ALL), where conventional therapies often fail to eradicate leukemia stem cells (LSCs) responsible for disease persistence and recurrence. Targeted therapies, such as inhibitors of the phosphatidylinositol 3-phosphate kinase (PI3K)/Akt/mTOR pathway, are being investigated for their ability to maximize survival with minimal side effects, as demonstrated in preclinical research on B-ALL (Capitani et al., 2018). In addition, the discovery of distinctive regulatory pathways, such as the function of PRL-3 in LSC self-renewal in T-ALL, provides novel targets for therapy, which necessitates the development of innovative intervention strategies for effectively treating and predicting relapse (Haney et al., 2021).

A CLOSER LOOK

CYTOGENETIC ABNORMALITIES

Cytogenetic aberrations are defined as alterations or modifications of the number or structure of chromosomes in cells. They include deletions, duplications, translocations, inversions, or aneuploidy (gaining or losing entire chromosomes). They are usually a primary factor contributing to the production of many diseases, particularly cancers such as leukemia and lymphoma.

Detecting cytogenetic abnormalities through techniques like karyotyping, fluorescence in situ hybridization (FISH), or chromosomal microarray analysis helps in diagnosing diseases, determining prognosis, and guiding treatment decisions. For example, the Philadelphia chromosome—a translocation between chromosomes 9 and 22—is a well-known cytogenetic abnormality associated with chronic myeloid leukemia (CML).

SUMMARY

Acute leukemias present a complex challenge that necessitates a multifaceted approach to treatment and patient care. The unique social and economic environment surrounding medical care plays a crucial role in decision-making processes, particularly when innovative therapies emerge to combat these life-threatening conditions (Kenneth). As advancements in treatment options, including inhibitors targeting the mammalian target of rapamycin (mTOR), appear, understanding their implications is vital for enhancing clinical outcomes (Bianchi et al., 2018). Furthermore, ongoing research into the molecular mechanisms underlying leukemogenesis is imperative, as it lays the groundwork for developing targeted therapies and improving patient quality of life. In general, the treatment of acute leukemias requires a strong partnership among medical experts, scientists, and policymakers to ensure that therapeutic advancements not only yield economic benefits but also support the dignity and well-being of individuals suffering from the disease.

The intricacies of acute leukemias revolve around the underlying properties of HSCs, specifically their self-renewal properties. The self-renewal is highly regulated by multiple signaling pathways that regulate the HSC self-renewal vs. differentiation balance within the bone marrow niche (Copland et al., 2013). As research continues to unravel, understanding these processes illuminates potential therapeutic methods that may inhibit leukemic stem cell proliferation and, hence, cure myeloid malignancies more effectively. Secondly, the cancer stem cell hypothesis has been studied to understand how self-renewal affects cancer development, to the extent of developing mathematical models that investigate interactions between cancer and normal cells (Busse et al., 2016). These models, which incorporate cell dynamics feedback loops, offer a platform for understanding leukemic cell proliferation and imply that regulatory processes will ultimately direct therapeutic strategies in the future. The integration of these findings highlights the pivotal convergence of stem cell biology and the therapy of leukemia.

REFERENCES

1. Khawaja, M. R., Allana, S. S., Akbaral, N. N., Adil, S. N., Khurshid, M., & Pervez, S. (2006). Flow cytometric and demographic analysis of t cell acute lymphoblastic leukemia in Pakistani population. *PubMed, 17*(4), 3–8. https://pubmed.ncbi.nlm.nih.gov/16599024Agurto, A., Amigo, R., Andreu-Heredia, A., Caprile, L., et al. (2024). The role of epithelial-to-mesenchymal transition transcription factors (EMT-TFs) in acute myeloid leukemia progression. https://core.ac.uk/download/630472596.pdf (accessed on 12th June 2025).

2. Al-Anazi, K. A. (2015). Update on leukemia in pregnancy. https://core.ac.uk/download/322425344.pdf (accessed on 12th June 2025).

3. Aljabali, A. A., El-Tanani, M., Hromić-Jahjefendić, A., Lee, C., et al. (2024). The impact of the BCR-ABL oncogene in the pathology and treatment of chronic myeloid leukemia. https://core.ac.uk/download/638996109.pdf (accessed on 12th June 2025).

4. Anderson, G., Bell, M., Borland, G., Cameron, E., et al. (2018). RUNX-mediated growth arrest and senescence are attenuated by diverse mechanisms in cells expressing RUNX1 fusion oncoproteins. https://core.ac.uk/download/132211224.pdf (accessed on 12th June 2025).

5. Arber, D. A., Hasserjian, R. P., Orazi, A., Mathews, V., Roberts, A. W., Schiffer, C. A., Roug, A. S., et al. (2022). Classification of myeloid neoplasms/acute leukemia: Global perspectives and the international consensus classification approach. *American Journal of Hematology, 97*, 514–518. https://doi.org/10.1002/ajh.26503 (accessed on 12th June 2025).

6. Aroso, R. (2017). Oral considerations in pediatric patients with acute lymphoblastic leukemia. https://core.ac.uk/download/154025937.pdf (accessed on 12th June 2025).

7. Askin, R., Bresters, D., Buck, S., Drazen, J., Ferrari, A., Gigliotti, M., Isaacs, H., et al. (2017). Neonates with cancer and causes of death; lessons from 615 cases in the SEER databases. https://core.ac.uk/download/199426024.pdf (accessed on 12th June 2025).

8. Attarbaschi, A., Barzilai, S., Escherich, G., Frandsen, T., et al. (2016). Consensus definitions of 14 severe acute toxic effects for childhood lymphoblastic leukemia treatment: A Delphi consensus. https://core.ac.uk/download/42370388.pdf (accessed on 12th June 2025).

9. Badura, S., Falkenburg, J. H. F., Liebermann, M., Nijmeijer, R., et al. (2013). Differential effects of selective inhibitors targeting the PI3K/AKT/mTOR pathway in acute lymphoblastic leukemia. https://core.ac.uk/download/18326051.pdf (accessed on 12th June 2025).

10. Bandieri, E., Bigi, S., Borelli, E., Bruera, E., et al. (2022). Early palliative care in acute myeloid leukemia. https://core.ac.uk/download/512041204.pdf (accessed on 12th June 2025).

11. Bassan, R., Bourquin, J. P., Chiaretti, S., DeAngelo, D. J., et al. (2025). New approaches to the management of adult acute lymphoblastic leukemia. https://core.ac.uk/download/159268742.pdf (accessed on 12th June 2025).

12. Basso, G., Bicciato, S., & te Kronnie, G. (2004). Acute leukemia subclassification: A marker protein expression perspective. https://core.ac.uk/download/53964878.pdf (accessed on 12th June 2025).

13. Basso, G., Boscolo, V., Calore, E., Cattelan, M., et al. (2017). Quality of life and psychopathology in adults who underwent hematopoietic stem cell transplantation (HSCT) in childhood: A qualitative and quantitative analysis. https://core.ac.uk/download/154330751.pdf (accessed on 12th June 2025).

14. Bianchi, M. P., Gianfelici, V., Mirabilii, S., Piedimonte, M., et al. (2018). Biological aspects of mTOR in leukemia. https://core.ac.uk/download/188824881.pdf (accessed on 12th June 2025).

15. Blair, A., Cox, C. V., Diamanti, P., Moppett, J., et al. (2013). Parthenopid eliminates leukemia-initiating cell populations and improves survival in xenografts of childhood acute lymphoblastic leukemia. https://core.ac.uk/download/29026690.pdf (accessed on 12th June 2025).

16. Borate, U., Welkie, R., Huang, Y., Swords, R., Traer, E., Stein, E., Lin, T. L., et al. (2024). Demographics, characteristics, survival and outcomes in older, untreated, acute myeloid leukemia patients with NPM1 mutations or KMT2A rearrangements from the Beat AML Master Clinical Trial. *Blood*. https://www.semanticscholar.org/paper/b34460f668e0ea0df7b1442e5435ed6814dbbd20 (accessed on 12th June 2025).

17. Braun, S., Duell, T., Gerhartz, H. H., Mittermueller, J., et al. (2000). Gene rearrangements in bone marrow cells of patients with acute myelogenous leukemia. https://core.ac.uk/download/16432953.pdf (accessed on 12th June 2025).

18. Brys, A. K., Sheth, M. R., Sohn, D. D., Sweidan, R., et al. (2015). Diagnostic and therapeutic considerations in idiopathic hyper eosinophilia with warm autoimmune hemolytic anemia. https://core.ac.uk/download/323075654.pdf (accessed on 12th June 2025).

19. Buccisano, F., Del Principe, I., Maurillo, L., Palmieri, R., et al. (2023). Therapy-related myeloid neoplasms: Considerations for patients' clinical evaluation. https://core.ac.uk/download/587465726.pdf (accessed on 12th June 2025).

20. Busse, J. E., Gwiazda, P., & Marciniak-Czochra, A. (2016). Mass concentration in a nonlocal model of clonal selection. http://arxiv.org/abs/1401.6043 (accessed on 12th June 2025).

21. Butler, J. T., Yashar, W. M., & Swords, R. (2025). Breaking the bone marrow barrier: Peripheral blood as a gateway to measurable residual disease detection in acute myelogenous leukemia. *American Journal of Hematology, 100*, 638–651. https://www.semanticscholar.org/paper/784b2ee291d991beb09c29678c930bcfea440c26 (accessed on 12th June 2025).

22. Capitani, S., Martelli, A. M., McCubrey, J. A., Neri, L., et al. (2018). Targeting the phosphatidylinositol 3-kinase/Akt/mechanistic target of rapamycin signaling pathway in B-lineage acute lymphoblastic leukemia: An update. https://core.ac.uk/download/155242119.pdf (accessed on 12th June 2025).

23. Chan, T. S., Hwang, Y., & Tse, E. (2020). Risk assessment of venous thromboembolism in hematological cancer patients: A review. *Expert Review of Hematology, 13*, 471–480. https://www.semanticscholar.org/paper/59f447d8fa5006878b31ed3ab5bdaa1dabd0fb98 (accessed on 12th June 2025).

24. Charalambous, G., Argyriadi, A., Patelarou, A., Paoullis, P., Laliotis, A., Patelarou, E., Katsarou, D., et al. (2024). The impact of leukemia on quality of life and mental health: Insights from a case study examining physical, social, and cultural implications. *International Journal of Science and Research Archive*. https://www.semanticscholar.org/paper/1853eed7735abcde3a672ae30e92b98277f605ae (accessed on 12th June 2025).

25. Chen, R., Cheng, T., Xie, S., Sun, X., Chen, M., Zhao, S., Ruan, Q., et al. (2024). Effective prevention and treatment of acute leukemias in mice by activation of thermogenic adipose tissues. *Advanced Science, 11*. https://www.semanticscholar.org/paper/dca8479a9d76cdab54c0750926ca7f0bad74273a (accessed on 12th June 2025).

26. Cheuk, D. K. L. (2013). Optimal stem cell source for allogeneic stem cell transplantation for hematological malignancies. https://core.ac.uk/download/38046057.pdf (accessed on 12th June 2025).

27. Copland, M., Sands, W. A., & Wheadon, H. (2013). Targeting self-renewal pathways in myeloid malignancies. https://core.ac.uk/download/16460116.pdf (accessed on 12th June 2025).

28. Couturier, R., Vasseur, L., Boissel, N., Dombret, H., Chevret, S., & Lambert, J. (2024). Handling of allograft as an intercurrent event in randomized controlled trials in acute leukemias: A systematic review. *Blood*. https://www.semanticscholar.org/paper/108a17c01ed28c76112ee91c73bc82cfbbffaccf (accessed on 12th June 2025).

29. Czajka, A., Piaszczyński, S., Płeska, K., Reguła, J., et al. (2024). The impact of chemotherapy dose adjustment and delay in patients with leukemias and lymphomas who exercise. https://core.ac.uk/download/613192446.pdf (accessed on 12th June 2025).

30. Davoren, M., Rivina, L., & Schiestl, R. H. (2014). Radiation-induced myeloid leukemia in murine models. https://core.ac.uk/download/323078927.pdf (accessed on 12th June 2025).

31. de Lima, M., Hourigan, C. S., & McCarthy, P. (2014). Back to the future! The evolving role of maintenance therapy after hematopoietic stem cell transplantation. https://core.ac.uk/download/pdf/82270718.pdf (accessed on 12th June 2025).

32. Delgado-Martin, C., Hermiston, M. L., Maude, S. L., Meyer, J. A., et al. (2019). CRLF2 rearrangement in Ph-like acute lymphoblastic leukemia predicts relative glucocorticoid resistance that is overcome with MEK or Akt inhibition. https://core.ac.uk/download/323073025.pdf (accessed on 12th June 2025).

33. Devi, J. R., Kadiyala, P. S., Lavu, S., Kasturi, N., & Kosuri, L. (2024). Enhancing acute lymphoblastic leukemia classification with a rapid and effective CNN model. *2024 Third International Conference on Distributed Computing and Electrical Circuits and Electronics (ICDCECE)*. https://www.semanticscholar.org/paper/4d2b0cc30325041b4751f63ca970e0a99796f96d (accessed on 12th June 2025).

34. Dworzak, M., Grosu, R., Lygizou, E. M., Maurer-Granofszky, M., et al. (2024). Automated immunophenotyping assessment for diagnosing childhood acute leukemia using set-transformers. http://arxiv.org/abs/2406.18309 (accessed on 12th June 2025).

35. Fernández Alfonso, A., Guevara Suárez, K. M., Proaño Bautista, C. X., Cantos Cantos, R. M., & Calvache Cañar, G. N. (2024). New perspectives on advances in diagnosis through imaging in chronic respiratory diseases: A systematic literature review. *Sapienza: International Journal of Interdisciplinary Studies*. https://www.semanticscholar.org/paper/9442044f883de919dadff943d7c3c7c45ed09ef7 (accessed on 12th June 2025).

36. Ferrando, A., Bash, R. O., Chen, Y., Condorelli, G., Dube, I., Fisch, P., et al. (2012). The molecular basis of T cell acute lymphoblastic leukemia. https://core.ac.uk/download/55802201.pdf (accessed on 12th June 2025).

37. Friedenson, B. (2011). Preventing hereditary cancers caused by opportunistic carcinogens. https://core.ac.uk/download/pdf/290483.pdf (accessed on 12th June 2025).

38. Genescà, E., & La Starza, R. (2022). Early T-cell precursor ALL and beyond: Immature and ambiguous lineage T-ALL subsets. https://core.ac.uk/download/574344737.pdf (accessed on 12th June 2025).

39. Gurbuxani, S., Larson, R. A., & Platzbecker, U. (2025). Diagnosis and treatment of AML in the context of WHO and ICC 2022 classifications: Divergent nomenclature converges on common therapies. https://core.ac.uk/download/637042911.pdf (accessed on 12th June 2025).
40. Han, H., Choi, K., & Suh, H. S. (2024). Impact of aging on acute myeloid leukemia epidemiology and survival outcomes: A real-world, population-based longitudinal cohort study. *PLOS ONE, 19*. https://www.semanticscholar.org/paper/3a19c54503b65dc934b3077967d99bb330c4105f (accessed on 12th June 2025).
41. Han, M., Chang, T., Chun, H., Jo, S., Jo, Y., Yu, D., Yoo, S., et al. (2024). Symptoms and conditions in children and adults up to 90 days after SARS-CoV-2 infection: A retrospective observational study utilizing the common data model. *Journal of Clinical Medicine, 13*. https://www.semanticscholar.org/paper/82dc79fea3b5df775bb234c5190678667ce47e0f (accessed on 12th June 2025).
42. Haney, M. G. (2021). Therapeutic targeting of leukemia stem cells to prevent T-cell acute lymphoblastic leukemia relapse. https://core.ac.uk/download/428350590.pdf (accessed on 12th June 2025).
43. Kabera, B., Macharia, W. M., Pamnani, R., Riyat, S., et al. (2014). Acute leukemias immunophenotypes at Aga Khan University Hospital, Nairobi. https://core.ac.uk/download/478296746.pdf (accessed on 12th June 2025).
44. Kjellander, C. (2016). Bloodstream infections in patients with hematological malignancies. https://core.ac.uk/download/70343959.pdf (accessed on 12th June 2025).
45. Larson, R. A., & Le Beau, M. M. (2011). Prognosis and therapy when acute promyelocytic leukemia and other "good risk" acute myeloid leukemias occur as a therapy-related myeloid neoplasm. https://core.ac.uk/download/pdf/8604634.pdf (accessed on 12th June 2025).
46. Lee, W. H., Lin, C. C., Tsai, C. H., Tien, F., Lo, M. Y., Tseng, M. H., Kuo, Y. Y., et al. (2024). Comparison of the 2022 World Health Organization classification and International Consensus Classification in myelodysplastic syndromes/neoplasms. *Blood Cancer Journal, 14*. https://www.semanticscholar.org/paper/423386c19b0f59d2b433eeb26abda54f6be02957 (accessed on 12th June 2025).
47. Li, X., Hao, T., Li, H., Lu, C., Cheng, S., Xu, X., Luo, H., et al. (2025). Abstract 1752: SY-13380, a novel menin-MLL inhibitor, exhibits efficacy against resistant mutations and anti-tumor activity for MLL-rearranged and NPM1-mutant acute myeloid leukemia in pre-clinical models. *Cancer Research*. https://www.semanticscholar.org/paper/60934520c15d825415eeefda0d67b22e264a0fbf (accessed on 12th June 2025).
48. Luo, B., Li, W., Zeng, J., Mao, Y., He, S., Hu, N., Guo, Q., et al. (2025). FHL1 as a prognostic biomarker and therapeutic target in acute promyelocytic leukemia. *Discover Oncology, 16*. https://www.semanticscholar.org/paper/9a3d5358d2ed3c8b21d1efd60b849653de4d1fc4 (accessed on 12th June 2025).
49. Martsenyuk, V., Sadiq, A. U., Sverstiuk, A., Dimitrov, G., & Gancarczyk, T. (2024). Stochastic machine learning models for mutation rate analysis of malignant cancer cells in patients with acute lymphoblastic leukemia. *International Journal of Circuits, Systems and Signal Processing*. https://www.semanticscholar.org/paper/0c3003ce399e57bfbeed0fdbd2dbe8c5d3c42c03 (accessed on 12th June 2025).

50. Matar, A. I., Obadiel, Y., & Jowah, H. (2025). Acute mechanical bowel obstruction: A comprehensive analysis of clinical presentation, etiology, surgical management, and postoperative outcomes in a Yemeni cohort. *Journal of Emergency Medicine, Trauma and Acute Care*. https://www.semanticscholar.org/paper/4e4ba0eb04a4e54faf7a6fcd7248c3e16a78a3af (accessed on 12th June 2025).

51. Maturo, A., Castellaccio, E., Moretti, V., Nier, S., Martinelli, G., Marconi, G., Musuraca, G., et al. (2024). Impact-AML: A European project for optimizing treatment and assessing quality of life in relapsed/refractory acute myeloid leukemia patients. *Blood*. https://www.semanticscholar.org/paper/09ff771e47e5300a3dc6b6118930187826b39218 (accessed on 12th June 2025).

52. Mencarini, L., Vestito, A., Zagari, R., & Montagnani, M. (2024). The diagnosis and treatment of acute cholecystitis: A comprehensive narrative review for a practical approach. *Journal of Clinical Medicine, 13*. https://www.semanticscholar.org/paper/2521f3d30eb4b1d29050a82ba5c7605f0671a78c (accessed on 12th June 2025).

53. Michalek, A. M., Pierce, D. A., Preston, D. L., Ron, E., Boice, J. D., Boice, J. D. J., Folley, J. H., et al. (2004). The Chernobyl childhood leukemia study: Background & lessons learned. https://core.ac.uk/download/pdf/3548874.pdf (accessed on 12th June 2025).

54. Mishra, S., & Rai, S. (2024). A comparative study of bone marrow aspiration and bone marrow biopsy in hematological diseases in a tertiary care center of Central India–A retrospective study. *Global Journal for Research Analysis*. https://www.semanticscholar.org/paper/e32467f0383bd8f3dea6eb9da2a6f6b19cc3ebae (accessed on 12th June 2025).

55. Naiel, A., Andreasson, H., Beverloo, H. B., Cho, K. H., Fleischman, E., Tsaur, G., Hollington, L., et al. (2013). A novel three-color fluorescence *in situ* hybridization approach for the detection of t(7;12)(q36;p13) in acute myeloid leukemia reveals new cryptic three-way translocation t(7;12;16). https://core.ac.uk/download/18488545.pdf (accessed on 12th June 2025).

56. Oppong, A. F., Nwozichi, C., Boakye, E. O., & Kyei, E. (2024). Characterizing the patterns of cervical cancer symptom recognition, symptom response, and associated factors among patients treated in a teaching hospital in Ghana. *Cancer Nursing*. https://www.semanticscholar.org/paper/381faab6a8dd864a747f63ea0574546acf0bd189 (accessed on 12th June 2025).

57. Shatilova, A., Budaeva, I., Matvienko, Y., Mirolyubova, Y., Ryzhkova, D., Grozov, R., Bogdanov, K., et al. (2024). Myeloid sarcoma or extramedullary acute myeloid leukemia: Experience in managing single-center patients' cohort. *Blood*. https://www.semanticscholar.org/paper/32b6646d16e6362c4cbb218a32fa8dfcd9bb8871 (accessed on 12th June 2025).

58. Siegel, R. L., Giaquinto, A. N., & Jemal, A. (2024). Cancer statistics, 2024. *CA: A Cancer Journal for Clinicians, 74*, 12–49. https://doi.org/10.3322/caac.21820 (accessed on 12th June 2025).

59. Smith, M. T., & Zhang, L. (1998). Biomarkers of leukemia risk: Benzene as a model. https://core.ac.uk/download/323068049.pdf (accessed on 12th June 2025).

60. Tang, X., Mai, H., Wang, L., Chen, S., Chen, F., Li, T., Liu, Y., et al. (2024). Diagnostic significance of cerebrospinal fluid flow cytometry in Chinese children with B lineage acute lymphoblastic leukemia. *BMC Pediatrics, 24*. https://www.semanticscholar.org/paper/100f3b4ea65da45b5ea7736ec340ba650e1fea0e (accessed on 12th June 2025).

61. Valiev, T. T., Shirin, A., Kokhno, A., Antipova, A., Baranova, O., Frenkel, M. A., Palladina, A., et al. (2025). Acute myeloid leukemias and myelodysplastic syndromes associated with previous cytotoxic therapy: Characteristic features, prognosis, and treatment approaches. *Russian*

Journal of Hematology and Transfusiology. https://www.semanticscholar.org/paper/43086d5d1ec7f2a92860609d9e013f0955628565 (accessed on 12th June 2025).

62. Venkatasubramanian, M., Schwartz, L., Ramachandra, N., Bennett, J., Subramanian, K. R., Chen, X., Gordon-Mitchell, S., et al. (2025). Splicing regulatory dynamics for precision analysis and treatment of heterogeneous leukemias. *Science Translational Medicine, 17*(797), eadr1471. https://www.semanticscholar.org/paper/1aeda1499d6d8469d7bfb136f75e4a1564756260 (accessed on 12th June 2025).

63. Warner, K. E. (2025). Treatment decision-making in catastrophic illness. https://core.ac.uk/download/pdf/6587141.pdf (accessed on 12th June 2025).

64. Yoshimura, S., Li, Z., Gocho, Y., Yang, W., Crews, K. R., Lee, S., Roberts, K., et al. (2024). Impact of age on pharmacogenomics and treatment outcomes of B-cell acute lymphoblastic leukemia. *Journal of Clinical Oncology, 42*, 3478–3490. https://www.semanticscholar.org/paper/367f6c5ff99506aea5419a6b28d014f326c51021 (accessed on 12th June 2025).

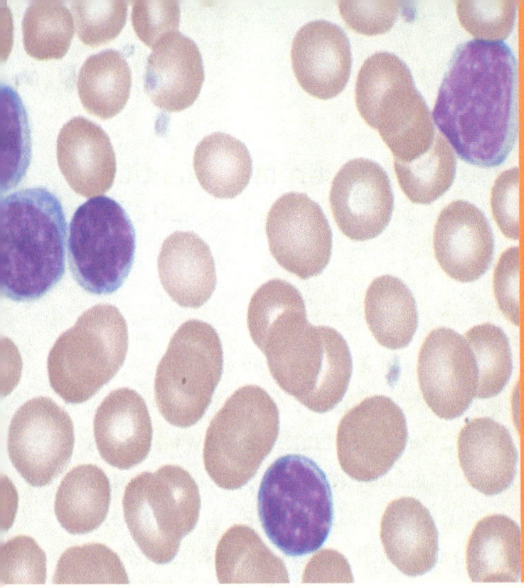

Chapter 12

CHRONIC LEUKEMIAS

Contents

Introduction....295
12.1. Types of Chronic Leukemias....296
12.2. Pathophysiology of Chronic Leukemias....300
12.3. Diagnosis and Monitoring....305
12.4. Treatment Options and Management....309
Summary....316
References....317

Introduction

This discipline has experienced significant progress in the understanding and management of chronic leukemias, most prominently with CLL, where continually evolving treatment paradigms have dramatically transformed patient outcomes. Patients have historically been treated mainly with chemoimmunotherapies, including regimens such as fludarabine and cyclophosphamide combined with rituximab. Despite this, the introduction of targeted agents, such as Bruton's TKI and B-cell lymphoma 2 antagonists, has transformed treatment strategies with resultant improved efficacy and safety profiles in patients (Korycka-WoAłowiec et al., 2025). Interestingly, the clinical variability of CLL requires patient- and disease-directed individualized treatment practices. As these innovations unfold, a critical area of exploration remains the impact of these therapies on patients' quality of life, an aspect that has received limited attention in the literature (Korycka-Wo Ałowiec et al., 2025). Understanding these factors is essential for providing the best care to patients with chronic leukemia (Figure 12.1).

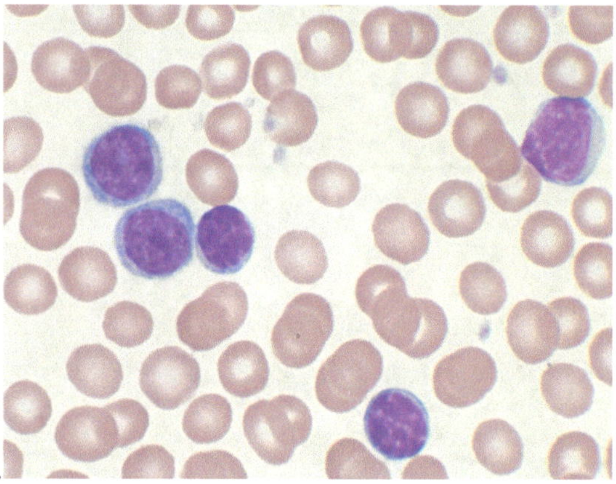

Figure 12.1. Chronic lymphocytic leukemia (CLL).

Source: https://upload.wikimedia.org/wikipedia/commons/0/0d/Chronic_lymphocytic_leukemia.jpg.

12.1. Types of Chronic Leukemias

Chronic leukemias are classified primarily into two main types: chronic lymphocytic leukemia (CLL) and chronic myeloid leukemia (CML). CLL is mostly found in older adults and involves the buildup of cancerous B lymphocytes in the blood, bone marrow, and lymphatic tissues, which results in a weakened immune system and an increased risk of getting infections. On the other hand, CML occurs when myeloid cells multiply excessively and is usually associated with the Philadelphia chromosome, which is caused by a genetic translocation. Due to this genetic change, the tyrosine kinase becomes more active, leading to uncontrolled cell growth and survival. Understanding the unique processes involved in CLL and CML is crucial for designing targeted treatments and achieving better outcomes. Recent advancements in diagnostic methods, including the application of hybrid AI models for classifying leukemia subtypes based on bone marrow cell images, hold promise for enhancing clinical decision-making in managing these chronic conditions (Hossain et al., 2024; Schweiger et al., 2025)

12.1.1. Chronic Lymphocytic Leukemia (CLL)

CLL is increasingly recognized for its diverse prognostic groups, largely determined by various genetic and molecular factors. The mutational status of the immunoglobulin heavy variable (IGHV) gene plays a crucial role in categorizing patients into three groups: mutated (M-IGHV), unmutated (U-IGHV), and borderline (BL-IGHV). Notably, the BL-IGHV subgroup, encompassing approximately 5% of cases, has sparked interest due to its unique clinical characteristics, such as a time to first treatment (TTFT) that aligns more closely with U-IGHV patients, yet a survival rate reminiscent of M-IGHV patients (Angotzi et al., 2024). Furthermore, advancements in targeted therapies, including Bruton TKI, emphasize the necessity for refined prognostic markers that can guide treatment decisions more effectively (Arcari et al., 2024). As new research is conducted, understanding these molecular differences may enhance the management of patients with CLL and their outcomes (Figure 12.2).

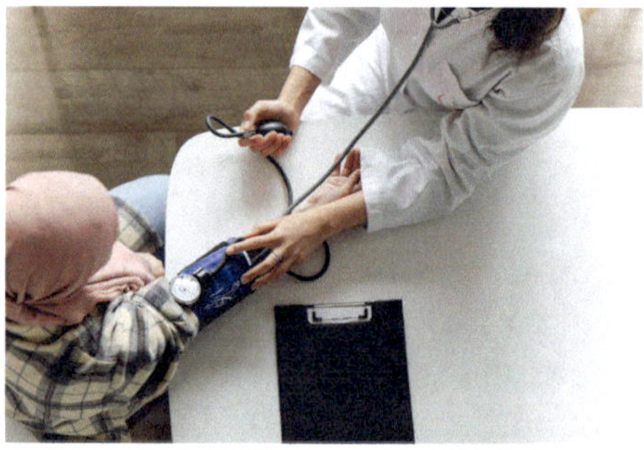

Figure 12.2. Chronic lymphocytic leukemia (CLL) is increasingly recognized for its diverse prognostic groups, largely determined by various genetic and molecular factors.

Source: https://annals.edu.sg/wp-content/uploads/2025/01/V54N1p36_pexels-thirdman-7659567.jpg.

12.1.2. Chronic Myeloid Leukemia (CML)

The emergence of targeted therapies has significantly transformed the management of CML, particularly with the introduction of tyrosine kinase inhibitors (TKIs) such as imatinib. Thanks to this innovation, more patients can receive treatment, and the survival rate has gone up, especially for those with CML in India and similar regions. Most patients present in the chronic phase, emphasizing the importance of timely and accurate risk stratification using scoring systems like Sokal and EUTOS, which inform treatment decisions and help predict clinical outcomes (Elango, 2024). However, treatment challenges persist, notably in cases resistant to TKIs, such as those harboring the T315I mutation, which complicates management strategies and impacts prognosis adversely (Kaleem et al., 2024). For this reason, keeping a close eye on the patient and following the treatment plan closely helps prevent the disease from worsening.

12.1.3. Rare Types of Chronic Leukemias

There are rare chronic leukemias that make it difficult to diagnose and treat them. Among these, chronic myelomonocytic leukemia (CMML) stands out as a malignancy that exhibits both myeloid and monocytic characteristics, complicating its classification and treatment protocols. Because CMML can cause symptoms such as tiredness and an enlarged spleen, these symptoms may be mistaken for those of other illnesses, and treatment is often delayed. The prognosis for CMML is particularly concerning, as noted in cases where karyotypic evolution plays a significant role in disease progression, leading to acute transformation and increased mortality rates (JM et al., 2006). Besides, adolescents are less often diagnosed with leukemia, yet they also have distinct types, including those that are not common in adults. It is essential to understand these uncommon forms to advance treatment and enhance outcomes for patients with chronic leukemia (Figure 12.3).

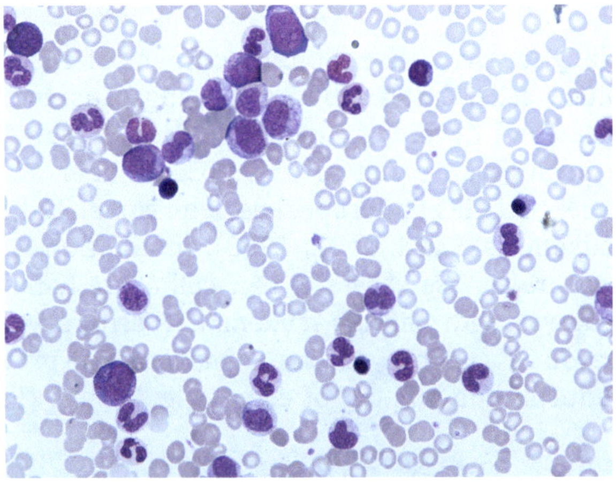

Figure 12.3. Chronic myelomonocytic leukemia (CMML).

Source: https://upload.wikimedia.org/wikipedia/commons/4/47/CMML.jpg.

12.1.4. Genetic Mutations Associated with Chronic Leukemias

Knowing the gene mutations found in chronic leukemias is important to improve therapeutic opportunities and patient outcomes. CLL, for instance, typically develops from a sequence of genetic changes, including somatic mutations and chromosomal lesions, that propel the malignancy's progression from asymptomatic monoclonal B-cell lymphocytosis to a more advanced and aggressive stage. Specific mutations in signal transduction and chromatin remodeling genes have been linked to the phenotypic heterogeneity observed in CLL, underscoring the importance of genetic context in disease expression. Likewise, CMML follows a complicated pattern of mutation, most of which affect epigenetic regulators and transcription factors (Ami et al., 2020). The interaction between these genetic mutations and the clinical phenotypes highlights the need for targeted therapy, particularly since patients with chronic leukemias also have increased risks of secondary primary cancers complicating their prognosis (Zheng et al., 2019).

12.1.5. Risk Factors for Developing Chronic Leukemias

Many factors cause the development of chronic leukemias and involves the abnormal growth of blood cells. Being exposed to dangerous chemicals, such as benzene, can significantly raise the chance of developing hematologic malignancies. Research has shown that occupational benzene exposure can result in chromosome aberrations in lymphocytes, a phenomenon that, based on recent studies in Europe, has been correlated with an increased cancer risk, particularly in chronic leukemias (Smith et al., 1998). In addition, genetic risks are important; some genetic mutations can predispose a person to T-cell acute lymphoblastic leukemias, which share some overlapping features with chronic leukemias (Ferrando et al., 2012). If these risk factors are understood, it becomes easier to develop measures that prevent and detect leukemia early, helping patients and reducing the number of chronic leukemias (Figure 12.4).

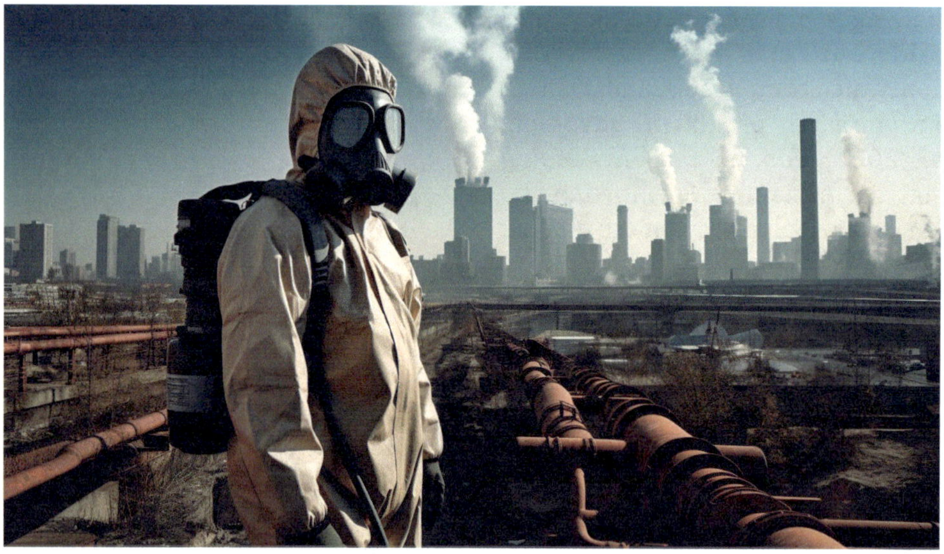

Figure 12.4. Environmental exposures, particularly to hazardous chemicals such as benzene, have been strongly linked to an increased risk of hematologic malignancies.

Source: https://brio-medical.com/wp-content/uploads/2023/07/benzene-exposure-cancer.jpg.

12.1.6. Age and Gender Distribution

The age and gender distribution of chronic leukemias, particularly CML, reveals significant insights into epidemiological trends. A study conducted in Iraq highlighted that the mean age of CML patients was approximately 47.3 years, indicating a prevalence among middle-aged adults, which is consistent with findings from other regions. Additionally, although the data showed variation in platelet counts according to gender, the overall hematological parameters did not exhibit significant differences between male and female CML patients, suggesting that age factors contribute more significantly to disease presentation than gender. Consequently, an occupational benzene poisoning study, which is an established risk factor for leukemia, revealed no distinctive age or duration of exposure differences between genders but noteworthy gender distribution differences to time. Generally, these findings stress the importance of taking gender and age into account in the pathogenesis and effects understanding of chronic leukemias (Mohammad et al., 2025; Gou et al., 2025).

12.1.7. Geographic Variations in Incidence

It is essential to understand how the rate of chronic leukemias varies by geography to guide the right actions and public health plans. The incidence of leukemia varies significantly between regions due to genetic factors, environmental exposures, and access to medical care. For instance, an analysis comparing incidence rates between Japan and England revealed that while certain leukemia types were more prevalent in Japan, others, such as Hodgkin lymphoma (HL) and renal tumors, showed markedly higher rates in England (Bonaventure et al., 2017). Similarly, disparities in cancer mortality rates among American Indian and Alaska Native populations highlight the importance of regional analysis to address health inequities (Cobb et al., 2003). As a result, it is crucial to organize cancer data by regions to design better public health strategies and use resources wisely to reduce the effects of chronic leukemias on people in different areas.

12.1.8. Prognosis for Different Types

Since the results for chronic leukemias vary with the subtype, it demonstrates that chronic leukemias are pretty complex. CLL, for instance, often presents with an indolent course and a relatively favorable overall survival rate, especially in early-stage cases. In contrast, CML is characterized by the presence of the Philadelphia chromosome, which can significantly influence treatment strategies and outcomes.

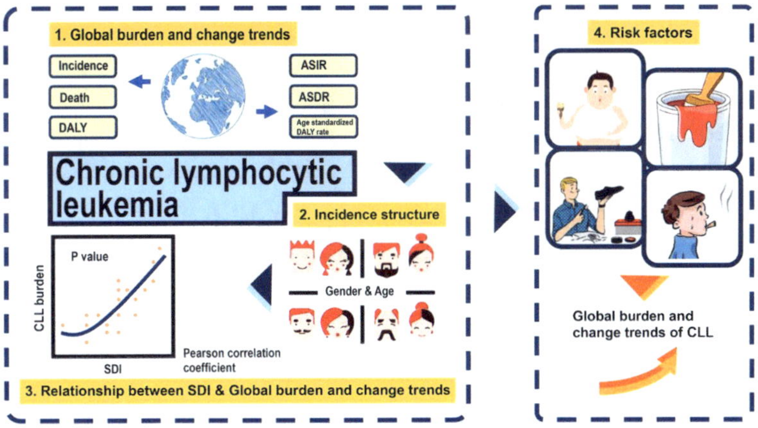

Figure 12.5. Chronic lymphocytic leukemia (CLL), for instance, often presents with an indolent course and a relatively favorable overall survival rate, especially in early-stage cases.

Source: https://media.springernature.com/lw1200/springer-static/image/art%3A10.1186%2Fs12938-021-00973-6/MediaObjects/12938_2021_973_Figa_HTML.png.

Because of advances in TKI, chances of survival for CML patients are much higher, which makes it a good choice for treating chronic leukemia. However, cytogenetic abnormalities, such as the ring chromosome 1 noted in the acute transformations of chronic diseases, may signal a poor prognosis, as evidenced in certain patient cases where disease progression occurs. Additionally, the dysregulation of pathways like the mammalian target of rapamycin (mTOR) has emerged as a critical factor in leukemogenesis, offering insights into potential therapeutic avenues (Bianchi et al., 2018) (Figure 12.5).

12.2. Pathophysiology of Chronic Leukemias

Chronic leukemias are mainly caused by abnormal hematopoietic stem cells (HSCs) that cause the uncontrolled growth of leukocytes. For instance, CML is notably driven by the Philadelphia chromosome, which results in the BCR-ABL1 oncoprotein that constitutively activates tyrosine kinase, fostering unrestrained cell division and survival. Unlike acute leukemias, chronic leukemias typically progress through distinct phases. CML transitions from a chronic phase to an accelerated phase and eventually a blast phase if untreated (Rinaldi et al., 2023). Moreover, complications such as leukostasis, reflective of high leukemic cell concentrations, can result in significant morbidity, necessitating urgent cytoreductive interventions (Macaron et al., 2022). The development of targeted therapies, mainly TKIs, has made CML manageable, allowing patients to expect the same life expectancy as healthy individuals, highlighting the importance of understanding the disease's causes.

12.2.1. Mechanisms of Leukemogenesis

The leukemogenesis process is complex and consists of a sequence of genetic, epigenetic, and environmental alterations that converge to convert normal hematopoietic cells into their malignant forms. The dysregulation of signaling pathways, such as NF-κB, is a crucial factor that drives this process, and it has been implicated in the pathogenesis of chronic leukemias, including CML. NF-κB facilitates cell proliferation and survival, with its activation linked to BCR-ABL signaling, further underscoring its role in leukemogenesis (Carr Gá et al., 2016). Additionally, CLL exemplifies the significance of epigenetic alterations, where aberrant DNA methylation patterns have been associated with distinct subtypes of the disease, notably influencing prognostic outcomes (Fong et al., 2012). These findings highlight the essential interplay between genetic mutations and epigenetic modifications, elucidating the intricate landscape of leukemogenic mechanisms that drive chronic leukemias (Figure 12.6).

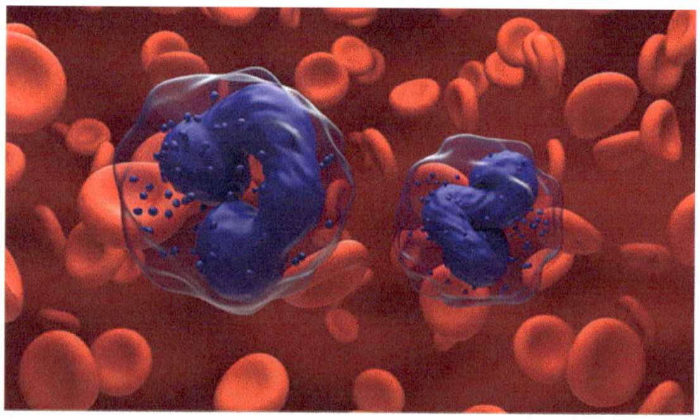

Figure 12.6. Chronic myeloid leukemia (CML).

Source: https://www.hopkinsmedicine.org/-/media/images/health/1_-conditions/leukemia/chronic-myelogenous-leukemia-symptoms-teaser.jpg.

12.2.2. Role of the Bone Marrow in Chronic Leukemias

The bone marrow plays a pivotal role in the pathogenesis and progression of chronic leukemias, particularly CLL, where malignant B cell clones proliferate within this hematopoietic environment. Notably, chromosomal abnormalities such as deletions at 13q14.3 have been identified as significant factors in CLL development, implicating microRNAs in the disease's etiology and progression (Javandoost et al., 2019). Another characteristic of the bone marrow immune landscape changes related to leukemia is the emergence of regulatory T cells, which, in some studies, have been shown to influence disease outcomes. Tregs in the bone marrow have been found to correlate directly with the level of leukemia blasts and have become a marker for predicting response to treatment (Niedźwiecki et al., 2018). Thus, understanding the dynamic interplay between bone marrow's cellular components and the leukemic processes is crucial for developing effective therapeutic strategies in chronic leukemias.

12.2.3. Impact of the Immune System

The immune system plays a crucial role in the development of chronic leukemias and in determining patient outcomes. Aberrant signaling pathways, such as NOTCH1, are frequently activated in leukemias, thereby disrupting normal immune functions and promoting malignant cell survival (Amadori et al., 2018). This error enables cancer cells to grow and also alters the immune system, allowing cancer cells to evade detection. It was discovered that the chemokine pathways that direct leukocyte movement are linked to the unusual infiltration in chronic leukemias, which complicates the disease. Recent studies have shown that specific chemokine axes, such as CCL25/CCR9, can direct leukemic cells to various niches within the body, thereby enhancing their ability to persist and proliferate (Brehme et al., 2016). All in all, these findings demonstrate the close relationship between the immune system and chronic leukemias, making immunotherapies a necessary target (Figure 12.7).

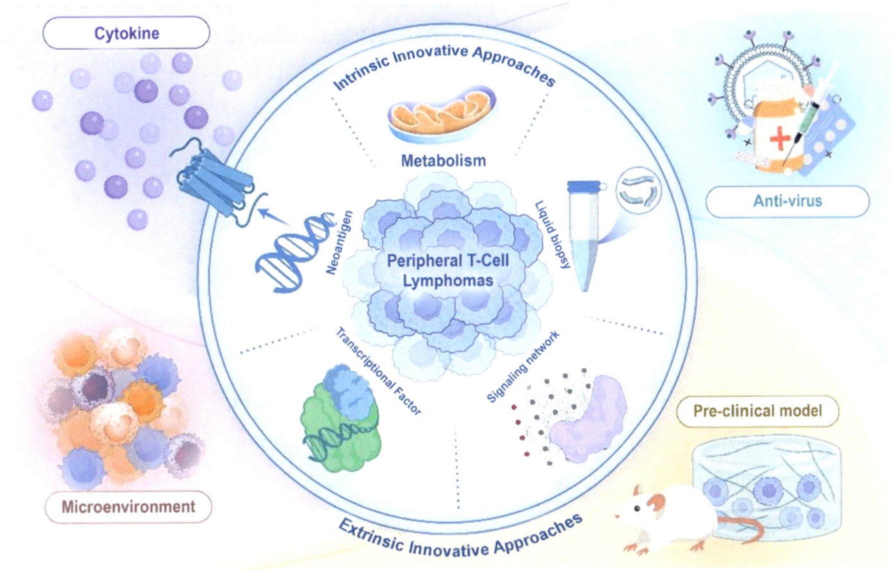

Figure 12.7. Aberrant signaling pathways, such as NOTCH1, are frequently activated in leukemias, thereby disrupting normal immune functions and promoting malignant cell survival

Source: https://data.the-innovation.org//innovation-data/medicine/2024/1/PIC/XINNMEDICINE-2023-0091-Abstract.jpg.

12.2.4. Genetic and Epigenetic Changes

The investigation of genetic and epigenetic alterations plays a vital role in the understanding of the pathogenesis of chronic leukemias because these changes play an important role in disease initiation and progression. Oncogenes and tumor suppressor genes' mutations are major initiators of malignancy but are complemented by epigenetic modifications, more so DNA methylation patterns. Notably, alterations in the methylation status have been identified as hallmarks of leukemias, with studies revealing that hypermethylation of gene promoters is more prevalent in lymphoid malignancies than in myeloid ones. By characterizing the DNA methylation profiles across various hematologic neoplasms, researchers have uncovered specific genes, such as DBC1, DIO3, and MYOD1, that exhibit significant hypermethylation across multiple subtypes, suggesting their potential role in the pathogenesis of these diseases (Agirre et al., 2011). Additionally, the interplay of chromatin modifications reinforces the importance of epigenetic mechanisms in cancer progression (Brown et al., 2006).

12.2.5. Microenvironmental Influences

The environment around the leukemia cells is very important for its development and the patient's response to treatment. Recent studies have revealed that tumors create environments that suppress the immune system's activity, making it more challenging for CAR-T cell therapy to function effectively. For instance, the application of a human bone marrow organoid platform demonstrated that the tumor microenvironment (TME) in chronic myeloproliferative neoplasms (MPNs) can limit the efficacy of targeting strategies, even when potent therapies, such as anti-CD33 antibody-drug conjugates, are employed. Additionally, TKIs used in CML treatment have exhibited nuanced interactions with immune cells, affecting outcomes based on their effects on dendritic cell function and T-cell responses. Such microenvironmental influences underscore the necessity for tailored therapeutic approaches that account for both leukemic cellular dynamics and the surrounding stroma (Zoë et al., 2024; Naik et al., 2024) (Figure 12.8).

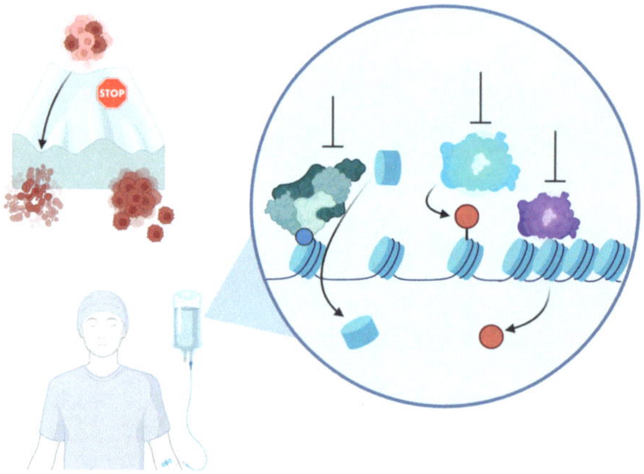

Figure 12.8. The microenvironment plays a crucial role in the progression and treatment response of chronic leukemias, significantly influencing patient outcomes.

Source: https://onlinelibrary.wiley.com/cms/asset/c13d51c6-487c-4fc5-ae76-d8e64134810d/ijc35389-toc-0001-m.jpg.

12.2.6. Clonal Evolution in Chronic Leukemias

The phenomenon of clonal evolution in chronic leukemias, particularly illustrated in CML, emphasizes the complexity underlying disease progression and therapeutic resistance. The changing and expanding populations of leukemic stem cells exhibit a range of clonal heterogeneity due to their hierarchical nature. New studies that utilized population dynamic modeling and examined CML patient biopsies revealed that similarity in CD34+ cells can indicate the progression of the disease. This approach not only delineates established stages of CML but also shows additional intricacies within each phase (Brehme et al., 2016). Furthermore, the immunophenotypic characterization of hematopoietic precursor cells highlights the interconnected nature of different leukemic forms, underscoring that similar clonal origins may underpin varied manifestations of leukemia (Gluzman et al., 2008). Because of this, the way chronic leukemias are managed and their outcomes can be improved..

12.2.7. Interaction with Other Diseases

The way chronic leukemia interacts with various diseases is an essential factor in choosing the treatment and outcomes for patients. For instance, the presence of autoimmune conditions, such as rheumatoid arthritis, can exacerbate the pathophysiology of CLL, leading to increased inflammation and further complicating treatment regimens. Studies indicate that inflammatory mediators released in conditions such as oligoarticular juvenile idiopathic arthritis can activate monocytes, thereby enhancing their ability to induce T-cell activation and promote chronic inflammation (Schmidt et al., 2023). Additionally, the genetic mutations associated with CLL, particularly those in immunoglobulin genes, have been found to influence disease prognosis and treatment response, demonstrating that interactions at the genetic level can also affect comorbid conditions (Datta et al., 2022). Understanding these relationships is crucial for developing therapies that address both chronic leukemia and related health issues (Figure 12.9).

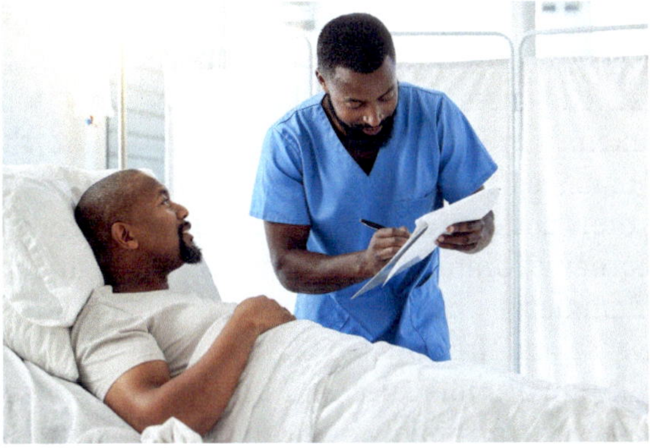

Figure 12.9. The interaction of chronic leukemias with other diseases plays a significant role in shaping the clinical management and outcomes for affected patients.

Source: https://d2jx2rerrg6sh3.cloudfront.net/images/news/ImageForNews_754391_16901834089405843.jpg.

12.2.8. Biomarkers for Chronic Leukemias

It is now crucial to identify and describe biomarkers for chronic leukemias to enhance both diagnosis and patient care. Biomarkers, such as genetic mutations, proteins, and metabolites, are used to diagnose, predict prognosis, and guide treatment of diseases. For instance, mutations in the TP53 gene are frequently observed in CLL and have been associated with poorer outcomes, underscoring the importance of genetic profiling in treatment stratification. Immunophenotyping has also found specific cell markers on the surface of cells that allow for the differentiation of chronic leukemias, for example, CD5 and CD23 in CLL. Additionally, new developments in metabolomics and lipidomics may provide us with fresh insights into the chemical changes that occur in these disorders, thereby improving our understanding of leukemic pathology. Further investigation into these emerging biomarkers could lead to more personalized treatment approaches in chronic leukemias (Wang et al., 2024; Veldi et al., 2025).

12.2.9. Current Research on Pathophysiology

Gaining a deeper understanding of pathophysiology in chronic leukemias is now crucial for developing new treatment options. Studies now examine the molecular and cellular changes that lead to the disease, elucidating how genetic alterations and epigenetic factors contribute to leukemia in blood cells. It has been found through studies that when signaling pathways are out of balance, it can cause these cancer cells to grow faster and live longer, illustrating the complexity of their actions. In addition to genetic factors, researchers are investigating the role of the immune microenvironment in promoting leukemia progression, a finding that parallels those in other inflammatory conditions, such as rheumatoid arthritis, where immune dysregulation exacerbates disease manifestation (Chatterjee et al., 2024). Innovations in therapeutic strategies, including novel small molecules and targeted biologics, are being scrutinized for their potential to mitigate these aberrant pathways while minimizing adverse effects (Magagnoli et al., 2024). It is essential to continue researching, as this helps doctors enhance the treatment of chronic leukemias and improve patient outcomes (Figure 12.10).

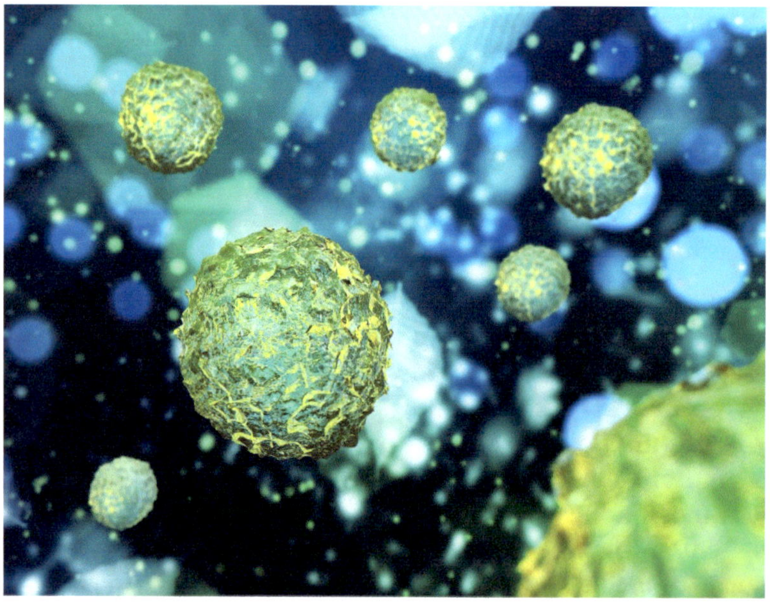

Figure 12.10. Current research delves into the molecular and cellular mechanisms driving the disease, revealing how genetic mutations and epigenetic alterations contribute to the leukemic transformation of hematopoietic cells.

Source: https://d2jx2rerrg6sh3.cloudfront.net/images/news/ImageForNews_758299_16940994355954918.jpg.

12.3. Diagnosis and Monitoring

The diagnosis and monitoring of chronic leukemias present significant challenges due to their complex pathophysiology and heterogeneous clinical manifestations. For instance, CML, which has an annual incidence of two cases per 100,000 and accounts for approximately 15% of newly diagnosed adult leukemia cases, necessitates regular monitoring to assess disease progression and treatment response (Jabbour et al., 2024). Diagnostic tools, such as complete blood counts (CBCs), cytogenetic analyses, and molecular testing for specific genetic markers, including the BCR-ABL fusion gene, are crucial for the accurate identification and stratification of the disease. As treatment regimens evolve, leveraging advanced technologies, including machine learning approaches, offers promising avenues for enhancing patient monitoring. These techniques enable healthcare providers to analyze comprehensive datasets, thus improving early detection and tracking of disease progression, an aspect critical for optimizing patient outcomes in chronic leukemias (Goel, 2024).

12.3.1. Initial Diagnostic Tests

Initial diagnostic tests are crucial in assessing chronic leukemias, particularly in distinguishing between various subtypes, such as CML. Flow cytometry serves as an essential tool for immunophenotyping. In a study involving 500 CML patients, significant differences in specific markers were identified between the CML and non-CML groups, yielding high sensitivity and specificity for diagnosis (Ma et al., 2024). Furthermore, the identification of the BCR::ABL1 fusion gene through cytogenetic testing plays a pivotal role in confirming CML, as this alteration underpins the diseases pathophysiology (Lee et al., 2024). Applying all these tests simultaneously improves the accuracy of diagnosing CML and also guides doctors on how to treat patients who do not respond to TKIs. Therefore, the results of initial testing play a big role in managing and treating chronic leukemia patients (Figure 12.11).

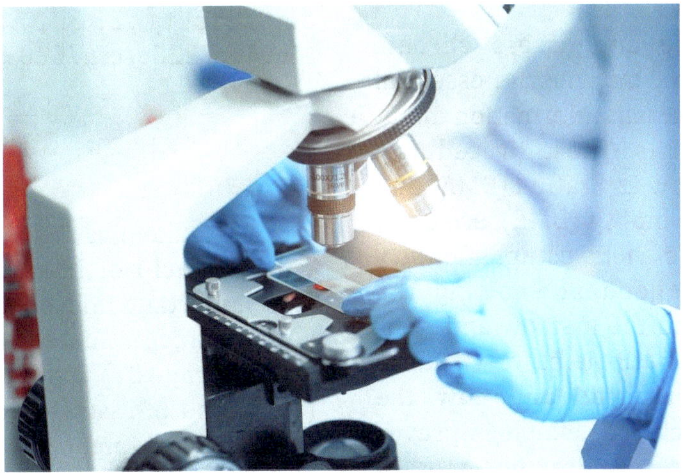

Figure 12.11. Initial diagnostic tests are crucial in the assessment of chronic leukemias, particularly in distinguishing between various subtypes such as chronic myeloid leukemia (CML).

Source: https://www.rockymountaincancercenters.com/hubfs/Understanding%20the%20Difference%20Between%20Acute%20and%20Chronic%20Leukemia.jpeg.

12.3.2. Role of Blood Tests in Diagnosis

Blood tests are crucial for identifying and managing chronic leukemias, as they reveal both blood abnormalities and genetic mutations. Techniques such as fluorescence in situ hybridization (FISH) and Optical Genome Mapping (OGM) are instrumental in identifying chromosomal abnormalities that characterize these malignancies, including deletions and translocations, which influence treatment decisions and prognostic outcomes. For instance, the detection of the del(17p) mutation in CLL can indicate a more aggressive disease course and necessitate alternative therapeutic approaches (Erdem et al., 2024). Similarly, in CML, cytogenetic analysis is crucial for detecting the BCR-ABL1 fusion gene, which informs treatment strategies and risk stratification (Elango, 2024). As a result, combining several blood tests helps with accurate diagnosis and enables doctors to provide more effective treatments to patients with chronic leukemia.

12.3.3. Bone Marrow Biopsy Procedures

In order to diagnose and assess chronic leukemias, bone marrow biopsies are essential because they give important information about the patient's blood cells. These procedures, specifically bone marrow aspiration (BMA) and bone marrow trephine biopsy (BMB), are often performed together to yield complementary information. BMA is good at showing the types of cells present in the marrow and their characteristics, while BMB helps to visualize how the cells are arranged and how the bone marrow is structured, which improves the accuracy of diagnosis. Previous studies have indicated that the combined analysis of BMA and BMB can significantly enhance the understanding of conditions such as CML, which is characterized by distinct cellular patterns and changes in marrow structure (Mishra et al., 2024). Moreover, the correlation between findings from both procedures has been shown to positively influence treatment planning and disease monitoring, underscoring the importance of these diagnostic techniques in the realm of chronic leukemias (Jawed et al., 2024) (Figure 12.12).

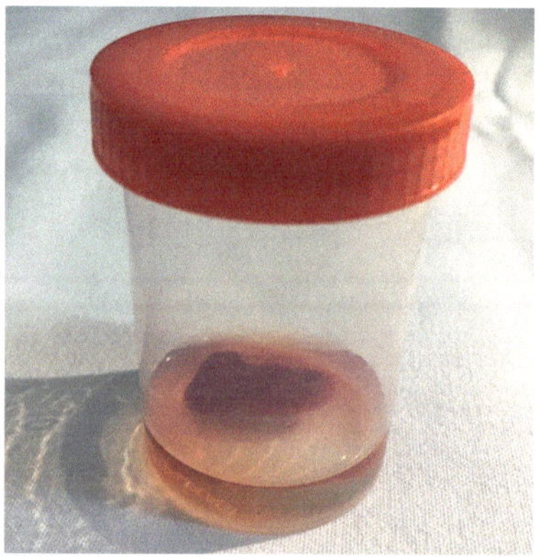

Figure 12.12. Bone marrow biopsy procedures are critical in the diagnosis and evaluation of chronic leukemias, providing necessary insights into the hematological landscape of affected patients.

Source: https://onlinelibrary.wiley.com/cms/asset/4236b071-a8eb-449f-897b-1fe94bc7326c/crh7590948-fig-0001b-m.jpg.

12.3.4. Imaging Studies in Chronic Leukemias

Chronic leukemias are managed and diagnosed with the help of imaging studies, since they give important information about the disease and treatment. Techniques such as computed tomography (CT), magnetic resonance imaging (MRI), and ultrasound are employed to assess the extent of splenomegaly, lymphadenopathy, and potential extramedullary involvement, enabling clinicians to tailor therapeutic strategies effectively. For example, CLL patients usually have enlarged lymph nodes, which can be seen on imaging and help in assessing the disease and predicting its outcomes. Advanced imaging methods enable doctors to assess how the disease is responding to treatment, which helps them determine the most effective course of action. The integration of innovative radiotracers, such as those used in renal imaging studies, could enhance the sensitivity of evaluating malignant cellular infiltration in chronic leukemias, as demonstrated in recent studies (Zhou et al., 2021; Ozturk et al., 2024). For this reason, imaging is a key element of treating leukemia.

12.3.5. Molecular Testing and Genetic Profiling

Testing at the molecular and genetic levels has dramatically changed the way chronic leukemias are diagnosed, treated, and monitored. The identification of specific genetic markers, such as the BCR-ABL1 fusion gene in CML, has been pivotal in tailoring therapeutic strategies to individual patient profiles, ultimately improving outcomes.

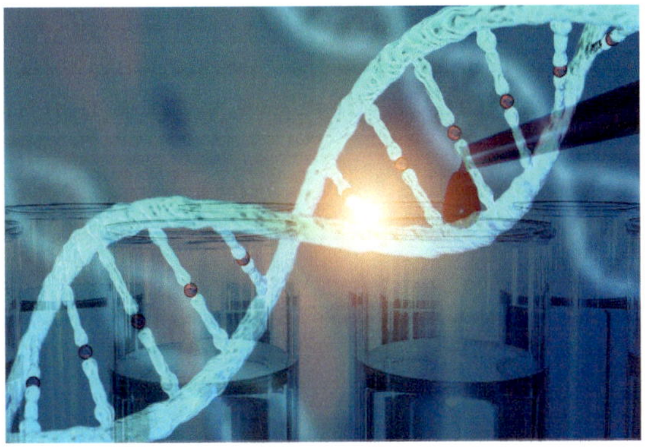

Figure 12.13. Molecular testing and genetic profiling have revolutionized the landscape of chronic leukemias, particularly in their diagnosis, treatment, and monitoring.

Source: https://www.targetedonc.com/_next/image?url=https%3A%2F%2Fcdn.sanity.io%2Fimages%2F0vv8moc6%2Ftargetedonc%2F94868741e43ada60e10c4e697d605da4799de401-3000x2000.jpg%3Ffit%3Dcrop%26auto%3Dformat&w=3840&q=75.

For example, cytogenetic analysis plays a crucial role in diagnosing CML and monitoring patient response to treatment, allowing clinicians to adjust therapies based on mutational profiles, especially for those showing resistance to TKI (Elango, 2024). In the context of CLL, detailed genetic profiling enables the characterization of refractory disease by identifying detrimental mutations, such as NOTCH1 and 11q deletions, which are indicative of a poor prognosis (Kurucova et al., 2024). For this reason, the use of molecular testing in medical practice is necessary to improve the treatment of chronic leukemias and enhance the quality of care provided to patients (Figure 12.13).

12.3.6. Staging of Chronic Leukemias

The staging of chronic leukemias, notably Chronic Myelomonocytic Leukemia (CMML) and B-cell CLL, plays a pivotal role in guiding treatment strategies and predicting patient outcomes. In CMML, for instance, classification is heavily reliant on the integration of immunophenotypic and genetic data to accurately delineate disease subtypes and stages, thereby enabling tailored therapeutic approaches that address the specific clonal architecture of the disease (Piñero et al., 2024). Likewise, the Rai-Binet system used in CLL groups patients based on their medical symptoms and the amount of β2-microglobulin in their blood, which is an essential sign of how the disease will progress. This approach to staging highlights the challenges of leukemias and emphasizes the importance of using advanced tools for diagnosis, which leads to better care and outcomes for patients with different types of leukemia.

12.3.7. Monitoring Disease Progression

It is imperative to regularly monitor the development of chronic leukemias to improve patient outcomes and choose the best treatment.

It requires doctors to check blood, chromosomes, and molecular markers regularly to monitor the patient's response to treatment and find out if resistance is occurring. For instance, in chronic myelogenous leukemia (CML), achieving cytogenetic remission requires ongoing surveillance of BCR-ABL transcript levels through reverse transcription polymerase chain reaction (RT-PCR), enabling clinicians to detect minimal residual disease (MRD) and adjust treatment as necessary (Branford et al., 2007). Furthermore, cytogenetic analysis provides insights into clonal evolution, which is crucial for predicting disease progression and informing subsequent therapeutic strategies (JM et al., 2006). With these monitoring methods, healthcare providers can identify changes in the disease state promptly, making it easier to provide timely care and improve the patient's outlook. This approach highlights the importance of close attention when dealing with these challenging cancers (Figure 12.14).

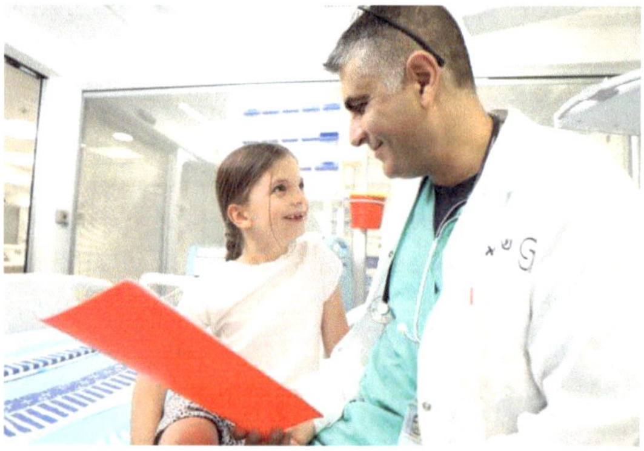

Figure 12.14. Effective monitoring of disease progression in chronic leukemias is crucial for optimizing patient outcomes and tailoring therapeutic interventions.

Source: https://www.shebaonline.org/wp-content/uploads/2022/07/pediatric-cml.jpg.

12.3.8. Challenges in Diagnosis

The diagnosis of chronic leukemias, particularly B-cell CLL and small lymphocytic lymphoma (SLL), is fraught with complexities that impede timely and accurate treatment interventions. Because these diseases are not the same, their symptoms and development can vary significantly from one person to another. For instance, the emergence of Richter transformation (RT), a condition characterized by the transformation of CLL/SLL into high-grade diffuse large B-cell lymphoma, complicates the diagnostic landscape. This advanced stage of the disease is often associated with specific genetic mutations, such as alterations in NOTCH1 and TP53, which complicates diagnosis further by requiring advanced molecular techniques to establish clonal relationships between the diseases (Broadway-Duren et al., 2022; Jacqueline, 2022). It is essential for health care providers to watch out for these signs, since early detection can help patients overcome the difficulties caused by chronic leukemias.

12.3.9. Importance of Early Detection

Early detection of chronic leukemias is crucial for the success of treatment and the patient's future. When the disease is detected early, doctors can utilize effective treatments that enhance the chances of survival and improve the quality of life for patients. Research has shown that certain biomarkers, such as MIAT, are upregulated in aggressive forms of CLL, indicating a potential avenue for early detection and monitoring (Croce et al., 2016).

Similarly, in CML, the identification of specific leukemic stem cell markers, such as CD26, aids in recognizing the disease's presence early, making it possible to initiate therapy before severe complications arise (Bilban et al., 2014). As a result, when advanced tools are used and people are aware of the symptoms, healthcare professionals can detect chronic leukemias early, which helps achieve better results (Figure 12.15).

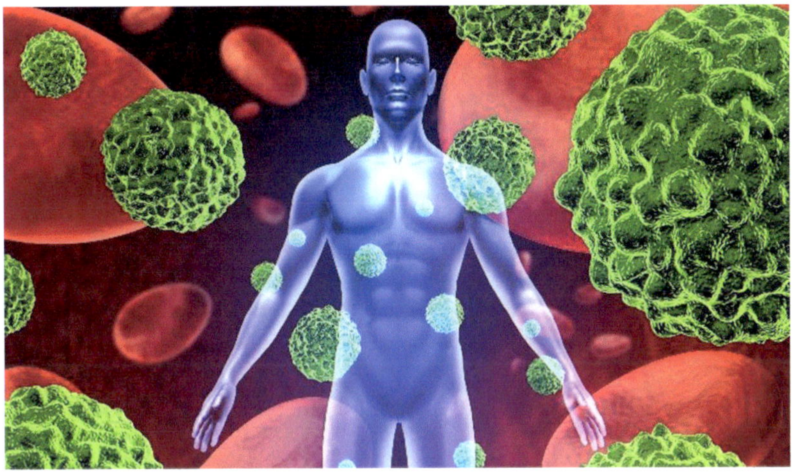

Figure 12.15. The early detection of chronic leukemias plays a crucial role in patient prognosis and treatment efficacy.

Source: https://www.nfcr.org/wp-content/uploads/2020/09/blood1-1-e1505328721283.jpg.

12.4. Treatment Options and Management

Since every type of chronic leukemia is different, a combination of treatments is used that is tailored to each patient. For CLL, traditional therapies have evolved to include novel approaches such as targeted therapies and immunotherapies, like Chimeric Antigen Receptor (CAR) T-cell therapy. While CAR T-cell therapy has revolutionized the treatment landscape for many B-cell malignancies, its efficacy in CLL has been tempered by challenges such as reduced T-cell fitness and suppressive TMEs, which contribute to treatment resistance (Borogovac et al., 2024). Additionally, the burden of resistant hypertension, particularly among high-risk patients, underscores the need for comprehensive management strategies that may involve leveraging new pharmacological advancements to enhance overall treatment outcomes (Flack et al., 2024). As researchers continue to discover new therapies, the treatment options for chronic leukemia are continually advancing, offering hope for improved patient outcomes.

12.4.1. Overview of Treatment Modalities

The treatment modalities for chronic leukemias, specifically CML, have evolved significantly with advances in targeted therapies. The cornerstone of CML treatment involves the use of TKIs, such as imatinib, which directly inhibit the activity of the BCR-ABL fusion protein that drives the disease pathology. This approach to treating cancer represents a shift from traditional chemotherapy to newer treatments that cause less harm to healthy cells. Ongoing research aims to address resistance mechanisms that arise from mutations in the BCR-ABL gene, underscoring the need for ongoing innovation in treatment strategies (Aljabali et al., 2024). Additionally, researchers are developing new therapies and combining multiple drugs to enhance effectiveness and mitigate drug resistance. Understanding the molecular landscape of chronic leukemias is thus critical for developing personalized treatment regimens that optimize clinical outcomes (Bano et al., 2024) (Figure 12.16).

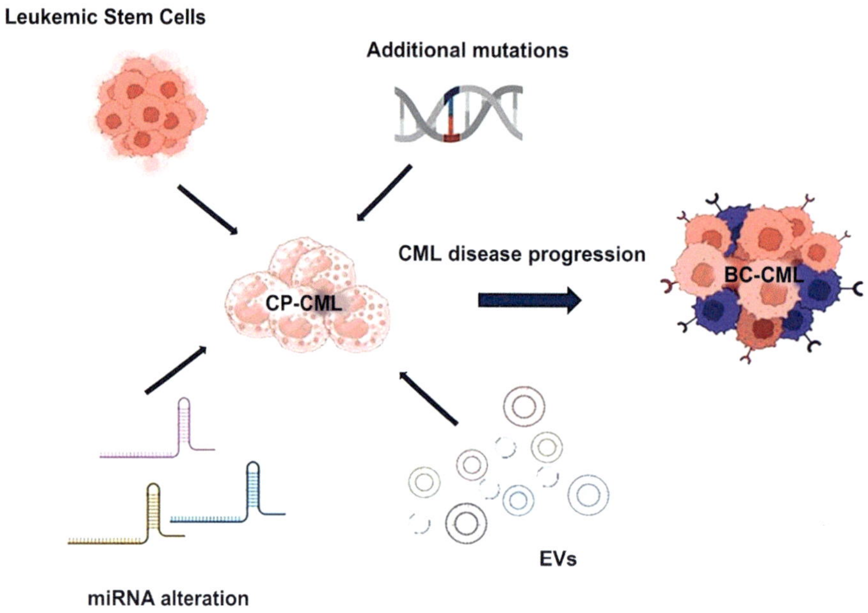

Figure 12.16. The cornerstone of CML treatment involves the use of tyrosine kinase inhibitors (TKIs), such as imatinib, which directly inhibit the activity of the BCR-ABL fusion protein that drives the disease pathology.

Source: https://www.frontiersin.org/files/Articles/1546813/fonc-15-1546813-HTML/image_m/fonc-15-1546813-g001.jpg.

12.4.2. Chemotherapy Regimens

For patients with chronic leukemia, chemotherapy is a central part of the treatment that helps control the disease and improve results. It is critical to adjust these regimens based on what is unique to each patient, since this can significantly improve the treatment's success and reduce harmful side effects. The literature emphasizes the need for innovation in chemotherapy protocols, suggesting that a nuanced approach could lead to better adherence and overall quality of life for patients undergoing treatment (Czajka et al., 2024). Moreover, recent studies indicate that additional consolidation chemotherapy before transplant does not yield a statistically significant improvement in overall survival, prompting a reevaluation of its routine application in clinical practice (Paulson et al., 2016). So, by perfecting chemotherapy and helping patients with complete education and support, more effective ways to treat chronic leukemia can be achieved.

12.4.3. Targeted Therapies and Their Mechanisms

The development of targeted therapies has revolutionized the treatment landscape for chronic leukemias, particularly CML and CLL. The central part of CML is the BCR–ABL1 fusion gene, which results in the activation of tyrosine kinase and uncontrolled cell multiplication. Targeted TKIs effectively suppress this activity, offering a focused approach to therapy that minimizes collateral damage to normal cells (Vysochinskaya et al., 2024). At the same time, the use of BTK inhibitors and Bcl-2 inhibitors in CLL has improved survival, so it is now essential to learn about resistance. Advanced sequencing technologies have revealed that mutations in key genes, such as BTK and PLCG2, emerge during therapy, affecting treatment efficacy and guiding future strategies (David et al., 2023). As time passes, incorporating molecular knowledge will become necessary to aid patients and overcome resistance in chronic leukemias (Figure 12.17).

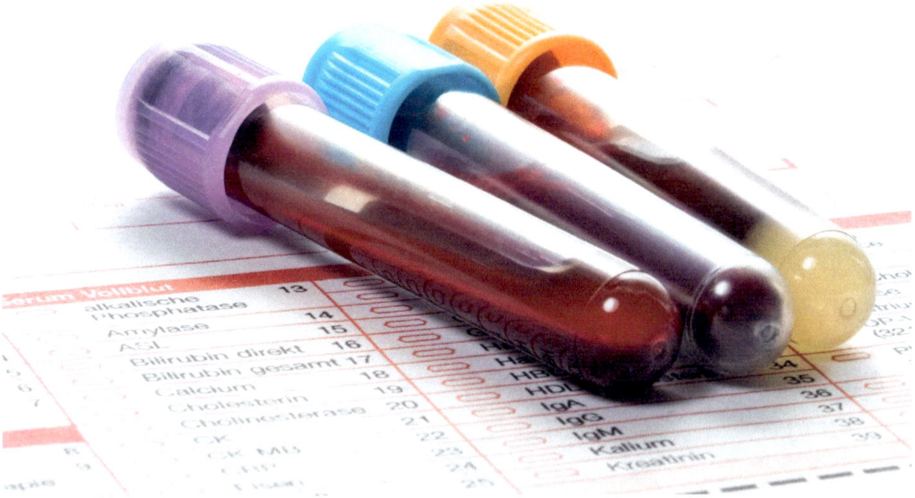

Figure 12.17. The development of targeted therapies has revolutionized the treatment landscape for chronic leukemias, particularly chronic myeloid leukemia (CML) and chronic lymphocytic leukemia (CLL).

Source: https://images.ctfassets.net/yixw23k2v6vo/61CM0JDiYUADqX0EVw5wt0/494b0f0fa9053c72da9332f1c38fac66/iStock-512298876.jpg.

12.4.4. Role of Immunotherapy

Immunotherapy significant difference in treating chronic leukemia, leading to better outcomes for patients. Advances in therapies, particularly for CLL, have led to prolonged progression-free survival, underscored by recent clinical trial data that validate the efficacy of these treatments in real-world settings (Roeker et al., 2025). Notably, venetoclax-based therapies and covalent Bruton TKI have shown substantial promise, as these regimens not only extend the duration of treatment but also facilitate a more favorable response compared to traditional therapies (Roeker et al., 2025). Additionally, the relationship between how the system treats the cancer and the tumor's environment underscores the role of immunology in combating cancer. Promoting inflammation in the tumor area can make chemotherapy more effective, which shows that knowing about immune activity is an essential factor for better results in chronic leukemias.

12.4.5. Stem Cell Transplantation

Stem cell transplantation is a key treatment for chronic leukemias since it can cure the disease by restoring the hematopoietic system and getting rid of cancer cells. HSC transplant (HSCT) can be sourced from bone marrow, peripheral blood, or cord blood, each presenting unique advantages and disadvantages. While randomized controlled trials indicate no significant survival advantage of peripheral blood stem cells (PBSC) over bone marrow-derived sources in matched sibling transplants, PBSC can lead to lower relapse rates and improved disease-free survival in high-risk patients, albeit with an increased risk of graft-versus-host disease (GVHD) (Basso et al., 2017). Moreover, the long-term psychological implications of HSCT must also be acknowledged, as survivors may experience significant distress and diminished quality of life, emphasizing the need for comprehensive post-transplant care and support strategies (Basso et al., 2017). When these medical factors are balanced, the source of stem cells is selected to match each patient's specific situation (Figure 12.18).

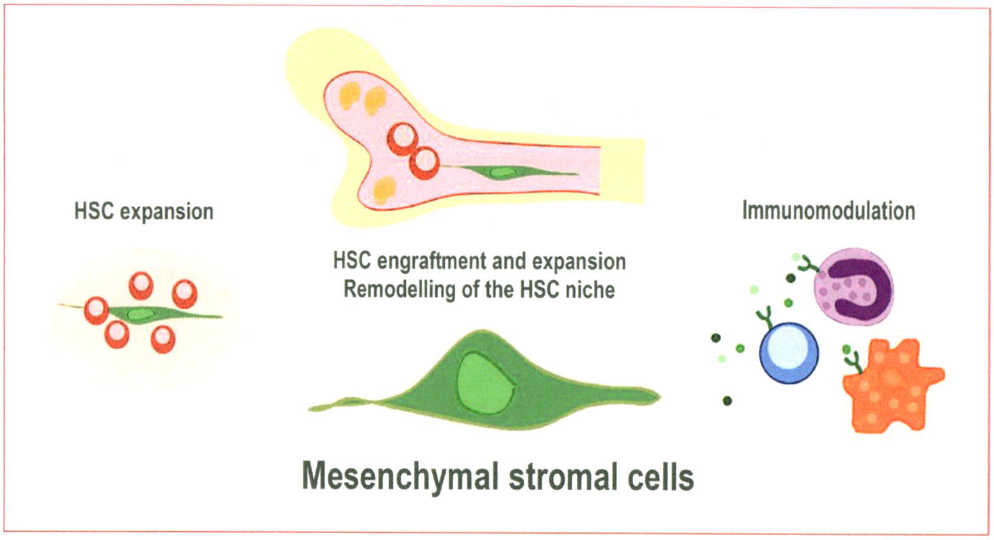

Figure 12.18. As a pivotal therapeutic intervention for chronic leukemias, stem cell transplantation offers a potential cure by replenishing the hematopoietic system and enabling the eradication of malignancies.

Source: https://www.mdpi.com/cancers/cancers-14-00580/article_deploy/html/images/cancers-14-00580-g001.png.

12.4.6. Supportive Care and Symptom Management

Since chronic leukemia patients usually experience challenging emotions and symptoms, it is essential to provide them with comprehensive support. Effective symptom management is paramount, involving the alleviation of pain, nausea, and psychological distress, which are commonly experienced during various stages of therapy, including BMT. Research indicates that integrating palliative care into the treatment regimens significantly enhances the quality of life for these patients by fostering open communication among healthcare providers and families and facilitating critical end-of-life discussions (Basso et al., 2017). Furthermore, survivors of pediatric hematopoietic stem cell transplantation (HSCT) have reported lower quality of life and increased psychological distress, highlighting the necessity for targeted interventions that address both the socio-demographic and medical variables influencing their care experiences (Basso et al., 2017). For this reason, a complete approach to supportive care is necessary to help people with chronic leukemia.

12.4.7. Clinical Trials and Emerging Therapies

Clinical trials investigating new therapies are leading to significant changes in the treatment of chronic leukemias. Recent advancements in targeted treatments, particularly for CML, have demonstrated the potential for more effective patient outcomes through precision medicine. Trials focusing on inhibitors that specifically disrupt the BCR-ABL fusion protein's activity have shown promise in overcoming resistance mechanisms associated with traditional therapies like imatinib, which targets the tyrosine kinase activity of the fusion protein (Aljabali et al., 2024). Moreover, innovative strategies, such as combination therapies, are being evaluated to address the heterogeneity of leukemic cells, thereby enhancing overall efficacy while minimizing side effects (Bano et al., 2024). When these trials gather vital information, they elucidate the biology of chronic leukemias and inform the development of new treatment guidelines, underscoring the need for ongoing research in this area (Figure 12.19).

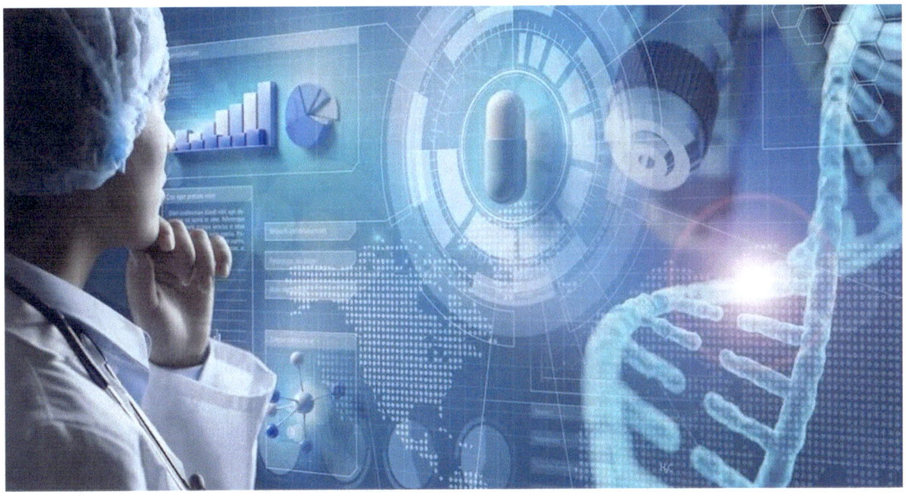

Figure 12.19. Clinical trials and emerging therapies for chronic leukemias.

Source: https://healthtree.org/images-resize?width=970&height=545&imageUrl=https%253A%252F%252Ffirebasestorage.googleapis.com%252Fv0%252Fb%252Fhealthtree-production.appspot.com%252Fo%252Fgallery%25252Fpublic%25252Fshutterstock_2217767129_1652f050-3d3e-4276-83ee-1b8444c7ce62.jpg%253Falt%253Dmedia.

12.4.8. Long-Term Management Strategies

Effective long-term management plans play a crucial role in enhancing the quality of life for patients with chronic leukemia. Survivors of pediatric HSCT often report long-lasting psychological distress and decreased quality of life, necessitating comprehensive follow-up care that addresses both physical and emotional health (Basso et al., 2017). Therapies such as counseling and support groups are helpful for survivors and can encourage them to join a supportive group. Furthermore, targeting specific molecular pathways, such as the PI3K/AKT/mTOR signaling cascade, presents promising therapeutic avenues for enhancing treatment efficacy and overcoming challenges associated with drug resistance (Badura et al., 2013). The best way to treat chronic leukemia is for clinicians to use a combination of medical, psychological, and social services, making sure each patient receives what they need to manage the disease in the long run.

12.4.9. Patient Education and Involvement in Treatment

Involving patients and teaching them properly is essential for managing chronic leukemias, as it encourages them to be actively involved in their care. When patients participate in specialized educational programs, they gain a deeper understanding of their condition, its treatment, and the importance of adhering to the doctor's instructions. When patients are involved in their treatment, the results are better, and they enjoy a higher quality of life, as they feel more responsible for their choices. Moreover, when patients are included in their care, they receive better psychosocial support and feel less alone due to their leukemia diagnosis. As highlighted in recent studies, the implementation of educational strategies and supportive care frameworks can ensure that patients are equipped with the necessary tools to navigate their treatment journey effectively, addressing not only the physical aspects of care but also the emotional needs accompanying chronic conditions like leukemia (Hameed et al., 2023; AlMusaileem et al., 2025) (Figure 12.20).

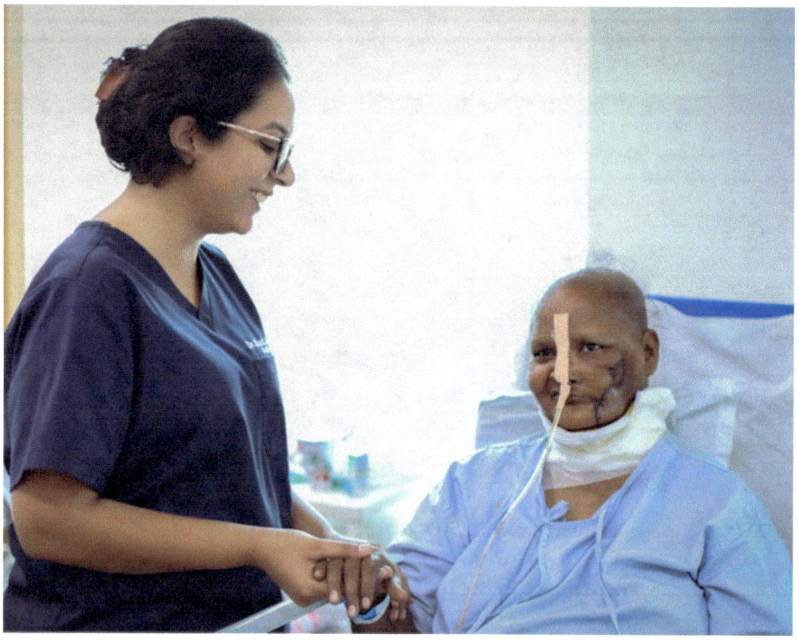

Figure 12.20. Effective patient education and involvement are critical components in managing chronic leukemias, as they empower patients to actively participate in their care.

Source: https://www.mgmch.org/images/oncology-about.jpg.

A CLOSER LOOK

B LYMPHOCYTES

B lymphocytes, or B cells, are a kind of WBC that helps the adaptive immune system. They primarily function by producing antibodies that can bind to foreign substances called antigens, which can include bacteria, viruses, or toxins. The binding process helps stop the invaders or identifies them for destruction by other parts of the immune system.

B cells are formed in the bone marrow, and when they encounter an antigen, they can either differentiate into plasma cells that produce large quantities of antibodies or become memory B cells to maintain long-lasting immunity. B lymphocytes are involved in balancing the immune system and presenting antigens to other immune cells.

SUMMARY

Treatment for chronic leukemias is greatly improved by the use of new strategies that help patients and reduce the risks of side effects. It is shown by studies that acalabrutinib and Obinutuzumab therapy leads to better outcomes than the previous standard chemoimmunotherapy. Specifically, the ELEVATE-TN study highlighted that 87% of patients receiving the novel combination maintained disease stability over four years, a stark contrast to just 25% of those undergoing conventional treatment, emphasizing the potential of targeted therapies in improving survival rates (Sharman et al., 2025). With time, learning about the effects of comorbidities, such as iron deficiency, helps improve the management of chronic leukemia. Such insights underscore the necessity for individualized treatment approaches that not only focus on disease control but also consider the overall health of patients to optimize therapeutic effectiveness (Mohamed et al., 2025).

Chronic leukemias involve many biological and medical factors that call for thorough understanding to handle them properly. A crucial aspect is epidemiology, which highlights that age, genetics, and lifestyle choices influence the risk of diseases. As discussed in the literature, treatment adherence emerges as a critical factor in achieving successful outcomes, necessitating multifaceted support strategies, including education and side-effect management (Czajka et al., 2024). Additionally, creating chemotherapy plans based on a person's genetic information may lead to improved outcomes and reduced side effects. This personalized approach aligns with innovative strategies aimed at enhancing immunotherapies, as evidenced by studies on bryostatin analogs that boost targeted treatment responses in leukemias by increasing the cell surface expression of key markers (Hardman et al., 2020). When all these elements are combined, they help improve treatment strategies and outcomes in patients with chronic leukemia..

REFERENCES

1. Abdalla, E., Fadul, A., Osman, A. E., Mohamed, G., Soliman, D. S., Shawayli, H., Abuasab, T., Almahmood, M., Saied, A., Mohamed, M., Ahmed, S., Singh, K., & Mohamed, S. (2024). Review of Rare Association between Chronic Lymphocytic Leukemia and Chromic Myeloid Leukemia. *Blood*, *144*(Supplement 1), 6805. https://doi.org/10.1182/blood-2024-205929Abuelfadol, E., Abdalla, M., Elsayid, M., & Agabeldour, A. (2024). Are chronic lymphocytic leukemia blood parameters differing from other leukemias subtypes? *Medical Research Updates Journal*. https://www.semanticscholar.org/paper/3cc5614704fe16a9c37542422138cb2f4430236c (accessed on 12th June 2025).

2. Agirre, X., Alvarez, S., Ammerpohl, O., Bibikova, M., et al. (2011). A comprehensive microarray-based DNA methylation study of 367 hematological neoplasms. https://core.ac.uk/download/14522607.pdf (accessed on 12th June 2025).

3. Aljabali, A. A., El-Tanani, M., Hromić-Jahjefendić, A., Lee, C., et al. (2024). The impact of the BCR-ABL oncogene in the pathology and treatment of chronic myeloid leukemia. https://core.ac.uk/download/638996109.pdf (accessed on 12th June 2025).

4. AlMusaileem, S., Almatter, E., Bourusly, M., AlMusaileem, W., Alabdulhadi, M. A., & Alsharidah, S. (2025). Hemolacria in children with hematological disorders: Case reports. *New Emirates Medical Journal*. https://www.semanticscholar.org/paper/7d7f2ffcdaea19b6b40ae2dca3eff2c4f84d5c33 (accessed on 12th June 2025).

5. Amadori, A., Piovan, E., Tosello, V., Zanovello, P., et al. (2018). Chemotactic cues for NOTCH1-dependent leukemia. https://core.ac.uk/download/154331808.pdf (accessed on 12th June 2025).

6. Angotzi, F., Cellini, A., Ruocco, V., Cavarretta, C. A., Zatta, I., Serafin, A., Pravato, S., et al. (2024). Chronic lymphocytic leukemia (CLL) with borderline immunoglobulin heavy chain mutational status, a rare subgroup of CLL with variable disease course. *Cancers, 16*. https://www.semanticscholar.org/paper/043167d733a5a0bd94640424668eb01260f1d96e (accessed on 12th June 2025).

7. Arcari, A., Morello, L., Borotti, E., Ronda, E., Rossi, A., & Vallisa, D. (2024). Recent advances in the molecular biology of chronic lymphocytic leukemia: How to define prognosis and guide treatment. *Cancers, 16*. https://www.semanticscholar.org/paper/a3c13c68ecb506ccc3f3b3f0d7d44f962adc11fb (accessed on 12th June 2025).

8. Badura, S., Falkenburg, J. H. F., Liebermann, M., Nijmeijer, R., et al. (2013). Differential effects of selective inhibitors targeting the PI3K/AKT/mTOR pathway in acute lymphoblastic leukemia. https://core.ac.uk/download/18326051.pdf (accessed on 12th June 2025).

9. Balan, Y., Sundaramurthy, R., Gaur, A., Varatharajan, S., & Raj, G. M. (2024). Impact of high-salt diet in health and diseases and its role in pursuit of cancer immunotherapy by modulating gut microbiome. *Journal of Family Medicine and Primary Care, 13*, 1628–1635. https://www.semanticscholar.org/paper/2e7578d82a95fb63e7bbbf1b897ac16206a7ec06 (accessed on 12th June 2025).

10. Bano, N., Gupta, Y., Khan, S., Rai, A., et al. (2024). Targeted therapies in cancer treatment: Unveiling the latest breakthroughs and promising approaches. https://core.ac.uk/download/597862456.pdf (accessed on 12th June 2025).

11. Basso, G., Boscolo, V., Calore, E., Cattelan, M., et al. (2017). Quality of life and psychopathology in adults who underwent hematopoietic stem cell transplantation (HSCT) in childhood: A qualitative and quantitative analysis. https://core.ac.uk/download/154330751.pdf (accessed on 12th June 2025).

12. Bennett, J. M., Wunderlich, B., Poleck-Dehlin, B., Chen, Z., Schmid, C., Cutler, C. S., De Witte, T., et al. (2006). Clonal karyotype evolution involving ring chromosome 1 with myelodysplastic syndrome subtype RAEB-t progressing into acute leukemia. https://core.ac.uk/download/16432948.pdf (accessed on 12th June 2025).

13. Bianchi, M. P., Gianfelici, V., Mirabilii, S., Piedimonte, M., et al. (2018). Biological aspects of mTOR in leukemia. https://core.ac.uk/download/188824881.pdf (accessed on 12th June 2025).

14. Bilban, M., Blatt, K., Cerny-Reiterer, S., Herndlhofer, B., et al. (2014). Dipeptidyl peptidase IV (CD26) defines leukemic stem cells (LSC) in chronic myeloid leukemia. https://core.ac.uk/download/42356265.pdf (accessed on 12th June 2025).

15. Bonaventure, A., Ito, Y., Katanoda, K., Magadi, M., et al. (2017). Childhood cancer incidence and survival in Japan and England: A population-based study (1993–2010). https://core.ac.uk/download/141439211.pdf (accessed on 12th June 2025).

16. Borogovac, A., & Siddiqi, T. (2024). Advancing CAR T-cell therapy for chronic lymphocytic leukemia: Exploring resistance mechanisms and the innovative strategies to overcome them. *Cancer Drug Resistance, 7*. https://www.semanticscholar.org/paper/e77ca6593c88f48f89a3c87864b922db6550843f (accessed on 12th June 2025).

17. Branford, S., Burger, H., Burgess, M. R., Cortes, J., Crossman, L. C., Donato, N. J., Druker, B. J., et al. (2007). Management of imatinib-resistant CML patients. https://core.ac.uk/download/16432346.pdf (accessed on 12th June 2025).

18. Brehme, M., Brümmendorf, T. H., Copland, M., et al. (2016). Combined population dynamics and entropy modelling supports patient stratification in chronic myeloid leukemia. https://core.ac.uk/download/42370689.pdf (accessed on 12th June 2025).

19. Broadway-Duren, J. B. (2022). An approach to diagnosis of Richter transformation in chronic lymphocytic leukemia. *Journal of the Advanced Practitioner in Oncology, 13*, 535–538. https://www.semanticscholar.org/paper/770d8063af3f030775c8cbd2482b1af855b9ab37 (accessed on 12th June 2025).

20. Brown, M. A., & Ducasse, M. (2006). Epigenetic aberrations and cancer. https://core.ac.uk/download/14502004.pdf (accessed on 12th June 2025).

21. Carrá, G., Torti, D., Crivellaro, S., Panuzzo, C., Taulli, R., Cilloni, D., Guerrasio, A., et al. (2016). The BCR-ABL/NF-κB signal transduction network: A long-lasting relationship in Philadelphia positive leukemias. *Oncotarget, 7*, 66287–66298. https://www.semanticscholar.org/paper/edac29d1f024f3b0fc568faf0173d9207b9ba737 (accessed on 12th June 2025).

22. Chatterjee, A., Jayaprakasan, M., Chakrabarty, A. K., Lakkaniga, N. R., Bhatt, B., Banerjee, D., Narwaria, A., et al. (2024). Comprehensive insights into rheumatoid arthritis: Pathophysiology, current therapies and herbal alternatives for effective disease management. *Phytotherapy Research, 38*, 2764–2799. https://www.semanticscholar.org/paper/3277199307711eb2cdf7412b2c2e6a23b704f1b2 (accessed on 12th June 2025).

23. Cheuk, D. K. L. (2013). Optimal stem cell source for allogeneic stem cell transplantation for hematological malignancies. https://core.ac.uk/download/38046057.pdf (accessed on 12th June 2025).

24. Cobb, N., Espey, D. K., & Paisano, R. E. (2003). Cancer mortality among American Indians and Alaska Natives: Regional differences, 1994–1998. https://core.ac.uk/download/151599885.pdf (accessed on 12th June 2025).

25. Croce, C. M., Kipps, T. J., Moshiri, F., Nakamura, M., et al. (2016). Upregulation of long noncoding RNA MIAT in aggressive form of chronic lymphocytic leukemias. https://core.ac.uk/download/323065221.pdf (accessed on 12th June 2025).

26. Czajka, A., Piaszczyński, S., Płeska, K., Reguła, M., et al. (2024). The impact of chemotherapy dose adjustment and delay in patients with leukemias and lymphomas who exercise. https://core.ac.uk/download/613192446.pdf (accessed on 12th June 2025).

27. Datta, M., & Jumaa, H. (2022). Immunoglobulin gene sequence as an inherited and acquired risk factor for chronic lymphocytic leukemia. *Cancers, 14*. https://www.semanticscholar.org/paper/bb0d1d26fcfd3140b583b3f5c64545a684a05429 (accessed on 12th June 2025).

28. Elango, A. (2024). Genetic diversity and variation in chronic myeloid leukemia patients of Indian origin—Implications for treatment response and prognosis. *International Journal of Molecular and Immune Oncology*. https://www.semanticscholar.org/paper/63bc12b0c9c501291848d54861b2b3a4498fa500 (accessed on 12th June 2025).

29. Erdem, S., Bayrak Tokaç, A. G., Aday, A., Karaca, D., Öztürk, Ş., Çefle, K., Yenerel, M., et al. (2024). Optical genome mapping in newly diagnosed chronic lymphocytic leukemia. *Blood*. https://www.semanticscholar.org/paper/aa397610d0135d3462a2464cdb5ddd401b025e51 (accessed on 12th June 2025).

30. Ferrando, A., Bash, H., Chen, X., Condorelli, G., Dube, I., Fisch, C., et al. (2012). The molecular basis of T cell acute lymphoblastic leukemia. https://core.ac.uk/download/55802201.pdf (accessed on 12th June 2025).

31. Flack, J., Buhnerkempe, M. G., & Moore, K. T. (2024). Resistant hypertension: Disease burden and emerging treatment options. *Current Hypertension Reports, 26*, 183–199. https://www.semanticscholar.org/paper/a268a53723a0ca76b9c3bbef50d1fba6ae4e7626 (accessed on 12th June 2025).

32. Gluzman, D. F., Ivanovskaya, T. S., Koval, S. V., Nadgornaya, V., et al. (2008). Study of morpho cytochemical and immunophenotypic features of acute leukemia stem cells.

33. Goel, V. (2024). Employability of the machine learning tools and techniques in the early detection and diagnosis of chronic kidney disease. *International Journal of Research in Medical Sciences and Technology*. https://www.semanticscholar.org/paper/cfea762f531edd999ce6c53656e57f343b6f892c (accessed on 12th June 2025).

34. Gou, L., Ma, X., Huang, L., Qiu, M., Guo, R., Jia, J., Xu, P., et al. (2025). The characteristics of chronic benzene poisoning in 176 Chinese occupational population cases. *Frontiers in Public Health, 12*. https://www.semanticscholar.org/paper/84ccad9e4678de72c7c6259f652c6cf0bed292c4 (accessed on 12th June 2025).

35. Hameed, M., Garcia, G., Yaseen, L., Sohail, I., Effendi, I., Amin, A., Ashraf, A., et al. (2023). Cancer survivorship in Gulf countries: An updated systematic review. *Blood*. https://www.

semanticscholar.org/paper/34a072740f574a586dd2845aa09a11da52fe4429 (accessed on 12th June 2025).

36. Hardman, C., Ho, S., Luu-Nguyen, Q., Marsden, M., et al. (2020). Synthesis and evaluation of designed PKC modulators for enhanced cancer immunotherapy. https://core.ac.uk/download/323075886.pdf (accessed on 12th June 2025).

37. Hossain, M. S., Ul, M., Asif, K., Rasham, R., Saaduzzaman, D. M., Maruf, M. H., Hasan, M. A., et al. (2024). Hybrid AI classification techniques for multi-class leukemia sub-types classification with bone marrow cells. *2024 6th International Conference on Sustainable Technologies for Industry 5.0 (STI).* https://www.semanticscholar.org/paper/56c1d6e48ea21cafe2e0d41698f55189449a19e0 (accessed on 12th June 2025).

38. Jabbour, E., & Kantarjian, H. (2024). Chronic myeloid leukemia: 2025 update on diagnosis, therapy, and monitoring. *American Journal of Hematology, 99*, 2191–2212. https://www.semanticscholar.org/paper/b3d30f2dce8b128df4350064a2a5963ef0768280 (accessed on 12th June 2025).

39. Javandoost, E., Firoozi-Majd, E., Rostamian, H., Khakpoor-Koosheh, M., & Mirzaei, H. (2019). Role of microRNAs in chronic lymphocytic leukemia pathogenesis. *Current Medicinal Chemistry*. https://www.semanticscholar.org/paper/1f3c7b0f4bf74a4ea886aee34ae4a3c73748d17b (accessed on 12th June 2025).

40. Jawed, M. A., Paswan, M. K., Mahto, S., Patra, S., Ashok, C., Ansari, M. A., Priya, A., et al. (2024). An extensive analysis and comparison of bone marrow aspiration and bone marrow trephine biopsy at a tertiary care hospital in Jharkhand for various hematological and non-hematological illnesses. *Cureus, 16*. https://www.semanticscholar.org/paper/32e696a7ca45fcbc8741ce86a244a19d63a9eb69 (accessed on 12th June 2025).

41. Johnson, M. (2024). Optimizing collaboration: A qualitative analysis of bone marrow transplant provider perceptions of palliative care roles. https://core.ac.uk/download/619714908.pdf (accessed on 12th June 2025).

42. Kaleem, B., Shahab, S., & Shamsi, T. S. (2024). T315I–a gatekeeper points mutation and its impact on the prognosis of chronic myeloid leukemia. *Advances in Laboratory Medicine, 5*, 412–417. https://www.semanticscholar.org/paper/9b3562de11dd39fe87cd931a47cd887c2451a0cc (accessed on 12th June 2025).

43. Korycka-Wołowiec, A., Wołowiec, D., Ławnicka, H., & Robak, T. (2025). Assessing adverse event burden in chronic lymphocytic leukemia treatment regimens: What's best for patient quality of life? *Expert Opinion on Drug Safety*. https://www.semanticscholar.org/paper/c12a6605ef121f59577f4a0826590ca34d8f4e63 (accessed on 12th June 2025).

44. Kuronuma, K., Shimokawahara, H., & Matsubara, H. (2025). An overview of balloon pulmonary angioplasty for chronic thromboembolic pulmonary hypertension. *Expert Review of Respiratory Medicine*. https://www.semanticscholar.org/paper/aeabc2f332f3d7911c488f68786b7ddaf5017d19 (accessed on 12th June 2025).

45. Kurucova, T., Reblova, K., Janovska, P., Porc, J., Navrkalova, V., Pavlova, S., Malcikova, J., et al. (2024). Unveiling the dynamics and molecular landscape of a rare chronic lymphocytic leukemia subpopulation driving refractoriness: Insights from single-cell RNA sequencing. *Molecular Oncology, 18*, 2541–2553. https://www.semanticscholar.org/paper/07a6a966875b5ea5d7794f14d6d61d330d5de332 (accessed on 12th June 2025).

46. Lee, M. H., Song, A., & Li, J. Y. (2024). Erythroid variant evolving from chronic myeloid leukemia resistant to multiple tyrosine kinase inhibitors: A rare case report. *Diagnostic Pathology, 19*. https://www.semanticscholar.org/paper/961fbe814e6befbde7774070599d6f2f5a6b4991 (accessed on 12th June 2025).

47. Ma, Y., Du, W., Shang, F., Song, L., Ma, B., He, S., Zheng, J., et al. (2024). A novel high-effective diagnostic model of chronic myelogenous leukemia by flow cytometry. *Blood*. https://www.semanticscholar.org/paper/d042cef29d53844139bb26a2af9dadfb30b79dfe (accessed on 12th June 2025).

48. Macaron, W., Sargsyan, Z., & Short, N. (2022). Hyperleukocytosis and leukocytosis in acute and chronic leukemias. *Leukemia & Lymphoma, 63*, 1780–1791. https://www.semanticscholar.org/paper/33ef569f99a093b8bcc061edb59c084f215857d8 (accessed on 12th June 2025).

49. Magagnoli, L., Ciceri, P., & Cozzolino, M. (2024). Secondary hyperparathyroidism in chronic kidney disease: Pathophysiology, current treatments and investigational drugs. *Expert Opinion on Investigational Drugs, 33*, 775–789. https://www.semanticscholar.org/paper/7806586389e4e34c00ae6c2ff4a57a268beaae0f (accessed on 12th June 2025).

50. Mishra, S., & Rai, S. (2024). A comparative study of bone marrow aspiration and bone marrow biopsy in hematological diseases in a tertiary care center of Central India—a retrospective study. *Global Journal for Research Analysis*. https://www.semanticscholar.org/paper/e32467f0383bd8f3dea6eb9da2a6f6b19cc3ebae (accessed on 12th June 2025).

51. Mohamed, A., Christensen, D. M., Mohammad, M., Torp-Pedersen, C., Koeber, L., Biering-Sørensen, T., Hansen, M. L., et al. (2025). Prognostic implications of iron deficiency in patients with atrial fibrillation, with and without chronic heart failure. *Heart*. https://www.semanticscholar.org/paper/1929b3cf82b8bb4a90388a60c16d6550f0a707ca (accessed on 12th June 2025).

52. Mohammad, F. I., & Nadim, A. R. (2025). Evaluating the correlation of age and gender with the hematological parameters of the chronic myeloid leukemia patients. *Journal of Biotechnology Research Center*. https://www.semanticscholar.org/paper/1e6d50897b6fa182929a7834d22be3c322da6546 (accessed on 12th June 2025).

53. Naik, J., Zuo, H., Kaspers, J., Karlsson-Parra, A., Rovers, J., Gjertsen, B. T., & Singh, S. (2024). *In vitro* interactions between TKIs and leukemic-derived dendritic cells as potential combination therapy for chronic myeloid leukemia. *Blood*. https://www.semanticscholar.org/paper/debcbeb1017ed6987fd63824fa97cbc22722bea9 (accessed on 12th June 2025).

54. Niedźwiecki, M., Budziło, O., Zieliński, M., Adamkiewicz-Drożyńska, E., Maciejka-Kembłowska, L., Szczepański, T., & Trzonkowski, P. (2018). CD4+CD25highCD127low/–FoxP3+ regulatory T cell subpopulations in the bone marrow and peripheral blood of children with ALL: Brief report. *Journal of Immunology Research, 2018*. https://www.semanticscholar.org/paper/9e6bbc4b0e09c8f61cc218e4c89585fba29f2f0e (accessed on 12th June 2025).

55. Ozturk, B., Celayir, A., Cibikci, A. O. G., Davulcu, C., & Kaynak, G. (2024). Surgical management of concurrent septic arthritis and forearm necrotizing fasciitis in an immunocompromised patient with a 20-year history of chronic lymphocytic leukemia: A case report. *Cureus, 16*. https://www.semanticscholar.org/paper/c3e70a3c59f55060a7d63f8791e51779173fd278 (accessed on 12th June 2025).

56. Patel, A. B., & Deininger, M. (2020). Genetic complexity of chronic myelomonocytic leukemia.

Leukemia & Lymphoma, 62, 1031–1045. https://www.semanticscholar.org/paper/9cdfec6a2cea92f083f593a10798239934eb50fd (accessed on 12th June 2025).

57. Paulson, C. (2016). The role of consolidation in reduced intensity transplantation for acute myeloid leukemia. https://core.ac.uk/download/644030421.pdf (accessed on 12th June 2025).
58. Piñero, P., Gonzalez, R., Díaz, V., Marin, E., Gonzalez, M., López, J., Manresa, P., et al. (2024). Single-tube flow cytometry 12-color combination for the screening, classification, and staging of chronic myelomonocytic leukemia. Correlation with NGS molecular data. *Blood*. https://www.semanticscholar.org/paper/7d48e16be1856295918b48697324a5f293b2107d (accessed on 12th June 2025).
59. Rinaldi, I., & Winston, K. (2023). Chronic myeloid leukemia, from pathophysiology to treatment-free remission: A narrative literature review. *Journal of Blood Medicine, 14*, 261–277. https://www.semanticscholar.org/paper/f303f105fac40b58fae95b1c9d270069a008946f (accessed on 12th June 2025).
60. Roeker, L., Burke, J., Rhodes, J. M., Emechebe, N., Jawaid, D., Manzoor, B. S., Jensen, C. E., et al. (2025). Real-world effectiveness of frontline treatments among patients with chronic lymphocytic leukemia: Results from ConcertAI. *Cancers, 17*. https://www.semanticscholar.org/paper/d2ad7d6ac71f3450c24a548ca4cb9aedf16a8091 (accessed on 12th June 2025).
61. Schmidt, T., Dahlberg, A., Berthold, E., Król, P., Arve-Butler, S., Rydén, E., Najibi, S. M., et al. (2023). Synovial monocytes contribute to chronic inflammation in childhood-onset arthritis via IL-6/STAT signaling and cell-cell interactions. *Frontiers in Immunology, 14*. https://www.semanticscholar.org/paper/e78e04562e7cabe6dacaaeaa0fecf74d66517a1f (accessed on 12th June 2025).
62. Schweiger, V., Cacciapuoti, M., Nizzero, M., Simari, S., Lombardi, G., Gottin, L., Stefani, L., et al. (2025). Exploring chronic pain in hemodialysis patients: An observational study based on the new IASP classification for ICD-11. *Pain and Therapy, 14*, 375–385. https://www.semanticscholar.org/paper/d2e63cf407468712e8b11eec93647c9a3c1b38b1 (accessed on 12th June 2025).
63. Sharman, J., & Hakre, S. (2025). Chemotherapy-free treatment with acalabrutinib can benefit patients with chronic lymphocytic leukemia/small lymphocytic lymphoma who were never treated before: A plain language summary of the ELEVATE-TN study. *Future Oncology, 21*, 737–748. https://www.semanticscholar.org/paper/2a144c4d6049239d9e077b68da01e411452107ae (accessed on 12th June 2025).
64. Smith, M. T., & Zhang, L. (1998). Biomarkers of leukemia risk: Benzene as a model. https://core.ac.uk/download/323068049.pdf (accessed on 12th June 2025).
65. Veldi, V. D. K., Gangahar, A., Kodapaka, L. N., Angara, S. S. P., Kaur, H., Sunil, A., Peela, S. T., et al. (2025). Emerging biomarkers in non-alcoholic fatty liver disease: A comprehensive narrative review of miRNA, lipidomic, and metabolomics for early detection and diagnosis. *Journal of Biomedical and Pharmaceutical Research*. https://www.semanticscholar.org/paper/98cf112aaebe31c25eb8996ed859c1a4d7dd289d (accessed on 12th June 2025).
66. Vysochinskaya, V., Dovbysh, O., Gorshkov, A., Brodskaia, A., Dubina, M., Vasin, A., & Zabrodskaya, Y. (2024). Advancements and future prospects in molecular targeted and siRNA therapies for chronic myeloid leukemia. *Biomolecules, 14*. https://www.semanticscholar.org/paper/bd8b52fa96af7f60aa6cda67c8d2af5fe1b9f458 (accessed on 12th June 2025).

67. Wang, Y., & Wang, F. (2024). Correlation of chronic periodontitis with Alzheimer's disease and research progress on salivary biomarkers. *Frontiers in Medical Science Research*. https://www.semanticscholar.org/paper/1c31a64ae784028a4dc0592a37d6889fb8470aba (accessed on 12th June 2025).

68. Wong, Z. C., Shen, Y., Rampotas, A., Gannon, I., Brierley, C. K., Benlabiod, C., Hayder, N., et al. (2024). Abstract C049: Implementing human bone marrow organoids to interrogate microenvironmental influences on the efficacy of blood cancer immunotherapies. *Cancer Research*. https://www.semanticscholar.org/paper/6aee8c91681fcd641874626a899d8a0762b404e9 (accessed on 12th June 2025).

69. Woolston, D. W., Lee, N. D., Shadman, M., Latorre-Esteves, E., Tee, X., Fredrickson, J., Kohrn, B. F., et al. (2023). Ultra-deep mutational landscape in chronic lymphocytic leukemia uncovers dynamics of resistance to targeted therapies. *Hematological, 109*, 835–845. https://www.semanticscholar.org/paper/34c30cbdff3d5098b499659aed6fc9e432fae082 (accessed on 12th June 2025).

70. Zheng, G., Chattopadhyay, S., Sud, A., Sundquist, K., Sundquist, J., Försti, A., Houlston, R., et al. (2019). Types of second primary cancers influence survival in chronic lymphocytic and hairy cell leukemia patients. *Blood Cancer Journal, 9*. https://www.semanticscholar.org/paper/1aeed0839963c0dfc0c354ade4eb5243257db8fa (accessed on 12th June 2025).

71. Zhou, Y., Yang, X., Liu, H., Luo, W., Liu, H., Lv, T., Wang, J., et al. (2021). Value of [^{68}Ga]Ga-FAPI-04 imaging in the diagnosis of renal fibrosis. *European Journal of Nuclear Medicine and Molecular Imaging, 48*, 3493–3501. https://www.semanticscholar.org/paper/8cc0e151d0dcd096397b7726f25e40e3a3c743f5 (accessed on 12th June 2025).

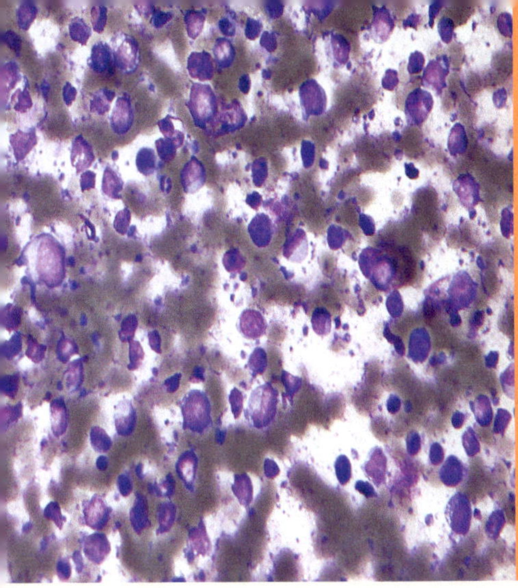

Chapter 13

LYMPHOMAS

Contents

Introduction.....325
13.1. Types of Lymphomas.....326
13.2. Causes and Risk Factors.....330
13.3. Diagnosis and Staging.....335
13.4. Treatment Options.....339
Summary.....346
References.....347

Introduction

Lymphomas are mostly found in the lymphatic system, which helps protect the body from infections. As these diseases are diverse, they are grouped into Hodgkin lymphoma (HL) and non-Hodgkin lymphoma (NHL), both of which have distinct characteristics, treatment approaches, and prognoses. Recent advancements in targeted therapies, including radionuclide treatments, have shown considerable promise in improving patient outcomes and minimizing harm to healthy tissues (Aquilina et al., 2008). Moreover, lymphomas can also exhibit secondary complications, such as hypereosinophilic syndrome, which presents diagnostic and therapeutic challenges due to its idiopathic nature (Brys et al., 2015). For this reason, examining lymphomas requires an understanding of their biology, as well as the latest approaches to treating them (Figure 13.1).

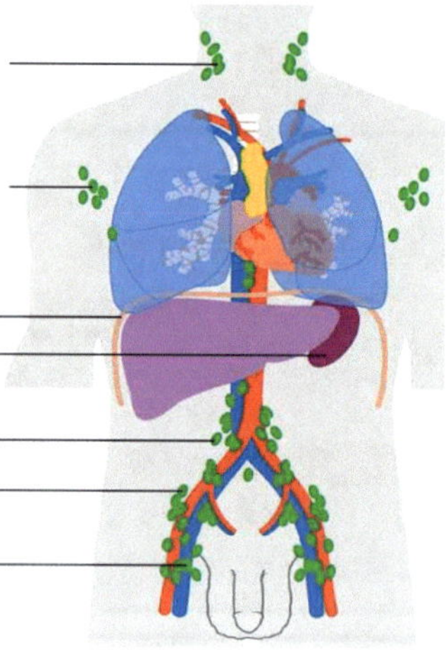

Figure 13.1. Lymphomas primarily originate in the lymphatic system, a vital component of the immune system responsible for combating infections.

Source: https://myhematology.com/wp-content/uploads/2024/02/Lymph-nodes.jpg.

13.1. Types of Lymphomas

Lymphomas, a diverse group of hematological malignancies, primarily fall into two main categories: Hodgkin lymphoma (HL) and non-Hodgkin lymphoma (NHL). HL is characterized by Reed-Sternberg cells and is known to spread from the lymph nodes in a typical manner, typically affecting younger individuals. However, NHLs are made up of more than 60 different types, which can also be classified as B-cell or T-cell neoplasms. The World Health Organization's system groups these lymphomas by looking at their appearance and immunology, which simplifies the process of diagnosis and treatment. Among the varieties of NHL, some, like primary non-Hodgkin lymphomas of the sinonasal tract, can be particularly challenging to differentiate from other malignancies due to their variable presentations, necessitating meticulous histopathological examination and immunohistochemistry for accurate diagnosis (Bhagat et al., 2009; Selvi et al., 2019).

13.1.1. Hodgkin Lymphoma (HL)

A form of lymphoid malignancy called Hodgkin lymphoma is characterized by Reed-Sternberg cells and is commonly classified into classic and nodular lymphocyte-predominant types. The pattern of HL's occurrence shows that it happens more often in young adults and in older people, which indicates that different factors may cause the disease at various ages. Data from the Golestan population-based cancer registry highlights that lymphomas, including HL, accounted for 4.67% of cancer cases diagnosed between 2004 and 2006, indicating a concerning trend in incidence in various geographical regions (Aarabi et al., 2011). Besides, since histological types are linked to the behavior of HLs, researchers are now looking into the complexities of its microenvironment. Studies indicate that the clinical behavior and prognosis may vary considerably, influenced by factors such as immune response and histopathological similarities with other lymphoid malignancies (Döring et al., 2013). It is crucial to understand these dynamics to enhance patient outcomes and select the most suitable treatment (Figure 13.2).

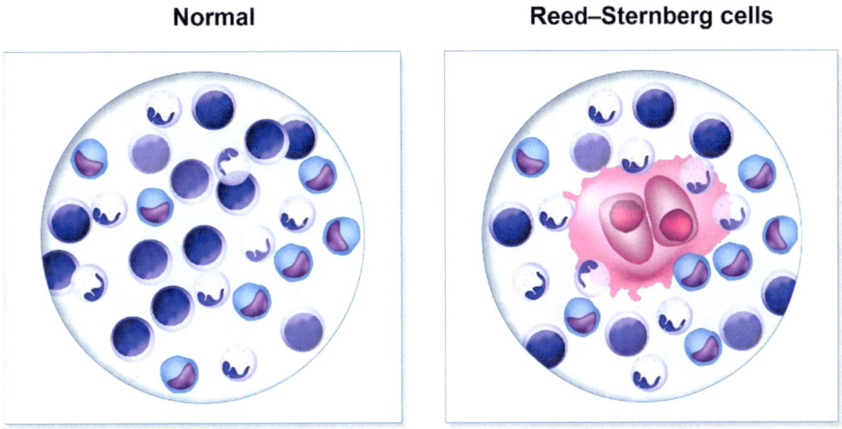

Figure 13.2. Hodgkin lymphoma classification.

Source: https://d2jx2rerrg6sh3.cloudfront.net/images/Article_Images/ImageForArticle_737_16637272234313617.jpg.

13.1.2. Non-Hodgkin Lymphoma (NHL)

As one of the most prevalent types of lymphoid malignancies, NHL encompasses a diverse group of hematological cancers primarily originating from B or T lymphocytes. NHL's complexity is demonstrated by its many subtypes, for example, diffuse large B-cell lymphoma and follicular lymphoma, which each have their own distinct clinical features and treatment challenges. The process of choosing a treatment is critical because there are many complex options. Decision aids have been proven beneficial in enhancing patient knowledge and satisfaction, as they guide individuals through weighing the pros and cons of treatment choices for conditions such as follicular lymphoma, thereby improving the overall decision-making experience (Lowery et al., 2007). Moreover, insights into lymphomas biology reveal remarkable similarities between specific subtypes of NHL and other lymphatic diseases, emphasizing the need for individualized treatment protocols (Diehl et al., 2011). All in all, this highlights the importance of patient involvement and the use of targeted methods by doctors.

13.1.3. Burkitt Lymphoma

Burkitt lymphoma is known to be very aggressive, as it causes tumors to develop quickly and mainly affects children and young adults. The MYC gene is often involved in chromosomal changes in this lymphoma, and these changes typically occur in conjunction with other cancer-causing mutations, which contribute to its severe behavior. Recent advancements in the classification of lymphoid neoplasms have refined our understanding of Burkitt lymphoma, as seen in the transition from earlier categorizations to a more hierarchical system in the 5th edition of the World Health Organization Classification (Alaggio et al., 2022). Additionally, genomic studies have shed light on the unique biological characteristics and clinical behavior of this malignancy, prompting updates to diagnostic criteria and treatment approaches (Elías Campo et al., 2022). These findings emphasize the importance of detecting lymphomas early and treating them effectively, as they grow rapidly and necessitate prompt action (Figure 13.3).

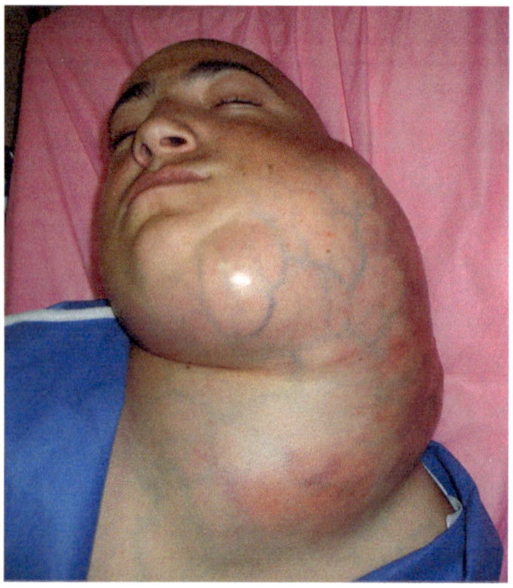

Figure 13.3. Burkitt lymphoma.

Source: https://www.bmj.com/content/bmj/351/bmj.h4545/F1.large.jpg?download=true.

13.1.4. Follicular Lymphoma

Follicular lymphoma is a specific type of NHL that originates in the germinal centers of B-lymphocytes. This slow-growing and unpredictable cancer is the second most usual type of lymphoma, showing the complexity of lymphoproliferative disorders. The pathology is closely associated with chromosomal translocations, particularly the (14;18) translocation, which leads to the overexpression of the BCL2 protein, promoting cell survival and contributing to immune evasion. Although follicular lymphoma develops slowly, it can become more aggressive, which is why it must be closely monitored and treated when necessary. Advances in therapy, for example PD-1 blockade, are helping to improve patient results, especially in the most challenging cases. The ongoing exploration of biomarkers, such as PD-1, in this context offers potential avenues for tailored treatment approaches, underscoring the critical need for continued research in the area of hematologic malignancies (Inan et al., 2023; Tateshita et al., 2025).

13.1.5. Diffuse Large B-Cell Lymphoma

Diffuse Large B-cell Lymphoma (DLBCL) represents the most common form of NHL, characterized by the rapid proliferation of large, malignant B cells. Since there are many kinds of cancer, it is essential to know about them to treat and manage the disease properly.

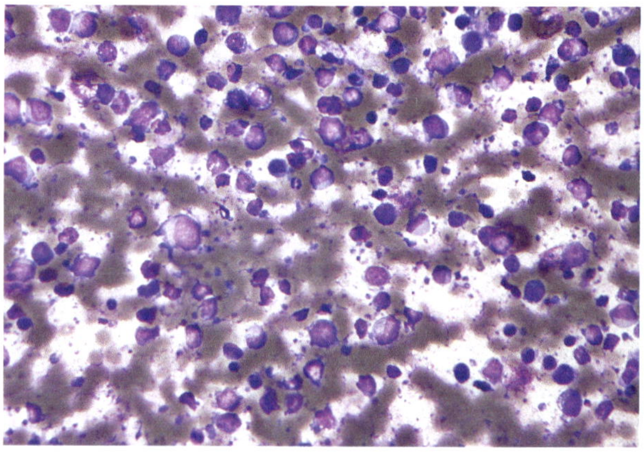

Figure 13.4. Diffuse large B-cell lymphoma (DLBCL).

Source: https://upload.wikimedia.org/wikipedia/commons/8/86/Diffuse_large_B_cell_lymphoma_-_cytology_low_mag.jpg.

Thanks to new research in genetics and molecular biology, experts have identified specific changes that cause DLBCL and have developed targeted treatments for it. For instance, distinct molecular profiles, such as activated B-cell-like (ABC) and germinal center B-cell-like (GCB) subtypes, indicate different prognoses and responses to treatment regimens. The role of diagnostic algorithms, as proposed by the Italian Group of Haematopathology, underscores the importance of integrating morphological and molecular assessments to optimize patient care, ensuring that those with aggressive forms receive intensified treatment reflective of their clinical needs (Agostinelli et al., 2019). This approach highlights a shift towards personalized medicine in tackling DLBCL and improving patient outcomes (Ansuinelli et al., 2017) (Figure 13.4).

13.1.6. Mantle Cell Lymphoma (MCL)

Mantle Cell Lymphoma (MCL) represents a distinct subgroup within the class of NHLs, characterized by a proliferation of neoplastic B-cells that typically express CD5 and BCL-1. MCL is more likely to affect older men, highlighting its common occurrence in this group, and is typically found at an advanced stage, which makes treatment more complicated. Current research is exploring innovative therapies, including chimeric antigen receptor T-cell (CAR-T) therapy, which has shown promise in managing relapsed or refractory cases of MCL.

A study on the efficacy of brexucabtagene autoleucel, a CAR-T treatment, illustrates the prognostic value of pre-treatment imaging, specifically FDG-PET/CT, in predicting patient outcomes after therapy. Patients achieving complete metabolic responses demonstrate significantly improved progression-free survival rates (Krauss et al., 2024). Additionally, the exploration of MCL within ocular adnexal lymphoma cases highlights its diverse manifestations, underscoring the need for tailored treatment approaches (Yu-ying Sun et al., 2024).

13.1.7. Peripheral T-Cell Lymphoma

Peripheral T-cell lymphoma (PTCL) represents a diverse category of NHLs that arise from mature T-cells, often exhibiting aggressive clinical behavior and a poor prognosis. Due to their variety, these lymphomas are challenging to diagnose and treat. The World Health Organization (WHO) classification system, which categorizes lymphoid neoplasms based on morphological and immunophenotypic characteristics, plays a crucial role in understanding these malignancies (Selvi et al., 2019). PTCLs are particularly notorious for their tendency to disseminate to extranodal sites, including the central nervous system (CNS), which occurs either at the time of initial diagnosis or upon relapse (Chiattone et al., 2021). Since the CNS is often involved, it is essential to closely monitor patients and employ various treatments, as finding effective ways to prevent CNS spread remains a major research goal. All in all, PTCL demonstrates that lymphoproliferative disorders are complicated and require special treatment plans for each patient (Figure 13.5).

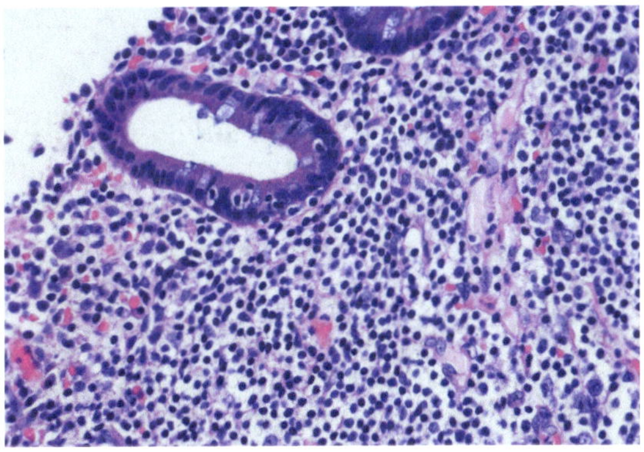

Figure 13.5. Peripheral T-cell lymphoma (PTCL) represents a diverse category of non-Hodgkin lymphomas that arise from mature T-cells, often exhibiting aggressive clinical behavior and a poor prognosis.

Source: https://www.cancertherapyadvisor.com/wp-content/uploads/sites/12/2019/07/nhlg618735906_1501199.jpg.

13.1.8. Anaplastic Large Cell Lymphoma

Anaplastic Large Cell Lymphoma (ALCL) represents a distinct subset of lymphomas characterized by the presence of large pleomorphic cells that typically express the CD30 marker. This characteristic feature distinguishes ALCL from other lymphoma types and highlights its unique pathology, making it a key consideration in the research and treatment of lymphoma. Evidence suggests a correlation between the expression of CD30 and potential therapeutic targeting, highlighting the importance of this biomarker in developing treatment strategies for ALCL patients (Garden et al., 2018). Furthermore, the understanding of ALCLs epidemiological features is exemplified through data from Kuwait, which illustrates that extranodal involvement occurs frequently within NHLs, including ALCL (Bamanikar et al., 2004). This indicates a strong need for further research and clinical trials to improve the care and outcomes of patients with this type of lymphoma.

13.1.9. Primary Mediastinal B-Cell Lymphoma (PMBCL)

Primary Mediastinal B-cell Lymphoma (PMBCL) represents a distinct subtype of Diffuse Large B-cell Lymphoma, characterized by its unique clinical presentation and biological behavior. Usually, this lymphoma starts in the mediastinum and is more common in young adults, mainly in females, often leading to symptoms such as chest pain, cough, and fever and weight loss. Recent studies suggest that PMBCL exhibits specific genetic alterations, including aberrations in the NOTCH signaling pathway, which play a crucial role in tumor development and progression (Zhou et al., 2022). The roles of these pathways in PMBCL show that the disease is complicated and encourage further research into new treatments. Since this type of lymphoma is very aggressive, the sooner it is found and managed, the better the patient's results. The integration of innovative therapeutic strategies alongside traditional approaches remains a pivotal area of exploration in enhancing the prognosis for individuals diagnosed with PMBCL (Alexander et al., 2022). (Figure 13.6).

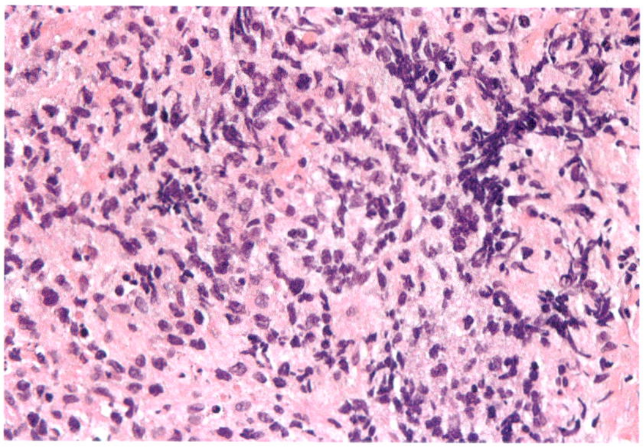

Figure 13.6. Primary mediastinal B-cell lymphoma (PMBCL).

Source: https://upload.wikimedia.org/wikipedia/commons/d/dd/Primary_mediastinal_large_B-cell_lymphoma_-_very_high_mag.jpg.

13.2. Causes and Risk Factors

To prevent and treat lymphomas well, it is essential to know their causes and risk factors. Lymphomas can develop due to both genetic factors and environmental factors. As an example, if a person has an inherited genetic condition, especially if their family has a history of blood cancers, they become more susceptible. Pesticides and solvents in the environment have been linked to a higher risk, primarily for individuals working in agriculture. Furthermore, research has shown that factors like age and sex play significant roles; younger patients and females tend to have better survival outcomes, as evidenced by studies indicating complete remission as a key determinant of survival (*see*

(Angrilli et al., 2019). Additionally, secondary malignancies due to prior treatments can complicate patient care and negatively impact prognosis, particularly in transplant recipients where immune suppression is necessary (Abu-Elmagd et al., 1995). All of these factors together indicate that lymphomas are complex, so each patient requires a personalized treatment plan.

13.2.1. Genetic Predisposition

Learning about genetic predisposition is crucial in lymphoma research, as some subtypes are often found in families. Research has shown that most lymphomas develop by chance; however, there are some cases where a family history suggests a genetic cause. For instance, in the evaluation of early-onset cancer risks among different racial and ethnic groups, significant variations in standardized incidence ratios (SIRs) were identified, hinting at genetic vulnerability based on familial lineage (de Smith et al., 2023). Specifically, studies on nodular lymphocyte-predominant Hodgkin lymphoma (NLPHL) and primary mediastinal large B-cell lymphoma have identified genetic alterations associated with predisposition in affected families. A compelling finding was a germline deletion in the NPAT gene associated with NLPHL susceptibility, indicating that genetic factors may contribute significantly to lymphoma risk in certain families (Saarinen et al., 2013). These discoveries enhance our understanding of lymphoma development and encourage further studies on families with a high risk of lymphoma (Figure 13.7).

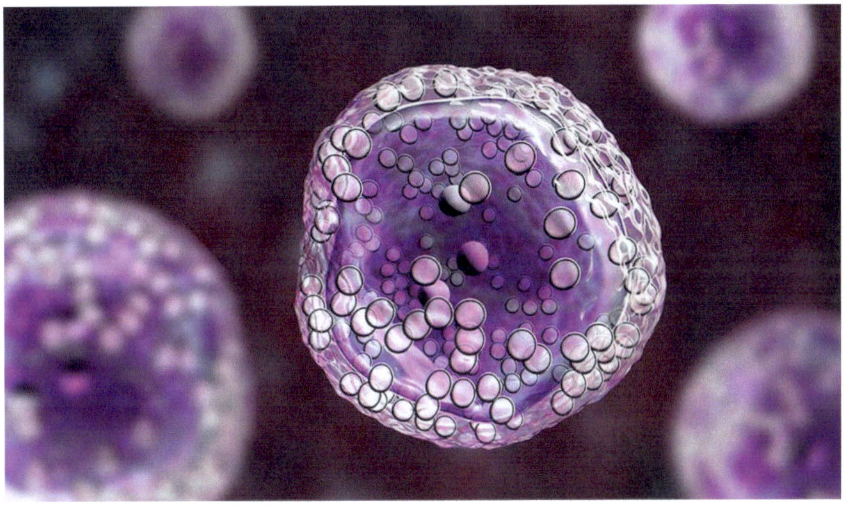

Figure 13.7. B-cell lymphoma.

Source: https://www.moffitt.org/contentassets/7431e4b707e44f768b878528b80502ef/b-cell-lymphoma.jpg.

13.2.2. Environmental Factors

Environmental factors play a pivotal role in the etiology of lymphomas, particularly influencing the incidence and progression of diffuse large B-cell lymphoma (DLBCL), the most prevalent type of NHL. Being exposed to certain chemicals, pesticides, and radiation may increase the risk of developing lymphomas, indicating that both environmental factors and genetics play a role. For instance, studies indicate that aberrant methylation patterns, such as those involving the GADD45γ gene, are associated with DLBCL progression, with methylation occurring more frequently in advanced-stage tumors compared to early-stage tumors (Barış et al., 2015). Furthermore, the landscape of immune signaling is altered by environmental stressors, such as pollutants, which can disrupt critical cellular processes, including those mediated by the ubiquitin system, thereby increasing susceptibility to lymphoma development (Fulda et al., 2012). To sum up, learning about these environmental factors is essential for designing effective prevention and therapy plans.

13.2.3. Viral Infections (e.g., EBV, HIV)

The interplay between viral infections and lymphomas is notably exemplified by the roles of Epstein-Barr Virus (EBV) and Human Immunodeficiency Virus (HIV). EBV, classified under the gammaherpesvirinae subfamily, is a well-established oncogenic virus implicated in various lymphoid tumors, including Burkitt's lymphoma (BL) and Hodgkin's disease. Notably, studies have demonstrated a significant association between elevated EBV levels in peripheral blood and the presence of non-Hodgkin lymphomas, as illustrated in research involving pediatric populations in northwestern Tanzania, where high EBV load correlated with lymphoma cases (Filipovich et al., 2013). Concurrently, while HIV is predominantly recognized for its immunosuppressive effects, its role in lymphomagenesis remains complex; however, evidence suggests that it does not significantly correlate with specific NHL subtypes when analyzed alongside EBV load (Abdel-Hamid et al., 2015). That is why it is essential to understand how viral infections contribute to lymphoma, both individually and in combination (Figure 13.8).

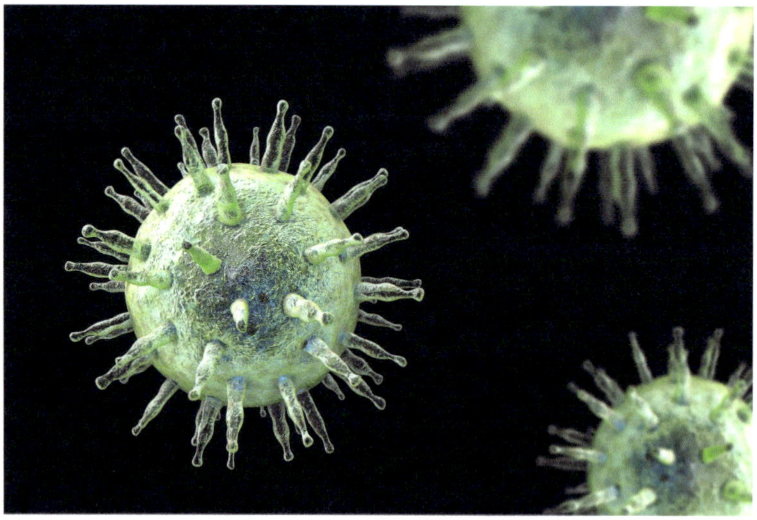

Figure 13.8. Epstein-barr virus (EBV).

Source: https://img.lb.wbmdstatic.com/vim/live/webmd/consumer_assets/site_images/article_thumbnails/BigBead/1800x1200_epstein_barr_bigbead.jpg.

13.2.4. Autoimmune Diseases

Autoimmune diseases are now considered important factors that increase the risk of developing lymphomas, which are many different types of cancer coming from lymphocytes. It is primarily due to the significant immune system issues in autoimmune diseases, which can lead to persistent inflammation and damage to cells. It is demonstrated that continuous inflammation facilitates the development of lymphoma and also impairs the body's ability to eliminate transformed cells. Certain autoimmune disorders are linked to particular types of lymphoma, showing that the kind of autoimmune disease might play a role in which lymphoma develops. Furthermore, as highlighted in recent studies, innovations in diagnostic techniques, such as the use of radiolabeled monoclonal antibodies, can enhance the assessment of malignancies associated with autoimmune diseases, offering new avenues for targeted therapy and patient management in this vulnerable population (Auletta et al., 2016; Kolijn et al., 2023).

13.2.5. Age and Gender Considerations

Understanding how a person's age and gender affect lymphoma epidemiology and prognosis is crucial. Research indicates that males are diagnosed at younger ages and exhibit significantly higher incidence rates compared to females across various lymphoma subtypes, with a noted male/female rate ratio of 2.2 in the under-15 age group for all subtypes combined (Fritz et al., 2015). Such a gap in healthcare can lead to more cases of these diseases and may also affect the way treatments are administered and their outcomes. Additionally, survival rates can vary significantly among lymphoma subtypes, with certain conditions, such as nodular lymphocyte-predominant Hodgkin lymphoma, achieving survival rates comparable to those of the general population, while others exhibit dramatically lower survival rates, particularly among less common B-cell and T-cell lymphomas (Fritz et al., 2015). That's why it is necessary to take both age and gender into account in treating and researching lymphoma to achieve the best results for patients (Figure 13.9).

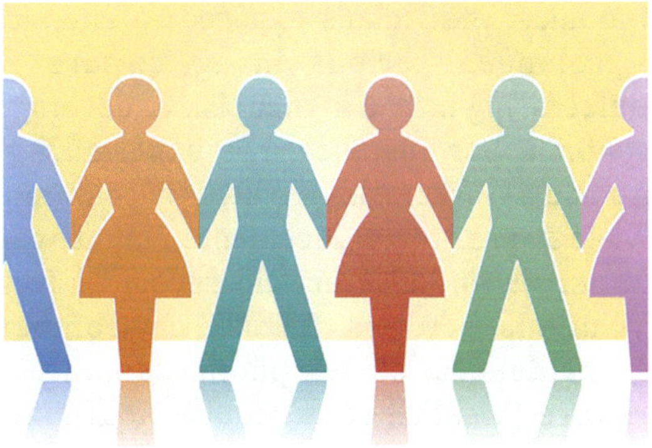

Figure 13.9. Age and gender are critical factors in understanding the epidemiology and prognosis of lymphomas.

Source: https://clf1.medpagetoday.com/assets/images/resource-center/cs-Patient-Demographics-Follicular-Lymphoma-61618.jpg.

13.2.6. Family History

Learning about family history is essential for lymphoma, since it is clear that genetics can play a role in causing the disease. It has been found that having family members with lymphoma suggests that certain genetic factors may play a significant role in its development. For instance, the association between human leukocyte antigen (HLA) variations and specific types of lymphomas underscores this connection. Research has shown that HL and NHL demonstrate varying associations with HLA polymorphisms, indicating that antigen presentation may influence disease development (Jarrett et al., 2015). Additionally, recent findings have highlighted the genetic underpinnings of conditions like Weaver syndrome, linking histone methylation to overgrowth syndromes that could indirectly relate to lymphoma predisposition, further emphasizing the importance of family history in the context of genetic research (Banka et al., 2011).

13.2.7. Occupational Exposures

Being exposed to specific jobs and workplaces can increase a person's chances of developing lymphomas. Individuals exposed to chemicals for prolonged periods in agriculture and manufacturing have a higher risk of developing lymphoma. For instance, the experiences of retired autoworkers, highlighted by community activists such as those documented in the works of Marshall (Mike) Westfall, reveal alarming correlations between factory environments and incidences of lymphoma among the workforce (Westfall et al., 2009). Additionally, environmental hazards from poorly managed landfill sites further accentuate these risks, where uncontrolled leachate and landfill gases may seep into nearby waters and air, potentially affecting the health of workers and surrounding communities (Bruen et al., 2004). So, it is essential to address these occupational risks to lessen the chances of lymphomas in those who are at risk (Figure 13.10).

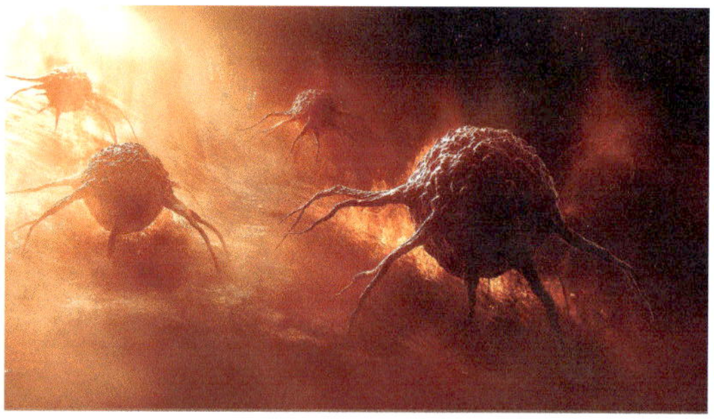

Figure 13.10. Occupational exposures play a significant role in the etiology of lymphomas, as certain industries and work environments present increased risk factors for these malignancies.

Source: https://assets.neurosurgicalatlas.com/aaroncohen-gadol-com/Patient_Education/Lymphoma/LymphomaBlog2Pic1.png.

13.2.8. Lifestyle Factors (e.g., Smoking, Diet)

Understanding how lifestyle affects the risk of lymphomas plays a crucial role in developing effective prevention methods. Smoking is known to increase the risk of lymphomas and other cancers since it weakens the immune system and leads to changes in genes. Furthermore, dietary choices play a crucial role; for instance, high consumption of processed foods and artificial sweeteners such as aspartame (APM) has been linked to adverse health outcomes, which raises concerns regarding their connection to cancer, including lymphomas. Although many individuals perceive APM as a harmless alternative for health improvement, emerging studies suggest that its consumption may be associated with various health issues, potentially increasing lymphoma risk (Majd et al., 2016). Additionally, the influence of environmental and lifestyle factors is significant, as evidenced by research indicating that such variables account for over 80% of certain cancers. However, the specific interactions with lymphoma risk remain less thoroughly understood (Park et al., 2020).

13.2.9. Previous Cancer Treatments

Over the years, new cancer treatments have significantly impacted the management of lymphomas, particularly in the field of immunotherapy. The introduction of monoclonal antibodies, including rituximab, has significantly improved the treatment of CD20+ lymphomas and increased survival rates among many patients. Because of this therapeutic approach, more monoclonal antibodies are now available for patients, even though their effectiveness is still being tested in clinical trials. In particular, a significant study found that survival outcomes were the same for high-dose chemotherapy, rituximab, and autograft as for conventional chemotherapy, indicating that CHOP-R is effective. Patients who achieved a complete remission also had significantly better survival rates, demonstrating that effective treatment outcomes substantially improve long-term outcomes. Overall, these advances reflect a dynamic shift in lymphoma treatment paradigms, paving the way for more tailored and effective management of these malignancies (Aurer et al., 2011; Angrilli et al., 2019) (Figure 13.11).

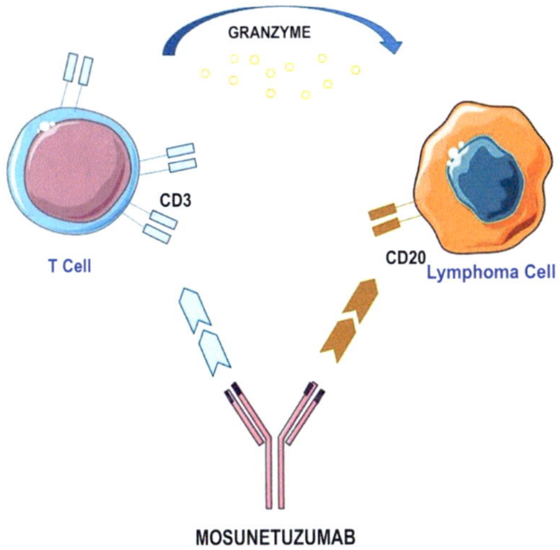

Figure 13.11. Mechanism of action of mosunetuzumab.

Source: https://pub.mdpi-res.com/cancers/cancers-17-01602/article_deploy/html/images/cancers-17-01602-g001.png?1746718028.

13.3. Diagnosis and Staging

It is crucial to accurately diagnose and stage lymphomas, as these steps significantly impact the type of treatment provided and the patient's outcome. Typically, a doctor will use clinical tests, examine tissue under a microscope, and perform imaging to determine the type of lymphoma. The extent of the disease and the chosen treatment depend largely on how staging is done using guidelines from research organizations. For instance, HL is known for its curability, with recent advancements emphasizing individualized treatment approaches that incorporate both chemotherapy and radiotherapy, tailored according to staging results (Su, 2019). In the context of NHL, studies indicate that factors such as the involvement of lymph nodes or the gastrointestinal tract can complicate the prognosis, affecting overall survival rates (Grégoire Marques et al., 2024). As a result, making a detailed diagnosis and accurate staging is crucial to inform therapies and improve outcomes for lymphoma patients.

13.3.1. Initial Symptoms and Clinical Evaluation

Spotting the first signs of lymphoma is very important for early treatment and a better outcome. Many patients exhibit symptoms such as fever, unexplained weight loss, and night sweats, which are similar to signs of infection. This clinical overlap necessitates thorough evaluation to distinguish between lymphomas and other conditions (Androutsos et al., 2011).

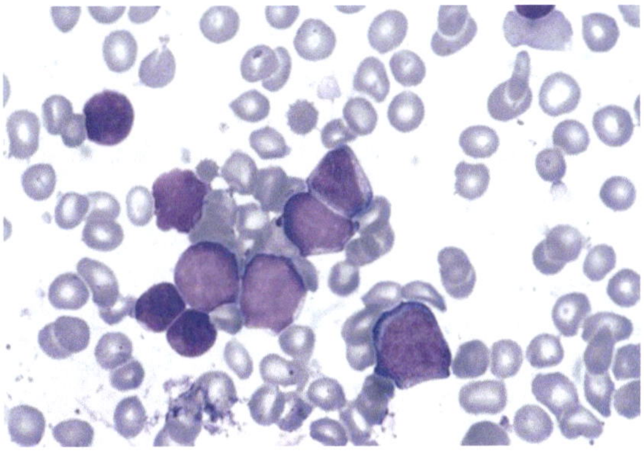

Figure 13.12. In cases where lymphomas are suspected, diagnostic techniques such as flow cytometry can provide crucial insights, especially when atypical cells are observed in blood or effusions.

Source: https://clinicalgate.com/wp-content/uploads/2015/03/B9780702031472000298_f029-013-9780702031472.jpg.

When lymphomas are suspected, flow cytometry provides important information, especially when unusual cells are detected in blood or fluid samples. It has been helpful in detecting aggressive lymphomas that at first are only noticed as fevers of unknown source. Moreover, the classification of these malignancies has been refined through techniques such as nuclear DNA content analysis, which correlates significantly with prognosis, thereby enhancing the accuracy of clinical evaluations (Abmayr et al., 1991). Assessing patients in such detail is very important for helping them and designing personalized treatment plans (Figure 13.12).

13.3.2. Imaging Techniques (e.g., CT, PET Scans)

Advancements in imaging techniques, particularly computed tomography (CT) and positron emission tomography (PET) scans, have substantially enhanced the diagnostic capabilities for lymphomas. They enable doctors to examine lymphatic tissues and assess the disease's progression, which is crucial for determining the next steps. Although CT scans enable doctors to visualize enlarged lymph nodes and structural changes, PET scans are crucial for distinguishing between active disease and residual masses by detecting metabolic alterations. Still, we should mention that these methods have some drawbacks, such as the potential for radiation exposure during CT and PET scans, which makes some people concerned about the patients' safety. Despite these drawbacks, early detection through these imaging methods remains vital, as it potentially improves patient outcomes through timely interventions, as highlighted by ongoing research in nuclear medicine (Baianu, 2011) and innovative approaches to diagnosis that continue to evolve in this field (Baianu et al., 2011).

13.3.3. Biopsy Procedures

Biopsies are crucial in diagnosing and treating lymphomas because they enable doctors to determine the most effective treatment based on precise tissue findings. Among these techniques, fine-needle aspiration (FNA) biopsy has emerged as a crucial method, particularly for evaluating lymphadenopathy, enabling pathologists to obtain cellular material with minimal invasiveness. The sensitivity of FNA in diagnosing head and neck lymphomas is notably high, with reported figures demonstrating a sensitivity of 90% and a specificity of 88% (Aurer et al., 2010). Therefore, FNA is very useful before other procedures, as it provides quick and helpful information for making decisions about a patient's care. Moreover, understanding the appearance of cells with immunocytochemistry is very important because it helps to sort lymphomas correctly. In cases where lymphoproliferative lesions arise post-transplantation, reducing immunosuppression has shown potential for regressing these lesions, highlighting the complexity and importance of biopsy procedures in lymphoma diagnostics (Atchison et al., 1984).

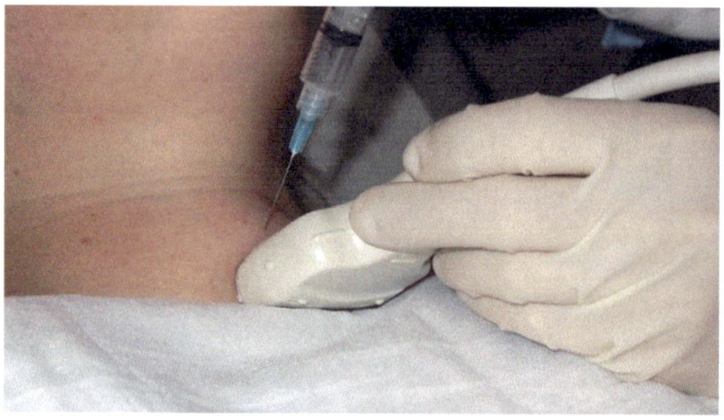

Figure 13.13. Fine-needle aspiration (FNA) biopsy has emerged as a crucial method particularly for evaluating lymphadenopathy, enabling pathologists to obtain cellular material with minimal invasiveness.

Source: https://www.fvhospital.com/wp-content/uploads/2020/02/fine-needle-aspiration-for-head-and-neck-conditions-1.jpg.

13.3.4. Blood Tests and Markers

Blood tests and markers are very important in diagnosing, monitoring, and predicting the outcome of lymphomas. Advances in global gene expression profiling enable the classification of tumors based on gene expression patterns, thereby enhancing the accuracy of lymphoma diagnosis, regardless of histological characteristics (Morris et al.,

2016). Proteomic studies have also been highly beneficial, identifying biomarkers in blood and other bodily fluids that aid in understanding tumors and how patients respond to therapy. For example, hypercalcemia in patients with high-grade lymphoma has been associated with immune reconstitution inflammatory syndrome, underscoring the dynamic interplay between lymphoma progression and metabolic changes (Bikle et al., 2019). They enable early diagnosis of conditions and the selection of the most effective treatment plan, ultimately benefiting the patient. As studies advance, it is expected that blood tests used in lymphoma treatment will become more sophisticated and tailored to each patient's specific needs.

13.3.5. Staging Systems (Ann Arbor, Lugano)

It is essential to be familiar with the Ann Arbor and Lugano staging systems to effectively manage lymphomas. They make it possible to measure the severity of the disease and inform the doctor on the most appropriate treatment. For instance, in localized cases of primary gastric diffuse large B-cell lymphoma (PG-DLBCL), the choice between surgery and chemotherapy options can profoundly affect patient outcomes, as evidenced by clinical characteristics revealing survival disparities associated with treatment approaches (Yu et al., 2015). Additionally, extranodal marginal zone lymphoma (EMZL), which often presents in various organs and is linked to chronic inflammatory processes, exemplifies the complexity of staging. The lack of consensus on the optimal staging system across different countries complicates treatment strategies, emphasizing the necessity for precise staging to tailor therapeutic interventions effectively (Bewarder et al., 2022). So, both approaches are essential in guiding the treatment of lymphoma patients (Figure 13.14).

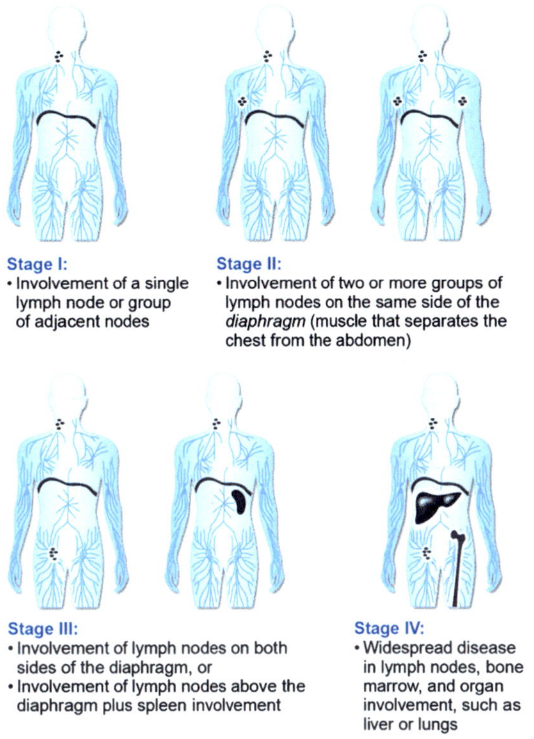

Figure 13.14. The staging systems.

Source: https://lymphoma.org/wp-content/uploads/2022/07/Lugano-Classification-793x1024.png.

13.3.6. Prognostic Factors

It is crucial in lymphoma research to identify factors that can predict a patient's outcome, allowing for customized treatment plans and improved results. Various studies have emphasized the significance of genetic aberrations, wherein C-MYC abnormalities have emerged as a notable, independent prognostic factor in DLBCL. Patients exhibiting these genetic changes face a markedly poorer prognosis, with overall survival rates significantly decreased (HR 2.22) compared to those without such aberrations (Zhou et al., 2014). Conversely, in Burkitt lymphoma, survival rates are intricately linked to demographic and disease characteristics, such as age, race, and disease stage, which influence overall survival outcomes

(Jorge et al., 2013). The evidence from these studies suggests that a clear understanding of prognostic factors helps explain the complexity of lymphoma and highlights the need for personalized care tailored to each patient's specific details for optimal outcomes.

13.3.7. Role of Pathologists

Pathologists help significantly in the diagnosis and treatment of lymphomas by identifying the different types of the disease using advanced tools. Thanks to their knowledge, they can review complex data from histology and immunology to differentiate between various types of lymphoid cancers.

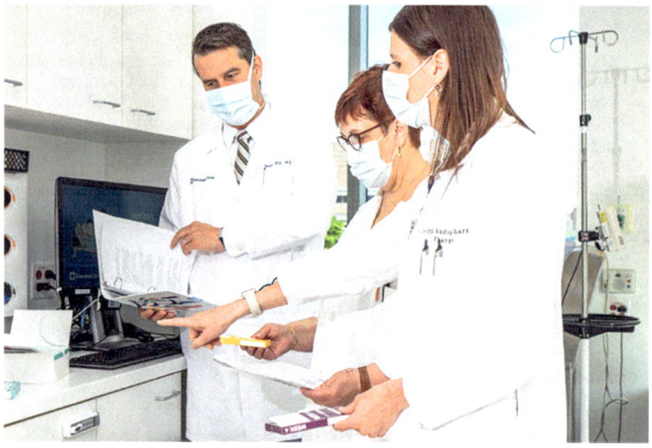

Figure 13.15. Pathologists play an indispensable role in the diagnosis and management of lymphomas.

Source: https://my.clevelandclinic.org/-/scassets/images/org/care-pages/cancer/non-hodgkin-lymphoma-feature.jpg?w=3840&q=75.

For instance, studies have shown that proteins such as B-cell maturation antigen (BCMA) and Netrin-1 exhibit sensitivity and specificity in specific lymphoma subtypes, notably plasmablastic and classical Hodgkin lymphomas, thereby aiding pathologists in making complex diagnoses that can inform therapeutic decisions (Donzel et al., 2025). Furthermore, in the context of cutaneous T-cell lymphomas, a multidisciplinary approach, which includes pathologists, is essential due to the multifaceted nature of these diseases and the limited treatment options available (Oliveira et al., 2024). Therefore, pathologists play a crucial role in designing personalized care and supporting patients with lymphoma (Figure 13.15).

13.3.8. Importance of Accurate Diagnosis

It is crucial to make an accurate diagnosis of lymphomas to effectively manage patients and achieve optimal treatment outcomes. It is crucial to recognize the various types of aggressive mature B cell lymphomas, as the treatment plan depends on the specific diagnosis. Current diagnostic protocols involve a combination of morphological, immunophenotypical, and cytogenetic analyses, which despite being resource-intensive, are essential for optimal disease management (Agostinelli et al., 2019). Furthermore, the significance of early and accurate diagnosis extends to other malignancies as well, as demonstrated by studies on salivary gland lesions wherein fine needle aspiration cytology (FNAC) achieved a diagnostic accuracy of 92%, thereby facilitating timely therapeutic interventions (Agravat et al., 2012). For this reason, using advanced diagnostic methods in hematopathology helps treat lymphoma and similar diseases more effectively, improving patient outcomes.

13.3.9. Challenges in Diagnosis

Lymphomas are challenging to diagnose, which has a significant effect on patients' outcomes and the methods used to treat them. A major obstacle lies in the diversity of health-related quality-of-life (HRQoL) instruments used to assess the experiences of patients with hematological malignancies, which can lead to inconsistencies in understanding and interpreting their symptoms and needs (Goswami et al., 2019).

Furthermore, primary diffuse large B-cell lymphoma (DLBCL) of the central nervous system illustrates additional diagnostic complications due to its aggressive nature and unique biological characteristics, complicating efforts to achieve timely and accurate diagnoses (Cwynarski et al., 2014). It is more difficult for older patients, those with weak immune systems, and people with relapsed or refractory disease, since there is not much clinical trial data available for them. For this reason, it is essential to utilize advanced techniques and collaborate with specialists to enhance the effectiveness of lymphoma diagnosis and treatment s(Figure 13.16).

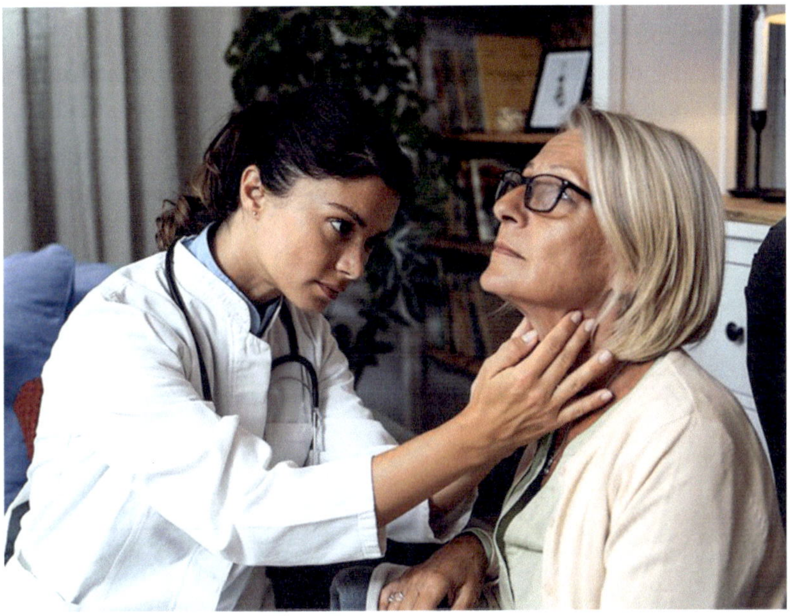

Figure 13.16. The diagnosis of lymphomas presents numerous challenges that significantly impact patient outcomes and treatment approaches.

Source: https://media.post.rvohealth.io/wp-content/uploads/sites/3/2023/11/female-doctor-patient-neck-732x549-thumbnail.jpg.

13.4. Treatment Options

Lymphoma treatment has undergone significant improvements, particularly with the introduction of targeted therapies, which have greatly benefited patients. Rituximab, a chimeric anti-CD20 monoclonal antibody, is now an important part of treating different B-cell cancers. Its effectivenesss in prolonging disease-free survival and overall survival has been well-documented across a range of conditions, including diffuse large B-cell lymphoma and chronic lymphocytic leukemia (CLL) (Abulayha et al., 2017). Moreover, innovative strategies, such as encapsulating rituximab within zwitterionic polymer layers for enhanced CNS delivery, are emerging to tackle metastatic challenges that traditional therapies struggle to address (Chen et al., 2019). These new approaches to treating lymphoma are expected to enhance the management of the disease and also reduce the number of side effects.

13.4.1. Chemotherapy Regimens

Managing lymphoma often depends on chemotherapy, which is the primary treatment given to patients with Hodgkin's and NHL. Choosing the right treatment plan depends on factors such as the severity of the illness, the patient's age, and their overall health. Studies have shown that a patient's unique risk factors significantly influence the effectiveness of treatment, suggesting that treatments should be tailored to each individual. In a hospital-based study, progressive disease was observed in 37.3% of patients undergoing chemotherapy, highlighting the variable efficacy of different regimens in managing this heterogeneous group of malignancies (Degala et al., 2025). Furthermore, while short-course chemotherapy has shown promise in other settings, it raises questions regarding efficacy and safety in lymphoma patients (Abramchenko et al., 2025). The results emphasize the need to adjust chemotherapy plans to enhance success rates and improve patient well-being, thereby making treatments more personalized in oncology (Figure 13.17).

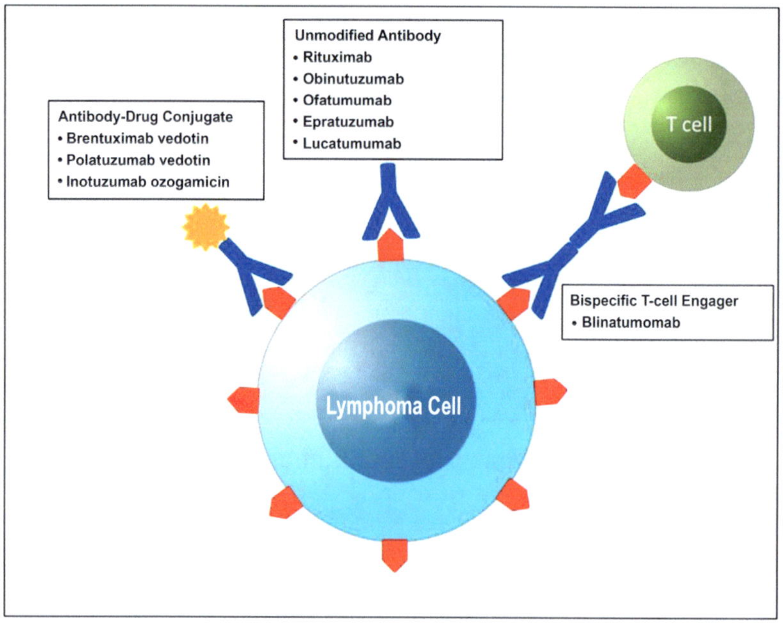

Figure 13.17. Chemotherapy regimens are critical in the management of lymphomas, serving as the cornerstone of treatment for both Hodgkin and non-Hodgkin lymphoma.

Source: https://www.mdpi.com/pharmaceuticals/pharmaceuticals-08-00607/article_deploy/html/images/pharmaceuticals-08-00607-g001.png.

13.4.2. Radiation Therapy

Radiation therapy is vital in treating lymphomas by reducing the tumor and easing symptoms. This treatment is beneficial for certain lymphomas, for example, primary cutaneous lymphomas, as low-dose radiotherapy is often used even though there are no controlled studies to determine the optimal radiation dose for each type of lymphoma. Consequently, radiation oncologists usually face the challenge of making individualized treatment decisions, a situation that underscores the need for more robust clinical evidence to guide therapies (Adeberg et al., 2024). Furthermore, the association of Epstein-Barr virus (EBV) with lymphoproliferative diseases complicates the landscape of lymphoma treatment, as EBV is known to influence the disease's aggressiveness and the patient's prognosis. Understanding these connections can enhance treatment strategies, ultimately aiming for more favorable outcomes in affected patients (Fox et al., 2011).

13.4.3. Targeted Therapies

Targeted therapies have made a big difference in lymphoma treatment by providing more accurate and effective options than the previous methods. They target specific processes that cause lymphoma cells to grow and live, which helps to keep normal cells safe. Recent advancements have revealed specific targets, such as the CCR4 receptor, which is crucial in cutaneous T-cell lymphoma (CTCL) due to its role in tumor immune evasion. Monoclonal antibodies, such as mogamulizumab, demonstrate the potential of targeting CCR4 to reduce tumor burden while enhancing patient outcomes through their ability to disrupt malignant T-cell functionality (Agostinelli et al., 2024). Furthermore, the growing understanding of genetic alterations in lymphomas has facilitated the development of personalized treatment strategies, thereby enhancing efficacy (Bano et al., 2024). However, since issues with drug resistance and identifying biomarkers persist, further research is needed to help lymphoma patients achieve better long-term outcomes (Figure 13.18).

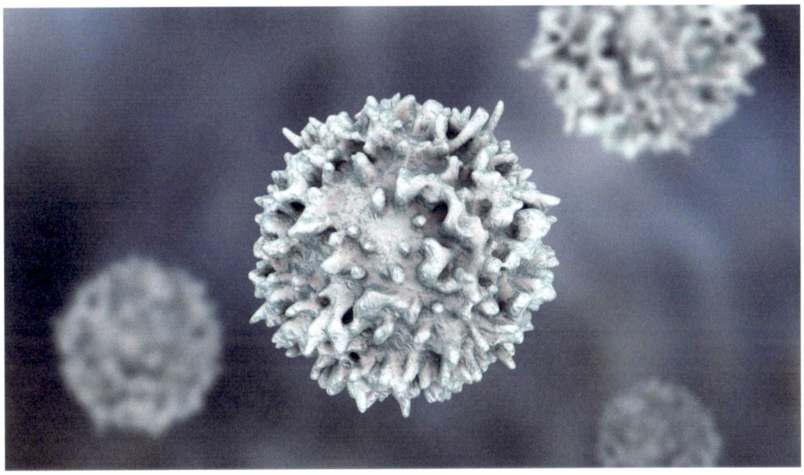

Figure 13.18. Recent advancements have revealed specific targets, such as the CCR4 receptor, which is crucial in cutaneous T-cell lymphoma (CTCL) due to its role in tumor immune evasion.

Source: https://d36dxcsn6kza9w.cloudfront.net/wp-content/uploads/2021/07/12102611/GettyImages-1159808506-scaled.jpg.

13.4.4. Immunotherapy

Immunotherapy is now an essential treatment for lymphomas and other malignancies because it uses the body's immune system to fight cancer cells. Notably, the advent of CAR (chimeric antigen receptor) T-cell therapy has demonstrated remarkable efficacy against B-cell malignancies, although its application in T-cell lymphomas has been less robust. Recent studies have explored innovative strategies, such as the development of CD5 CAR T cells, which have shown promise in targeting T-cell malignancies, particularly in cases involving CNS infiltration. CD5-IL15/IL15sushi CAR T cells rapidly reduced the number of lymphoblasts in the central nervous system, resulting in remission in a patient with refractory T-cell leukemia. This groundbreaking approach represents a significant advancement in immunotherapy, as it not only enhances patient outcomes but also suggests that targeted immunotherapies may evolve to address the complexities associated with T-cell cancers (Feng et al., 2021). Furthermore, the overall landscape of cancer treatment is undergoing a dynamic shift, with cancer mortality rates notably declining due to innovative therapies, including immunotherapy, which have led to improved survival rates and quality of life for patients (Rebecca et al., 2021).

13.4.5. Stem Cell Transplantation

Using stem cell transplantation is now a primary approach for treating lymphomas, especially when the disease recurs or does not respond to treatment. During the procedure, hematopoietic stem cells (HSCs) are given to help the body recover its blood-forming ability after intense chemotherapy or radiation treatments. The integration of stem cell transplantation in treatment protocols has enhanced outcomes, especially in aggressive forms such as DLBCL and lymphoblastic lymphoma. Notably, advancements in understanding the biology of lymphomas have opened avenues for more tailored approaches pre- and post-transplant, enhancing the efficacy of transplant outcomes (Aurer et al., 2011). Moreover, the transition toward using high-dose chemotherapy regimens coupled with stem cell support has been associated with improved survival rates among high-risk patients, even as challenges persist in managing associated complications and long-term effects on cognitive function (Cwynarski et al., 2014). All in all, stem cell transplantation remains a crucial component of evolving treatments for lymphomas (Figure 13.19).

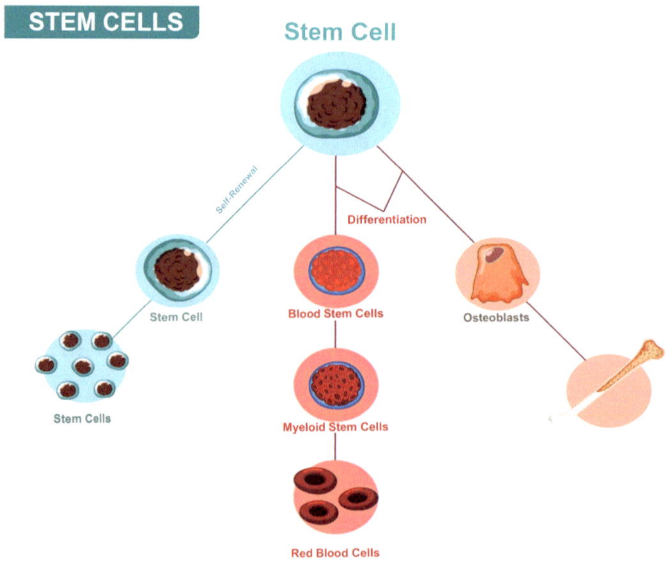

Figure 13.19. Stem cell transplantation has emerged as a pivotal strategy in the management of lymphomas, particularly for patients facing relapsed or refractory disease.

Source: https://www.mdpi.com/cells/cells-12-02855/article_deploy/html/images/cells-12-02855-g001.png.

13.4.6. Clinical Trials and Research

The field of lymphoma research and clinical trials is constantly evolving, primarily due to studies on targeted therapies that address the genetic causes of the disease. For example, the p53 transcription factor is often altered in many cancers, including lymphomas, and its missense mutations typically indicate that the treatment will not be effective and the patient's outcome will be poor. Novel agents aimed at restoring p53 function are under investigation, with studies indicating that approximately 50% of p53-mutant tumors exhibit heterogeneous responses to these therapies, implicating pathways such as TNF in treatment sensitivity (Larsson et al., 2017). Additionally, the addition of histone deacetylase inhibitors, such as vorinostat, has been shown to enhance the effectiveness of standard chemotherapy treatments. In a recent phase I trial, vorinostat combined with R-EPOCH yielded an impressive complete response rate of 83% in aggressive HIV-associated non-Hodgkin lymphoma patients, underscoring the potential for innovative approaches in lymphoma treatment (Aboulafia et al., 2018).

13.4.7. Palliative Care Approaches

When lymphoma treatments are no longer effective or unsuitable, palliative care is crucial in helping patients maintain a better quality of life. The approach focuses on alleviating symptoms and addressing the psychological, social, and spiritual needs of patients with life-limiting illnesses. Emerging therapies, such as low-dose radiotherapy, have demonstrated an increasing efficacy in managing localized symptoms associated with primary cutaneous lymphomas, despite the lack of standardized clinical trials defining optimal dosages for various lymphoma types (Adeberg et al., 2024). Additionally, novel radionuclide therapies are being integrated into palliative care, effectively delivering cytotoxic agents directly to cancerous cells while minimizing damage to healthy tissues, thus enhancing patient comfort and outcomes (Aquilina et al., 2008). Due to these new palliative approaches, it is evident that a whole-person approach is necessary for treating lymphoma patients, prioritizing their dignity and well-being (Figure 13.20).

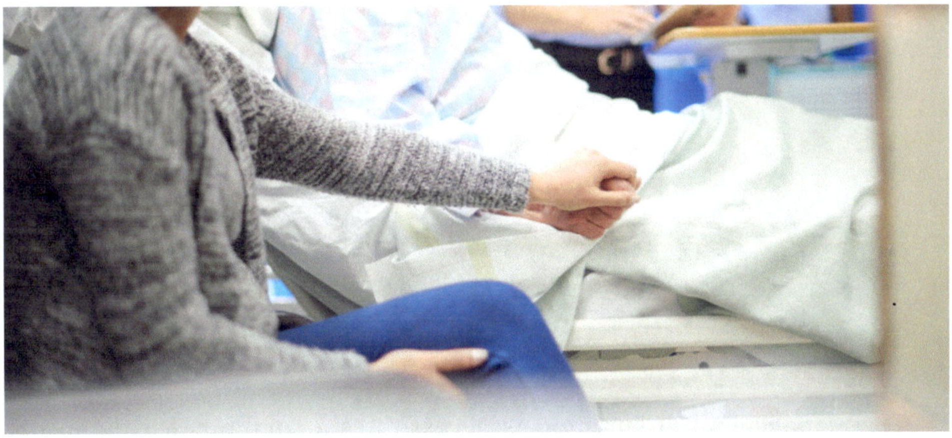

Figure 13.20. Palliative care approaches play a critical role in improving the quality of life for patients, particularly when curative treatments have been exhausted or deemed inappropriate.

Source: https://elderlycaremalaysia.com/wp-content/uploads/2023/10/What-is-Palliative-Care-for-the-Elderly.png.

13.4.8. Side Effects and Management

Managing the side effects associated with lymphoma treatments is crucial for patients' well-being and quality of life. A therapy called pixantrone has gained notice for how well it treats aggressive relapsed NHL, but it does have some risks. The panel of experts emphasized the importance of a favorable benefit/risk profile. It recommended periodic cardiac monitoring due to the potential for cardiotoxicity, despite its relatively low occurrence in clinical trials (Barosi et al., 2016). Also, a study about high-risk follicular lymphoma patients found that although several treatments are available, such as high-dose chemotherapy with rituximab and standard regimens, dealing with side effects is still essential. Notably, complete remission was associated with improved survival rates, reinforcing the importance of managing side effects to facilitate treatment adherence and enhance therapeutic efficacy (Angrilli et al., 2019). Dealing with side effects as a group is necessary for successful lymphoma treatment.

13.4.9. Role of Multidisciplinary Teams

The management of lymphomas necessitates a comprehensive approach, which is where multidisciplinary teams (MDTs) play a vital role. When specialists from hematology, oncology, and supportive care collaborate, they help the team understand the disease and what the patient experiences. For instance, hematology/hemato-oncology teams are often pivotal in managing lymphoma cases, accounting for a significant proportion of referrals in clinical settings (Carrard et al., 2021). By working together, doctors can ensure that the treatment plan meets the patient's needs and is accurate. Furthermore, engaging diverse expertise allows for the incorporation of mental health support, which is increasingly recognized as essential in oncology settings (Creese et al., 2013). Effective cooperation among MDT members helps improve outcomes for people with lymphoma, reduce risks, and enhance their quality of life (Figure 13.21).

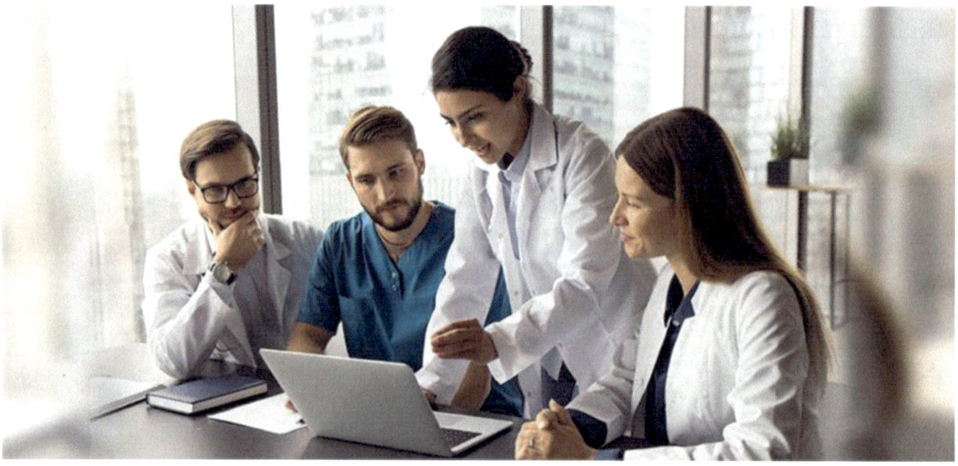

Figure 13.21. The management of lymphomas necessitates a comprehensive approach, which is where multidisciplinary teams (MDTs) play a vital role.

Source: https://www.riomed.com/wp-content/uploads/2025/02/MDT-Blog-Img-1.jpg2

A CLOSER LOOK

HYPEREOSINOPHILIC SYNDROME

Hypereosinophilic syndrome (HES) is a rare disorder characterized by a persistently high number of eosinophils—a type of WBC involved in allergic reactions and fighting parasites—in the blood and tissues. When eosinophil levels remain elevated for an extended period without a clear cause, they can accumulate and cause damage to organs such as the heart, lungs, skin, and nervous system.

Symptoms vary depending on which organs are affected but may include fatigue, rash, coughing, difficulty breathing, and heart problems. The exact cause of HES is often unknown, but it can sometimes be linked to genetic mutations or underlying cancers.

Treatment typically involves medications to reduce eosinophil levels and inflammation, such as corticosteroids, targeted therapies like TKIs, or other immunosuppressive drugs, depending on the cause and severity. Early diagnosis and management are crucial to prevent organ damage.

SUMMARY

Since lymphomas are very complex, it is essential to use detailed methods for both diagnosis and treatment. As highlighted, primary non-Hodgkin lymphomas of the sinonasal tract illustrate the diagnostic challenges faced in identifying this malignancy, as they can easily mimic other serious conditions, leading to potential misdiagnosis and delayed treatment (Bhagat et al., 2009). This highlights the importance of having a high level of suspicion and conducting a thorough histopathological analysis. Furthermore, the varied presentations of lymphoma necessitate an accurate classification of distinct subgroups, as this influences treatment approaches significantly (Agostinelli et al., 2019). It is essential to know the morphological, immunophenotypical, and molecular details to give patients the best care. Improvements in how lymphomas are diagnosed may lead to better outcomes, but more effort is needed in research and practice to effectively manage these diseases.

Lymphomas should be studied by examining their various types and the effects they have on patients. Key points include the significance of post-transplant lymphoproliferative disorders (PTLDs), which arise in immunocompromised conditions, illustrating how impaired T-cell function due to immunosuppressive therapy after transplantation can lead to significant lymphoid proliferations. In a study involving Parkinsonian Macaca fascicularis, nine out of 28 subjects developed masses indicative of PTLD, with a strong correlation to the presence of macaca lymphocryptovirus, highlighting the importance of viral load monitoring as a potential diagnostic tool for early PTLD intervention (Badin et al., 2016). Additionally, innovative treatment protocols such as the ImbruVeRCHOP trial emphasize the evolving nature of lymphoma treatment, combining conventional chemotherapy with targeted therapies to enhance outcomes for older patients with high-risk diffuse large B-cell lymphoma (Anagnostopoulos et al., 2019). They point out that lymphoma is a complicated disease that is constantly being studied and treated.

REFERENCES

1. Roshandel, G., Semnani, S., Aarabi, M., Keshtkar, A., Noohi, A., Najafi, L., Besharat, S., Moradi, A., & Kalavi, K. (2011). Lymphomas in Golestan province of Iran: results of a population-based cancer registry. *PubMed, 12*(1), 219–222. https://pubmed.ncbi.nlm.nih.gov/21517261Abdel-Hamid, M., Ali, A. S., Aboulola, M., Al-Hakami, A. M., Akiba, S., Aldoss, I. T., Allan, G. J., et al. (2015). Epstein-Barr virus: Clinical and epidemiological revisits and genetic basis of oncogenesis. https://core.ac.uk/download/42154478.pdf (accessed on 12th June 2025).
2. Abmayr, W., Braun-Falco, O., Burg, G., Dummer, R., et al. (1991). Prognostic significance of DNA cytometry in cutaneous malignant lymphomas. https://core.ac.uk/download/11538287.pdf (accessed on 12th June 2025).
3. Aboulafia, D., Ambinder, R. F., Cesarman, E., Henry, K., et al. (2018). Safety and preliminary efficacy of vorinostat with R-EPOCH in high-risk HIV-associated non-Hodgkin's lymphoma (AMC-075). https://core.ac.uk/download/212865067.pdf (accessed on 12th June 2025).
4. Abramchenko, A., Romanova, M. I., Gayda, A. I., Mozhokina, G., Samoylova, A. G., & Vasilyeva, I. A. (2025). Effectiveness and safety of short-course chemotherapy regimens for drug-resistant tuberculosis: Literature review and meta-analysis. *Tuberculosis and Lung Diseases*. https://www.semanticscholar.org/paper/16efaf4c54117323ce91c9b35524d11f50f6760b (accessed on 12th June 2025).
5. Abu-Elmagd, K., Furukawa, H., Lee, R. G., Rao, A., et al. (1995). Outcome analysis of 71 clinical intestinal transplantations. https://core.ac.uk/download/12205210.pdf (accessed on 12th June 2025).
6. Abulayha, A., Chanan-Khan, A., Davies, A., Prica, A., Rezvani, A. R., Bonavida, B., Coiffier, B., et al. (2017). Rituximab in B-cell hematologic malignancies: A review of 20 years of clinical experience. https://core.ac.uk/download/153370800.pdf (accessed on 12th June 2025).
7. Adeberg, S., Assaf, C., Bagot, M., Battistella, M., et al. (2024). Radiotherapy in cutaneous lymphomas: Recommendations from the EORTC cutaneous lymphoma tumor group. https://core.ac.uk/download/628399195.pdf (accessed on 12th June 2025).
8. Agostinelli, C., Ambrosio, M. R., Ascani, S., Carbone, A., et al. (2019). A practical algorithmic approach to mature aggressive B-cell lymphoma diagnosis in the double/triple hit era: Selecting cases, matching clinical benefit. A position paper from the Italian Group of Hematopathology (G.I.E.). https://core.ac.uk/download/231747395.pdf (accessed on 12th June 2025).
9. Agostinelli, C., Guglielmo, A., Motta, G., Mussi, M., Pileri, A., Piraccini, B. M., Sabattini, E., et al. (2024). A narrative review of the state of the art of CCR4-based therapies in cutaneous T-cell lymphomas: Focus on mogamulizumab and future treatments. https://core.ac.uk/download/620488925.pdf (accessed on 12th June 2025).
10. Agravat, A. H., Dhruva, G. A., Pujara, K. M., Sanghvi, A., et al. (2012). Role of fine needle aspiration cytology in salivary gland pathology and its histopathological correlation: A two-year prospective study in Western India. https://core.ac.uk/download/pdf/13598776.pdf (accessed on 12th June 2025).
11. Alaggio, R., Amador, C., Anagnostopoulos, I., Attygalle, A. D., Araújo, I., Berti, E., Bhagat, G., et al. (2022). The 5th edition of the World Health Organization Classification of Hematolymphoid Tumors: Lymphoid neoplasms. *Leukemia, 36*, 1720–1748. https://doi.org/10.1038/s41375-

022-01620-2 (accessed on 12th June 2025).

12. Anagnostopoulos, I., Bittner, A., Denker, S., Frick, M., et al. (2019). A Phase I/II first-line study of R-CHOP plus B-cell receptor/NF-κB-double-targeting to molecularly assess therapy response. https://core.ac.uk/download/288114089.pdf (accessed on 12th June 2025).
13. Androutsos, G., Chini, S., Galanopoulos, A., Gortzolidis, G., et al. (2011). Flow cytometry as a diagnostic tool in the early diagnosis of aggressive lymphomas mimicking life-threatening infection. https://core.ac.uk/download/pdf/8579289.pdf (accessed on 12th June 2025).
14. Angrilli, F., Barbui, A. M., Benedetti, F., Billio, A., et al. (2019). Prolonged survival in the absence of disease recurrence in advanced-stage follicular lymphoma following chemo-immunotherapy: 13-year update of the prospective, multicenter randomized GITMO-IIL trial. https://core.ac.uk/download/287849315.pdf (accessed on 12th June 2025).
15. Ansuinelli, M., De Angelis, F., Di Rocco, A., Foa, R., et al. (2017). Is now the time for molecular driven therapy for diffuse large B-cell lymphoma? https://core.ac.uk/download/98349167.pdf (accessed on 12th June 2025).
16. Aquilina, M. A. (2008). The expanding role of nuclear medicine in therapeutic strategies. https://core.ac.uk/download/46602172.pdf (accessed on 12th June 2025).
17. Atchison, R. W., Bahnson, H. T., Griffith, B. P., Hakala, T. R., et al. (1984). Reversibility of lymphomas and lymphoproliferative lesions developing under cyclosporin-steroid therapy. https://core.ac.uk/download/12203970.pdf (accessed on 12th June 2025).
18. Auletta, S., Carideo, L., Galli, F., Lauri, C., et al. (2016). Immunoscintigraphic for therapy decision making and follow-up of biological therapies. https://core.ac.uk/download/153364883.pdf (accessed on 12th June 2025).
19. Aurer, I. (2011). Changing therapeutic landscape–The last decade. https://core.ac.uk/download/11700019.pdf (accessed on 12th June 2025).
20. Aurer, I., Bašić-Kinda, S., Gjadrov Kuveždić, K., Ilić, I., et al. (2010). FNA based diagnosis of head and neck nodal lymphoma [Citomorfološka dijagnoza limfoma u području glave i vrata]. https://core.ac.uk/download/11699836.pdf (accessed on 12th June 2025).
21. Badin, R. A., Cavicchioli, L., Cozzi, E., Crossan, D., et al. (2016). Posttransplant lymphoproliferative disorders in neuronal Xeno transplanted macaques. https://core.ac.uk/download/293883125.pdf (accessed on 12th June 2025).
22. Baianu, I. C. (2011). Early diagnosis of Alzheimer's disease by NIRF spectroscopy and nuclear medicine. https://core.ac.uk/download/pdf/332860.pdf (accessed on 12th June 2025).
23. Baianu, I. C. (2011). Early diagnosis of Alzheimer's disease by NIRF spectroscopy and nuclear medicine. https://core.ac.uk/download/pdf/290230.pdf (accessed on 12th June 2025).
24. Bamanikar, S., D'Amore, F., Ducreux, M., Sinowatz, F., Freeman, C., Gospodarowicz, M. K., Amanguno, H., et al. (2004). Clinicopathological features of extranodal lymphomas: Kuwait experience. https://core.ac.uk/download/16432410.pdf (accessed on 12th June 2025).
25. Banka, S., Childhood Overgrowth Collaboration, Clericuzio, C., Cole, T., et al. (2011). Germline mutations in the oncogene EZH2 cause Weaver syndrome and increased human height. https://core.ac.uk/download/29469464.pdf (accessed on 12th June 2025).

26. Bano, N., Gupta, Y., Khan, S., Rai, R., et al. (2024). Targeted therapies in cancer treatment: Unveiling the latest breakthroughs and promising approaches. https://core.ac.uk/download/597862456.pdf (accessed on 12th June 2025).

27. Barış, İ. C., Bağcı, G., Can, Ö., Caner, A., et al. (2015). Possible role of GADD45γ methylation in diffuse large B-cell lymphoma: Does it affect the progression and tissue involvement? https://core.ac.uk/download/227072632.pdf (accessed on 12th June 2025).

28. Barosi, G., Corradini, P., Martelli, M., Minotti, C., et al. (2016). Critical concepts, practice recommendations, and research perspectives of pixantrone therapy in non-Hodgkin lymphoma: A SIE, SIES, and GITMO consensus paper. https://core.ac.uk/download/80310806.pdf (accessed on 12th June 2025).

29. Bewarder, M., Christofyllakis, K., Kaddu-Mulindwa, D., Kos, F., et al. (2022). Management of extranidal marginal zone lymphoma: Present and upcoming perspectives. https://core.ac.uk/download/521112052.pdf (accessed on 12th June 2025).

30. Bhagat, S., Bist, S. S., Gupta, N., Singh, A., et al. (2009). Primary non-Hodgkin's malignant lymphoma of the sinonasal tract. https://core.ac.uk/download/pdf/87268.pdf (accessed on 12th June 2025).

31. Bikle, D., Kim, S., Kim, S. J., Peluso, J., et al. (2019). Rapid onset of hypercalcemia from high-grade lymphoma in the setting of HIV-related immune reconstitution inflammatory syndrome. https://core.ac.uk/download/323067318.pdf (accessed on 12th June 2025).

32. Bruen, M., Crowley, D., O'Connor, P., Staines, A., et al. (2004). Public health and landfill sites. https://core.ac.uk/download/11309293.pdf (accessed on 12th June 2025).

33. Brys, A. K., Sheth, M. R., Sohn, D. D., Sweidan, R., et al. (2015). Diagnostic and therapeutic considerations in idiopathic hypereosinophilia with warm autoimmune hemolytic anemia. https://core.ac.uk/download/323075654.pdf (accessed on 12th June 2025).

34. Campo, E., Jaffe, E. S., Cook, J. R., Quintanilla-Martínez, L., Swerdlow, S. H., Anderson, K. C., Brousset, P., et al. (2022). The International Consensus Classification of mature lymphoid neoplasms: A report from the Clinical Advisory Committee. *Blood, 140*, 1229–1253. https://doi.org/10.1182/blood.2022015851 (accessed on 12th June 2025).

35. Carrard, V. C., Martins, M. D., Martins, M. A. T., Neves, A. C., et al. (2021). Analysis of referrals to the stomatology service in a Southern Brazilian hospital: A retrospective study. https://core.ac.uk/download/548518305.pdf (accessed on 12th June 2025).

36. Castillo, J. J., Winer, E. S., & Olszewski, A. J. (2013). Population-based prognostic factors for survival in patients with Burkitt lymphoma: An analysis from the Surveillance, Epidemiology, and End Results database. *Cancer, 119*, 3672–3679. https://doi.org/10.1002/cncr.28264 (accessed on 12th June 2025).

37. Chen, I. S. Y., Guan, X., Kamata, M., Kranz, D. M., et al. (2019). Sustained delivery and molecular targeting of a therapeutic monoclonal antibody to metastases in the central nervous system of mice. https://core.ac.uk/download/323077415.pdf (accessed on 12th June 2025).

38. Chiattone, C., Federico, M., Ferreri, A. J. M., Fischer, T., & Zing, N. (2021). Diagnosis, prevention and treatment of central nervous system involvement in peripheral T-cell lymphomas. https://core.ac.uk/download/543266457.pdf (accessed on 12th June 2025).

39. Creese, A., Jaquet, A., Van Rie, A., Thota, A. B., Owe-Larsson, B., Sherbourne, C. D., Gilks,

C. F., et al. (2013). Grand challenges: Improving HIV treatment outcomes by integrating interventions for co-morbid mental illness. https://core.ac.uk/download/pdf/16666900.pdf (accessed on 12th June 2025).

40. Cwynarski, K., Fox, C. P., & Phillips, E. H. (2014). Primary CNS lymphoma. https://core.ac.uk/download/29412338.pdf (accessed on 12th June 2025).

41. de Smith, A. J., Feng, Q., Gauderman, W. J., Godley, L. A., et al. (2023). Increased burden of familial-associated early-onset cancer risk among minority Americans compared to non-Latino whites. https://core.ac.uk/download/595483481.pdf (accessed on 12th June 2025).

42. Degala, R. P., Kamala, G. R., Ratna Priya, G., Manne, J., Nagumantri, H. T., & Nakkina, V. N. L. (2025). A prospective study of risk factor analysis and treatment outcomes of chemotherapy in cancer patients. *Journal of Pharma Insights and Research*. https://www.semanticscholar.org/paper/2000b44e385e4a53c0d856c1210e69029af29411 (accessed on 12th June 2025).

43. Diehl, V., Fanale, M. A., Hasenclever, D., Farrell, K., Leach, M., Orlandi, E., McKay, P., et al. (2011). Nodular lymphocyte predominant Hodgkin lymphoma behaves as a distinct clinical entity with good outcome: Evidence from 14-year follow-up in the West of Scotland Cancer Network. https://core.ac.uk/download/110461.pdf (accessed on 12th June 2025).

44. Donzel, M., Trécourt, A., Ghesquières, H., Nguyen, T. T. T., Dandash, S., Denis, M., Cros-Perrial, E., et al. (2025). Netrin-1 and B-cell maturation antigen expression in a large cohort of 361 lymphomas: Sensitive and specific staining in plasmolysis lymphomas, and therapeutic perspectives. *The Journal of Pathology: Clinical Research, 11*. https://www.semanticscholar.org/paper/a6b65128ada118d8076b35eea633bfa1126d8cc4 (accessed on 12th June 2025).

45. Döring, C., Facchetti, F., Gascoyne, R., Hansmann, M. L., et al. (2013). Nodular lymphocyte predominant Hodgkin lymphoma and T cell/histiocyte rich large B-cell lymphoma: Endpoints of a spectrum of one disease? https://core.ac.uk/download/18325970.pdf (accessed on 12th June 2025).

46. Feng, J., Xu, H., Cinquina, A., Wu, Z., Chen, Q., Zhang, P., Wang, X., et al. (2021). Treatment of aggressive T cell lymphoblastic lymphoma/leukemia using anti-CD5 CAR T cells. *Stem Cell Reviews and Reports, 17*, 652–661. https://doi.org/10.1007/s12015-020-10092-9 (accessed on 12th June 2025).

47. Filipovich, A. H., De Rossi, A., Cavdar, A. O., Kidenya, B., Klumb, C. E., Kim, D., Mwizamuholya, D., et al. (2013). Relationship between non-Hodgkin's lymphoma and blood levels of Epstein-Barr virus in children in North-Western Tanzania: A case control study. https://core.ac.uk/download/pdf/11307798.pdf (accessed on 12th June 2025).

48. Fox, C. P., Rowe, M., & Shannon-Lowe, C. (2011). Deciphering the role of Epstein-Barr virus in the pathogenesis of T and NK cell lymphoproliferations. https://core.ac.uk/download/pdf/1631278.pdf (accessed on 12th June 2025).

49. Fritz, A., Jack, A., Mohd Noor, A., Smith, A., Smith, A., Smith, A., Michallet, A. S. A., et al. (2015). Lymphoma incidence, survival and prevalence 2004–2014: Sub-type analyses from the UK's Hematological Malignancy Research Network. https://core.ac.uk/download/83942712.pdf (accessed on 12th June 2025).

50. Fulda, S., Rajalingam, K., & Dikic, I. (2012). Ubiquitylation in immune disorders and cancer: From molecular mechanisms to therapeutic implications. https://core.ac.uk/download/14528498.pdf (accessed on 12th June 2025).

51. Garden, O. A., Pittaway, R., Polton, G., Priestnall, S. L., et al. (2018). Diagnosis of anaplastic large-cell lymphoma in a dog using CD30 immunohistochemistry. https://core.ac.uk/download/151393667.pdf (accessed on 12th June 2025).

52. Goswami, P., Khatib, Y., & Salek, S. (2019). Hematological malignancy: Are we measuring what is important to patients? A systematic review of quality-of-life instruments. https://core.ac.uk/download/287582202.pdf (accessed on 12th June 2025).

53. Inan, M., Ogut, B., Gurer, M., & Erdem, O. (2023). CD30 and PD-1 in mycosis fungoides. *Turkish Journal of Dermatology, 17*, 93–99. https://www.semanticscholar.org/paper/b4bd75be2337055c491493b0665784544446693a9 (accessed on 12th June 2025).

54. Jarrett, R. F., & McAulay, K. A. (2015). Human leukocyte antigens and genetic susceptibility to lymphoma. https://core.ac.uk/download/46558899.pdf (accessed on 12th June 2025).

55. Kolijn, P. M., & Langerak, A. W. (2023). Immune dysregulation as a leading principle for lymphoma development in diverse immunological backgrounds. https://core.ac.uk/download/588754331.pdf (accessed on 12th June 2025).

56. Krauss, S., Seiffert, S., Perez Fernandez, C., Georgi, T., Kirchberg, J., Bach, E., Brueckner, M., et al. (2024). Prognostic value of baseline and early response FDG-PET/CT combined with cellular dynamics in patients with refractory and relapsed mantle cell lymphoma (MCL) undergoing chimeric antigen receptor (CAR)-T cell therapy. *Blood*. https://www.semanticscholar.org/paper/ebc184c3ecb078ddc9412a786d29b1aec4672a66 (accessed on 12th June 2025).

57. Larsson, C. A. (2017). Evaluating the therapeutic efficacy of restoring wild-type P53 activity in P53-mutant tumors. https://core.ac.uk/download/151746094.pdf (accessed on 12th June 2025).

58. Lleras-Muney, A., & Glied, S. (2025). Health inequality, education and medical innovation. https://core.ac.uk/download/pdf/6605133.pdf (accessed on 12th June 2025).

59. Lowery, A. J. (2007). Evaluation of a guided decision aid for treatment selection in follicular non-Hodgkin's lymphoma. https://core.ac.uk/download/230462175.pdf (accessed on 12th June 2025).

60. Lyon, A. R., López-Fernández, T., Couch, L. S., Asteggiano, R., Aznar, M. C., Bergler-Klein, J., Boriani, G., et al. (2022). 2022 ESC guidelines on cardio-oncology developed in collaboration with the European Hematology Association (EHA), the European Society for Therapeutic Radiology and Oncology (ESTRO), and the International Cardio-Oncology Society (IC-OS). *European Heart Journal, 43*, 4229–4361. https://doi.org/10.1093/eurheartj/ehac244 (accessed on 12th June 2025).

61. Majd, N. (2016). The truth behind aspartame: An examination of the adverse health effects associated with its consumption. https://open.bu.edu/bitstream/2144/16058/1/Majd_bu_0017N_11073.pdf (accessed on 12th June 2025).

62. Marques, G. B., Ponce, F., Beaudu-Lange, C., Béguin, J., Boissy, L., Chavalle, T., Denoeux, P., et al. (2024). Feline high-grade and large granular lymphocyte alimentary lymphomas treated with COP- or CHOP-based chemotherapy: A multi-centric retrospective study of 57 cases. *Veterinary and Comparative Oncology*. https://www.semanticscholar.org/paper/e0096298d63a27c1bf2a64da27f7405f049a4875 (accessed on 12th June 2025).

63. Morris, J. S. (2016). Genomic and proteomic profiling for cancer diagnosis in dogs. https://core.ac.uk/download/46559176.pdf (accessed on 12th June 2025).

64. Oliveira, A. L., Fischer, T., Balthazar, J. A., Abrantes, L. L., Schmidt Filho, J., & Silveira, T. B. (2024). Allogenic transplant in mycosis fungoides: Never or never too late? Brazilian single center experience. *Blood*. https://www.semanticscholar.org/paper/2e836b53a8f57a911b89ddf850dd5dfe4ed8b05e (accessed on 12th June 2025).
65. Park, H. L. (2020). Epigenetic biomarkers for environmental exposures and personalized breast cancer prevention. https://core.ac.uk/download/323075287.pdf (accessed on 12th June 2025).
66. Saarinen, S. (2013). Genetic basis of familial lymphoma predisposition. https://core.ac.uk/download/14928057.pdf (accessed on 12th June 2025).
67. Selvi, S. K., Shrinuvasan, S., & Srinivas, B. H. (2019). B-cell lymphomas. https://core.ac.uk/download/322445477.pdf (accessed on 12th June 2025).
68. Siegel, R. L., Miller, K. D., Fuchs, H. E., & Jemal, A. (2021). Cancer statistics, 2021. *CA: A Cancer Journal for Clinicians, 71*, 7–33. https://doi.org/10.3322/caac.21654 (accessed on 12th June 2025).
69. Su, W. (2019). Diagnosis and treatment progress of Hodgkin lymphoma. *Cancer Research and Clinic, 31*, 213–216. https://www.semanticscholar.org/paper/777616743f7b6e88b8eb9da5c8a1498a8d32e2bc (accessed on 12th June 2025).
70. Sun, Y., Luo, S., & Huang, C. (2024). Clinical analysis of 94 cases of ocular adnexal lymphomas. *Precision Medical Sciences, 13*, 43–51. https://www.semanticscholar.org/paper/c435456db810128e4b435803a739c00ec6d1e2c1 (accessed on 12th June 2025).
71. Tateshita, N., Watanabe, N., Shimbo, T., Morimoto, A., Takeda, K., & Tanihiro, T. (2025). Abstract 7324: ONO-4685: A novel PD-1/CD3 bispecific T-cell engager (TCE) for the treatment of T-cell malignancies. *Cancer Research*. https://www.semanticscholar.org/paper/f6c5917c91e3f4a7f29b6a71a9bf862b85962a58 (accessed on 12th June 2025).
72. Westfall, M. (2009). Toxic time bomb: The true legacy cost of the auto industry. https://core.ac.uk/download/5132496.pdf (accessed on 12th June 2025).
73. Yu, D., Wang, L., Zhang, L., Li, Q., Zhang, S., Cheng, S., Zhao, W., et al. (2015). Localized primary gastrointestinal diffuse large B-cell lymphoma received a surgical approach: An analysis of prognostic factors and comparison of staging systems in 101 patients from a single institution. https://core.ac.uk/download/pdf/81848332.pdf (accessed on 12th June 2025).
74. Zhou, B., Lin, W., Long, Y., Yang, Y., Zhang, H., Wu, K., & Chu, Q. (2022). Notch signaling pathway: Architecture, disease, and therapeutics. *Signal Transduction and Targeted Therapy, 7*. https://doi.org/10.1038/s41392-022-00934-y (accessed on 12th June 2025).
75. Zhou, K., Xu, D., Cao, Y., Wang, J., Yang, Y., & Huang, M. (2014). C-MYC aberrations as prognostic factors in diffuse large B-cell lymphoma: A meta-analysis of epidemiological studies. *PLoS ONE, 9*, e95020–e95020. https://doi.org/10.1371/journal.pone.0095020 (accessed on 12th June 2025).

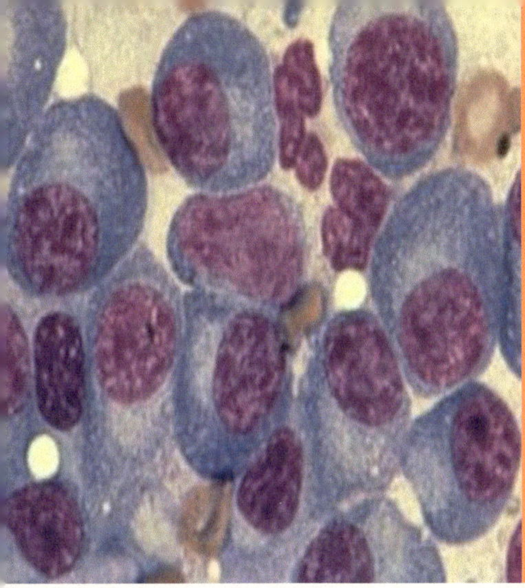

Chapter 14
PLASMA CELL DYSCRASIAS

Contents

Introduction....353
14.1. Types of Plasma Cell Dyscrasias....354
14.2. Pathophysiology of Plasma Cell Dyscrasias....358
14.3. Diagnosis and Evaluation....363
14.4. Treatment Options and Management....367
Summary....374
References....375

Introduction

Plasma cell dyscrasias are a group of hematologic malignancies with aberrant plasma cell growth in the bone marrow and numerous clinical syndromes and staggering health issues. Multiple myeloma (MM) is the most prevalent among these illnesses and results in considerable morbidity and mortality in the population. Plasma cell biology and their role in antibody production underscore the complexity of these conditions. Evolutions in the treatments in recent times, particularly the advent of immunomodulatory therapy, monoclonal antibodies, and targeted therapies, have significantly improved the outcomes of patients and revolutionized treatment paradigms. As noted in recent publications, the amalgamation of traditional treatment modalities with innovative therapies, such as bispecific antibodies and CAR T-cell therapy, highlights the dynamic shift in current modalities for managing MM and related disorders (Jurczyszyn et al., 2025). This chapter provides a summary of plasma cell dyscrasias, with an emphasis on their pathophysiology, diagnostic issues, and emerging treatment paradigms (Cooper et al., 2011) (Figure 14.1).

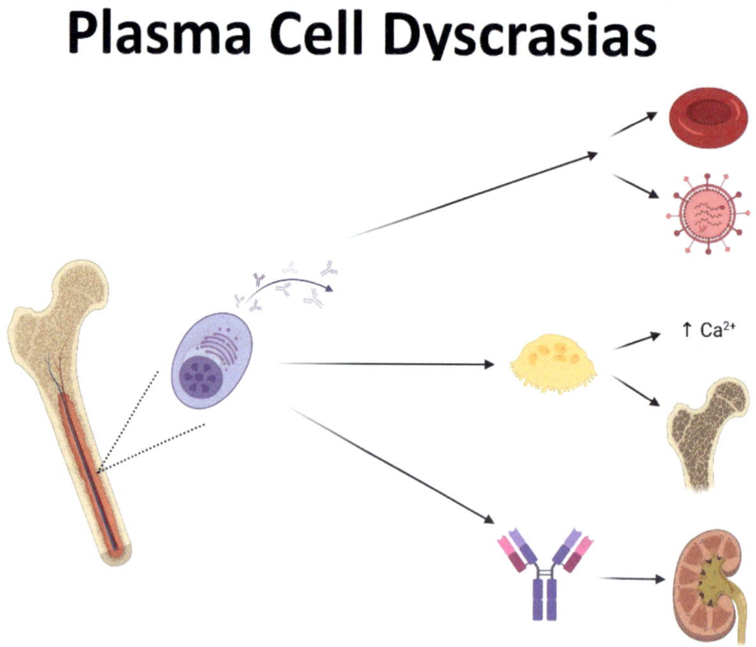

Figure 14.1. Plasma cell dyscrasias.

Source: https://teachim.org/wp-content/uploads/2023/02/Plasma-cell-dyscrasia-scaled.jpg.

14.1. Types of Plasma Cell Dyscrasias

Plasma cell dyscrasias encompass various disorders in which plasma cells, crucial for producing antibodies, proliferate abnormally. Of all the types, MM is a serious condition characterized by the overgrowth of neoplastic plasma cells in the bone marrow. As a result, patients may develop bone problems, low blood, and kidney dysfunction. In addition to MM, other disorders such as monoclonal gammopathy of undetermined significance (MGUS) and plasmacytoma represent variations of plasma cell dyscrasia. MGUS is usually harmless, but it can progress into a malignant disease, whereas plasmacytoma typically appears as a single mass in a specific area. Advances in the pathobiology of conditions, particularly through the investigation of non-coding RNAs, have therapeutic value for both therapy and diagnosis, underscoring the importance of appropriate clinical monitoring and research into new therapeutic techniques (Babarović et al., 2010; Azab et al., 2020).

14.1.1. Multiple Myeloma (MM)

MM is one of the plasma cell dyscrasias distinguished by its complex pathophysiology and clinical importance. The MM disorder itself is caused by the uncontrolled proliferation of monoclonal plasma cells in the bone marrow, which interferes with normal hematopoiesis and can lead to various consequences, including anemia and renal dysfunction. Further testing of the disease's complexity comes from emerging research on non-coding RNAs, which reveals novel pathways of gene regulation often disrupted in MM. These non-coding molecules not only enhance our understanding of the mechanisms underlying disease but also suggest promising avenues for targeted therapies and prognostic markers. For example, notable findings highlight the role of dysregulation of these RNAs in the malignant transformation of plasma cells, underscoring the need for novel treatment approaches to enhance patient outcomes (Azab et al., 2020). Additionally, the ocular manifestations of MM also warrant attention, as they frequently indicate underlying hematological issues, emphasizing the importance of comprehensive evaluations in affected patients (Suhasini et al., 2017) (Figure 14.2).

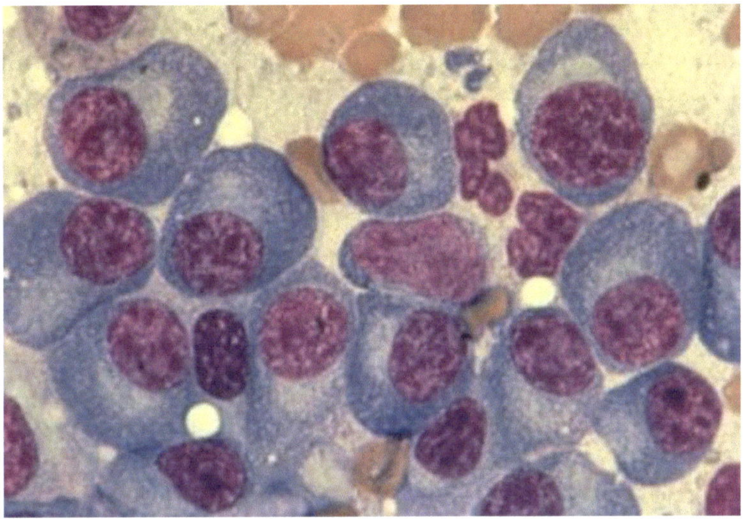

Figure 14.2. Multiple myeloma (MM).

Source: https://img.medscapestatic.com/pi/meds/ckb/10/36610tn.jpg.

14.1.2. Monoclonal Gammopathy of Undetermined Significance (MGUS)

Monoclonal Gammopathy of Undetermined Significance (MGUS) serves as a foundational concept within the spectrum of plasma cell dyscrasias, representing a pre-malignant state characterized by the presence of monoclonal protein in the bloodstream. Although its innocuous-sounding appellation, MGUS is a dangerous condition; approximately 25% of patients with the disease will ultimately develop more aggressive disease, such as plasma cell myeloma (PCM) or other associated diseases, and close monitoring and assessment of disease markers is essential. Recent studies have shown that plasma cells in MGUS differ from those in PCM. For instance, MGUS typically presents with both regular and aberrant plasma cell subpopulations. At the same time, PCM exhibits a predominance of cells lacking regular phenotypic markers such as CD19, indicating a potential progression pathway that these immunophenotypic changes may influence (Rawstron et al., 2008; Azab et al., 2020). Having knowledge of MGUS helps doctors predict the course of the disease and improve patient outcomes with plasma cell dyscrasias.

14.1.3. Waldenström Macroglobulinemia

Waldenström Macroglobulinemia (WM) represents a unique entity within the spectrum of plasma cell dyscrasias, characterized primarily by the infiltration of lymphoplasmacytic cells in the bone marrow and the subsequent overproduction of monoclonal immunoglobulin M (IgM) antibodies. Although traditionally challenging to diagnose, advances in genetic characterization have significantly enhanced diagnostic accuracy. Genetic mutations, such as L265P in the MYD88 gene, are found in over 90% of patients, providing critical insights into disease behavior and treatment response (Askari et al., 2021). WM is viewed in the clinic as a combination of signs from high blood viscosity, low blood count, and organ enlargement. In addition, the risk of complications extends to ocular complications, which warrant a multidisciplinary approach to management to avoid systemic consequences and enhance patient outcomes (Singh et al., 2023). Therefore, understanding the molecular specifics of WM is essential for developing novel therapies, which have the potential to reshape the diagnosis and prognosis of plasma cell dyscrasias (Figure 14.3).

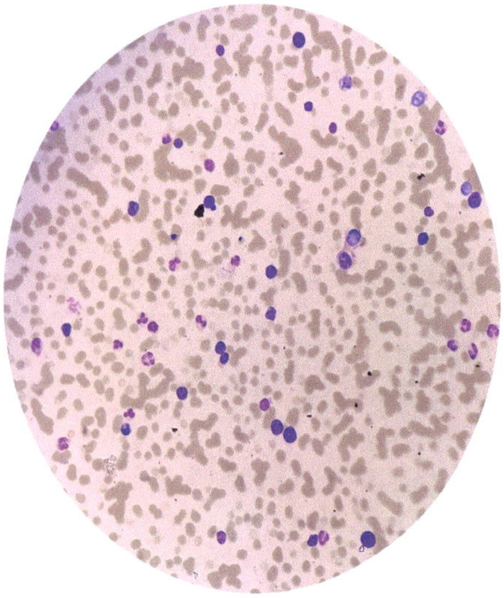

Figure 14.3. Waldenström Macroglobulinemia (WM).

Source: https://www.cancertherapyadvisor.com/wp-content/uploads/sites/12/2023/07/GettyImages-1365890537-scaled.jpg.

14.1.4. Primary Amyloidosis

Primary Amyloidosis, or immunoglobulin light chain (AL) amyloidosis, emerges as a significant complication arising from plasma cell dyscrasias, particularly MM. As a result of this condition, the monoclonal light chains made by cancerous plasma cells are deposited in several organs, causing significant damage and problems to those organs. The precise mechanisms of light chain aggregation and subsequent amyloid fibril formation remain incompletely understood, yet they are closely linked to the dysregulated behavior of plasma cells, particularly the CD138/38 positive subset, which is actively involved in light chain production (Baldovino et al., 2020). Additionally, recent studies have shown that non-coding RNA molecules play a role in controlling gene activity in plasma cell malignancies, suggesting potential new treatments. It would therefore become essential to examine how such information might possibly enhance the prognosis and also the treatment modalities for patients suffering from this multi-factorial disorder, the possibility of employing non-coding RNA as therapeutic targets or biomarkers being envisioned (Azab et al., 2020).

14.1.5. Light Chain Deposition Disease

Light Chain Deposition Disease (LCDD) represents a significant manifestation of plasma cell dyscrasias, characterized by the abnormal accumulation of light chains produced by malignant plasma cells, primarily impacting renal function. The pathophysiology of LCDD involves the filtration of free light chains (FLC) through the glomerular basement membrane, leading to their deposition in the renal tubules and glomeruli, which results in tubulointerstitial injury and ultimately acute kidney injury (AKI) in many patients. Recent studies highlight that renal involvement occurs in nearly 50% of individuals diagnosed with MM, with 12-20% presenting with acute kidney injury requiring dialysis (Antolino et al., 2018). Treatments focusing on reducing the circulating burden of FLC are essential, as novel apheretic techniques demonstrate the potential to mitigate the effects of renal deposition diseases, suggesting that timely intervention may improve renal outcomes and overall patient prognosis (Festuccia et al., 2022) (Figure 14.4).

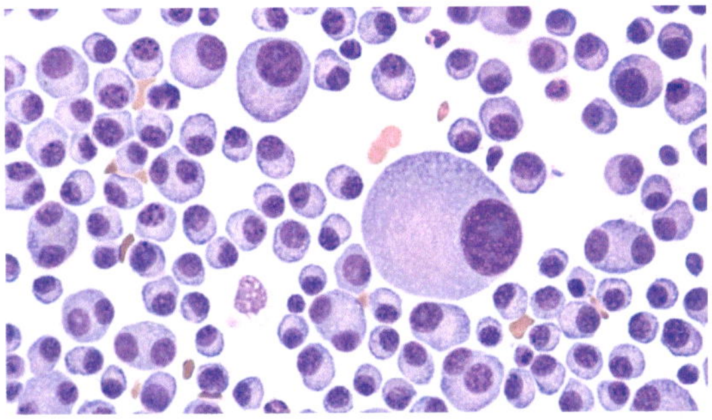

Figure 14.4. Light Chain Deposition Disease (LCDD) represents a significant manifestation of plasma cell dyscrasias, characterized by the abnormal accumulation of light chains produced by malignant plasma cells, primarily impacting renal function.

Source: https://img.medscapestatic.com/thumbnail_library/920799.jpg.

14.1.6. Plasma Cell Leukemia (PCL)

Plasma cell leukemia (PCL) represents one of the most aggressive manifestations of plasma cell dyscrasias, characterized by a significant increase of neoplastic plasma cells in the peripheral blood. This condition can present in two forms: primary PCL (pPCL), which occurs at initial diagnosis, and secondary plasma cell leukemia (sPCL), which arises from preexisting MM. The survival outcomes for patients with PCL remain poor, with median overall survival rates markedly lower than those for MM, with approximately 6.9 months compared to 26.0 months for pPCL (Broughton et al., 2024). Although advances in therapy, including the application of novel agents and autologous stem cell transplant, have been promising, the malignancy of PCL, as well as the rapidity of tumor growth and insensitivity to standard treatment, necessitate investigation into innovative therapies, such as CAR T-cell therapies, to improve patient outcomes (Heather et al., 2025).

14.1.7. Solitary Plasmacytoma

Solitary plasmacytoma is a localized neoplasm of monoclonal plasma cells, representing a distinct entity within the spectrum of plasma cell dyscrasias.

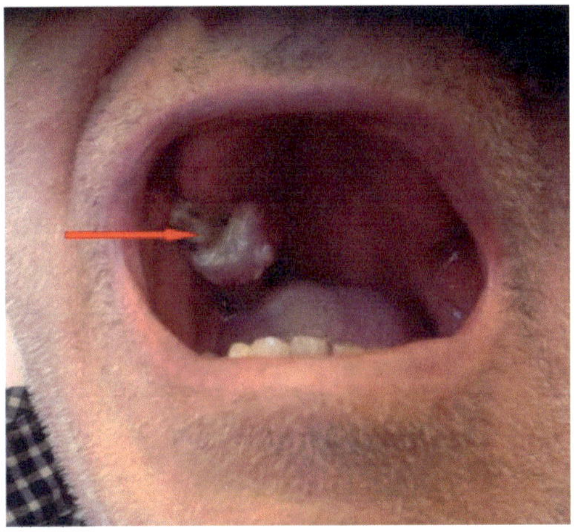

Figure 14.5. Solitary plasmacytoma.

Source: https://www.researchgate.net/publication/279955815/figure/fig1/AS:284553106214916@1444854155408/An-image-showing-solitary-plasmacytoma-in-the-oral-cavity.png.

Unlike its more aggressive counterparts, such as MM, solitary plasmacytoma typically presents as a solitary bone lesion or an extramedullary manifestation, which can vary significantly in its clinical expression. Such a diagnosis often relies on a combination of imaging techniques, histological examination, and cytogenetic analysis to distinguish it from other plasma cell disorders and evaluate the degree of bone marrow involvement. Advances in the field, driven by the advent of next-generation sequencing, have uncovered critical insights, revealing that approximately 71% of patients harbor somatic mutations correlated with disease progression, underscoring the importance of genetic profiling in management strategies (Andres et al., 2022).

Additionally, ocular complications in patients with plasma cell dyscrasias, including solitary plasmacytoma, may present unique challenges that necessitate a multidisciplinary approach to optimize patient outcomes (Agarwal et al., 2023) (Figure 14.5).

14.1.8. Non-Secretory Multiple Myeloma (MM)

Non-secretory MM represents a distinct and challenging subtype of plasma cell dyscrasias, characterized by the absence of detectable monoclonal proteins in serum or urine. Patients often present with typical symptoms of MM, such as anemia, bone lesions, and renal dysfunction, complicating diagnosis due to the lack of secretory markers.

The complexity of this condition is illustrated by case studies revealing atypical presentations, such as gastrointestinal symptoms originating from plasma cell infiltration of the colon, as seen in a 74-year-old patient whose diagnosis was confirmed through bone marrow biopsy and imaging techniques (Delicata et al., 2013).

The diverse clinical presentations and underlying pathophysiology of non-secretory types underscore the need for meticulous diagnostic approaches, such as bone marrow aspiration to detect plasmacytosis, which can occur due to both neoplastic and non-neoplastic pathology (Neema et al., 2023). Knowledge of this subtype is crucial for directing appropriate treatment and management planning.

14.2. Pathophysiology of Plasma Cell Dyscrasias

Knowledge of the pathophysiology of the plasma cell dyscrasias is crucial in defining the complexities of diseases like MM and associated disorders. These disorders result from the malignant proliferation of plasma cells that are intended to produce antibodies. Dysregulation usually leads to the overproduction of a specific type of antibody, resulting in monoclonal gammopathy. This abnormality may be due to several pathological processes, such as tissue deposition of paraproteins, which compromise organ function. The clinical presentation may vary from anemia, renal impairment, to immunosuppression, ultimately manifesting with detrimental clinical outcomes. Moreover, ocular involvement is now increasingly valued and represents a significant feature of these hematological conditions. A survey reported that 31 patients initially reported to ophthalmologists with visual symptoms and were later diagnosed with blood dyscrasias, emphasizing the importance of thorough ocular examination in such patients (Suhasini et al., 2017). A proper understanding of these pathophysiological processes is crucial for accurate diagnosis and effective management approaches (Estes et al., 1962).

14.2.1. Normal Plasma Cell Function

Knowledge of the pathophysiology of the plasma cell dyscrasias is critical in delineating the nature of diseases like MM and its associated disorders. These disorders result from the neoplastic proliferation of plasma cells that are programmed to secrete antibodies. Overproduction of a single class of antibody due to dysregulation results in monoclonal gammopathy. This abnormality is the result of a wide range of pathological processes, including the deposition of paraproteins in tissue, which disrupts organ function. The clinical presentation may vary from anemia to renal dysfunction and immunosuppression, ultimately leading to unfavorable clinical results. Ocular involvement is increasingly identified and constitutes a prominent feature of such hematological abnormalities. Thirty-one patients presenting to ophthalmologists with vision-related symptoms were actually diagnosed with blood dyscrasias, highlighting the role of a detailed ocular examination in such patients (Suhasini et al., 2017). Adequate knowledge about the pathophysiological processes involved is crucial for the correct diagnosis and management strategies (Estes et al., 1962) (Figure 14.6).

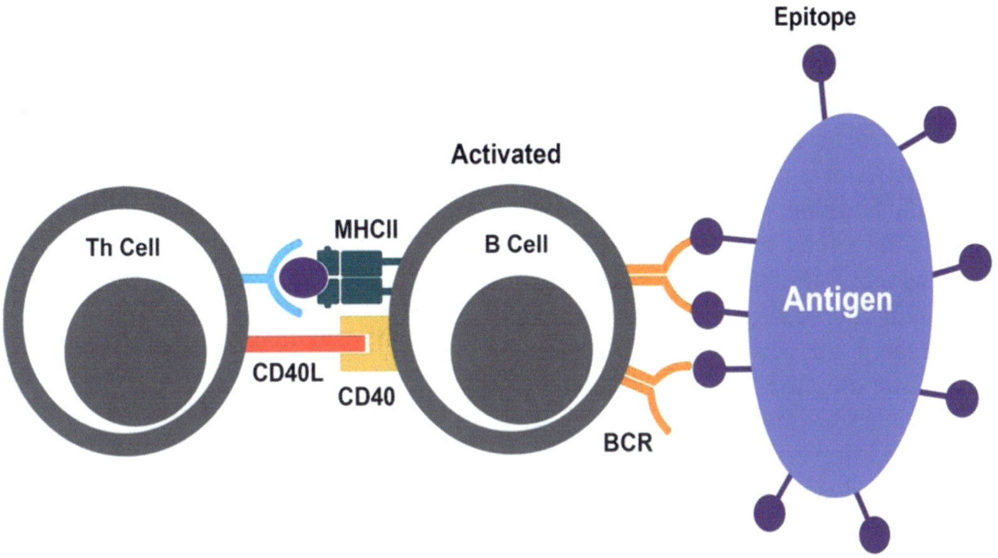

Figure 14.6. Plasma cells, derived from B lymphocytes, play a pivotal role in the adaptive immune response by producing high-affinity antibodies specific to antigens.

Source: https://www.thermofisher.com/sa/en/home/life-science/cell-analysis/cell-analysis-learning-center/immunology-at-work/b-cell-overview/_jcr_content/MainParsys/image_2e02/backgroundimg.img.png/1671800560919.png.

14.2.2. Genetic Mutations and Abnormalities

Genetic mutations and abnormalities characterize plasma cell dyscrasias generally, especially in MM and MGUS. Recent studies have revealed that numerically and structurally, chromosomal abnormalities are present among these patients. The deletions on chromosome 13 are particularly noteworthy. These deletions, notably monosomy 13, are found in 10-20% of MM cases and serve as a crucial predictor of patient survival, as indicated in research that employed high-resolution genomic techniques to analyze tumor samples. Moreover, the interplay between genetic factors and immune responses is emerging as a critical area of research, as the balance of lymphocyte subsets and cytokines may influence the progression from MGUS to malignant states (Allegra et al., 2019). Understanding these genetic underpinnings is essential for developing targeted therapies and improving patient outcomes in plasma cell dyscrasias.

14.2.3. Role of the Bone Marrow Microenvironment

The bone marrow microenvironment is pivotal to plasma cell dyscrasias and particularly MM pathogenesis and progression. It is not only structurally supportive but also enhances interactions between plasma cells and cellular components, exerting an impact on their survival and proliferation. The relationship between various subsets of lymphocytes and numerous cytokines in this environment has been revealed with greater precision, sustaining the equilibrium impaired in cancer. The discovery of non-coding RNAs within this system has revealed new mechanisms for the control of gene expression pertinent to the pathological plasma cell behavior and therefore to therapeutic perspectives. With increasingly sophisticated therapies predicated on modulating immune responses, understanding the intricate dynamics within the bone marrow microenvironment is the linchpin to creating effective strategies to manage plasma cell dyscrasias (Allegra et al., 2019; Azab et al., 2020) (Figure 14.7).

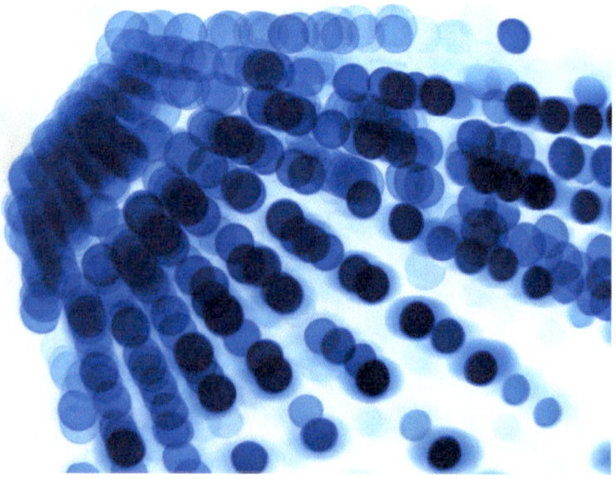

Figure 14.7. The characterization of non-coding RNAs within this ecosystem has unveiled new mechanisms of gene expression regulation that significantly contribute to the aberrant behavior of plasma cells, thus highlighting potential therapeutic targets.

Source: https://www.twistbioscience.com/sites/default/files/2024-07/RNA%20Sequencing.jpg.

14.2.4. Mechanisms of Monoclonal Antibody Production

A significant aspect of plasma cell dyscrasias, the manufacture of monoclonal antibodies is intrinsically based on the characteristics and function of plasma cells. Plasma cells are long-lived and arise from activated B lymphocytes and undergo a process of differentiation that enables them to secrete one type of antibody, but one that is directed against antigens. In diseases like MGUS and MM, chromosomal changes like deletions of chromosome 13 are significant in dysregulated synthesis of such antibodies, which ultimately result in pathological effects. More significantly, processes related to the polymerization of the immunoglobulin light chains, a characteristic of light chain amyloidosis, highlight the involvement of CD138+ plasma cells in such situations. These plasma cells not only produce monoclonal light chains but also play a role in modulating immune responses, which can be therapeutically targeted using anti-CD38 monoclonal antibodies (Baldovino et al., 2020). Knowledge of these mechanisms is therefore crucial in managing the multifactorial nature of plasma cell dyscrasias.

14.2.5. Immune Dysregulation

Immune dysregulation is a key feature in the pathogenesis of plasma cell dyscrasias, and most notably in MM. Regulation of different subsets of lymphocytes as well as the cytokine milieu is vital in whether benign diseases, for instance, MGUS, can potentially develop into malignancy. Notably, immune dysregulation generally results from alterations in the levels and functions of cytokines and lymphocytes, leading to the neoplastic transformation of plasma cells. The discovery of non-coding RNAs has led to the identification of new pathways of gene expression control that frequently become aberrant in such cancers, thus opening up potential for therapeutic targeting and prognostic applications in MM treatment, as outlined by Azab et al. (2020). In addition, understanding the immune context of benign and malignant gammopathies is crucial to optimize treatment modalities, as novel immunotherapeutic methods are increasingly employed in clinical practice (Allegra et al., 2019) (Figure 14.8).

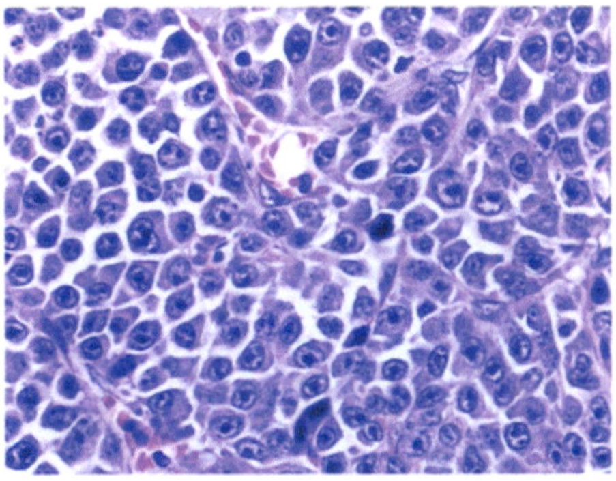

Figure 14.8. The phenomenon of immune dysregulation plays a crucial role in the pathogenesis of plasma cell dyscrasias, particularly as it relates to multiple myeloma (MM).

Source: https://static.cambridge.org/binary/version/id/urn:cambridge.org:id:binary-alt:20180930180927-67500-mediumThumb-04123fig11_1.jpg?pub-status=live.

14.2.6. Cytokine Involvement

Cytokines are pivotal in the pathophysiology of plasma cell dyscrasias, impacting both the proliferation of malignant plasma cells and the immune response against neoplasms. In addition, pro-inflammatory cytokines such as interleukin-6 (IL-6), tumor necrosis factor-alpha (TNF-α), and transforming growth factor-beta (TGF-β) play a role in the microenvironment that promotes plasma cell proliferation and survival. Of specific note, IL-6 has been determined to play a role in plasma cell proliferation and differentiation, driving monoclonal proliferation that is common in diseases like MM. Moreover, emerging evidence suggests that NK cells, known for their anti-tumor capabilities, can also release tumor-promoting cytokines through mechanisms such as AREG production, potentially enhancing plasma cell survival (Zhao et al., 2024). In addition, pyroptosis, whereby pro-inflammatory cytokines such as IL-1β and IL-18 are secreted, also highlights the complex association between cytokines in a role to alter immune dynamics within plasma cell dyscrasias (Chen et al., 2022).

14.2.7. Tumor Microenvironment Interactions

The tumor microenvironment (TME) plays a crucial role in the progression and treatment resistance of plasma cell dyscrasias, particularly MM. These numerous cellular and non-cellular components in the TME play a significant role in influencing tumor behavior and evading detection by the immune system. Notably, the communication between plasma cells and the surrounding tissue can lead to the release of substances that suppress the immune system and attract immune cells that facilitate the growth of cancer cells. For instance, there is growing recognition of how non-coding RNAs within the TME can regulate gene expression pathways pivotal to the survival of malignant plasma cells, thus presenting potential therapeutic targets (Azab et al., 2020). Additionally, the intricate interplay between lymphocyte subsets and cytokines, especially during the transition from MGUS to malignant states, underscores the importance of understanding the TME for effective treatment strategies in plasma cell disorders (Allegra et al., 2019) (Figure 14.9).

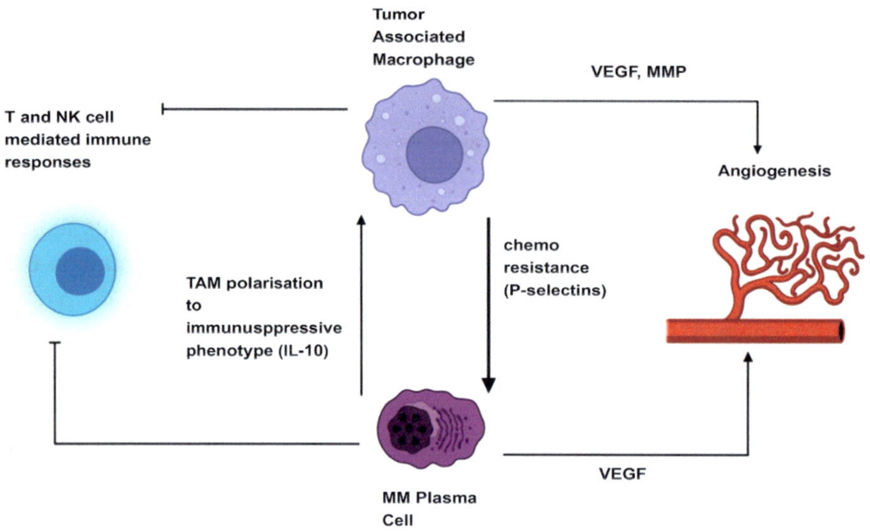

Figure 14.9. The tumor microenvironment (TME) plays a crucial role in the progression and treatment resistance of plasma cell dyscrasias, particularly multiple myeloma (MM).

Source: https://www.mdpi.com/cancers/cancers-14-05654/article_deploy/html/images/cancers-14-05654-g001.png.

14.2.8. Progression from Monoclonal Gammopathy of Undetermined Significance (MGUS) to Multiple Myeloma (MM)

The progression from MGUS to MM represents a critical transition within the spectrum of plasma cell dyscrasias. Even though MGUS includes monoclonal protein and a few symptoms, recent research shows that nearly all cases of MM develop from this condition. However, despite this established link, specific predictive markers that could indicate which patients with MGUS are likely to develop malignancy remain elusive (Allegra et al., 2019). During this transition, the communication between lymphocyte subsets and cytokines plays a crucial role in illustrating how the immune microenvironment influences the disease. Additionally, advancements in understanding non-coding RNAs offer promising insights into therapeutic and prognostic strategies for MM, underscoring the need for effective monitoring of patients with MGUS to facilitate timely intervention (Azab et al., 2020). For this reason, it is essential to understand the processes involved in this progression to effectively support patients.

14.2.9. Impact of Pathophysiology on Treatment Strategies

Understanding the pathophysiology of plasma cell dyscrasias, particularly of MM, is crucial in the planning of the optimal treatment modalities. The condition is characterized by the proliferation of malignant plasma cells with subsequent complications of anemia, bone pain, and renal failure. These reports significantly influence treatment modalities, which need to consider treatments to the cancer cells as well as systemic effects on the patient itself (Nicholas et al., 2024). For instance, how interleukin-6 promotes myeloma cell growth and survival identifies a possible targeted therapy that could inhibit the activity of this cytokine (Khorasani et al., 2024). In addition, the pathophysiologic background dictates the application of standard treatments, including chemotherapy and immunotherapy, which, although enhancing patient prognosis, tend to be limited by issues of drug resistance and adverse side effects. As research advances, a deeper understanding of these mechanisms may lead to new treatment strategies that enhance patient quality of life while reducing disease severity (Figure 14.10).

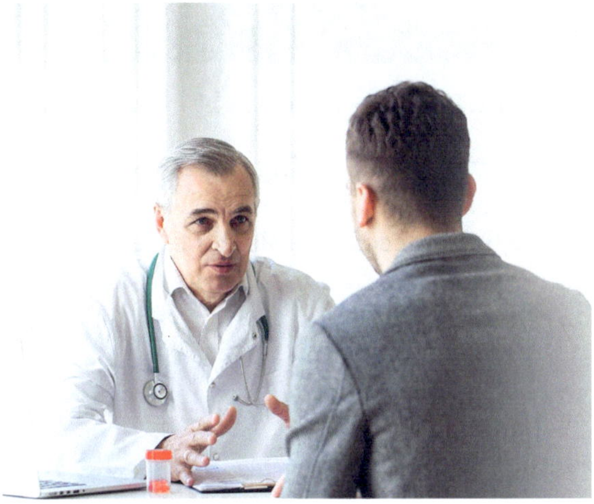

Figure 14.10. Understanding the pathophysiology of plasma cell dyscrasias, particularly multiple myeloma, is crucial for developing effective treatment strategies.

Source: https://www.lifeextension.com/-/media/lifeextension/scienceresearch/protocols/p_hero_cancer.jpg?rev=e74c1043f08347b98e22a0d68c4914de&h=800&w=1920&la=en&hash=AD66615C68D2B967CBF855FA80A195D7.

14.3. Diagnosis and Evaluation

It is essential to diagnose and evaluate plasma cell dyscrasias to manage patients well and plan the right treatment. Typically, clinicians inquire about the patient's medical history and conduct a physical examination, which can reveal symptoms of anemia, renal impairment, or bone-related issues. In addition, laboratory studies, for example, serum protein electrophoresis and immunofixation, play a key role in finding monoclonal proteins that are signs of plasma cell disorders. Also, doctors use X-rays or MRIs to check for lesions in the bones and signs of organ involvement. Notably, ocular manifestations can also serve as significant diagnostic clues; as outlined in (Suhasini et al., 2017), up to 31 patients initially presenting to ophthalmologists for vision defects were later diagnosed with blood dyscrasias, emphasizing the need for heightened awareness among healthcare providers. As laboratory results are linked to a patient's symptoms during the evaluation process, it leads to a more accurate diagnosis and a better assessment of the outcome (Figure 14.11).

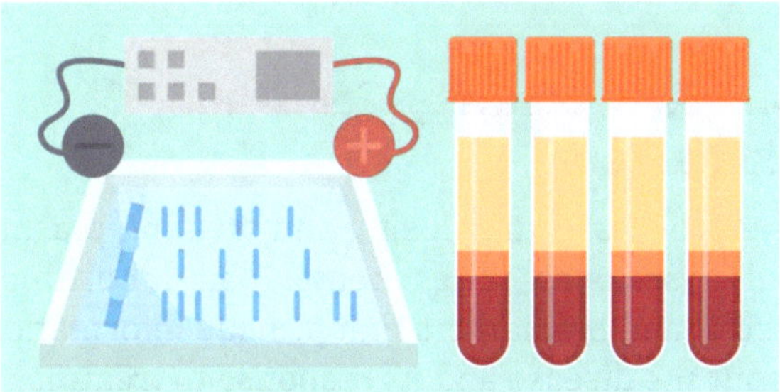

Figure 14.11. Laboratory tests, such as serum protein electrophoresis and immunofixation, are essential in identifying the presence of monoclonal proteins indicative of plasma cell disorders.

Source: https://cdn.myhealthteams.com/graphic/615cd87af53528150f1dac85/woriginal/Myeloma_-_Understanding_Serum_Protein_Electrophoresis_%28SPEP%29_for_Multiple_Myeloma_1200x630-7f8f476ff9dc8ba053487ad371edcb82.webp?1729535408.

14.3.1. Clinical Assessment and History Taking

A detailed history is crucial in assessing patients with plasma cell dyscrasias to identify both the symptoms and the underlying causes of the illness. Weakened immune systems in these individuals make them more susceptible to infections, so this should be given special attention during consultations. For example, the SHIVERING 1 and SHIVERING 2 trials underscore the need for tailored vaccination strategies, showing that a boosted high-dose influenza vaccine can significantly enhance seroprotection in this population (Duffy et al., 2018). Beyond immune status, clinicians must also consider comorbid conditions, such as those found in a case of a 62-year-old female with systemic lupus erythematosus who presented with a solitary pulmonary nodule that was later diagnosed as an amyloidoma (Anić et al., 2015). Therefore, a thorough evaluation, based on a detailed medical history, is necessary for the proper management and treatment of individuals with plasma cell dyscrasias.

14.3.2. Laboratory Tests and Biomarkers

The process of diagnosing and treating plasma cell dyscrasias relies heavily on laboratory results and biomarkers that provide information about the disease and its response to treatment. Among these, the measurement of serum-free light chains (FLC) has emerged as a cornerstone in evaluating patients with suspected plasma cell disorders due to its higher sensitivity compared to traditional urine-based electrophoretic assays. Since their introduction in 2001, serum FLC assays have been incorporated into international guidelines and risk stratification scores for conditions such as MGUS and light chain amyloidosis (AL amyloidosis) (Giles et al., 2024). Additionally, innovative markers like soluble mannose receptor (sMR) have shown promise in correlating with clinical features and other biomarkers, thereby enhancing our understanding of conditions like Gaucher disease, where macrophage function is altered (Beaton et al., 2024). They demonstrate that laboratory tests and biomarkers play a crucial role in enhancing the management of plasma cell dyscrasias (Figure 14.12).

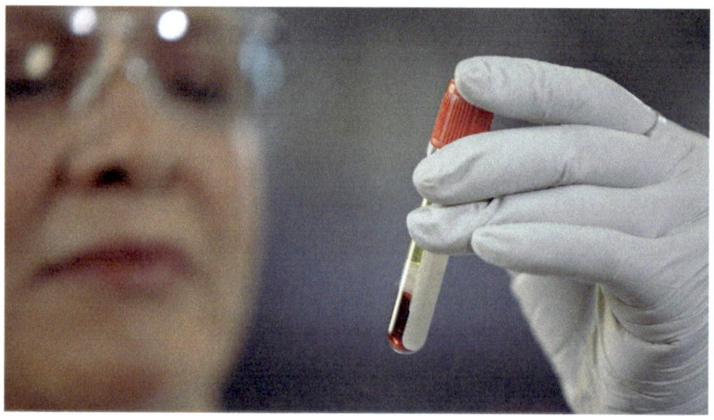

Figure 14.12. Serum-free light chains (FLC).

Source: https://marketing.webassets.siemens-healthineers.com/656ca6516121401b/18f236b2be6f/v/b8840ccc5694/siemens-healthineers_plasma-proteins_flc-monitoring-monoclonal-gammopathies.jpg.

14.3.3. Imaging Studies in Diagnosis

Imaging examinations play a crucial role in the diagnosis and management of plasma cell dyscrasias, particularly in the diagnosis of disease-related complications and determination of the extent of disease. Imaging modalities such as magnetic resonance imaging (MRI) and computed tomography (CT) are extremely useful in imaging the bone marrow and associated structures so that physicians can diagnose lytic lesions that may be indicative of underlying malignancies such as MM. For instance, individuals with plasma cell disorders manifesting retinopathy, as highlighted in a report with striking ocular manifestations, can be evaluated by imaging, which underscores the need for thorough evaluations (Suhasini et al., 2017). In addition, unusual presentations, such as thyroid lesions mimicking plasma cell malignancies, highlight the need for extensive imaging studies to ensure that the specificity of diagnosis and the corresponding treatment protocol are not compromised (Mo et al., 2020). Thus, imaging not only aids in diagnosis but also provides essential information regarding patient management in this complex spectrum of disorders.

14.3.4. Bone Marrow Biopsy Techniques

The process of bone marrow biopsy is very important for diagnosing plasma cell dyscrasias, especially when looking for MM. Usually, bone marrow aspiration and trephine biopsy are done at the same time to give a clear picture of the bone marrow's cells and their functions.

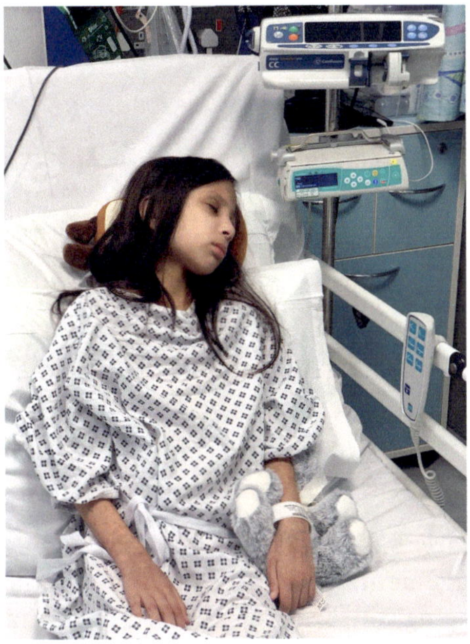

Figure 14.13. Trephine biopsy.

These techniques not only elucidate the presence of abnormal plasma cells but also help assess the overall hematological condition of the patient, with aspiration yielding cytological details and trephine providing histological context (Anem et al., 2017). Furthermore, advancements in imaging techniques, such as MRI, have enhanced diagnostic accuracy by assessing bone marrow infiltration patterns and vascularization, crucial for staging MM and monitoring treatment response (Baur et al., 2016). All in all, using both traditional biopsy and advanced imaging methods leads to better management of patients suffering from plasma cell dyscrasias (Figure 14.13). *Source:* https://pbs.twimg.com/media/GQBr7VMXkAEEJoG.jpg:large.

14.3.5. Role of Flow Cytometry

Flow cytometry (FCM) has increasingly been employed in the diagnosis and treatment of plasma cell dyscrasias because it is susceptible and specific. FCM technology enables the correct identification and characterization of aberrant plasma cells, which is key to understanding several conditions, such as MM and associated disorders. New studies demonstrate the strength of FCM in detecting neoplastic plasma cells in cerebrospinal fluid, thereby dramatically increasing diagnostic sensitivity in the meningeal localization of MM, as classical cytological methods often fail in most cases (Carulli et al., 2018). Moreover, the sophisticated application of FCM for immunophenotyping facilitates the measurement of surface antigen expression, which is crucial in determining the clonal status of plasma cell populations and in making treatment decisions (Balasubramanian et al., 2017). Thus, FCM is a technological advancement that not only aids diagnosis but also affects prognostic evaluation and therapeutic intervention in the management of plasma cell dyscrasias.

14.3.6. Genetic Testing and Prognostic Factors

Genetic testing is now vital in determining the outcome and treatment of patients with plasma cell dyscrasias. The intricate genetic landscape of conditions such as MM highlights the variability in treatment responses linked to specific genetic alterations. Studies suggest that genetic heterogeneity within myeloma cases can lead to differences in how patients respond to therapies, emphasizing the importance of personalized medicine in treatment planning (Tripathi et al., 2020). Additionally, certain genetic traits, including chromosomal translocations, may indicate that a patient is less likely to respond well to specific treatments, providing doctors with a better understanding of how to approach the patient's care. For instance, identifying patterns that correlate with resistance or sensitivity to treatments such as venetoclax can guide clinicians in crafting tailored therapeutic strategies (Mo et al., 2020). For this reason, the use of genetic testing in medicine helps doctors improve their ability to forecast a disease and select the most effective treatment for each patient (Figure 14.14).

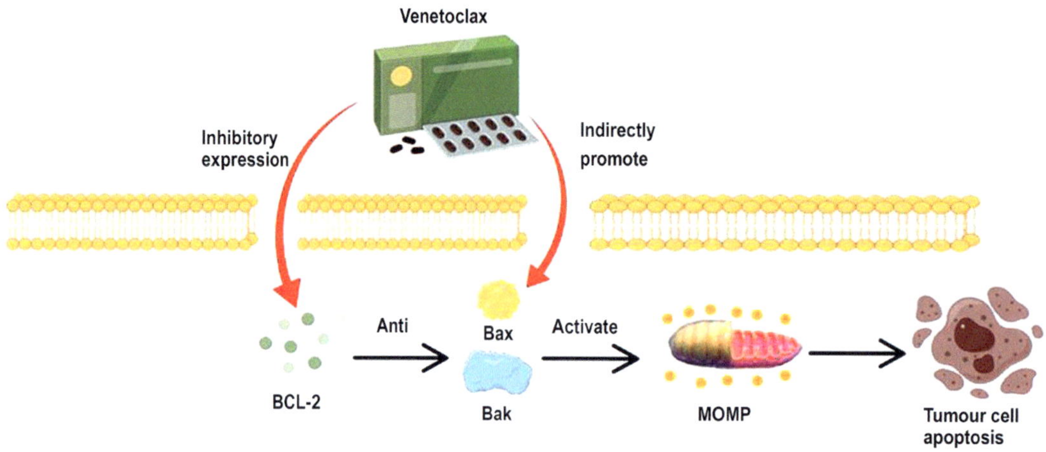

Figure 14.14. Venetoclax.

Source: https://www.frontiersin.org/files/Articles/1291920/fphar-14-1291920-HTML/image_m/fphar-14-1291920-g001.jpg.

14.3.7. Differential Diagnosis Considerations

In the clinical evaluation of plasma cell dyscrasias, particularly MM and MGUS, differential diagnosis plays a crucial role in determining treatment and management. The association of MGUS with the progression into MM often makes diagnosis challenging since no clear, predictive markers exist to identify which patients with MGUS are likely to develop malignancies (Allegra et al., 2019). Overlapping presentations with other diseases, including acute kidney injury caused by cast nephropathy, require cautious assessment to separate malignant and benign conditions. Cast nephropathy itself illustrates how myeloma kidney can initiate renal complications, where proteins filtered into the renal tubules complicate symptoms in patients and further blur diagnostic borders (Festuccia et al., 2022). Therefore, the strategy must be responsive to facilitate accurate diagnoses, ultimately leading to effective therapeutic measures.

14.3.8. Staging Systems for Plasma Cell Dyscrasias

The assessment and classification of plasma cell dyscrasias depend significantly on staging systems, as they help determine the prognosis and the most effective course of treatment. The International Staging System (ISS) remains a cornerstone, stratifying MM patients based on serum albumin and beta-2 microglobulin levels, thus providing crucial insights into overall survival outcomes. Recent studies highlight that approximately 39% of patients present with ISS stage III at diagnosis, emphasizing the need for early identification of high-risk patients to optimize therapeutic strategies (Iftikhar et al., 2024). Moreover, advancements in genetic profiling have introduced additional complexities to staging, particularly with the identification of gene mutations associated with myelodysplastic syndromes (MDSs), which can complicate the clinical picture in plasma cell disorders (Kirk et al., 2023). That is why it is necessary to merge traditional staging with molecular findings to better manage patients in all healthcare settings (Figure 14.15).

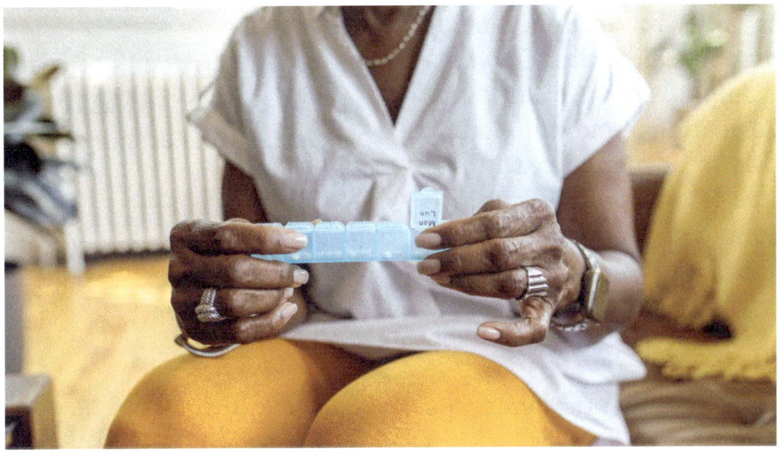

Figure 14.15: The International Staging System (ISS) remains a cornerstone, stratifying multiple myeloma patients based on serum albumin and beta-2 microglobulin levels, thus providing crucial insights into overall survival outcomes.

Source: https://res.cloudinary.com/sharecare/image/upload/ar_16:9,c_scale,w_828/f_webp,q_auto/dpr_3.0/v1698414482/taxonomy/How-is-multiple-myeloma-treated.

14.3.9. Importance of Multidisciplinary Approach

In MM and similar plasma cell dyscrasias, it is crucial to employ a team approach to ensure accurate diagnosis and treatment. Since these disorders have many symptoms, doctors from hematology, cardiology, and neurology may be needed to fully understand the patient's needs. In managing MM, doctors should also pay close attention to heart problems, since high-output heart failure affects around 8% of patients. This interrelation underscores the importance of collaboration among healthcare professionals in navigating the complexities of treatment, as hemodynamic abnormalities and enhanced angiogenesis can exacerbate existing conditions, necessitating tailored therapeutic strategies (Caimi et al., 2022). Additionally, addressing rare syndromes such as POEMS, which often co-occur with plasma cell neoplasms, requires further interdisciplinary synergy to improve patient outcomes and enhance overall care (Agrawal, 2025).

14.4. Treatment Options and Management

Managing plasma cell dyscrasias, mainly MM, has improved a lot, making it possible to use more effective treatments that help patients. New findings have revealed that non-coding RNAs play a key part in these disorders, which suggests they could be helpful for treatment. Studies have suggested that dysregulated non-coding transcripts may influence gene expression in malignant plasma cells, offering novel avenues for treatment strategies that could enhance the efficacy of existing therapies (Azab et al., 2020). Moreover, specific conditions such as cryoglobulinaemia associated with plasma cell dyscrasias necessitate a multifaceted approach, often incorporating antiviral treatments for underlying infections, like hepatitis C, which can provoke these complications (Braun et al., 2007). This new information about non-coding RNAs and the need to treat related conditions demonstrates that precision medicine can help improve outcomes and quality of life for people with plasma cell dyscrasias.

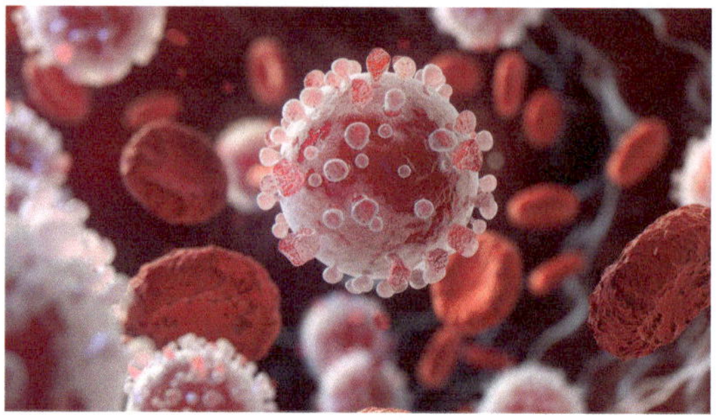

Figure 14.16. The treatment landscape for plasma cell dyscrasias has evolved significantly, particularly concerning chemotherapy regimens.

Source: https://s3.amazonaws.com/production.scholastica/article/125804/large/adobestock_854356781.jpeg?1731324929.

14.4.1. Chemotherapy Regimens

Much, however, in the therapeutic landscape of plasma cell dyscrasias, has changed with a specific focus lying on chemotherapy regimens. Such regimens drive the treatment for diseases like MM, systemic AL amyloidosis, and PCL – each of them with specific therapeutic challenges. Generally, conventional therapy is always an association of newer drugs and chemotherapy induction followed by autologous stem cell transplantation; however, these aggressive treatment modalities are hugely variable among patients. For instance, only 20% or even fewer of AL amyloidosis patients are transplant-eligible, so other combination induction regimens have to be employed.

They can be undermined by pre-existing organ dysfunction. In addition, relapse in PCL patients after intensive treatment implies the deficiencies of current chemotherapy regimens. New therapies, such as the novel CAR T-cell therapies that target plasma cells, are promising; however, clinical evidence remains limited in these same challenging plasma cell disorders (Heather et al., 2025; Gao et al., 2025) (Figure 14.16).

14.4.2. Targeted Therapies

The evolution of targeted therapies has dramatically changed the landscape of plasma cell dyscrasias, particularly in the treatment of MM. Targeted therapies differ from traditional chemotherapy in that the latter indiscriminately targets proliferating cells, while the former specifically targets unique molecular mechanisms responsible for the disease, thereby optimizing therapeutic benefit with minimal associated side effects. Agents include proteasome inhibitors, such as bortezomib, and immunomodulatory drugs, such as lenalidomide, which have achieved remarkable clinical benefits through their novel mechanisms of interfering with cellular processes critical to myeloma cell survival and growth. In addition, recent studies highlight the role of genetic markers in the evaluation of the treatment effects; for instance, the use of patterns of gene expression can direct treatment decisions with BCL2 inhibitors such as venetoclax that show differential effectiveness based on patients' genetic profiles (Tripathi et al., 2020; Adadzi et al., 2024). These innovations in targeted therapy are, therefore, not only personalizing treatment protocols but also offering significantly improved patient outcomes in this challenging situation.

14.4.3. Immunotherapy Approaches

With advancements in treatment for plasma cell dyscrasias, immunotherapy has become a crucial tool for physicians. In particular, anti-CD38 monoclonal antibodies, for example daratumumab, have been effective in treating light chain amyloidosis and MM. They not only fight malignant plasma cells but also boost the immune system to eliminate more abnormal cells. The dual action of these antibodies facilitates both direct depletion of neoplastic cells and rejuvenation of the immune system, promising a multifaceted approach to combating disease progression (Baldovino et al., 2020). Moreover, advancements in immunomodulatory drugs and CAR T-cell therapy have begun to reshape the treatment paradigm, offering tailored solutions that align with individual patient profiles (Adadzi et al., 2024). Using immunotherapeutic approaches in plasma cell dyscrasias is a significant advancement that may help patients live better and healthier lives (Figure 14.17).

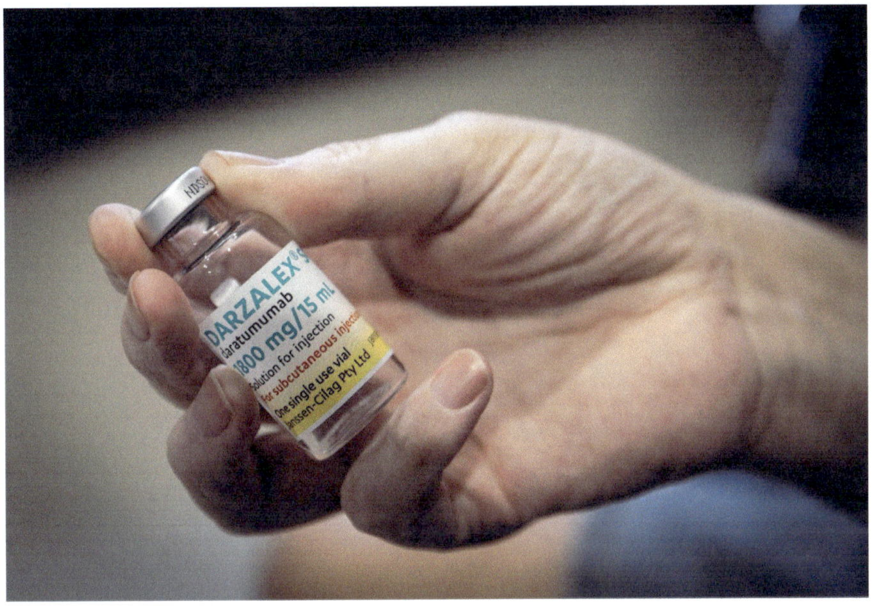

Figure 14.17. Daratumumab.

Source: https://cloudfront-ap-southeast-2.images.arcpublishing.com/nzme/N7WHNAA7ANB2FMYXCHPCD2JYZM.JPG.

14.4.4. Stem Cell Transplantation

Treatment with stem cell transplantation is now a main approach in the management of plasma cell dyscrasias, mainly when the condition results in permanent damage to organs, as in AL amyloidosis. High-dose melphalan followed by stem cell transplantation has been shown to significantly improve survival rates among patients affected by this condition, challenging prior assumptions about the limited feasibility of these treatments due to associated risks of disease relapse and graft failure (Wiest et al., 2018). Additionally, the treatment of these disorders has been evolving due to new insights into their causes. Research into non-coding RNAs has revealed their potential both as biomarkers and therapeutic targets, offering new avenues for clinical application in treating conditions like MM (Azab et al., 2020). As a result, stem cell transplantation for plasma cell dyscrasias highlights its major role in treatment and also shows the progress in managing these diseases.

14.4.5. Supportive Care and Symptom Management

Treatment of plasma cell dyscrasias relies heavily on good supportive care and symptom management, as patients typically experience multiple symptoms. As a result of MM and similar conditions, people may experience kidney problems, neurological symptoms, and intense pain. In cases of central nervous system (CNS) infiltration, for example, symptomatic management becomes crucial; treatments may include intrathecal chemotherapy and radiation, along with comprehensive supportive strategies that address the patient's holistic needs (Issa et al., 2025). Furthermore, complications arising from overlapping syndromes such as vanishing bile duct syndrome (VBDS) and hemophagocytic lymphohistiocytosis (HLH) underscore the necessity for tailored approaches in symptom management (Sukhija et al., 2024). When palliative care, pain management, and psychosocial support are all integrated, providers can significantly enhance the quality of life for these patients by addressing both their physical and emotional needs (Figure 14.18).

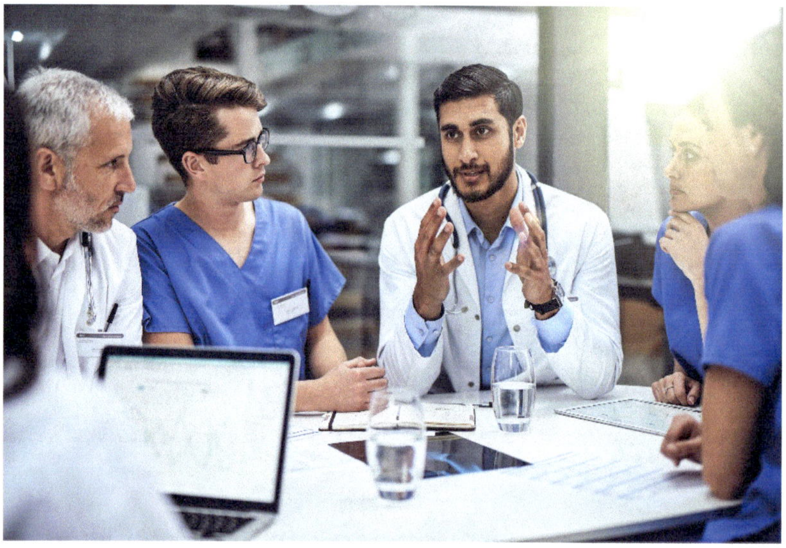

Figure 14.18. Effective supportive care and symptom management are crucial components in the treatment of plasma cell dyscrasias, particularly as patients often experience complex symptomatology.

source: https://images.ctfassets.net/tytuahdkbx9m/7IljI8WXncY4ip3muVV5mC/759a31d64cfd88a3921a0c639b557f1d/GettyImages-638646884.jpg.

14.4.6. Role of Clinical Trials

Clinical trials are essential in helping patients with plasma cell dyscrasias by testing new therapies in a well-organized way. Due to the SHIVERING 1 and SHIVERING 2 trials, researchers have improved the management of these conditions, primarily by focusing on vaccine effectiveness and infection risk. In these studies, a double high-dose influenza vaccine was administered to patients, demonstrating significantly higher rates of seroprotection compared to conventional regimens, underscoring the potential for tailored approaches in care (Duffy et al., 2018). Furthermore, the development of innovative treatment modalities, such as high-flux hemodialysis techniques, is crucial in managing complications like acute kidney injury in MM patients, underscoring the need for clinical trials to optimize therapeutic strategies and improve outcomes (Antolino et al., 2018). Pursuing evidence through clinical trials is a key part of the ongoing battle against plasma cell dyscrasias.

14.4.7. Long-term Management Strategies

Proper management strategies over time play an essential role in helping patients with plasma cell dyscrasias live better and healthier. Since these cancers are complicated, it is necessary to keep looking for new treatments and interventions. One promising avenue involves targeting non-coding RNAs, which have emerged as pivotal players in regulating gene expression and may offer both prognostic and therapeutic potential in MM (Azab et al., 2020). Also, it is now essential to use innovative vaccination methods to protect these patients from infections. Trials such as the SHIVERING study have demonstrated that high-dose influenza vaccinations can significantly improve seroprotection rates, thereby reducing the incidence of flu infections among patients with plasma cell dyscrasias (Duffy et al., 2018). Further research will necessitate the use of long-term management approaches to assist those affected (Figure 14.19).

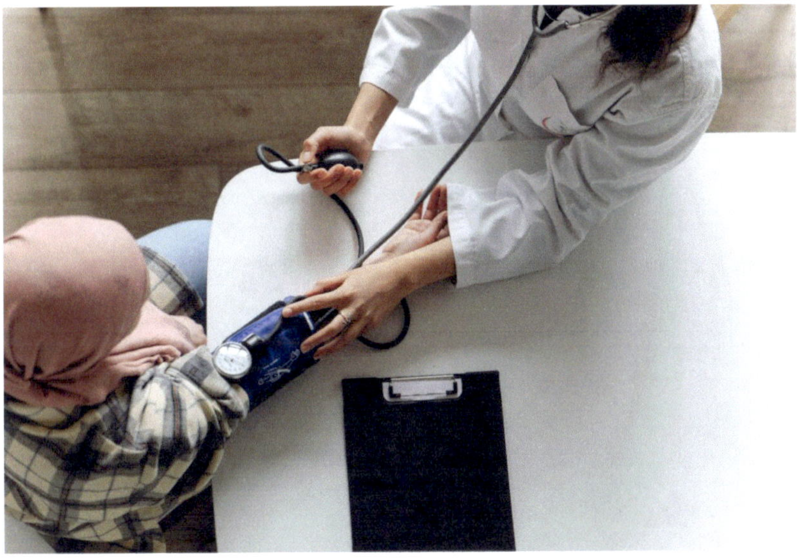

Figure 14.19. Long-term management strategies for plasma cell dyscrasias are critical in optimizing patient outcomes and enhancing quality of life.

Source: https://annals.edu.sg/wp-content/uploads/2023/11/07_RA_AAMS_2023_101-pexels-thirdman-7659567-1-e1701246122921.jpg.

14.4.8. Challenges in Treatment Adherence

Following the treatment plans for plasma cell dyscrasias can be very challenging and may result in less favorable outcomes for patients. Patients experiencing MM often face a complex therapeutic landscape characterized by a combination of chemotherapy, corticosteroids, and emerging therapies such as monoclonal antibodies and targeted agents (Adadzi et al., 2024). Still, many patients do not follow their treatment plans because of problems like side effects, mental stress, and the cost of long-term care. The presence of debilitating symptoms—such as anemia, bone pain, and fatigue—can lead to non-compliance as patients may prioritize immediate comfort over complex regimens (Andrea et al., 2013). Additionally, if patients are not well-informed about the importance of adhering to their treatment, it can exacerbate these issues and reduce the effectiveness of the therapy. As a result, improving adherence calls for special interventions that tackle the various issues patients face during their treatment period.

14.4.9. Future Directions in Treatment Research

As new research is done in plasma cell dyscrasias, it is essential to focus on new treatments that improve patient results. Recent studies have identified the regulatory T (Treg) and Th17 cell equilibrium as critical factors influencing disease progression and survival in MM and other plasma cell disorders, highlighting potential targets for immunotherapy (Aklilu et al., 2013). Furthermore, the introduction of high-dose influenza vaccination regimens has shown promise in significantly increasing seroprotection rates among patients with plasma cell dyscrasias, suggesting that tailored vaccination strategies may help mitigate infection risks in these vulnerable individuals (Duffy et al., 2018). As future studies advance, bringing together immunological findings and personalized vaccine development may lead to improved approaches for managing plasma cell diseases. New therapies, when used in conjunction with improved vaccination methods, could lead to better outcomes and a higher quality of life for patients.

A CLOSER LOOK

NON-CODING RNAS

Non-coding RNAs (ncRNAs) are RNA molecules that do not encode proteins but play key roles in regulating gene expression and cellular functions. Unlike messenger RNA (mRNA), which serves as a template for protein synthesis, ncRNAs help control how genes are turned on or off and how genetic information is processed. Common types of ncRNAs include microRNAs (miRNAs), which regulate gene expression by blocking or degrading mRNA, and long non-coding RNAs (lncRNAs), which can influence gene activity at many levels. A typical development process requires non-coding RNAs, and if their functions are disrupted, they can lead to different diseases.

SUMMARY

Managing plasma cell dyscrasias is challenging, primarily because they affect the immune system and increase the risk of infections. As evidenced by the SHIVERING trials, a boosted high-dose influenza vaccine regimen not only enhances seroprotection rates but also reduces the incidence of influenza among vulnerable patients, highlighting an essential advancement in patient care (Duffy et al., 2018). Moreover, understanding conditions such as POEMS syndrome reinforces the necessity for tailored treatment strategies, as these patients exhibit a complex interplay of symptoms that can complicate diagnosis and management (Agrawal, 2025). All in all, these results highlight the need for further research and large-scale studies to confirm their promising findings and aid in developing more effective treatments for patients with plasma cell disorders. It will be essential to address both short-term and long-term care to effectively face the complex challenges posed by these diseases.

Plasma cell dyscrasias are disorders characterized by the excessive growth of plasma cells, resulting in severe clinical symptoms. A critical understanding of these conditions includes recognizing MM as the second most common hematologic malignancy, emphasizing the importance of early intervention for improving patient survival rates. As highlighted, imaging techniques play a crucial role in both diagnosing and monitoring MM, with low-dose whole-body CT currently considered the primary modality for initial assessments due to its ability to detect bone lesions. At the same time, new features in diffusion-weighted MRI have made it easier to assess the severity of the disease and its response to treatment. Additionally, light chain (AL) amyloidosis demonstrates the complexities of plasma cell disorders, with unique pathways related to mutant antibody light chains that form harmful fibrils in various organs, signifying the need for targeted therapeutic approaches to manage these diverse conditions (Víctor et al., 2024; Georg et al., 2023).

REFERENCES

1. Issa, J. A., Vusqa, U., Behling, E. M., Budak-Alpdogan, T., & Ghimire, S. (2025). Multiple Myeloma with leptomeningeal involvement: A study of three cases exploring diagnosis and treatment challenges. *Cureus*. https://doi.org/10.7759/cureus.81602Adadzi, J., Alozie, U. G., Anderson II, J., Azi, A., et al. (2024). Current strategies and future directions in multiple myeloma: Disease overview and pathophysiology, conventional treatments and emerging therapies, challenges and innovations in management. https://core.ac.uk/download/621451768.pdf (accessed on 12th June 2025).
2. Agarwal, A., Cho, J. S., Dhingra, L. S., Kaur, K., et al. (2023). Ocular complications of plasma cell dyscrasias. https://core.ac.uk/download/612050555.pdf (accessed on 12th June 2025).
3. Agrawal, S. S. (2025). Case series on POEMS syndrome–a rare paraneoplastic disorder. https://core.ac.uk/download/640070983.pdf (accessed on 12th June 2025).
4. Aklilu, E. (2013). Immune regulation in plasma cell myeloma. https://opus.lib.uts.edu.au/bitstream/10453/28068/1/01front.pdf (accessed on 12th June 2025).
5. Allegra, A., Allegra, A. G., Di Salvo, E., Gangemi, S., Innao, V., Musolino, C., Pugliese, M., et al. (2019). Lymphocyte subsets and inflammatory cytokines of monoclonal gammopathy of undetermined significance and multiple myeloma. https://core.ac.uk/download/224993590.pdf (accessed on 12th June 2025).
6. Andres, M., Bacher, U., Banz, Y., Legros, M., et al. (2022). Correlation of plasma cell assessment by phenotypic methods and molecular profiles by NGS in patients with plasma cell dyscrasias. https://core.ac.uk/download/541130684.pdf (accessed on 12th June 2025).
7. Anem, V., Atla, B. L., & Dasari, A. (2017). Prospective study of bone marrow in hematological disorders. https://core.ac.uk/download/539912932.pdf (accessed on 12th June 2025).
8. Anić, B., Barešić, M., Brčić, L., Hećimović, A., et al. (2015). Solitary pulmonary amyloidal mimicking lung cancer on 18F-FDG PET-CT scan in systemic lupus erythematosus patient. https://core.ac.uk/download/130165593.pdf (accessed on 12th June 2025).
9. Antolino, G., Festuccia, F., Fofi, C., Giammarioli, A., et al. (2018). Serum free light chains removal by HFR hemodiafiltration in patients with multiple myeloma and acute kidney injury: A case series. https://core.ac.uk/download/188822815.pdf (accessed on 12th June 2025).
10. Askari, E., Rodríguez, S., & García-Sanz, R. (2021). Waldenström's macroglobulinemia: An exploration into the pathology and diagnosis of a complex B-cell malignancy. *Journal of Blood Medicine, 12*, 795–807. https://www.semanticscholar.org/paper/c381a76d440ff31c18eddf04dabd3bfe2a9e83c4 (accessed on 12th June 2025).
11. Azab, K. A., Morelli, E., Rocca, A., et al. (2020). The non-coding RNA landscape of plasma cell dyscrasias. https://core.ac.uk/download/287888008.pdf (accessed on 12th June 2025).
12. Babarović, E., Jonjić, N., Lučin, K., Načinović, A., et al. (2010). Combined evaluation of bone marrow aspirate and biopsy is superior in the prognosis of multiple myeloma. https://core.ac.uk/download/pdf/8418331.pdf (accessed on 12th June 2025).
13. Balasubramanian, S. K., Sadaps, M., Thota, S., Aly, M., Przychodzen, B., Hirsch, C. M., Visconte, V., et al. (2017). Rational management approach to pure red cell aplasia. *Hematological, 103*, 221–230. https://doi.org/10.3324/haematol.2017.175810 (accessed on 12th June 2025).

14. Baldovino, S., Barreca, A., Fenoglio, R., Ferro, M., et al. (2020). CD38 and anti-CD38 monoclonal antibodies in AL amyloidosis: Targeting plasma cells and beyond. https://core.ac.uk/download/351122522.pdf (accessed on 12th June 2025).

15. Baur, A., Baur-Melnyk, A., Stabler, A., Padhani, A. R., et al. (2016). MRI in multiple myeloma: A pictorial review of diagnostic and post-treatment findings. https://core.ac.uk/download/55803399.pdf (accessed on 12th June 2025).

16. Beaton, B., & Hughes, D. A. (2024). Soluble mannose receptor: A potential biomarker in Gaucher disease. https://core.ac.uk/download/598038632.pdf (accessed on 12th June 2025).

17. Braun, G. S., Horster, S., Ihrler, S., Schmid, C., et al. (2007). Cryoglobulinemic vasculitis: Classification and clinical and therapeutic aspects. https://core.ac.uk/download/12175185.pdf (accessed on 12th June 2025).

18. Broughton, M., Bhatta, S., Sharma, N., Umyarova, E., Khan, A. M., Devarakonda, S., Bumma, N., et al. (2024). Evaluation of characteristics and outcomes of patients with primary and secondary plasma cell leukemia treated with modern therapies. *Blood*. https://www.semanticscholar.org/paper/ccbf75a787336152f2eab0798597cf69b44e4325 (accessed on 12th June 2025).

19. Caimi, G., Carlisi, M., Lo Presti, R., Mancuso, D., et al. (2022). High output heart failure in multiple myeloma: Pathogenetic considerations. https://core.ac.uk/download/491502059.pdf (accessed on 12th June 2025).

20. Carulli, G., Caracciolo, F., Sammuri, P., Domenichini, C., Tarasco, A., Rousseau, M., Ottaviano, V., et al. (2018). Leptomeningeal myelotomies diagnosed by an eight-color single tube in dried formulation: A case report. *Cytometry Part B Clinical Cytometry, 94*, 721–723. https://doi.org/10.1002/cyto.b.21620 (accessed on 12th June 2025).

21. Chen, M., Rong, R., & Xia, X. (2022). Spotlight on proptosis: Role in pathogenesis and therapeutic potential of ocular diseases. *Journal of Neuroinflammation, 19*. https://www.semanticscholar.org/paper/544710d7e6d65d45d3308704312159ae261f5a84 (accessed on 12th June 2025).

22. Cooper, M., & Mayr, L. (2011). Label-free technologies for drug discovery. https://www.semanticscholar.org/paper/c680f9ae2aceb56146779560e911aae3f1840f0d (accessed on 12th June 2025).

23. Delicata, J., & Farrugia, D. (2013). An unusual case of multiple myeloma. https://core.ac.uk/download/46603947.pdf (accessed on 12th June 2025).

24. Duffy, E. (2018). The S.H.I.V.E.R.I.N.G. Trials: A novel vaccine strategy and analysis of serologic durability in patients with plasma cell dyscrasias. https://core.ac.uk/download/232776417.pdf (accessed on 12th June 2025).

25. Egyed, M., Kovács, Á., Moizs, M., Rajnics, P., et al. (2020). Can 18F-FDG PET/MR imaging contribute to the assessment of bone lesions in patients with plasma cell dyscrasias? https://core.ac.uk/download/323164860.pdf (accessed on 12th June 2025).

26. Estes, J. W. (1962). Modern concepts of the platelet in health and disease. https://open.bu.edu/bitstream/2144/26002/1/Estes_J.%20Worth_1962_web.pdf (accessed on 12th June 2025).

27. Festuccia, F., Lai, S., Mene,' P., Stoppacciaro, A., et al. (2022). Light chain cast nephropathy in multiple myeloma: Prevalence, impact and management challenges. https://core.ac.uk/download/566517062.pdf (accessed on 12th June 2025).

28. Gao, L., & Liu, B. (2025). Clinical significance of the peripheral blood neutrophil-to-lymphocyte ratio in predicting chemotherapy outcomes for small cell lung cancer. *Cancer Management and Research, 17*, 113–119. https://www.semanticscholar.org/paper/43422adbaf1553dc44caa0e363494891afd5c4fc (accessed on 12th June 2025).

29. Giles, H. V., & Karunanithi, K. (2024). Performance characteristics and limitations of the available assays for the detection and quantitation of monoclonal free light chains and new emerging methodologies. https://core.ac.uk/download/603470365.pdf (accessed on 12th June 2025).

30. Iftikhar, R., Ghani, D., Chaudhary, A., Ali, N., Anwar, N., Bokhari, S. W., Mahnoor, M., et al. (2024). Real world outcomes of autologous stem cell transplant in multiple myeloma: A study on behalf of Plasma Cell Dyscrasia Working Party of Pakistan Blood and Marrow Transplant Group. *Blood.* https://www.semanticscholar.org/paper/59c4e57abe377241cf2bc64cc037192c3306c7fe (accessed on 12th June 2025).

31. Jurczyszyn, A., Bator, M., Vesole, D. H., Salman, T., Richardson, P. G., & Anderson, K. C. (2025). New therapies in multiple myeloma: Benefits and limitations. *Polish Archives of Internal Medicine.* https://www.semanticscholar.org/paper/16aaced26b32f931b3840006d2495c27eadd92a7 (accessed on 12th June 2025).

32. Kerna, N. A., Pruitt, K. D., Carsrud, N. V., Ngwu, D. C., Kadivi, K., Holets, H. M., Flores, J. V., et al. (2024). Current strategies and future directions in multiple myeloma: Disease overview and pathophysiology, conventional treatments and emerging therapies, challenges and innovations in management. *European Journal of Medical and Health Research.* https://www.semanticscholar.org/paper/1730f55e3e34fd349359cbe350e58f88a2f4d061 (accessed on 12th June 2025).

33. Khorasani, A. B. S., Soufizomorrod, M., & Bashash, D. (2024). Unleashing the impact of exosomes derived from human placental mesenchymal stem cells (hPMSCs) on U-266 myeloma cell line. *International Journal of Hematology-Oncology and Stem Cell Research, 18*, 274–284. https://www.semanticscholar.org/paper/269e639bf5c9b5ef1b592625b8f7bb00c1177f2f (accessed on 12th June 2025).

34. Kirk, K., Hooper, K., Vankina, R., & Kumar, S. (2023). A retrospective review assessing the development of myelodysplastic syndromes in patients with plasma cell dyscrasias. *Blood.* https://www.semanticscholar.org/paper/177cfd4825037953dabdf1ff9defc4b36e533c64 (accessed on 12th June 2025).

35. Mo, J. H., Tan, D., Tjoa, T., Wang, J., et al. (2020). Anaplastic thyroid carcinoma histologically mimicking a plasmacytoma. https://core.ac.uk/download/323075504.pdf (accessed on 12th June 2025).

36. Morgan, H. T., Derman, B., Ma, H., & Kumar, S. K. (2025). Changing lanes: Extending CAR T-cell therapy to high-risk plasma cell dyscrasias. *Frontiers in Immunology, 16.* https://www.semanticscholar.org/paper/a436057f10981b9b33ec1fdd6d1d2ced7d11a543 (accessed on 12th June 2025).

37. Rawstron, A. C., Seegmiller, A. C., Joshua, D., Perez-Persona, E., et al. (2008). Immunophenotypic studies of monoclonal gammopathy of undetermined significance. https://core.ac.uk/download/pdf/8231774.pdf (accessed on 12th June 2025).

38. Rodriguez Laval, V., Lumbreras-Fernández, B., Aguado-Bueno, B., & Gómez León, N. (2024).

Imaging of multiple myeloma: Present and future. *Journal of Clinical Medicine, 13*, 264–264. https://doi.org/10.3390/jcm13010264 (accessed on 12th June 2025).

39. Rottenaicher, G. J., Absmeier, R. M., Meier, L., Zacharias, M., & Büchner, J. (2023). A constant domain mutation in a patient-derived antibody light chain reveals principles of AL amyloidosis. *Communications Biology, 6*. https://doi.org/10.1038/s42003-023-04574-y (accessed on 12th June 2025).
40. Singh, R., Singhal, S., Sinha, S., Cho, J., Nguyen, A. X., Dhingra, L., Kaur, S., et al. (2023). Ocular complications of plasma cell dyscrasias. *European Journal of Ophthalmology, 33*, 1786–1800. https://www.semanticscholar.org/paper/a31c6bb52dad1f587e2152f128e4505ba53b5ace (accessed on 12th June 2025).
41. Suhasini, S. (2017). Ocular manifestations of blood dyscrasias. https://core.ac.uk/download/288215952.pdf (accessed on 12th June 2025).
42. Sukhija, G., Baldwin, C., Elfar, E., Thoroughgood, J., Rutherford, A., Wincup, C., & Mahto, A. (2024). P08 Vanishing bile duct syndrome in hemophagocytic lymph histiocytosis precipitated by Stevens-Johnson syndrome: A rare case report. *Rheumatology Advances in Practice, 8*. https://www.semanticscholar.org/paper/5104de139cae57625c31e9f85a66384d233f4714 (accessed on 12th June 2025).
43. Tiwari, N., Sharma, R., Goyal, S., Mittal, S., & Gupta, V. (2023). Varied presentation of plasmacytosis seen in bone marrow at a tertiary care set-up. https://core.ac.uk/download/588567083.pdf (accessed on 12th June 2025).
44. Tripathi, S. (2020). Identifying gene expression biomarkers for venetoclax and bortezomib resistance in multiple myeloma. https://core.ac.uk/download/328856032.pdf (accessed on 12th June 2025).
45. Wiest, A. T. (2018). Single-center outcomes of renal transplantation in patients with AL amyloidosis. https://open.bu.edu/bitstream/2144/33020/5/Wiest_bu_0017N_14036.pdf (accessed on 12th June 2025).
46. Zendrini, A., Caimi, L., Di Noto, G., Paolini, L., et al. (2013). C-src enriched serum microvesicles are generated in malignant plasma cell dyscrasia. https://core.ac.uk/download/53617484.pdf (accessed on 12th June 2025).
47. Zhao, Y., Wei, Q., Zeng, R., Wang, Y., Yang, Y., & Wang, Y. (2024). Natural killer cell dysfunction drives keloid pathogenesis. *bioRxiv*. https://www.semanticscholar.org/paper/4b52b68005464978fcec084aa34c2729be7e6fde (accessed on 12th June 2025).

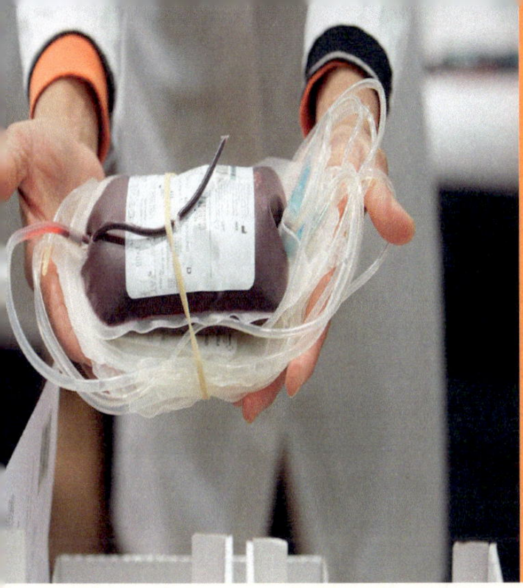

Chapter 14

TRANSFUSION MEDICINE AND BONE MARROW TRANSPLANTATION

Contents

Introduction...379

15.1. Fundamentals of Transfusion Medicine...380

15.2. Bone Marrow: Structure and Function...384

15.3. Bone Marrow Transplantation Procedures...388

15.4. The Intersection of Transfusion Medicine and Bone Marrow Transplantation (BMT)...392

Summary...399

References...400

Introduction

Bone marrow transplantation (BMT) and transfusion medicine are essential components of healthcare today, helping to treat many blood diseases and increasing the chances of survival for patients. The main advantage of these therapies is that they assist patients with leukemia and other malignancies by restoring their blood and immune systems. With new developments in stem cell technology, innovative therapies are being developed to address diseases that were once considered untreatable. Notably, the versatility of human pluripotent stem cells (hPSCs) and multipotent mesenchymal stem cells (MSCs) has garnered significant attention within regenerative medicine, indicating their potential in treating a wide range of conditions, as discussed in Duc et al. (2022). Furthermore, transfusion practices have evolved, emphasizing the importance of donor compatibility and the management of transfusion reactions, thereby enhancing the therapeutic efficacy and safety of blood products (Alexander et al., 2022). All these elements demonstrate how transfusion medicine and BMT have significantly transformed the way patients are treated.

15.1. Fundamentals of Transfusion Medicine

In the healthcare system, transfusion medicine is critical, especially when it comes to bone marrow transplantation (BMT). Proper and effective blood transfusions enable practitioners to significantly improve patient outcomes, particularly for those undergoing hematopoietic stem cell transplants. Red blood cells (RBCs) and platelets in the blood are essential for treating anemia and thrombocytopenia, which can occur during intense cancer treatments. Additionally, the challenges in transfusion medicine extend beyond providing blood; they also necessitate rigorous testing and screening to prevent infections. Better technology and methods have greatly helped, as evidenced by improved methods for screening pathogens that protect immunocompromised patients from infections during transfusions. This increasing focus on safety and efficacy is especially pertinent given the unique vulnerabilities faced by patients in a BMT setting, underscoring the integral role of transfusion medicine in modern health care (Udvardy et al., 2023; Anasiz et al., 2024) (Figure 15.1).

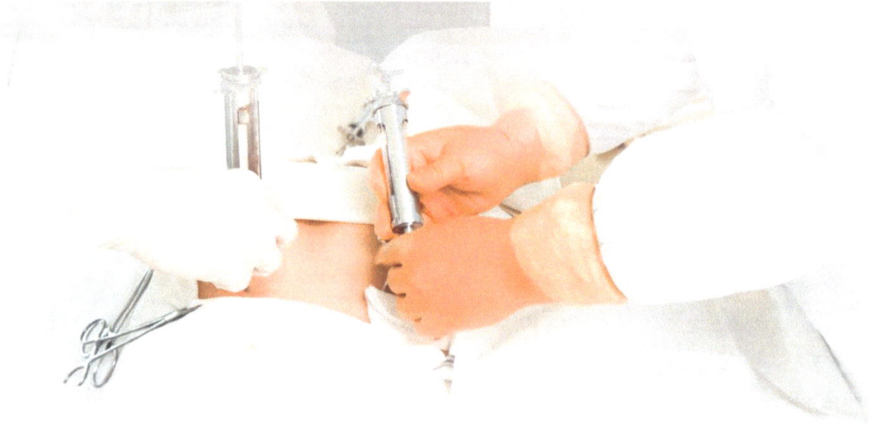

Figure 15.1. Transfusion medicine serves as a critical cornerstone within the healthcare system, particularly in the context of BMT.

Source: https://aiio.asterhospitals.in/sites/default/files/2022-11/bone-marrow-transplant-procedure-and-types.jpg.

15.1.1. Types of Blood Components Used in Transfusions

Blood components play a significant role in transfusion medicine to support various medical treatments. RBCs are the most commonly transfused component, essential for replenishing oxygen-carrying capacity in patients with anemia, trauma, or surgery. Patients receiving chemotherapy or those with blood disorders rely on platelets for their crucial role in blood clotting. Plasma is administered to individuals with coagulopathies and during massive transfusions, as it contains clotting factors. Additionally, cryoprecipitate, derived from plasma, is beneficial in managing fibrinogen deficiency. Innovations in blood component therapies, such as those involving umbilical cord blood, are also expanding treatment options; these hematopoietic stem cells (HSCs) are increasingly recognized for their potential beyond traditional uses and could play a significant role in future therapeutic interventions (Pateraki et al., 2024). This critical understanding of blood components highlights the complexity and significance of transfusion practices in modern medicine (Sophia et al., 2024).

15.1.2. Indications for Blood Transfusion

Blood transfusions are typically administered based on the medical conditions that necessitate them. Blood transfusion is usually recommended for severe anemia, a lot of blood loss from trauma or surgery, and certain hematological diseases, mainly thalassemia and sickle cell disease (SCD). For instance, patients with β thalassemia often require regular transfusions to alleviate chronic anemia resulting from ineffective erythropoiesis and to maintain hemoglobin levels for optimal physiological functioning (Lal et al., 2021). Additionally, in cases such as SCD, RBC exchange transfusions are a standard therapeutic approach to mitigate the risk of stroke and manage acute complications, emphasizing the importance of clinical context in determining transfusion strategies (Güssi et al., 2019). For these reasons, it is essential to understand the various applications of blood transfusion to effectively assist patients and tailor treatments to each person's unique needs (Figure 15.2).

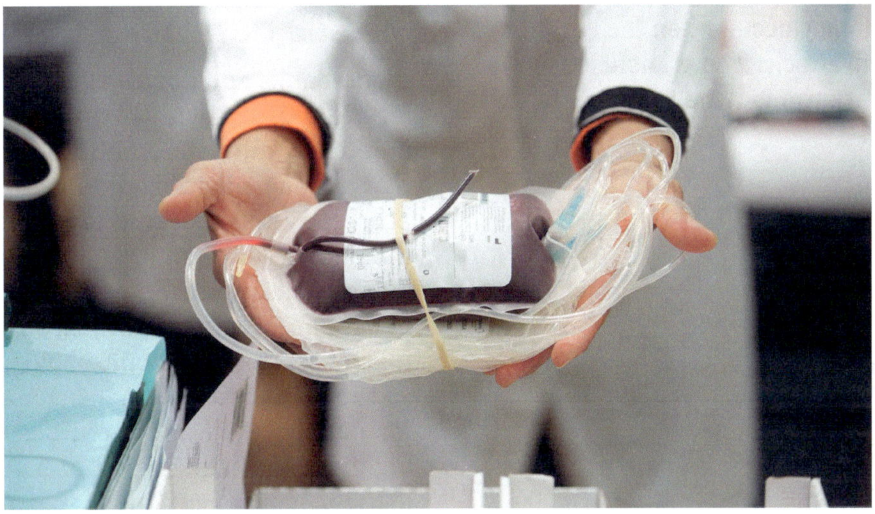

Figure 15.2. Indications for blood transfusion typically encompass severe anemia, significant blood loss from trauma or surgery, and specific hematological disorders, most notably thalassemia and sickle cell disease.

Source: https://post.healthline.com/wp-content/uploads/2020/08/Healthcare-worker-holding-out-blood-bag-1296x728-header.jpg.

15.1.3. Blood Typing and Crossmatching Procedures

One of the most essential parts of transfusion medicine is carrying out blood typing and crossmatching to make sure the blood is compatible. Accurate blood typing involves both forward and reverse typing methods; however, discrepancies can arise due to various factors, including the influence of monoclonal immunoglobulins and the presence of blood type subtypes, which can complicate interpretation and necessitate additional testing methods, such as physiological saline, polyamine, and anti-human globulin approaches (Qiu et al., 2023). Moreover, crossmatching is essential to prevent immune reactions, particularly in the context of BMT, where patients may require antigen-matched RBCs to minimize the risk of complications (Karim et al., 2023). With improved blood typing methods, it is essential to regularly screen for homologous antibodies, taking into account a patient's medical history and previous transfusions, to ensure optimal results and effective transfusion practices in various medical situations.

15.1.4. Risks and Complications Associated with Transfusions

Transfusions are essential for many patients, but they may also bring risks and possible problems that can happen during or after the procedure. A significant worry is the chance of hemolytic reactions, which may occur when the recipient's immune system attacks the transfused blood, especially in situations where there is ABO incompatibility.

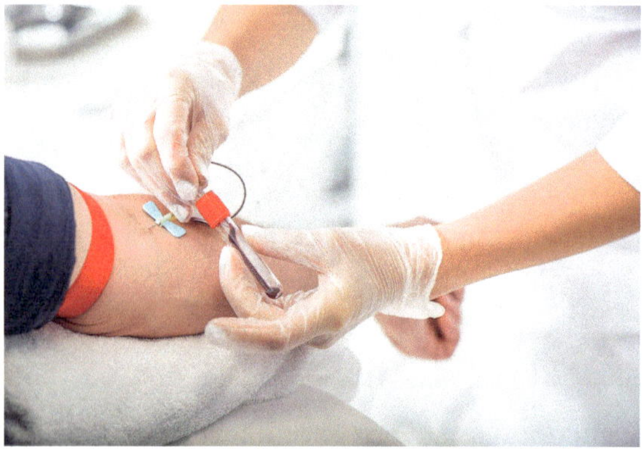

Figure 15.3. Transfusions, while often life-saving, are not without inherent risks and complications that can arise during or after the procedure.

Source: https://www.broadgategp.co.uk/wp-content/uploads/2021/10/Blood-Transfusion-1800x1202.jpeg.

However, the possibility of infections, including those from bloodborne pathogens, remains a significant concern despite thorough screening. Furthermore, complications such as transfusion-related acute lung injury (TRALI) can pose severe challenges to patient recovery post-transfusion. In specific cases, particularly within the context of BMT, RBC exchange transfusions can mitigate specific risks, such as iron overload, although they come with increased costs and resource demands (Güssi et al., 2019). The advancement of adoptive T cell transfer presents an innovative approach that may enhance transfusion efficacy while addressing some of these complications, thus demonstrating the dynamic evolution within transfusion medicine (Carl et al., 2018) (Figure 15.3).

15.1.5. Role of Blood Banks and Donation Centers

Blood banks and donation centers are essential for healthcare, mainly in the areas of transfusion medicine and BMT. These centers ensure that blood and its components are collected, processed, and delivered to patients who require them for transfusions. Besides providing blood, blood banks conduct thorough testing to prevent infections from spreading through transfusions. In transfusion medicine, advancements such as the use of recombinant factor VIIa (rFVIIa) for patients with inherited bleeding disorders highlight the importance of blood products in managing complex clinical scenarios. Moreover, ongoing efforts to reduce reliance on bovine-derived serum in cell cultures, as evidenced by the exploration of human platelet lysates as alternatives, underscore the need for innovation within donation centers to enhance the quality of therapeutic applications (Jan van der Valk, 2017; Revel et al., 2013).

15.1.6. Advances in Blood Preservation Techniques

Advances in blood preservation methodologies have significantly impacted the efficiency and safety of bone marrow transplant and transfusion medicine. Emerging technologies, including the development of synthetic substitutes for blood and sophisticated cryopreservation methods, have enhanced the viability of long-term stored blood products. Such improvements enable better management of donor blood supply, particularly in regions with limited access to fresh donations. Furthermore, the intersection of blood preservation and regenerative medicine is depicted by stem cell technologies, whose role is increasingly viewed as having therapeutic applications within the context of regenerative medicine and transplantation (Duc et al., 2022). Furthermore, combining such innovations with new immunological processing can contribute to reduced tissue transplantation complications, thereby opening up new directions for patient treatment and transfusion practice outcomes (Padula et al., 2022). Better preservation methods not only optimize blood storage but also maximize the overall efficacy of transfusion therapy (Figure 15.4).

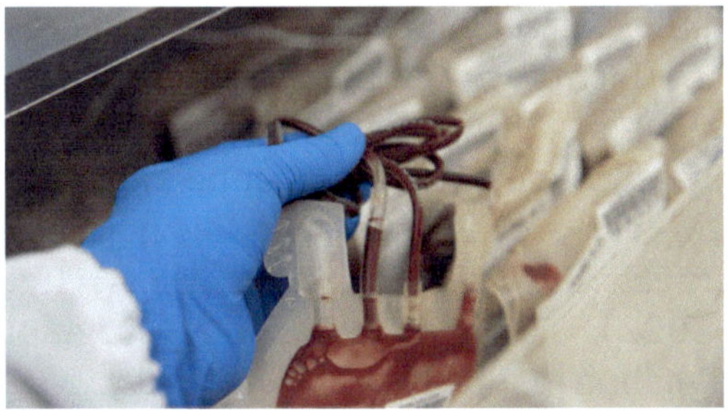

Figure 15.4.The evolution of blood preservation techniques has significantly impacted the efficiency and safety of transfusion medicine and bone marrow transplantation.

Source: https://www.froilabo.com/wp-content/uploads/2022/12/bllod-bank.png.

15.1.7. Ethical Considerations in Blood Donation

Advances in blood preservation technology have had a significant impact on the efficacy and safety of transfusion medicine and BMT. New technologies, such as the production of artificial blood substitutes and sophisticated cryopreservation methods, have improved viability of long-stored blood products. These developments allow better management of the donor blood supply, particularly for regions with remote access to fresh donations. In addition, the convergence of blood preservation and regenerative medicine is illustrated by stem cell technology, whose therapeutic applications are increasingly recognized within the framework of regenerative medicine and transplantation (Duc et al., 2022). In addition, integrating such innovations together with emerging immunological processing will lead to fewer tissue transplantation complications and thus new avenues for patient treatment and transfusion practice outcomes (Padula et al., 2022). Enhanced preservation methods not only optimize storage of blood but also optimize the overall efficiency of transfusion therapy.

15.1.8. Regulations Governing Transfusion Practices

Following the regulations for transfusion is crucial for patient safety, especially in BMT, where patients may be at a greater risk. These regulations mandate rigorous screening processes and pathogen inactivation strategies to mitigate the transmission of infections, a concern exacerbated by the emergence of novel pathogens in recent years, as highlighted in the assessment of transfusion-transmitted agents (Udvardy et al., 2023). Research has demonstrated a significant correlation between transfusion volume and complications, such as graft-versus-host disease (GvHD) and infection rates, among patients undergoing allogeneic hematopoietic stem cell transplantation (AHSCT) (Nabih et al., 2019). That is why adhering to strict rules enhances the effectiveness of transfusions and underscores the importance of vigilance in identifying potential risks associated with blood products. For this reason, these rules are crucial for enhancing the outcomes of transfusions administered to patients undergoing BMT (Figure 15.5).

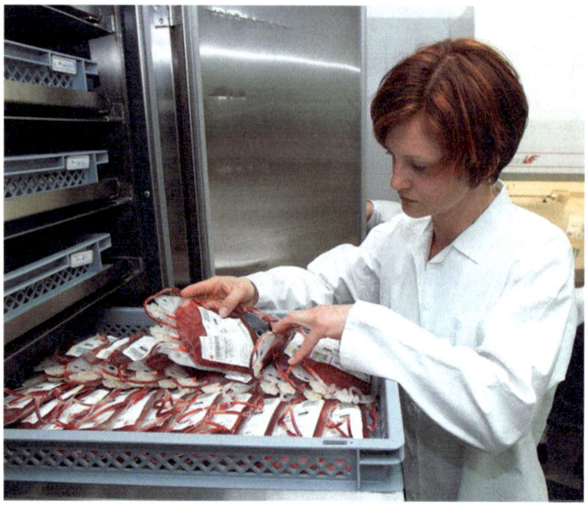

Figure 15.5. The regulations governing transfusion practices are pivotal for ensuring patient safety, particularly in the context of bone marrow transplantation, where immunocompromised patients face heightened risks.

Source: https://cdn.britannica.com/09/147309-050-70516926/Blood-bank-employee-blood.jpg.

15.1.9. Future Directions in Transfusion Medicine

As transfusion medicine continues to evolve, future trends hold promise in the form of advanced patient care and enhanced treatment effectiveness. The use of adeno-associated virus (AAV) in gene therapy represents a revolutionary step with great promise for the treatment of hematological conditions that are frequently treated with transfusion therapy. Recent research on the use of recombinant AAV (rAAV) has revealed its potential for administering genetic therapies, particularly in conditions such as hemophilia and SCD, for which traditional transfusions prove insufficient (Wang et al., 2024). Concurrently, the integration of regenerative medicine approaches, such as stem cell therapy, is revolutionizing treatment planning in transfusion medicine and BMT, allowing for more effective ways to address several hematologic issues (Liang et al., 2024). As they develop, they not only hold the promise of enriching the therapeutic space but also highlight the value placed on adaptability and futurism within the profession, ultimately seeking better results in patient care.

15.2. Bone Marrow: Structure and Function

Bone marrow is essential in the hematopoietic system since it is the principal place where blood cells are produced and mature. This spongy tissue, located within the central cavities of bones, contains a diverse array of stem cells, particularly HSCs and MSCs. Because HSCs produce RBCs, white blood cells (WBCs), and platelets, they help keep the body's balance and defend it from infections. At the same time, MSCs play a crucial role in repairing and regenerating tissues, making them highly valuable in regenerative medicine. Recent advancements in the understanding of these cells suggest potential therapeutic avenues using MSCs derived from bone marrow for treating various diseases, including neurological disorders and metabolic conditions (Duc et al., 2022). Furthermore, the dysregulation of signaling pathways, such as the JAK/STAT pathway, can adversely affect hematopoiesis, highlighting the need for research into targeted therapies in transplant settings (Hu et al., 2021).

15.2.1. Anatomy of Bone Marrow

The bone marrow anatomy is quite critical in comprehending the way it functions in transfusion medicine and BMT. Bone marrow is housed within the cavities of long bones and serves as a significant site of hematopoiesis, the process of producing blood cells. It occurs in two primary forms: red marrow, which is actively involved in the production of RBCs, WBCs, and platelets, and yellow marrow, which is essentially a fat depot. Clinicians and scientists must grasp this distinction when determining the nature of bone marrow failure in most hematologic disorders. In addition, the bone marrow complex microenvironment facilitates mutual interactions between stromal cells and supportive HSCs, which are essential for successful bone marrow transplants. The technical sophistication of bone marrow justifies its importance not only in normal physiology but also in the therapeutic approaches that address cancer and its complication due to its treatment, according to the NCCN Guidelines for Survivorship (Crystal et al., 2018) and the issues raised in recent cancer treatment methods (Maeda et al., 2018) (Figure 15.6).

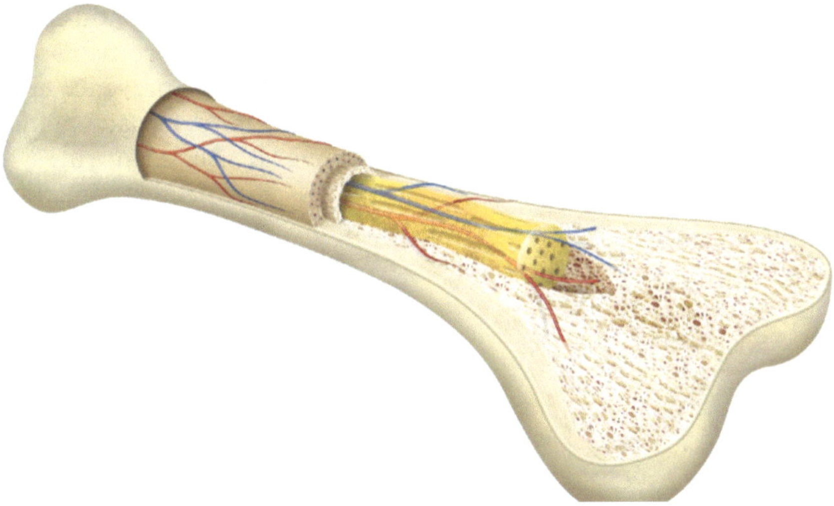

Figure 15.6. The anatomy of bone marrow plays a crucial role in understanding its function within the framework of transfusion medicine and bone marrow transplantation.

Source: https://stgaccinwbsdevlrs01.blob.core.windows.net/newcorporatewbsite/blogs/october2023/detail-main-Bone-Marrow.jpeg.

15.2.2. Types of Cells Produced in Bone Marrow

Bone marrow is responsible for producing various blood cells that are essential for the proper functioning of the immune and circulatory systems. Among these, HSCs give rise to multiple cell lineages, including RBCs (erythrocytes), which are essential for oxygen transport; WBCs (leukocytes), which are crucial for immune response; and platelets (thrombocytes), which are involved in clotting mechanisms. The process of HSCs differentiating into various cell types is closely regulated by the growth factors and cytokines present in the bone marrow. Recent advancements in transfusion medicine emphasize the importance of high-quality cell production for therapeutic purposes, particularly in the context of BMT, where engineered cells, such as chimeric antigen receptor (CAR) T cells, can significantly enhance the efficacy of treatment against conditions like leukemia and lymphoma (Carl et al., 2018; Bieback et al., 2019).

15.2.3. Role of Bone Marrow in Hematopoiesis

In the system that produces blood cells, the bone marrow is essential for creating all blood components, including RBCs, WBCs, and platelets. As the primary site of hematopoiesis, the bone marrow provides a specialized microenvironment that supports the proliferation and differentiation of HSCs. The stem cells develop inside the marrow and eventually become mature blood cells that enter the peripheral circulation. The connection between HSCs and stromal cells in the bone marrow is necessary to maintain the proper balance between renewing blood cells and making new ones. As advancements in transfusion medicine and techniques in BMT evolve, understanding the intricacies of hematopoiesis remains vital for improving therapeutic strategies in treating hematological disorders (Chocholata et al., 2019; Iolascon et al., 2021) (Figure 15.7).

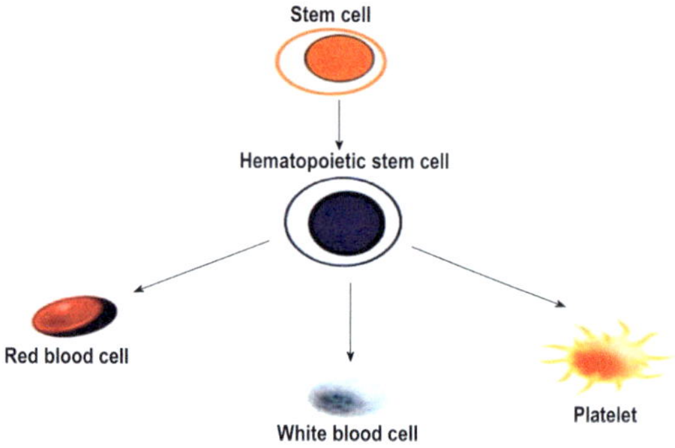

Figure 15.7. Within the complex hierarchy of blood cell production, bone marrow plays an indispensable role in hematopoiesis, the process through which all blood components, including RBCs, white blood cells, and platelets, are generated.

Source: https://f6publishing.blob.core.windows.net/2626da25-cc43-4110-b898-98a43ed245ad/87532-g001.png.

15.2.4. Factors Affecting Bone Marrow Function

Several factors influence the function of bone marrow, including the source of stem cells, the conditioning treatment, and the recipient's age and other underlying health issues. Recent studies have highlighted the role of donor traits, such as thalassemia trait status, in determining post-transplant hematological outcomes, revealing that recipients of stem cells from thalassemia trait donors exhibit lower hemoglobin levels compared to those from normal donors, emphasizing the importance of donor selection in transplantation success (Khan et al., 2024). Additionally, factors like the intensity of pre-transplant conditioning regimens and the presence of acute GVHD have been shown to impact platelet engraftment and overall survival rates post-transplant (Andrew et al., 2024). Understanding all these factors is crucial for developing more effective transplantation methods and improving patient outcomes in transfusion medicine and associated therapies.

15.2.5. Diseases Affecting Bone Marrow Health

Since blood cells are produced in the bone marrow, its health is crucial. Diseases that harm the bone marrow, such as leukemia, aplastic anemia, and myelodysplastic syndromes, reduce the production of blood cells and impact the health of the immune and cardiovascular systems. Chronic myeloid leukemia (CML), for example, leads to the uncontrolled proliferation of abnormal WBCs, which can infiltrate and disrupt normal marrow function, thereby increasing susceptibility to infections and anemia (Alexander et al., 2022). The latest progress in stem cell technology may help solve these issues. Stem cell therapies using bone marrow-derived mesenchymal stem cells (BM-MSCs) have shown potential in regenerating damaged tissues and correcting hematological disorders, thereby enhancing patients' quality of life and recovery outcomes (Duc et al., 2022). Using a variety of therapeutic methods, the outlook for treating bone marrow diseases is looking better (Figure 15.8).

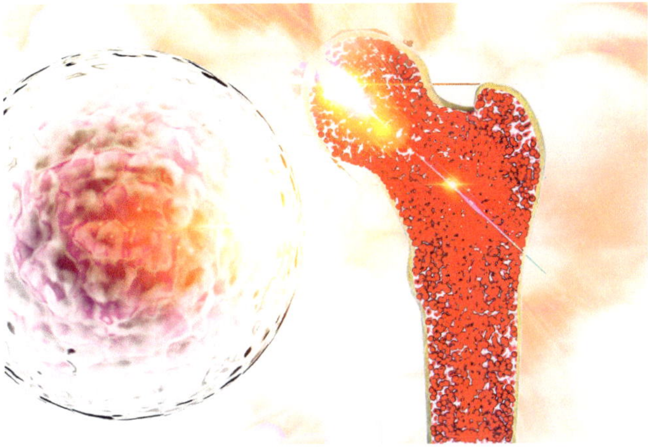

Figure 15.8. The health of bone marrow is critically significant, as it is the site of hematopoiesis—the process of blood cell formation.

Source: https://nyulangone.org/news/sites/default/files/2019-07/press-release-scientists-define-set-of-bone-marrow-cells.jpg.

15.2.6. Diagnostic Techniques for Bone Marrow Disorders

Bone marrow disorders are usually diagnosed by using both traditional and advanced methods. In the beginning, bone marrow aspiration and biopsy helped pathologists examine the cells and identify several types of blood cancers. However, the use of molecular methods has significantly improved both the accuracy and understanding in diagnosis. Techniques such as fluorescence in situ hybridization (FISH) and polymerase chain reaction (PCR) are crucial in detecting genetic abnormalities characteristic of specific disorders, including translocations indicative of leukemias and lymphomas. These studies enhance the classification of diseases and inform treatment plans, guiding therapy based on the patient's response to treatment, primarily in the field of hematopoietic stem cell transplantation (HSCT). As demonstrated in pioneering programs, such as those developed in resource-constrained settings, these advanced diagnostics are crucial for improving patient outcomes in transfusion medicine and transplant services (Veillon, 2002; Albert et al., 2016).

15.2.7. Importance of Bone Marrow Microenvironment

The environment within the bone marrow is crucial for hematopoiesis, as it facilitates the development and proper functioning of blood cells, thereby maintaining the body's balance. This complex niche not only provides structural support but also engages in dynamic signaling processes, crucial for the survival and differentiation of HSCs. This microenvironment is critical when it comes to progress in transfusion medicine and BMT. As recent research suggests, stem cell-based therapies, including those utilizing bone marrow-derived multipotent MSCs, hold promise for treating a wide array of disorders stemming from dysfunctional hematopoiesis (Duc et al., 2022). Additionally, the regulation of pathways such as JAK/STAT within the bone marrow microenvironment can significantly impact cell proliferation and function, suggesting that targeting these pathways may enhance therapeutic outcomes in both transplantation and regenerative medicine contexts (Hu et al., 2021) (Figure 15.9).

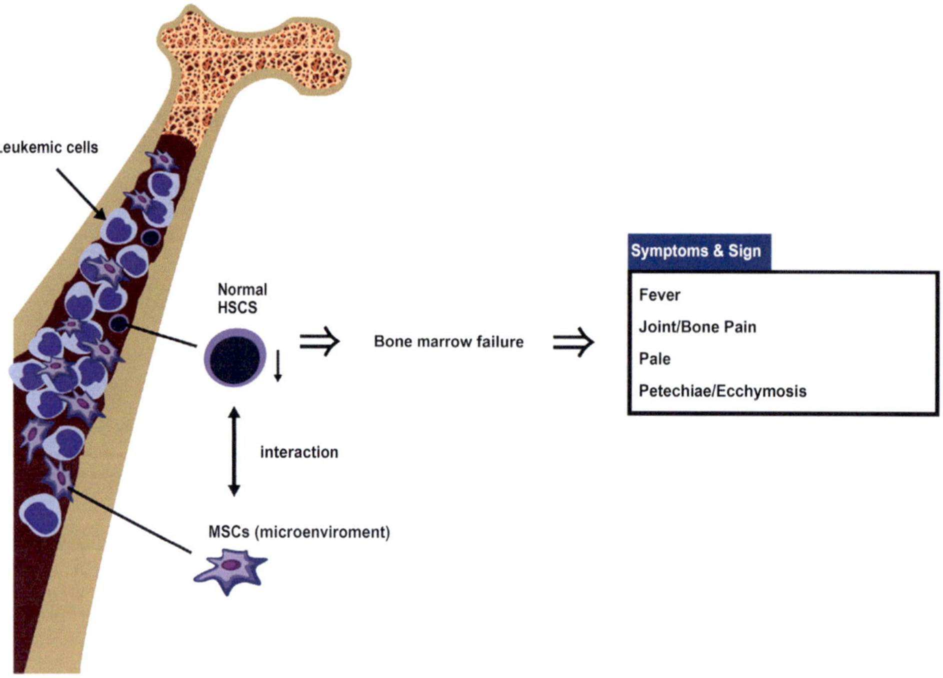

Figure 15.9. The bone marrow microenvironment plays a critical role in hematopoiesis, influencing the development and function of various blood cell lineages essential for maintaining systemic homeostasis.

Source: https://www.mdpi.com/ijms/ijms-25-02527/article_deploy/html/images/ijms-25-02527-g001.png.

15.2.8. Genetic Factors Influencing Bone Marrow Function

Genetic factors play a significant role in how bone marrow works, which is vital for blood transfusion and BMT. Genetic disorders, such as severe combined immunodeficiency (SCID) and β-thalassemia, highlight the essential role of specific genes in the development and maintenance of HSCs. For instance, in β-thalassemia, mutant alleles lead to ineffective erythropoiesis and alterations in the bone marrow microenvironment, thereby compromising HSC quiescence and self-renewal abilities, ultimately affecting transplant outcomes (Vinchi et al., 2020). Similarly, inborn errors of immunity (IEI), encompassing a variety of genetic mutations, can disrupt immune function, necessitating HSCT as a corrective measure (Fernandes et al., 2021). Understanding these genetic factors is crucial for developing more effective treatments and supporting patients with genetic hematological disorders.

15.3. Bone Marrow Transplantation Procedures

BMT is an integral part of treating different blood disorders, both malignant and non-malignant. The treatment involves administering HSCs to help patients with bone marrow failure or abnormal blood cell production. The procedure begins by collecting stem cells from the bone marrow or from the blood circulating outside the bone marrow. It is crucial to carefully match the donor and recipient to minimize the risk of GVHD, a significant complication following allogeneic transplants. Additionally, strategies such as anti-CD19 CAR T-cell therapy are being explored to enhance treatment efficacy by targeting specific antigens in malignant cells. However, these therapies present their challenges, including complex manufacturing and potential toxic effects (Liu et al., 2020). Furthermore, apheresis techniques, including RBC exchange transfusions, may be helpful in managing complications associated with bone marrow transplants, such as those arising from sickle cell disease (Güssi et al., 2019).

15.3.1. Types of Bone Marrow Transplants (Autologous vs. Allogeneic)

Using BMT is important for treating both malignant and non-malignant blood disorders. Doctors give HSCs to patients who have trouble with bone marrow or unusual blood cell production.

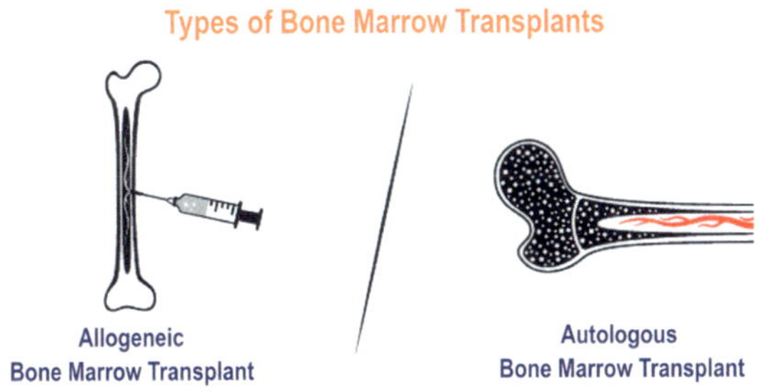

Figure 15.10. Bone marrow transplants, a critical therapeutic intervention in transfusion medicine, are classified into two primary types: autologous and allogeneic.

Source: https://www.yashodahospitals.com/wp-content/uploads/2024/09/Types-of-Stem-Cell-and-Bone-Marrow-Transplants_Body-1-1200x675.png.

First, the procedure involves obtaining stem cells from the bone marrow or from the blood, which is not contained within the bone marrow. It is necessary to find a good match between the donor and the recipient to prevent GVHD, which is a big issue after allogeneic transplants. Additionally, strategies such as anti-CD19 CAR T-cell therapy are being explored to enhance treatment efficacy by targeting specific antigens in malignant cells, although these therapies present their challenges, including complex manufacturing and potential toxic effects (Liu et al., 2020). Furthermore, apheresis techniques, including RBC exchange transfusions, may be helpful in managing complications associated with bone marrow transplants, such as those arising from SCD (Güssi et al., 2019) (Figure 15.10).

15.3.2. Pre-Transplant Evaluation and Preparation

A thorough evaluation and preparation before the transplant are crucial in BMT, as they help avoid complications and make the treatment process more efficient. At this time, the team reviews the patient's previous medical records, assesses their current condition, and determines if they are a suitable candidate for transplantation. In particular, tests may include imaging studies, laboratory exams, and assessments of organ function to check

if the patient is ready for the transplant. This meticulous preparation is particularly relevant in the context of stem cell therapies, where advancements in technologies, including the use of multipotent MSCs, are explored for their applications in regenerative medicine and the treatment of various disorders (Duc et al., 2022). As noted, the efficacy of MSCs derived from different tissues underscores the importance of personalized approaches in transplantation outcomes (Alexander et al., 2022).

15.3.3. The Transplant Procedure: Step-by-Step

The procedure for transplanting organs is very important in today's medicine, especially when it comes to transfusion medicine and BMT. Before proceeding, the process involves thoroughly reviewing patients to determine if they are suitable for transplantation. When the donor is selected, the next part is to take stem cells, which is vital for the success of the transplant. The recipients are then put through conditioning programs that ready their bodies for the transplanted cells, usually including chemotherapy and radiation to get rid of any diseased cells. After harvesting, the infusion of stem cells is a major step because it allows the cells to settle and become active within the patient's bone marrow. Recent advancements in bone tissue engineering and regenerative applications, as outlined in the current literature, underscore the evolving landscape of transplantation methods in promoting healing and recovery from severe injuries or chronic diseases (Mahla, 2016; Chocholata et al., 2019) (Figure 15.11).

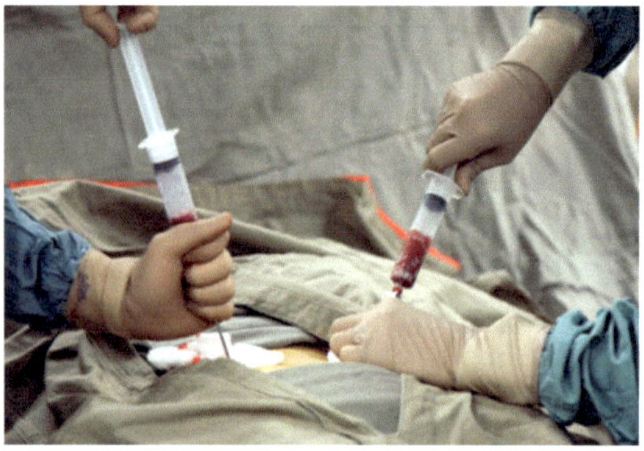

Figure 15.11. The transplant procedure represents a critical aspect of modern medical practice, particularly in the context of transfusion medicine and bone marrow transplantation.

Source: https://www.alafiyameditour.com/wp-content/uploads/2020/10/marrow-1.jpg.

15.3.4. Post-Transplant Care and Monitoring

After a bone marrow transplant, careful monitoring and support are very important because they can significantly affect the patient's condition and health. After transplantation, patients are at heightened risk for complications such as infections, GVHD, and relapsed malignancy. It is essential to regularly assess a patient's condition using clinical evaluations, laboratory tests, and imaging studies to identify and manage these complications promptly. Post-transplant care relies on the teamwork of oncologists, hematologists, transplant coordinators, and nurses to properly look after the patient. Additionally, advancements in gene therapy—particularly involving retroviral vectors—have shown potential benefits in enhancing engraftment and reducing complications, although they also raise concerns related to genotoxicity and insertional mutagenesis (Biasco et al., 2017; Alexander et al., 2022). For this reason, reviewing and evaluating different treatments and therapies is important for better results and improved care after transplant.

15.3.5. Complications and Management Strategies

Since there are many challenges in transfusion medicine and BMT, it is essential to use complete strategies to keep patients safe and improve their outcomes. Common complications such as infections, GVHD, and transplant rejection pose significant risks that require vigilant monitoring and timely interventions. In particular, proper training in the administration of transfusions and the management of post-transplant therapies is crucial for healthcare providers, as evidenced by programs focused on building clinical competencies in these areas (Albert et al., 2016). Furthermore, the development of specialized treatments for various blood disorders indicates that management methods are continually advancing. For instance, advancements in pharmacological therapies and personalized medicine are reshaping the landscape of treatment effectiveness for conditions like acute lymphoblastic leukemia (Varma et al., 2015). Dealing with complications using precise methods will help patients recover more effectively and improve the success of transplantation plans (Figure 15.12).

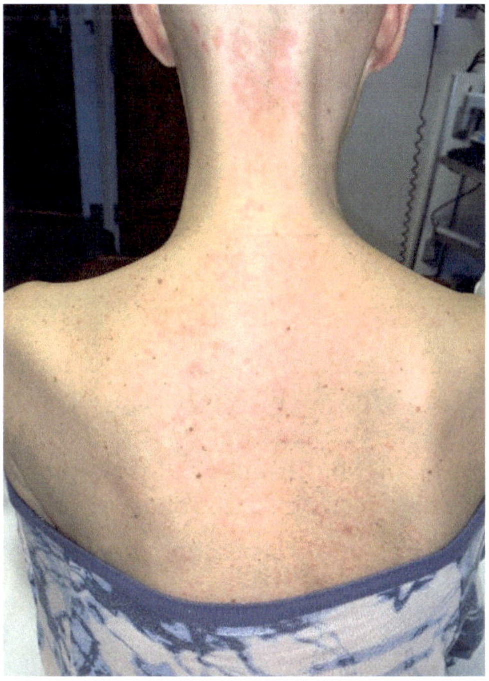

Figure 15.12. Common complications such as infections, graft-versus-host disease (GVHD), and transplant rejection pose significant risks that require vigilant monitoring and timely interventions.

Source: https://media.springernature.com/lw1200/springer-static/image/art%3A10.1007%2Fs13671-024-00461-9/MediaObjects/13671_2024_461_Fig1_HTML.jpg.

15.3.6. Role of Graft-versus-Host Disease (GVHD)

GVHD is a significant complication following allogeneic BMT, where donor immune cells attack the recipient's tissues, leading to variable clinical manifestations. The way GVHD develops points out that careful matching of the donor and recipient is essential to avoid the risk. Although GVHD may help prevent tumors, it is still a significant reason for illness and death in patients who have transplants. Recent advancements in cell-based therapies, including the use of MSCs, have shown promise in modulating immune responses and potentially alleviating GVHD symptoms. Studies indicate that MSCs may foster a more favorable immunological environment, reducing the severity of GVHD while maintaining the graft's efficacy against malignancies (Squillaro et al., 2016). As research progresses, integrating GVHD management strategies into routine transfusion medicine practices is essential for improving patient outcomes after transplant (Hayden et al., 2021).

15.3.7. Long-term Outcomes of Bone Marrow Transplantation (BMT)

The long-term outcomes of BMT reveal critical insights into patient recovery, survival rates, and quality of life. After transplantation, managing thrombocytopenia is very important, especially for people with blood cancers. Updated guidelines propose a shift from prophylactic platelet transfusions to therapeutic strategies, emphasizing the importance of individualized treatment plans based on patient outcomes, as demonstrated in recent studies that show no substantial difference in bleeding events between approaches (Patricia et al., 2021). Additionally, ongoing research indicates that BMT can effectively correct inborn errors of immunity, making it the treatment of choice for several genetic disorders (Fernandes et al., 2021). As the field advances, using evidence-based approaches in BMT will help patients survive and also improve their well-being as they recover from the procedure (Figure 15.13).

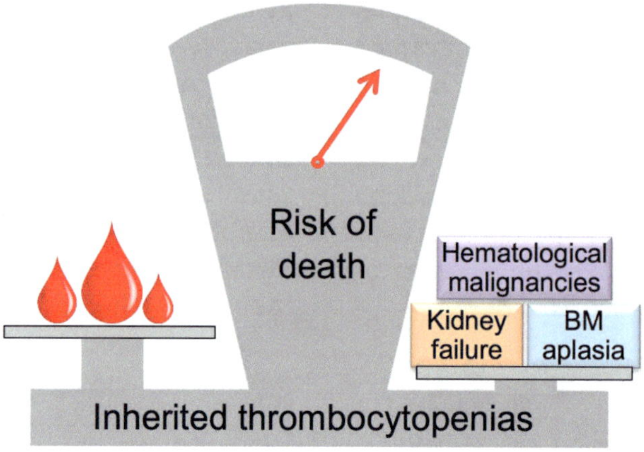

Figure 15.13. One of the significant concerns post-transplantation is the management of thrombocytopenia, particularly in patients with hematological malignancies.

Source: https://haematologica.org/article/download/haematol.2022.280856/74521/78311.

15.3.8. Psychosocial Aspects of Bone Marrow Transplantation (BMT)

The psychosocial aspects of BMT are critical to understanding the overall efficacy and patient well-being associated with this life-saving procedure. Many patients who get BMT experience emotional and psychological issues like anxiety and depression because they are unsure about their recovery, and the procedure is very invasive. Having support from family and friends helps patients deal with their illness and improves their quality of life. Research has shown that robust psychosocial interventions can lead to improved emotional outcomes and even positively influence physical recovery during the transplantation process (Alexander et al., 2022). Furthermore, emerging evidence highlights the importance of understanding the role of stem cell technologies in regenerative medicine, pointing to their potential implications for both psychological and physical healing, thus broadening the scope of support provided to these patients (Duc et al., 2022). All in all, focusing on psychosocial needs is essential to support a more effective approach to BMT.

15.4. The Intersection of Transfusion Medicine and Bone Marrow Transplantation (BMT)

Both transfusion medicine and BMT are essential in clinical practice because they both depend on handling blood products and stem cells for better patient results. During BMT, transfusion medicine helps by providing packed RBCs and platelets to manage anemia and thrombocytopenia. Moreover, advancements in stem cell research, as highlighted in recent studies, demonstrate the evolving understanding of stem cells' clinical applications in regenerative medicine, which is paramount for improving transplant efficacy and patient recovery (Meerim et al., 2024). When these areas are combined, they support the need for treatments that utilize both blood transfusions and stem cell therapies, which in turn help individuals with hematological disorders.

15.4.1. Role of Blood Products in Transplantation

For transplantation to be successful, many blood products are needed to ensure the patient's recovery and proper engraftment. During surgery, doctors rely on the blood components RBCs, platelets, and plasma to handle possible anemia, coagulopathy, and thrombocytopenia that patients may develop due to their health conditions or the operation. Also, blood products are essential not only for surgery; they are necessary for the hematopoietic system during BMT. As noted, HSCs, which are fundamental for regenerating blood lineages post-transplant, rely on robust and compatible blood donation frameworks to ensure adequate supply and availability of products necessary for patient recovery (Yavor et al., 2023). Furthermore, understanding the genetic distribution of blood types and hematological factors, as illustrated in studies of ABO and Rh groups, is critical for personalized care in transplantation settings (Onaiwu et al., 2018) (Figure 15.14).

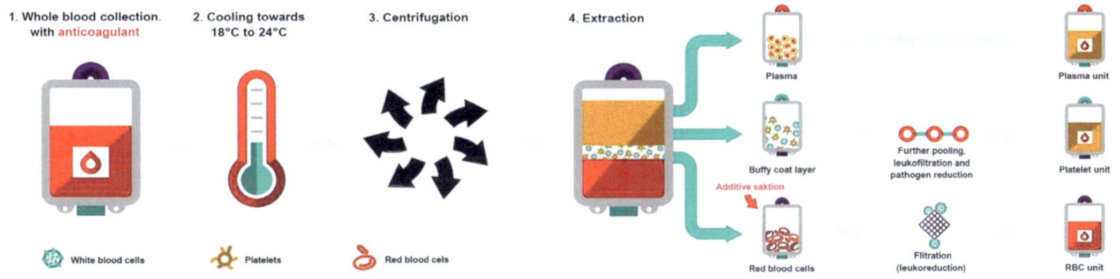

Figure 15.14. Blood components, including red blood cells, platelets, and plasma, are critical during perioperative management to address issues such as anemia, coagulopathy, and thrombocytopenia, which patients may experience due to underlying conditions or surgical interventions.

Source: https://professionaleducation.blood.ca/sites/default/files/2025-04/M4559-EN-MAI-CGTT_Chp2%202025_Figure1_PlateletChange.jpg.

15.4.2. Pre-Transplant Blood Management Strategies

Effective pre-transplant blood management strategies are essential in promoting positive outcomes for patients undergoing BMT. Among these strategies, it is crucial to closely monitor and adjust a patient's hemoglobin levels to prevent complications associated with the transplant. Studies indicate that patients with inflammatory conditions, such as ulcerative colitis (UC), experience worse outcomes, including increased mortality and higher rates of blood transfusions during BMT procedures (Chandani et al., 2024).

The presence of many comorbidities in these patients indicates that special care should be given before the transplant. Additionally, in the context of the COVID-19 pandemic, which poses significant risks to immunocompromised individuals, implementing rigorous transfusion protocols and infection prevention measures is vital to enhance patient safety (Anurathapan et al., 2020). All in all, effective blood management plans before transplant help patients get ready and reduce the risk of complications after surgery.

15.4.3. Impact of Transfusion on Transplant Outcomes

In the field of transfusion medicine, it is essential to study the impact of blood transfusions on the results of BMT. Giving many blood transfusions to control anemia can sometimes cause problems that reduce the chance of a successful transplant. For instance, excessive transfusions may precipitate iron overload, which is known to contribute to organ damage, particularly in pediatric patients with conditions like thalassemia, further complicating their treatment pathways (Yousuf et al., 2022). Additionally, transfusion-associated thrombotic microangiopathy (TA-TMA) has emerged as a significant complication following hematopoietic cell transplantation, with its diagnostic criteria still evolving, affecting morbidity and mortality rates (Schoettler et al., 2022). Thus, it is crucial to manage and monitor patients before and after transplantation to ensure their survival and better quality of life (Figure 15.15).

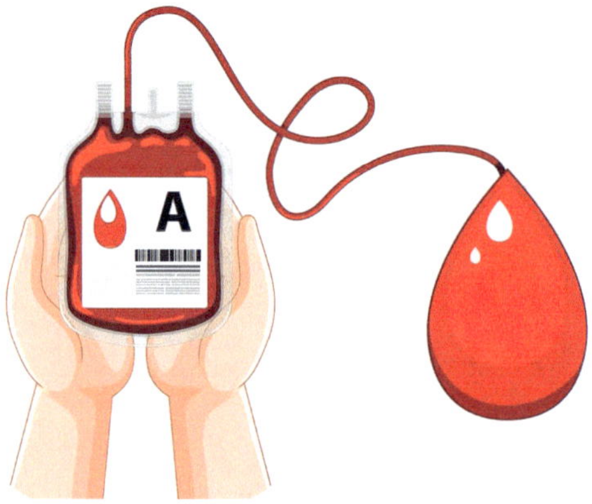

Figure 15.15. Repeated blood transfusions, while often necessary for managing severe anemia, can lead to complications that adversely affect transplant survival rates.

Source: https://www.apexhospitals.com/_next/image?url=https%3A%2F%2Fbed.apexhospitals.com%2Fuploads%2Fblood_transfusion_2_79e4cddec4.jpg&w=1920&q=75.

15.4.4. Immunological Considerations in Transfusion and Transplantation

Learning about immunology in transfusion and transplantation helps improve patient outcomes and prevent many complications. The immune response plays a critical role in the rejection of transplanted tissues, where mismatched human leukocyte antigens (HLAs) can trigger robust alloreactivity. During transfusions, similar mechanisms can lead to transfusion-related acute lung injury (TRALI) or hemolytic reactions if donor and recipient blood types are incompatible. Recent advancements in regenerative medicine, particularly stem cell therapies utilizing hPSCs and MSCs, offer promising avenues for managing these immunological challenges. Research suggests that the origin of MSCs—whether from bone marrow, adipose tissue, or the umbilical cord—can impact their therapeutic efficacy, particularly in regenerative applications (Duc et al., 2022). In parallel, techniques such as adoptive T cell transfer (ACT) have been introduced in transfusion medicine, expanding the possibilities for treatment in oncology and autoimmune conditions (Carl et al., 2018). All these points highlight that immunology plays a crucial role in the clinical work of transfusion and transplantation.

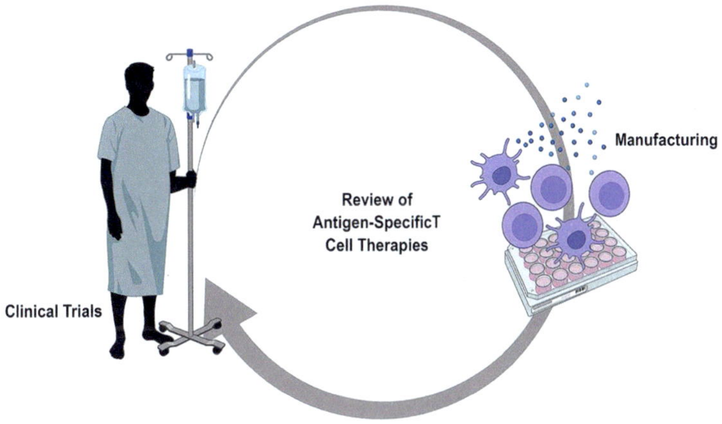

Figure 15.16. Techniques like adoptive T cell transfer (ACT) have been introduced in transfusion medicine, expanding possibilities for treatment in oncology and autoimmune conditions

Source: https://www.cell.com/cms/10.1016/j.ymthe.2022.02.002/asset/c6a74e3b-e5d1-4206-b26c-1d55a64fb10d/main.assets/fx1_lrg.jpg.

15.4.5. Case Studies of Transfusion in Bone Marrow Recipients

Several case studies illustrate the numerous challenges that can arise during and after BMT for patients. For instance, one detailed case illustrated a patient who developed pure red cell aplasia (PRCA) following an ABO-mismatched allogeneic stem cell transplantation. Since the patient had severe reticulocytopenia and needed regular blood transfusions, a course of daratumumab was given after the first treatments did not work. This demonstrates that successful transplantation outcomes depend on the timely application of transfusion medicine to address issues such as PRCA. Furthermore, innovative practices in regions like Bangladesh demonstrate an expanding horizon for HSCT, with centers recording significant milestones in patient care and transfusion management, as seen in their 65 completed transplant cases, which reinforces the role of transfusions in optimizing patient recovery (Karim et al., 2023; Gulied et al., 2024).

15.4.6. Research on Transfusion-Related Transplant Complications

Problems related to transfusion are essential in the outcomes of BMT, so they need to be studied in transfusion medicine. Research indicates that patients undergoing this procedure often experience hemostatic disturbances due to chronic conditions, such as cirrhosis, which can complicate transfusion strategies and lead to increased bleeding risks during and after the transplant process (Patrick et al., 2020). Furthermore, innovative treatments, such as ivosidenib for relapsed acute myeloid leukemia patients, are being explored to mitigate these complications, illustrating the intricate relationship between transfusion practices and transplant success (Courtney et al., 2018). As we learn more about hemostatic changes in patients with specific characteristics, it is clear that customized transfusion protocols are necessary. Taking care of these complications is essential for better managing patients and getting better outcomes in BMT and transfusion medicine (Figure 15.17).

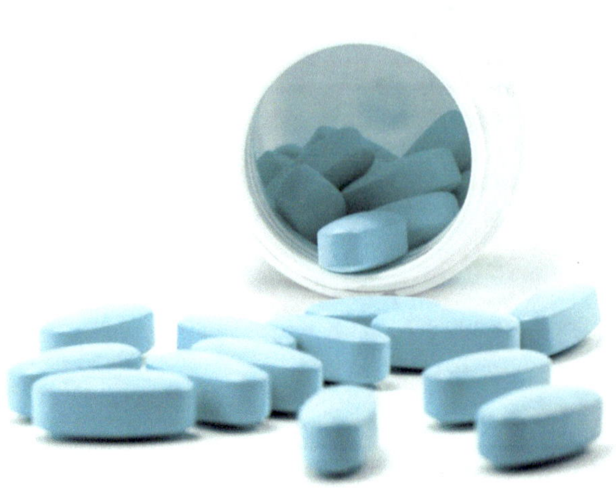

Figure 15.17. Ivosidenib.

Source: https://www.bjh.be/app/uploads/2022/06/GettyImages-588395678-blauwe-pillen-IVOSIDENIB-e1654606451590.jpg.

15.4.7. Collaborative Approaches in Transfusion and Transplant Medicine

Transfusion and transplant medicine are now focusing more on teamwork to improve patient results and better use available resources. These methods enable hematologists, immunologists, and transfusion specialists to collaborate, ensuring that patients receive the best possible care. For instance, advancements in cell therapies, such as the use of human platelet lysate (hPL), underscore this collaboration; hPL serves as a promising alternative to fetal bovine serum in cell culture, minimizing risks associated with xenogeneic components and improving safety profiles (Bieback et al., 2019). Moreover, the recent approvals of gene therapy products exemplify the rapid progress facilitated by cooperative efforts among clinical researchers and regulatory bodies, highlighting a significant shift towards shared knowledge and innovation in treatment modalities (Katherine et al., 2019). Such partnerships help address clinical issues and also lead to the development of standard practices that make transfusion and transplantation therapies more effective and safe.

15.4.8. Education and Training for Healthcare Professionals

The right training and education of healthcare professionals help achieve the best results in transfusion medicine and BMT. Proper training programs provide clinicians with the necessary information about the challenges associated with HSCT and blood product transfusions. The programs put importance on careful donor selection and handling of any problems that arise after transfusion to ensure patient safety. Moreover, using different approaches together helps healthcare teams collaborate, which improves the way care is delivered in various settings. As evidenced during the COVID-19 pandemic, adapting educational curricula to address emerging challenges is vital for maintaining the continuity of care, particularly for vulnerable populations such as pediatric cancer patients, who require specialized attention during crises (Sullivan et al.,

2020). Consequently, ongoing education not only elevates clinical competency but also fosters resilience within healthcare systems to navigate both routine and extraordinary circumstances (Alexander et al., 2022) (Figure 15.18).

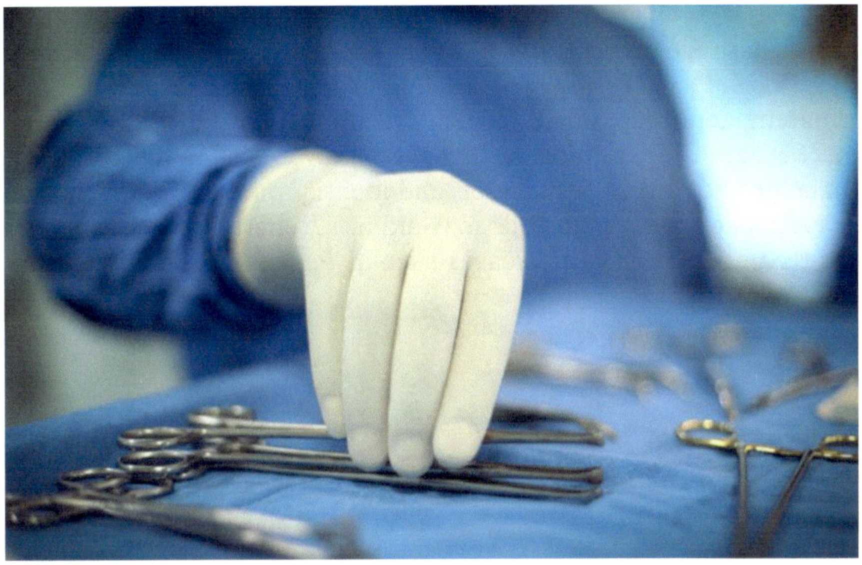

Figure 15.18. The education and training of healthcare professionals are critical components in ensuring optimal outcomes in transfusion medicine and bone marrow transplantation.

Source: https://www.mgmch.org/images/plastic-surgery-therapeutics.jpg.

15.4.9. Future Research Directions at the Intersection

The evolving field of transfusion medicine and BMT presents numerous new opportunities for research, particularly at the intersection of these two disciplines. For example, new findings in stem cell research could lead to improved regenerative therapies, as cellular sources are now recognized as crucial in clinical settings. A bibliometric review highlights the rapid advancements in this domain, emphasizing the necessity for stringent analyses to identify emerging trends and influential publications (Meerim et al., 2024). Also, being aware of the psychological side of patient care and the role of hope in medicine can make treatment in transfusion medicine and BMT more effective. Future studies should aim to integrate the latest scientific advancements with a deep understanding of patients' experiences, enabling the development of new and improved treatment methods that benefit patients more effectively.

A CLOSER LOOK

HUMAN PLURIPOTENT STEM CELLS (HPSCS)

hPSCs are unique cells with the remarkable ability to develop into nearly any cell type in the human body. This includes both embryonic stem cells (ESCs), which are derived from early-stage embryos, and induced pluripotent stem cells (iPSCs), which are adult cells that have been reprogrammed to a pluripotent state. Because they are flexible, hPSCs are now crucial in research, enabling scientists to study early human growth, simulate diseases, and identify potential remedies. Because they can differentiate into specialized cells, stem cells may aid in regenerative medicine and could be used to repair damaged tissues and address diseases such as Parkinson's, diabetes, and heart disease.

SUMMARY

Transfusion medicine and BMT have made a significant difference in treating hematological disorders, underscoring the importance of innovative treatments and patient care. The introduction of targeted therapies, such as ivosidenib for patients with IDH1 mutations, demonstrates the potential for improved outcomes in acute myeloid leukemia, with notable rates of remission and transfusion independence observed in clinical trials (Courtney et al., 2018). Moreover, the application of MSCs in regenerative medicine illustrates the evolving landscape of treatment options, as these cells exhibit promising properties for addressing a variety of diseases, including hematological conditions (Squillaro et al., 2016). Together with rigorous clinical trials, researchers are continually refining these therapies to make them better and safer. All in all, new developments in the field are expected to significantly impact the outcomes for patients who rely on transfusion and transplantation.

In this field, several important findings have highlighted the progress being made in hematological therapies. Advances in the understanding of disease-specific pathophysiology, particularly in conditions like CML, have paved the way for more targeted approaches to treatment. Recent clinical trials have highlighted the efficacy of novel drug combinations, such as ivosidenib and azacitidine, which demonstrate statistically significant improvements in event-free survival and overall survival rates in patients with IDH1-mutated acute myeloid leukemia (Montesinos et al., 2022). Furthermore, emerging data indicate that the risks associated with transfusion-related complications can be mitigated through enhanced screening and matching protocols, thereby improving patient outcomes and minimizing adverse effects (Alexander et al., 2022). All of these advances demonstrate a significant improvement in treatments, indicating that further research is necessary to continue enhancing them.

REFERENCES

1. Advani, R., Flinn, I., Popplewell, L., Forero, A., Bartlett, N. L., Ghosh, N., Kline, J., Roschewski, M., LaCasce, A., Collins, G. P., Tran, T., Lynn, J., Chen, J. Y., Volkmer, J., Agoram, B., Huang, J., Majeti, R., Weissman, I. L., Takimoto, C. H., . . . Smith, S. M. (2018). CD47 blockade by HU5F9-G4 and Rituximab in Non-Hodgkin's lymphoma. *New England Journal of Medicine, 379*(18), 1711–1721. https://doi.org/10.1056/nejmoa1807315Anasiz, Y., Ozgul, R., & Uçkan-Çetinkaya, D. (2024). Turning trash into treasure: A simple protocol for human mesenchymal stromal cell isolation from used bone marrow collection kits. *Current Protocols, 4*. https://www.semanticscholar.org/paper/69b64ef30a3fa1d7384168a6f78389b64c4ab899 (accessed on 12th June 2025).
2. Anurathapan, U., Apiwattanakul, N., Pakakasama, S., Pongphitcha, P., Thitithanyanont, A., Pasomsub, E., & Hongeng, S. (2020). Hematopoietic stem cell transplantation from an infected SARS-CoV2 donor sibling. *Bone Marrow Transplantation, 55*, 2359–2360. https://www.semanticscholar.org/paper/ae3ddd968b5f8bd09a30bc981cc902c24ff0329a (accessed on 12th June 2025).
3. Biasco, L., Rothe, M., Büning, H., & Schambach, A. (2017). Analyzing the genotoxicity of retroviral vectors in hematopoietic cell gene therapy. *Molecular Therapy–Methods & Clinical Development, 8*, 21–30. https://doi.org/10.1016/j.omtm.2017.10.002 (accessed on 12th June 2025).
4. Bieback, K., Fernández-Muñoz, B., Pati, S., & Schäfer, R. (2019). Gaps in the knowledge of human platelet lysate as a cell culture supplement for cell therapy: A joint publication from the AABB and the International Society for Cell & Gene Therapy. *Transfusion, 59*, 3448–3460. https://doi.org/10.1111/trf.15483 (accessed on 12th June 2025).
5. Bozhilov, Y. K., Hsu, I., Brown, E. J., & Wilkinson, A. (2023). *In vitro* human hematopoietic stem cell expansion and differentiation. *Cells, 12*. https://www.semanticscholar.org/paper/fe815a1e3aac9dd0dcf57a24c3540ca6f7300081 (accessed on 12th June 2025).
6. Chandani, K. U., Agrawal, S., Raval, M., Lotia, D., Nadeem, A., & Kelkar, A. H. (2024). Ulcerative colitis and adverse outcomes in hematopoietic stem cell transplantation: A nationwide analysis. *Blood*. https://www.semanticscholar.org/paper/fe0e8c75706ac3e5859bfbc2fbc43ef2ec8ac928 (accessed on 12th June 2025).
7. Chocholata, P., Kulda, V., & Babuška, V. (2019). Fabrication of scaffolds for bone-tissue regeneration. *Materials, 12*, 568–568. https://doi.org/10.3390/ma12040568 (accessed on 12th June 2025).
8. Delicou, S., Moraki, M., Papatheodorou, E., & Xydaki, A. (2024). Treatment options for congenital dyserythropoietic anemias (CDAs): Advances in bone marrow transplantation, gene therapy, and targeted therapies. *Journal of Hematology and Clinical Research*. https://www.semanticscholar.org/paper/84e44944d6dac1b2dce749ccd835b7751c2eeb73 (accessed on 12th June 2025).
9. Denlinger, C. S., Sanft, T., Baker, K. S., Broderick, G. A., Demark-Wahnefried, W., Friedman, D. L., Goldman, M., et al. (2018). Survivorship, version 2.2018, NCCN clinical practice guidelines in oncology. *Journal of the National Comprehensive Cancer Network, 16*, 1216–1247. https://doi.org/10.6004/jnccn.2018.0078 (accessed on 12th June 2025).

10. DiNardo, C. D., Stein, E. M., de Botton, S., Roboz, G. J., Altman, J. K., Mims, A. S., Swords, R. T., et al. (2018). Durable remissions with ivosidenib in *IDH1*-mutated relapsed or refractory AML. *New England Journal of Medicine, 378*, 2386–2398. https://doi.org/10.1056/nejmoa1716984 (accessed on 12th June 2025).

11. Fernandes, J. F. F., & Bonfim, C. (2021). Hematopoietic stem cell transplantation for inborn errors of immunity. *Journal of Bone Marrow Transplantation and Cellular Therapy*. https://www.semanticscholar.org/paper/11ce35a6f85f472bde6e73be2743c853622655ac (accessed on 12th June 2025).

12. Gulied, A., Fadul, A., Jacob, S., Soliman, D., Ganwo, I., Gameil, A., Hamad, A., et al. (2024). Pure red cell aplasia after ABO incompatible hematopoietic stem cell transplantation successfully treated with daratumumab: A case report. *Blood*. https://www.semanticscholar.org/paper/5ef80a4217a276e1a0bf4a6932d2e306b5ebe7f2 (accessed on 12th June 2025).

13. Hayden, P., Roddie, C., Bader, P., Basak, G., Bönig, H., Bonini, C., Chabannon, C., et al. (2021). Management of adults and children receiving CAR T-cell therapy: 2021 best practice recommendations of the European Society for Blood and Marrow Transplantation (EBMT) and the Joint Accreditation Committee of ISCT and EBMT (JACIE) and the European Hematology Association (EHA). *Annals of Oncology, 33*, 259–275. https://doi.org/10.1016/j.annonc.2021.12.003 (accessed on 12th June 2025).

14. High, K. A., & Roncarolo, M. G. (2019). Gene therapy. *New England Journal of Medicine, 381*, 455–464. https://doi.org/10.1056/nejmra1706910 (accessed on 12th June 2025).

15. Hoang, D. M., Pham, P. T., Bach, T. Q., Ngo, A. T., Nguyen, Q. T., Phan, T. K. T., Giang, N. H., et al. (2022). Stem cell-based therapy for human diseases. *Signal Transduction and Targeted Therapy, 7*. https://doi.org/10.1038/s41392-022-01134-4 (accessed on 12th June 2025).

16. Hu, X., Li, J., Fu, M., Zhao, X., & Wang, W. (2021). The JAK/STAT signaling pathway: From bench to clinic. *Signal Transduction and Targeted Therapy, 6*. https://doi.org/10.1038/s41392-021-00791-1 (accessed on 12th June 2025).

17. Iolascon, A., Rivella, S., Anagnou, N. P., Camaschella, C., Swinkels, D. W., Muckenthaler, M. U., Porto, G., et al. (2021). The EHA research roadmap: Anemias. *Hemisphere, 5*, e607–e607. https://doi.org/10.1097/hs9.0000000000000607 (accessed on 12th June 2025).

18. June, C. H., O'Connor, R. S., Kawalekar, O. U., Ghassemi, S., & Milone, M. C. (2018). CAR T cell immunotherapy for human cancer. *Science, 359*, 1361–1365. https://doi.org/10.1126/science.aar6711 (accessed on 12th June 2025).

19. Karim, M., Mahfuz, H., Uddin, M., Khan, A. K., & Akhter, S. (2023). Bone marrow transplantation: Pre and after care. *Bangladesh Journal of Medicine*. https://www.semanticscholar.org/paper/b6f90c15f853b6227a7ccfcb51ceeefdf41b707b (accessed on 12th June 2025).

20. Khan, K., O'Boyle, F., Lund, K., Petterson, T., Bremathas, S., Hennessy, K., Gassas, A., et al. (2024). Donor trait status determines hematological outcomes post-haemopoietic stem cell transplantation in transfusion dependent thalassemia independent of HLA matching and chimerism status. *Blood*. https://www.semanticscholar.org/paper/d7061af0e7881567f7125be75c47cb3b1aff0fcc (accessed on 12th June 2025).

21. Kumar, M. A., Baba, S. K., Sadida, H. Q., Al Marzooqi, S., Jerobin, J., Altemani, F. H., Algehainy,

N. A., et al. (2024). Extracellular vesicles as tools and targets in therapy for diseases. *Signal Transduction and Targeted Therapy, 9*. https://doi.org/10.1038/s41392-024-01735-1 (accessed on 12th June 2025).

22. La Padula, S., Pensato, R., Pizza, C., Coiante, E., Roccaro, G., Longo, B., D'Andrea, F., et al. (2022). Face transplant: Indications, outcomes, and ethical issues—Where do we stand? *Journal of Clinical Medicine, 11*, 5750–5750. https://doi.org/10.3390/jcm11195750 (accessed on 12th June 2025).

23. Lal, A., Wong, T. E., Keel, S., Pagano, M. B., Chung, J., Kamdar, A., Rao, L., et al. (2021). The transfusion management of beta thalassemia in the United States. *Transfusion, 61*, 3027–3039. https://doi.org/10.1111/trf.16640 (accessed on 12th June 2025).

24. Li, T., Yang, Y., Qi, H., Cui, W., Zhang, L., Fu, X., He, X., et al. (2023). CRISPR/Cas9 therapeutics: Progress and prospects. *Signal Transduction and Targeted Therapy, 8*. https://doi.org/10.1038/s41392-023-01309-7 (accessed on 12th June 2025).

25. Liang, W., Zhou, C., Bai, J., Zhang, H., Jiang, B., Wang, J., Fu, L., et al. (2024). Current advancements in therapeutic approaches in orthopedic surgery: A review of recent trends. *Frontiers in Bioengineering and Biotechnology, 12*. https://doi.org/10.3389/fbioe.2024.1328997 (accessed on 12th June 2025).

26. Liu, E., Marín, D., Banerjee, P. P., Macapinlac, H. A., Thompson, P. A., Başar, R., Kerbauy, L. N., et al. (2020). Use of CAR-transduced natural killer cells in CD19-positive lymphoid tumors. *New England Journal of Medicine, 382*, 545–553. https://doi.org/10.1056/nejmoa1910607 (accessed on 12th June 2025).

27. Locantore-Ford, P. A., Mistry, R. H., Patel, E., Chen, S., & Goodacre, R. (2021). Use of an antifibrinolytic agent and vitamin K as alternative to platelet transfusions in autologous hematopoietic cell transplantation. *Blood*. https://www.semanticscholar.org/paper/851e0a887a2d9ad71c2a29c794accbd8bf70befe (accessed on 12th June 2025).

28. Lyon, A. R., López-Fernández, T., Couch, L. S., Asteggiano, R., Aznar, M. C., Bergler-Klein, J., Boriani, G., et al. (2022). 2022 ESC guidelines on cardio-oncology developed in collaboration with the European Hematology Association (EHA), the European Society for Therapeutic Radiology and Oncology (ESTRO) and the International Cardio-Oncology Society (IC-OS). *European Heart Journal, 43*, 4229–4361. https://doi.org/10.1093/eurheartj/ehac244 (accessed on 12th June 2025).

29. Maeda, H., & Khatami, M. (2018). Analyses of repeated failures in cancer therapy for solid tumors: Poor tumor-selective drug delivery, low therapeutic efficacy and unsustainable costs. *Clinical and Translational Medicine, 7*. https://doi.org/10.1186/s40169-018-0185-6 (accessed on 12th June 2025).

30. Mahla, R. S. (2016). Stem cells applications in regenerative medicine and disease therapeutics. *International Journal of Cell Biology, 2016*, 1–24. https://doi.org/10.1155/2016/6940283 (accessed on 12th June 2025).

31. Montesinos, P., Récher, C., Vives, S., Zarzycka, E., Wang, J., Bertani, G., Heuser, M., et al. (2022). Ivosidenib and azacitidine in *IDH1*-mutated acute myeloid leukemia. *New England Journal of Medicine, 386*, 1519–1531. https://doi.org/10.1056/nejmoa2117344 (accessed on 12th June 2025).

32. Nabih, N., Elkorashy, S. A., & Magdy, R. (2019). Impact of blood transfusion on hematopoietic stem cell transplantation outcome. *Journal of Clinical and Diagnostic Research*. https://www.semanticscholar.org/paper/663203dd4622da5a64233e4021d553bce9a3d7b1 (accessed on 12th June 2025).

33. Northup, P. G., García-Pagán, J. C., García-Tsao, G., Intagliata, N. M., Superina, R., Roberts, L. N., Lisman, T., et al. (2020). Vascular liver disorders, portal vein thrombosis, and procedural bleeding in patients with liver disease: 2020 practice guidance by the American Association for the Study of Liver Diseases. *Hepatology, 73*, 366–413. https://doi.org/10.1002/hep.31646 (accessed on 12th June 2025).

34. Nurbaeva, M. K., & Dzhunushalieva, G. (2024). Bibliometric analysis of literature on stem cells in regenerative medicine and their clinical applications (2010 to 2024): A scoping review. *Precision and Future Medicine*. https://doi.org/10.23838/pfm.2024.00121 (accessed on 12th June 2025).

35. Ohiengbomwan, O. T., Idemudia, N., Owoicho, O., & Adeyanju, A. A. (2018). Gene frequencies of hemoglobin genotype, ABO and Rhesus blood groups among students' population of a private university in Nigeria—Implications for blood banking. *International Journal of Life-Sciences Scientific Research*. https://www.semanticscholar.org/paper/937e566a092983807 4c4a5f263e34c021804d5dd (accessed on 12th June 2025).

36. Pateraki, P., Latsoudis, H., Papadopoulou, A., Gontika, I., Fragiadaki, I., Mavroudi, I., Bizymi, N., et al. (2024). Perspectives for the use of umbilical cord blood in transplantation and beyond: Initiatives for an advanced and sustainable public banking program in Greece. *Journal of Clinical Medicine, 13*. https://www.semanticscholar.org/paper/d3b9450936531817645b4da3ebbfc1ad2a5f0101 (accessed on 12th June 2025).

37. Qiu, H., Wang, X., & Shao, Y. (2023). Forward and reverse typing discrepancy and crossmatch incompatibility of ABO blood groups: Cause analysis and treatment. *Hematology, 28*. https://www.semanticscholar.org/paper/d8033cd27778ee06c566d4f9c9b1bce390e2cdfe (accessed on 12th June 2025).

38. Revel-Vilk, S., Cox, P. N., Robitaille, N., & Blanchette, V. S. (2013). Hematological problems in pediatric intensive care. *Pediatric and Adolescent Medicine*. https://doi.org/10.1159/000350346 (accessed on 12th June 2025).

39. Sagar, R., Almeida-Porada, G., Blakemore, K. J., Chan, J. K. Y., Choolani, M., Götherström, C., Jaulent, A. M., et al. (2020). Fetal and maternal safety considerations for in utero therapy clinical trials: iFeTiS consensus statement. *Molecular Therapy, 28*, 2316–2319. https://doi.org/10.1016/j.ymthe.2020.10.012 (accessed on 12th June 2025).

40. Schoettler, M. L., Carreras, E., Cho, B. S., Dandoy, C. E., Ho, V. T., Jodele, S., Moissev, I., et al. (2022). Harmonizing definitions for diagnostic criteria and prognostic assessment of transplantation-associated thrombotic microangiopathy: A report on behalf of the European Society for Blood and Marrow Transplantation, American Society for Transplantation and Cellular Therapy, Asia-Pacific Blood and Marrow Transplantation Group, and Center for International Blood and Marrow Transplant Research. *Transplantation and Cellular Therapy, 29*, 151–163. https://doi.org/10.1016/j.jtct.2022.11.015 (accessed on 12th June 2025).

41. Squillaro, T., Peluso, G., & Galderisi, U. (2016). Clinical trials with mesenchymal stem cells: An update. *Cell Transplantation, 25*, 829–848. https://doi.org/10.3727/096368915x689622 (accessed on 12th June 2025).

42. Stüssi, G., Buser, A., & Holbro, A. (2019). Red blood cells: Exchange, transfuse, or deplete. *Transfusion Medicine and Hemotherapy, 46*, 407–416. https://doi.org/10.1159/000504144 (accessed on 12th June 2025).

43. Sullivan, M., Bouffet, É., Rodríguez-Galindo, C., Luna-Fineman, S., Khan, M. S., Kearns, P., Hawkins, D. S., et al. (2020). The COVID-19 pandemic: A rapid global response for children with cancer from SIOP, COG, SIOP-E, SIOP-PODC, IPSO, PROS, CCI, and St Jude Global. *Pediatric Blood & Cancer, 67*. https://doi.org/10.1002/pbc.28409 (accessed on 12th June 2025).

44. Trunk, A. D., Li, H., Kalaycio, M., Sobecks, R., Brunstein, C., Sauter, C., & Hamilton, B. (2024). Factors associated with platelet engraftment following allogeneic hematopoietic cell transplantation. *Blood*. https://www.semanticscholar.org/paper/91f28e0271a5111122bb8d6c00ae3480753133e9 (accessed on 12th June 2025).

45. Udvardy, M., Illés, Á., Gergely, L., Pinczés, L., Magyari, F., & Simon, Z. (2023). Transfusion-transmitted disorders 2023 with special attention to bone marrow transplant patients. *Pathogens, 12*. https://www.semanticscholar.org/paper/4e4e4b1717f2e484af2179e60475302e16c9ec5e (accessed on 12th June 2025).

46. van der Valk, J. (2017). Fetal bovine serum (FBS): Past–present–future. *ALTEX*. https://doi.org/10.14573/altex.1705101 (accessed on 12th June 2025).

47. Varma, N., & Sharma, P. (2015). Controversies in pediatric and adolescent hematology. *The Indian Journal of Medical Research, 141*, 848–849. https://www.semanticscholar.org/paper/a1d4f246921eb4cc1b16f87ae2ae704331c3712a (accessed on 12th June 2025).

48. Veillon, D. (2002). Impact of molecular genetics on the practice of pathology. *Pathology Case Reviews, 7*, 51–52. https://www.semanticscholar.org/paper/27a477f125228a09cb2117b26dc09c043d981051 (accessed on 12th June 2025).

49. Vinchi, F., & Vance, S. (2020). Challenging the erythropoiesis paradigm in β-thalassemia. *HemaSphere, 4*. https://www.semanticscholar.org/paper/9c4425df38b550604839e2e7604d3b27ff605f8e (accessed on 12th June 2025).

50. Wang, J. H., Gessler, D. J., Zhan, W., Gallagher, T. L., & Gao, G. (2024). Adeno-associated virus as a delivery vector for gene therapy of human diseases. *Signal Transduction and Targeted Therapy, 9*. https://doi.org/10.1038/s41392-024-01780-w (accessed on 12th June 2025).

51. Watson, N., Brandel, J. P., Green, A., Hermann, P., Ladogana, A., Lindsay, T., Mackenzie, J., et al. (2021). The importance of ongoing international surveillance for Creutzfeldt–Jakob disease. *Nature Reviews Neurology, 17*, 362–379. https://doi.org/10.1038/s41582-021-00488-7 (accessed on 12th June 2025).

52. Yeh, A. C., Khan, M., Khan, S., Harlow, J., Biswas, A., Akter, M., Ferdous, J., et al. (2016). Hematopoietic stem cell transplantation in the resource-limited setting: Establishing the first bone marrow transplant unit in Bangladesh and initial outcomes. *Blood, 128*, 2384–2384. https://www.semanticscholar.org/paper/3de3c7310e19571cc4f9f4e42a66d887ebcb9f0f (accessed on 12th June 2025).

53. Yousuf, R., Akter, S., Wasek, S. M., Sinha, S., Ahmad, R., & Haque, M. (2022). Thalassemia: A review of the challenges to the families and caregivers. *Cureus*. https://doi.org/10.7759/cureus.32491 (accessed on 12th June 2025).

INDEX

Symbols

β-thalassemia syndromes 81

A

aberrant hemoglobin S 108
Abnormalities 1, 17
Acquired disorders 83
Acquired Platelet Disorders 182
activated B-cell-like (ABC) 329
acute kidney injury (AKI) 356
acute lymphoblastic leukemia (ALL) 157
acute myeloid leukemia (AML) 157
adaptive immunity 151, 152, 153, 154, 155, 169, 170
adeno-associated virus (AAV) 384
adenosine diphosphate (ADP) 185
Africa 107, 110, 112
age group 207
agranulocytes 152
allogeneic hematopoietic stem cell transplantation (AHSCT) 383
allogeneic hematopoietic stem cell transplantation (allo-HSCT) 269
amyloid fibril formation 356
Anaplastic Large Cell Lymphoma (ALCL) 330
anemias 27, 28, 29, 30, 31, 32, 33, 34, 36, 37, 38, 39, 40, 41, 42, 43, 44, 45, 46, 49, 51, 52
ankylosing spondylitis 32, 54
antibiotics 84
antibody-activated platelets 238
antidiabetic 84
anti-human globulin 381
antiphospholipid antibodies (aPL) 210
antiphospholipid syndrome (APS), 208
Aplastic anemia 36
arterial events 240
arterial lumens 239
artificial intelligence 180
Asia 107, 109, 110, 112, 113, 127
atherosclerosis 239, 246
autism spectrum disorder (ASD) 162
autoantibody formation 83
autoimmune diseases 131
autoimmune hemolytic anemias (AIHAs) 28
autoimmune mechanisms 81, 91, 94

B

bacteria 85
basophils 152, 154
B-cell precursor ALL (B-ALL), 271
B cells 152, 153, 154, 169
benzene 298, 319
Bernard-Soulier Syndrome (BSS) 183
beta-thalassemia 27, 46, 53
biochemical constituents 2
bleeding 237, 242, 247, 248, 256, 261, 264
blood 1, 2, 3, 4, 5, 6, 7, 8, 9, 10, 11, 12, 13, 14, 15, 16,

17, 18, 19, 20, 21, 22, 23, 24
Blood 2, 3, 4, 5, 6, 17, 19, 21, 23, 25
blood cells 1, 2, 3, 6, 7, 8, 11, 12, 13, 15, 19, 22
blood clotting 182
blood coagulation 2, 4, 18
blood composition 2, 6
blood-producing organs 1
blood smear analysis 180
bloodstream 237
blood viscosity 356
bone marrow 1, 3, 4, 6, 7, 8, 10, 11, 12, 13, 17, 25
Bone marrow aspiration (BMA) 275
Bone marrow biopsy 161
bone marrow-derived mesenchymal stem cells (BM-MSCs) 386
bone marrow erythroblasts 29
bone marrow transplantation (BMT) 161
bone marrow trephine biopsy (BMB) 275
Burkitt lymphoma 327, 328, 337, 349

C

celiac disease 57
cells 1, 2, 3, 4, 5, 6, 7, 8, 10, 11, 12, 17, 19, 21, 22, 25
cell-to-cell communication 2
cellular growth control mechanisms 270
central nervous system (CNS) 329
Cerebral venous sinus thrombosis (CVST) 240
Chédiak-Higashi syndrome (CHS) 159
chemoimmunotherapies 295
chemokines 154
chimeric antigen receptor (CAR) 385
chromosome aberrations 298
chronic blood loss 55, 71
chronic diseases 27, 42
chronic inflammation 28, 43
chronic lymphocytic leukemia (CLL) 157, 165, 296, 311
chronic multisymptom illnesses (CMI) 215, 218
chronic myeloid leukemia (CML) 157, 296, 305, 311
clinical findings 27, 41
clinical syndromes 353
coagulopathies 181, 189
cobalamin deficiency 131
cobalamin serum levels 131
cold agglutinin disease 83, 89, 92, 102, 106
collagen 185
comorbidities 107
Complete Blood Count (CBC) 160
computed tomographic scans 275
congenital diseases 131
congenital dyserythropoietic anemias (CDAs) 130
congenital sideroblastic anemias (CSAs) 2
copper deficiency 59
correlation 31, 41
COVID-19 55, 78
CRLF2 overexpression 274
Crohn's disease 57
cytokine receptor-like factor 2 (CRLF2) 274, 281
cytokines 153, 154, 155
cytotoxic granules 154

D

dapagliflozin 84, 105
Decision 327
deep venous thrombosis (DVT) 184
dendritic cells (DCs) 155
development 268, 269, 270, 273, 280, 285, 286, 288
diacylglycerol (DAG) levels 185
diagnosis 27, 30, 34, 38, 39, 40, 41, 42, 43, 49, 50, 52, 53, 54
diagnostic methods 107, 118
dietary intake 56, 60, 71
dietary iron 56, 59, 71
Diffuse Large B-cell Lymphoma (DLBCL) 328
discrimination 27, 32
disorders 1, 4, 5, 6, 8, 9, 10, 11, 12, 13, 15, 16, 17, 18, 19, 20, 22, 25
Disseminated Intravascular Coagulation (DIC) 211
DNA synthesis 129, 130, 131, 132, 135, 142, 145
drug-induced hemolytic anemia (DIIHA) 84
dysfunctional cells 28

E

Education 107, 124, 128
electrolytes 2, 4
enterocytes 32
enzymatic deficits 82
eosinophils 152, 154, 164
Epstein-Barr Virus (EBV) 332
erythrocytes 2, 3, 4, 7, 8, 9, 21, 25
erythropoiesis 27, 28, 29, 31, 32, 33, 34, 35, 37, 40, 43, 44, 45
exercise
extramedullary acute myeloid leukemia (eAML) 270

F

Factor V Leiden mutation 210
Family history
fatigue 131, 133, 134, 136, 137, 139
ferroportin 29, 32
fetal well-being 56
fibrinolysis 241, 243, 246, 249, 260, 262
flow cytometry 159, 161
fluorescence in situ hybridization (FISH) 273, 287, 387
folate 129, 130, 131, 132, 133, 134, 135, 136, 137, 138, 141, 142, 143, 145, 146
folate deficiency 129, 132, 138, 143, 146
Follicular lymphoma 328
follow-up care 268, 284
free light chains (FLC) 356, 364

G

gastroenterological diseases 131
Gastrointestinal disorders 59
gastrointestinal symptoms 85
gene mutations 60, 75
genes 207, 213, 228, 230, 234
genetic abnormalities 387
genetic disorders 27, 42, 43
genetic etiology 182
genetic factors 2, 11
genetic predisposition 331
Genetic testing 162
genetic translocation 296
genetic versus 109
gestational diabetes Mellitus (GDM)
Glanzmann's thrombasthenia 180, 191, 198, 202, 203
globalization 107, 109, 111, 120
graft-versus-host disease (GvHD) 383
Granulocytes 152

H

haptoglobin levels 84
healthy eating
heavy menstrual bleeding (HMB) 184
hematological cancers 268, 269
hematological diseases 1, 9, 11, 16
hematological malignancies 1, 13
Hematology 1, 4, 14, 16, 19, 20, 23
hematopoiesis 1, 2, 3, 4, 5, 6, 7, 8, 9, 10, 11, 12, 13, 15, 17, 19, 20, 22, 23, 24, 25
hematopoietic progenitor cells 132
hematopoietic stem cells (HSCs) 1, 10, 380
heme biosynthesis 58, 59, 60, 61, 62, 63, 65, 69, 71, 76, 77, 79
Hemoglobin C Disease (HbC) 109
Hemoglobin D Disease 109
Hemoglobin E Disease 109
Hemoglobin H Disease 110
hemoglobinization 2
hemoglobinopathies 82, 108, 109, 110, 111, 112, 113, 114, 115, 116, 117, 118, 119, 120, 121, 122, 123, 124, 126, 127, 128
hemoglobinopathy patients 107, 121
hemolysis 27, 28, 30, 32, 39
hemolytic uremic syndrome 34, 51
hemophilia A 209, 212, 231, 234
Hemophilia B 209
heparin 154
Heparin-induced thrombocytopenia (HIT) 238
hepcidin 28, 30, 32, 37, 45, 54
hereditary spherocytosis 30
High-performance liquid chromatography (HPLC) 110

histamine 154
Hodgkin lymphoma (HL) 299, 325, 326
Human Immunodeficiency Virus (HIV) 332
human pluripotent stem cells (hPSCs) 379
hyperactivity 151
hypereosinophilic syndrome 325

I

illnesses 353
imatinib 297, 309, 310, 313, 318
immune response 151, 152, 155, 156, 158, 159, 172, 175
immune system abnormalities 27
immune thrombocytopenic purpura (ITP) 180, 191, 196, 211
immunity 2, 3
immunocompromised patients 380, 384
immunoglobulin heavy variable (IGHV) gene 296
immunomodulatory therapy 353
immunophenotyping 160, 161, 175
immunosuppressive therapy 134, 138, 140
infection 151, 152, 153, 156, 157, 158, 159, 169, 174
Inherited platelet disorders (IPDs) 181, 182
International Consensus Classification (ICC) 272, 286
in vivo models 272
iron 2, 5, 6, 8, 9, 11, 12, 20, 22, 28, 29, 30, 32, 34, 36, 37, 38, 39, 40, 41, 42, 43, 44, 45, 46, 50, 51, 52, 54
iron deficiency anemia (IDA) 32
ischemia 239, 241

J

Janus kinase (JAK) inhibitors 237, 258
jaundice 82, 84, 86

L

laboratory exams 39
lactate dehydrogenase (LDH) 84
lactate dehydrogenase levels 82
lactation 56, 58
lethargy 82
leukemia 1, 9, 10, 12, 13, 15, 19, 20
leukemic hematopoiesis 1
leukemic initiating cells (LIC) 273
leukemogenesis 300
Leukocyte Adhesion Deficiency type I (LAD-I) 159
leukopenia 151, 156, 158, 163
Leukopenia 156
liver 181, 185, 189, 190, 200, 203
lymphadenopathy 157
lymphatic tissues 296
lymphocytes 151, 152, 153, 157, 169
lymphoproliferative disorders 328, 329, 346, 348

M

Macrocytic anemia 34
macrophages 32, 37
macrothrombocytes 183
magnetic resonance imaging 275
malabsorption 55, 57, 58, 71
malaria 107, 108, 109, 110, 112, 127
malignancies 211, 220
Malnutrition 132
mammalian target of rapamycin (mTOR) 300
mammalian target of rapamycin (mTOR) signaling 269
management 130, 131, 134, 135, 136, 137, 138, 140, 141, 143, 147, 148
management plans 207
Mantle Cell Lymphoma (MCL) 329
maternal subnutrition 2
matrix Gla-protein 212
mean corpuscular volume (MCV) 132
measurable residual disease (MRD) 275
Mediterranean 107, 110
Megaloblastic anemia 129, 130, 132, 134, 135, 138, 145, 146
membrane dysfunction 82
Menstrual bleeding 59
metabolism 2, 5, 8, 20
Microcytic anemia 34
micronutrient deficiency disorders 59
mitochondria 55, 61, 62, 68, 72, 75, 77
mitochondrial function 59, 61, 68, 75, 76
molecular biology 328

molecular mechanisms 151
monoclonal antibodies 353, 360, 369, 371, 376
Monoclonal Gammopathy of Undetermined Significance (MGUS) 355, 362
monoclonal immunoglobulin M (IgM) antibodies 356
monocytes 151, 152, 153, 157
morbidity 353
mortality 353
multifactorial clotting abnormalities 181
multiple cell lineages 385
Multiple myeloma (MM) is 353
multiple sclerosis (MS) 214
musculoskeletal disorders 237, 264
mutations 2, 3, 5, 6, 7, 9, 11, 14, 15, 17, 19, 20, 22
myelodysplastic syndromes (MDSs) 157
myelodysplastic syndromes/neoplasms (MDS) 272
myeloid sarcoma (MS) 270
myeloproliferative neoplasms (MPNs) 157
Myocardial infarction 241

N

natural killer (NK) cells 153
NDUFB11 gene 56, 62, 64, 68
neonatal development 56
nerve damage
neutrophils 151, 152, 153, 157, 164, 174
nodular lymphocyte-predominant Hodgkin lymphoma (NLPHL) 331
non-coding RNA molecules 356
non-fatal
non-Hodgkin lymphoma (NHL) 325, 326
Non-specific Orbital Inflammation (NSOI) 154
Normocytic anemia 35
nutrient deficiencies 27
nutrients 2
nutrition 2
nutritional deficiency 2

O

obstetric emergencies 242
organ dysfunction 84
osmotic balance 2
osteocalcin 212
oxygen 2, 3, 4, 5, 6, 12, 14, 21
oxygen-carrying capacity 81, 93
oxygen transport 3, 5, 6, 12

P

pallor 131, 133, 134, 136, 137, 139
pathogens 380, 382, 383
pathophysiology 27, 29, 31, 32, 33, 36, 37, 38, 39, 40, 41, 43, 45, 49, 50, 51, 52, 53, 54
phagocytic mononuclear cells 153
phagocytosis 28
pharmacological treatments 237
Philadelphia chromosome 296, 299, 300
physiological saline 381
plasma cell dyscrasias 353, 354, 355, 356, 357, 358, 359, 360, 361, 362, 363, 364, 365, 366, 367, 368, 369, 370, 371, 372, 374, 375, 376, 377, 378
Plasma cell dyscrasias 353, 354, 374
plasma cell myeloma (PCM) 355
Platelet disorder 179
platelet-rich plasma (PRP) treatments 180
platelets 2, 4, 9, 13, 18
pleomorphic cells 330
polyamine 381
polymerase chain reaction (PCR) 387
postpartum hemorrhage (PPH) 184
pregnancy 2
Primary Amyloidosis 356
Primary Mediastinal B-cell Lymphoma (PMBCL) 330
proaggregatory substances 241
prognostic outcomes 268
pro-inflammatory cytokines 244
prophylactic emicizumab 212
protein C 240
protein S 240
P-selectin 185
public health
pulmonary embolism (PE) 210, 227

Q

qualitative disorders 180

R

radiation exposure 269
radionuclide therapy 179
RBC integrity 81, 84
red cells 2
Reed-Sternberg cells 326
regenerative medicine 379, 383, 384, 387, 389, 392, 394, 398, 399, 402, 403
renal tumors 299
Reticulocyte count 40
reticulocytosis 82
rituximab 295
Roux-en-Y gastric bypass surgery (RYGB) 57

S

screening 110, 111, 112, 115, 117, 118, 119, 120, 121, 126, 128
secondary plasma cell leukemia (sPCL) 357
self-perpetuating thromboinflammatory cycle 244
senescence 270, 289
sensitization 153, 155
sepsis 242
serum iron 40
sickle cell disease 27, 38, 50, 53
sideroblastic anemia 55, 56, 57, 58, 59, 60, 61, 62, 63, 64, 65, 66, 67, 68, 69, 70, 71, 72, 73, 76, 77, 78
sideroblastic-like anemia 55
single-nucleotide mutation 109
society
Solitary plasmacytoma 357
splanchnic vein thrombosis (SVT) 184
splenomegaly 109, 110
standardized incidence ratios (SIRs) 331
stem cell technology 379, 383, 386
stress 153, 156, 167, 172
stroke 237, 240, 241, 249, 250, 253, 254, 260, 264, 265
suboptimal intake 131
systemic hypoxia 55

T

tachycardia 82
T cell acute lymphoblastic leukemia (T-ALL) 268
T-cell (CAR-T) therapy 329
T cells 152, 153, 154, 155, 169, 176
Thalassemia Major 110
Thalassemia Minor 110
therapy 27, 30, 43, 44, 46, 47
thrombin 185, 187
thrombocytopathy 179, 180, 181, 196
thrombocytopenia 179, 180, 183, 185, 187, 189, 191, 195, 196, 201, 202, 204
thrombophilia 207, 232
thrombopoietin (TPO) 185
thrombosis 237, 238, 239, 240, 241, 242, 243, 244, 245, 246, 247, 248, 249, 250, 252, 256, 259, 261, 263, 264, 265
thrombotic thrombocytopenic purpura (TTP) 181, 202, 204
tissues 29, 31, 33, 48
total iron-binding capacity (TIBC) 40
toxic exposures 131
transfusion 379, 380, 381, 382, 383, 384, 385, 386, 387, 388, 389, 390, 391, 392, 393, 394, 395, 396, 397, 399, 401, 402, 403
transfusion reactions 379
transfusion-related acute lung injury (TRALI) 382, 394
trauma 211, 224
treatment 129, 130, 131, 133, 134, 135, 136, 137, 138, 139, 140, 141, 142, 143, 145, 146
treatment protocols 268, 280, 283
Type 2 diabetes
tyrosine kinase inhibitors (TKIs) 297, 310

U

umbilical cord blood 380, 403

V

vaso-occlusive crisis 108, 123
venous thromboembolism (VTE) 210
Vitamin B12 deficiency 37
vitamin K 211, 212, 222, 233
vitamins B6 59
von Willebrand factor (vWF) 186

W

Waldenström Macroglobulinemia (WM) 355, 356
water 2, 4
weakness 131
white cells 2
whole blood counts 272
World Health Organization 268, 272, 292

Z

zinc deficiency 59